# Pharmacotherapy Principles & Practice Study Guide: A Case-Based Care Plan Approach

**THIRD EDITION**

Editors

**Michael D. Katz, PharmD**
Professor
Department of Pharmacy Practice and Science
University of Arizona College of Pharmacy
Tucson, Arizona

**Kathryn R. Matthias, PharmD, BCPS (AQ-ID)**
Assistant Professor
Department of Pharmacy Practice and Science
University of Arizona College of Pharmacy
Tucson, Arizona

**Marie A. Chisholm-Burns, PharmD, MPH, FCCP, FASHP**
Dean and Professor
University of Tennessee College of Pharmacy
Memphis, Tennessee

New York   Chicago   San Francisco   Athens   London   Madrid   Mexico City
Milan   New Delhi   Singapore   Sydney   Toronto

**Pharmacotherapy Principles & Practice Study Guide: A Case-Based Care Plan Approach, Third Edition**

1 2 3 4 5 6 7 8 9 10   DOW/DOW   18 17 16 15 14 13

ISBN 978-0-07-180178-2
MHID 0-07-180178-2

This book was set in Minion Pro by Cenveo® Publisher Services.
The editors were Michael Weitz and Peter J. Boyle.
The production supervisor was Catherine Saggese.
Project management was provided by Harleen Chopra, Cenveo Publisher Services.
The designer was Alan Barnett; the cover designer was Thomas De Pierro.
RR Donnelley was printer and binder.

This book is printed on acid-free paper.

**Library of Congress Cataloging-in-Publication Data**

Pharmacotherapy principles & practice study guide : a case-based care plan approach/editors, Michael D. Katz, PharmD, professor, Department of Pharmacy Practice and Science, College of Pharmacy, Tucson, Arizona, Kathryn R. Matthias, PharmD, BCPS (AQ-ID), assistant professor, Department of Pharmacy Practice and Science, University of Arizona College of Pharmacy, Tucson, Arizona, Marie A. Chisholm-Burns, PharmD, MPH, FCCP, FASHP, dean and professor, University of Tennessee, College of Pharmacy, Memphis, Tennessee. —Third edition.
   pages cm
   ISBN 978-0-07-180178-2 (pbk.) — ISBN 978-0-07-180179-9 (ebook)   1. Chemotherapy—Problems, exercises, etc.   2. Drug utilization—Problems, exercises, etc.   I. Katz, Michael D., editor of compilation.   II. Matthias, Kathryn R., editor of compilation.   III. Chisholm-Burns, Marie A., editor of compilation.   IV. Title: Pharmacotherapy principles and practice study guide.
   RM262.P4754 2014
   615.5′8076—dc23                                                    2013030988

# CONTENTS

# CONTRIBUTORS

**Kimberly A. Ackerbauer, PharmD, BCPS**
Clinical Pharmacy Specialist, Cardiac Intensive Care Unit
Rush University Medical Center
Chicago, Illinois

**Sarah M. Adriance, PharmD, BCPS**
Specialty Practice Pharmacist, Critical Care
Ohio State University Medical Center
Columbus, Ohio

**Ronda L. Akins, PharmD**
Infectious Diseases Clinical Specialist
Methodist Charlton Medical Center
Dallas, Texas
Gratis Assistant Professor
Louisiana State University Health Sciences Center
Shreveport, Louisiana

**Rita R. Alloway, PharmD, FCCP**
Research Professor of Medicine
University of Cincinnati
Director, Transplant Clinical Research
University Hospital
Cincinnati, Ohio

**David A. Apgar, PharmD**
Assistant Professor
Department of Pharmacy Practice and Science
University of Arizona College of Pharmacy
Tucson, Arizona

**Katie E. Barber, PharmD**
Infectious Diseases Pharmacy Research Fellow
Detroit Medical Center
Detroit, Michigan

**Kim W. Benner, PharmD, BCPS, FASHP, FPPAG**
Professor of Pharmacy Practice
Samford University McWhorter School of Pharmacy
Birmingham, Alabama

**P. Brandon Bookstaver, PharmD, BCPS (AQ-ID), AAHIVE**
Vice-Chair and Associate Professor
Department of Clinical Pharmacy & Outcomes Sciences
South Carolina College of Pharmacy
University of South Carolina Campus
Clinical Pharmacy Specialist, Infectious Diseases
Palmetto Health Richland
Columbia, South Carolina

**Emily B. Borders, PharmD, BCOP**
Assistant Professor
University of Oklahoma College of Pharmacy
University of Oklahoma Health Sciences Center
Oklahoma City, Oklahoma

**Sheila R. Botts, PharmD, FCCP, BCPP**
Clinical Pharmacy Specialist, Behavioral Health
Kaiser Foundation Health Plan–Colorado
Westminster, Colorado

**Nicole J. Brandt, PharmD, CGP, BCPP, FASCP**
Associate Professor, Geriatric Pharmacotherapy
Department of Pharmacy Practice and Science, UMB School
of Pharmacy
Director, Clinical and Education Programs of Peter Lamy
Center Drug Therapy and Aging
Baltimore, Maryland

**Adam Bress, PharmD, MS-CTS**
Clinical Pharmacist
Department of Pharmacy Practice
University of Illinois Hospitals and Health Sciences System
University of Illinois at Chicago
Chicago, Illinois

**Ryan M. Brimeyer, DO**
Pulmonary and Critical Care Fellow
Creighton University Medical Center
Omaha, Nebraska

**Gretchen M. Brophy, PharmD, BCPS, FCCP, FCCM**
Professor of Pharmacotherapy & Outcomes Science and
Neurosurgery
Virginia Commonwealth University
Medical College of Virginia Campus
Richmond, Virginia

**Susan P. Bruce, PharmD, BCPS**
Professor and Chair
Northeast Ohio Medical University
Rootstown, Ohio

**Imad F. Btaiche, BS, PharmD, BCNSP**
Associate Dean for Academic Affairs and Professor
Lebanese American University School of Pharmacy
Byblos, Lebanon

**Christopher J. Campen, PharmD, BCPS**
Clinical Oncology Pharmacist
University of Arizona Cancer Center - Orange Grove Campus
Tucson, Arizona

**Diane M. Cappelletty, PharmD**
Associate Professor of Pharmacy Practice
University of Toledo College of Pharmacy
Toledo, Ohio

**Joshua C. Caraccio, PharmD, BCPS**
Antimicrobial Stewardship Clinical Pharmacist
Utah Valley Regional Medical Center
Provo, Utah

**Larisa H. Cavallari, PharmD, BCPS, FCCP**
Associate Professor
Department of Pharmacy Practice
University of Illinois at Chicago
Chicago, Illinois

**Juliana Chan, PharmD, BCACP, FCCP**
Clinical Associate Professor
Department of Pharmacy Practice College of Pharmacy
Department of Medicine, Sections of Digestive Diseases and
    Nutrition and Section of Hepatology
University of Illinois at Chicago
Clinical Pharmacist, GI/ Hepatology and Hepatology
    Telemedicine
University of Illinois Hospital & Health Sciences System
Chicago, Illinois

**Jack J. Chen, PharmD, FCCP, BCPS, CGP**
Associate Professor (Neurology)
Loma Linda University Schools of Medicine and Pharmacy
Loma Linda, California

**Allison A. Chilipko, PharmD, BCPS, CGP**
Clinical Assistant Professor
University of Maryland School of Pharmacy
Clinical Pharmacy Specialist, Internal Medicine
MedStar Union Memorial Hospital
Baltimore, Maryland

**Marie A. Chisholm-Burns, PharmD, MPH, FCCP, FASHP**
Dean and Professor
University of Tennessee College of Pharmacy
Memphis, Tennessee

**Holly Chiu, PharmD, BCACP**
Adjunct Faculty
Wayne State University Eugene Applebaum College of
    Health Science and Pharmacy
Detroit, Michagan

**Kevin W. Cleveland, PharmD, ANP**
Assistant Dean for Experiential Education and Special
    Projects
Associate Professor
Idaho State University College of Pharmacy
Meridian, Idaho

**Amanda H. Corbett, PharmD, BCPS, FCCP, CPP**
Clinical Associate Professor
University of North Carolina
Eshelman School of Pharmacy
Chapel Hill, North Carolina

**Susan Cornell, BS, PharmD, CDE, FAPhA, FAADE**
Assistant Director of Experiential Education
Associate Professor of Pharmacy Practice
Midwestern University Chicago College of Pharmacy

Clinical Pharmacist/ Diabetes Educator
Access DuPage Community Clinic
Downers Grove, Illinois

**Brian L. Crabtree, PharmD, BCPP**
Professor of Pharmacy Practice
Wayne State University Eugene Applebaum College of
    Pharmacy and Health Sciences
Detroit, Michigan

**Jean E. Cunningham, PharmD, BCPS**
Clinical Content Specialist
Truven Health Analytics
Greenwood Village, Colorado

**Clarence E. Curry, Jr., PharmD**
Associate Professor of Pharmacy Practice
College of Pharmacy, Howard University
Washington, DC

**Devra K. Dang, PharmD, BCPS, CDE**
Associate Clinical Professor
University of Connecticut School of Pharmacy
Clinical Faculty, Burgdorf Primary Care Clinic
Storrs, Connecticut

**Stephanie J. Davis, PharmD, BCACP**
Program Manager, Education and Clinical Services
Southern Arizona VA Healthcare System
Clinical Assistant Professor
University of Arizona College of Pharmacy
Tucson, Arizona

**Kristina De Los Santos, PharmD, BCPS**
Chief, Pharmacy Service Line
Southern Arizona VA Healthcare System
Adjunct Clinical Assistant Professor, Pharmacy
    Practice & Science
University of Arizona College of Pharmacy
Tucson, Arizona

**Robert J. DiDomenico, PharmD, BCACP**
Clinical Associate Professor
Department of Pharmacy Practice
University of Illinois at Chicago
Cardiovascular Clinical Pharmacist
University of Illinois Hospital & Health
    Sciences System
Chicago, Illinois

**Eric A. Dietrich, PharmD, BCPS**
Clinical Assistant Professor
Department of Family Medicine, College of Medicine
University of Florida
Gainesville, Florida

**Monica A. Donnelley, PharmD**
Infectious Diseases Pharmacist
University of California Davis Medical Center
Sacramento, California

**Leona Downey, MD**
Arizona Oncology
Tucson, Arizona

**Jeremiah J. Duby, PharmD, BCPS**
Senior Critical Care Pharmacist
University of California Davis Medical Center
Assistant Clinical Professor
University of California, Davis School of Medicine
Touro University
University of California San Francisco
Sacramento, California

**Colleen Clark Dula, PharmD**
Clinical Assistant Professor
Director, Professional Practice Laboratory
Pharmacy Practice and Administration
Ohio State University College of Pharmacy
Columbus, Ohio

**Christopher J. Edwards, PharmD, BCPS**
Clinical Assistant Professor
University of Arizona, College of Pharmacy
Clinical Staff Pharmacist, Emergency Medicine
University of Arizona Medical Center–University Campus
Tucson, Arizona

**Megan J. Ehret, PharmD, MS, BCPP**
Associate Professor
University of Connecticut
Clinical Psychopharmacologust
University of Connecticutt Health Center
Storrs, Connecticut

**Shareen Y. El-Ibiary, PharmD, BCPS, FCCP**
Professor of Pharmacy Practice
Department of Pharmacy Practice
Midwestern University College of Pharmacy-Glendale
Glendale, Arizona

**John Erramouspe, PharmD, MS**
Professor of Pharmacy Practice
Idaho State University College of Pharmacy
Pocatello, Idaho

**Brian L. Erstad, PharmD, BCPS, FASHP**
Head and Professor
Department of Pharmacy Practice and Science
University of Arizona College of Pharmacy
Program Director, Critical Care Residency
University of Arizona Medical Center- University Campus
Tucson, Arizona

**Nicole M. Even, PharmD, BCPS**
Clinical Staff Pharmacist, Pediatrics
University of Arizona Medical Center–University Campus
Diamond Children's Medical Center
Tucson, Arizona

**Ema Ferreira, BPharm, MSc, PharmD, FCSHP**
Clinical Professor
Faculty of Pharmacy - University of Montreal
Pharmacist, Obstetrics and Gynecology
Centre Hospitalier Sainte-Justine, Montreal
Quebec, Canada

**Melanie Foeppel, PharmD**
Assistant Professor
Pacific University School of Pharmacy
Hillsboro, Oregon

**Andrea S. Franks, PharmD, BCPS**
Associate Professor of Clinical Pharmacy
University of Tennessee Health Science Center
Associate Professor of Family Medicine
University of Tennessee Graduate School of Medicine
Knoxville, Tennessee

**Patty Ghazvini, PharmD**
Professor of Pharmacy Practice
Florida A&M University College of Pharmacy
Internal Medicine Clinical Preceptor
Tallahassee Memorial Hospital
Tallahassee, Florida

**Vijay Gogineni, MD**
Pulmonary and Critical Care Fellow
Creighton University
Omaha, Nebraska

**Lisa W. Goldstone, MS, PharmD, BCPS**
Assistant Professor
University of Arizona College of Pharmacy
Clinical Specialty Pharmacist, Psychiatry
University of Arizona Medical Center–South Campus
Tucson, Arizona

**Maqual R. Graham, PharmD**
Professor and Director of Applied Therapeutics and
    Professional Skills
Division of Pharmacy Practice and Administration
University of Missouri-Kansas City
Kansas City, Missouri

**Elaine M. Greifenstein, MD**
Staff Rheumatologist
Louis Stokes Cleveland Veterans Affairs Medical Center
Akron, Ohio

**William Joshua Guffey, PharmD, BCACP, BC-ADM**
Associate Director of Pharmacy Education
Charlotte Area Health Education Center
Clinical Assistant Professor
Eshelman School of Pharmacy
University of North Carolina
Charlotte, North Carolina

**John G. Gums, PharmD, FCCP**
Professor of Pharmacy and Medicine
Associate Chair, Department of Pharmacotherapy and
    Translational Research
Director of Clinical Research in Family Medicine
University of Florida
Gainesville, Florida

**Tracy M. Hagemann, PharmD, FCCP, FPPAG**
Professor
Director of Clinical Affairs
University of Oklahoma College of Pharmacy
Clinical Pediatric Pharmacy Specialist – Hematology/
    Oncology
Children's Hospital at OU Medical Center
Oklahoma City, Oklahoma

**Keri D. Hager, PharmD, BCPS**
Assistant Professor
Pharmacy Practice and Pharmaceutical Sciences Department
College of Pharmacy
University of Minnesota, Duluth
Duluth, Minnesota

**Julie Hasse, PharmD**
Pharmacist
Southeast Missouri Hospital
Girardeau, Missouri

**Nancy H. Heideman, PharmD, BCPS**
Clinical Pharmacy Specialist, Pediatrics
University of New Mexico Hospital
Albuquerque, New Mexico

**Richard L. Heideman, MD**
Professor of Pediatrics
Division of Pediatric Hematology/Oncology
University of New Mexico
Albuquerque, New Mexico

**Brett H. Heintz, PharmD, BCPS, (AQ ID), AAHIVE**
Associate Professor (Clinical)
University of Iowa, College of Pharmacy
Pharmacy Specialist, Internal Medicine and Infectious
    Diseases
Iowa City Veterans Affairs Health Care System
Iowa City, Iowa

**Brian A. Hemstreet, PharmD, BCPS, FCCP**
Associate Professor
Director, Pharmaceutical Care Learning Center
University of Colorado Skaggs School of Pharmacy and
    Pharmaceutical Sciences
Clinical Specialist in Adult Internal Medicine
University of Colorado Hospital
Aurora, Colorado

**Michelle L. Hilaire, PharmD, CDE, BCPS**
Clinical Associate Professor of Pharmacy Practice
University of Wyoming School of Pharmacy
Clinical Pharmacist
Fort Collins Family Medicine Residency Program
Fort Collins, Colorado

**Alexis E. Horace, PharmD**
Assistant Professor
University of Louisiana at Monroe College of Pharmacy
Clinical Pharmacist
University of Louisiana Mid-City Clinic
Baton Rouge, Louisiana

**Jaime R. Hornecker, PharmD, BCPS**
Clinical Associate Professor of Pharmacy Practice
University of Wyoming School of Pharmacy
Faculty Clinical Pharmacist and PGY1 Pharmacy Residency
    Director
University of Wyoming Family Medicine Residency
    Program
Casper, Wyoming

**Marcella Hoyland, PharmD, BCPS**
Assistant Professor, Department of Pharmacy Practice and
    Science
University of Arizona College of Pharmacy
University of Arizona Medical Center – University Campus
Tucson, Arizona

**Jamie Hwang, PharmD, CGP**
Ambulatory Care Clinical Specialist
Henry Ford Health System/ HAP
Grosse Pointe, Michigan

**Cherry W. Jackson, BS, PharmD, BCPP, FASHP**
Professor of Pharmacy
Department of Psychiatry and Neurology
Auburn University
Clinical Professor
Department of Psychiatry and Behavioral Neurobiology
University of Alabama, Birmingham
Birmingham, Alabama

**David M. Jacobs, PharmD**
PGY2 Pharmacy Resident in Infectious Diseases
University of Houston College of Pharmacy
Houston, Texas

**Jennifer Jordan, PharmD, BCPS**
Associate Professor
Pacific University School of Pharmacy
Hillsboro, Oregon

**Michael P. Kane, PharmD, FCCP, BCPS, BCACP**
Professor
Department of Pharmacy Practice
Albany College of Pharmacy and Health Sciences
Clinical Pharmacy Specialist
The Endocrine Group, LLP
Albany, New York

**Michael D. Katz, PharmD**
Professor
Director, International Programs
Department of Pharmacy Practice and Science
University of Arizona College of Pharmacy
Tucson, Arizona

**Deanna L. Kelly, PharmD, BCPP**
Director, Treatment of Research Program
Maryland Psychiatric Research Center
Professor of Psychiatry
University of Maryland Baltimore
Catonsville, Maryland

**Amy K. Kennedy, PharmD, BCACP**
Assistant Professor
University of Arizona College of Pharmacy
Clinical Pharmacist
El Rio Health Center
Tucson, Arizona

**Shelley A. Klochan, PharmD**
Clinical ICU Specialist
Cabell Huntington Hospital
Huntington, West Virginia

**Jacqueline M. Klootwyk, PharmD, BCPS, BCACP**
Assistant Professor
Clinical, Social and Administrative Sciences
Mylan School of Pharmacy
Duquesne University
Pittsburgh, Pennsylvania

**Michael D. Kraft, PharmD, BCNSP**
Clinical Associate Professor
University of Michigan College of Pharmacy
Assistant Director – Education and Research
University of Michigan Health System
Ann Arbor, Michigan

**Wallace G. Leader, PharmD (Deceased)**
Dean and Professor of Clinical Pharmacy Practice
University of Louisiana at
Monroe College of Pharmacy
Monroe, Louisiana

**Jeannie Kim Lee, PharmD, BCPS**
University of Arizona College of Pharmacy
University of Arizona College of Medicine
Clinical Faculty
Southern Arizona VA Health Care System
Tucson, Arizona

**Jiehyun Lee, PharmD**
Primary Care Resident
University of Connecticut
Storrs, Connecticut

**Mary Lee, PharmD, BCPS, FCCP**
Vice President and Chief Academic Officer
Pharmacy, Optometry & Health Sciences Education
Midwestern University Professor of Pharmacy Practice
Chicago College of Pharmacy
Downers Grove, Illinois

**Russell E. Lewis, PharmD, FCCP, BCPS**
Associate Professor of Medicine
Department of Medical Sciences and Surgery
University of Bologna
Clinical Pharmacologist
Infectious Diseases Unit
S'Orsola-Malpighi Hospital, University of Bologna
Bologna, Italy

**Amy M. Lugo, PharmD, BCPS, BC-ADM**
Clinical Pharmacy Specialist
Department of Defense Pharmacoeconomic Center
Fort Sam Houston, Texas

**Leigh V. Maine, PharmD**
Clinical Staff Pharmacist
University of Arizona Medical Center – University Campus
Tucson, Arizona

**Mark A. Malesker, PharmD, FCCP, FASHP, BCPS**
Professor of Pharmacy Practice and Medicine
Creighton University
Clinical Pharmacy Specialist
Creighton University Medical Center
Omaha, Nebraska

**Michelle T. Martin, PharmD, BCPS, BCACP**
Assistant Professor
University of Illinois at Chicago College of Pharmacy
Clinical Pharmacist
University of Illinois Hospital and Health Sciences System
Chicago, Illinois

**Kathryn R. Matthias, PharmD, BCPS (AQ-ID)**
Assistant Professor
University of Arizona College of Pharmacy
University of Arizona Medical Center–University Campus
Tucson, Arizona

**Lena M. Maynor, PharmD, BCPS**
Clinical Assistant Professor
West Virginia University School of Pharmacy
Morgantown, West Virginia

**Shelley King McIntire, PharmD, BCPS**
Pharmacist
DCH Regional Medical Center
Tuscaloosa, Alabama

**Yolanda B. McKoy-Beach, PharmD, CDE**
Assistant Professor
Howard University College of Pharmacy
Clinical Pharmacist
La Clinica Del Pueblo
Washington, DC

**Patrick J. Medina, PharmD, BCOP**
Associate Professor
University of Oklahoma College of Pharmacy
University of Oklahoma Health Science Center
Oklahoma City, Oklahoma

**Beverly C. Mims, PharmD**
Associate Professor of Pharmacy Practice
Howard University College of Pharmacy
Clinical Pharmacist
Howard University Hospital
Washington, DC

**Brice Labruzzo Mohondro, PharmD, BCACP**
Clinical Pharmacist—Population Management
Blue Cross and Blue Shield of Louisiana
Baton Rouge, Louisiana

**Caroline Morin, BPharm, MSc**
Clinical Associate, Faculty of Pharmacy
University of Montreal (QC) Canada
Pharmacist, Obstetrics and Gynecology, Centre IMAGe
CHU Sainte-Justine, Montreal (QC)
Quebec, Canada

**Lee E. Morrow, MD, MSc**
Associate Professor of Medicine
Associate Professor of Pharmacy Practice
Creighton University Medical Center
Omaha, Nebraska

**Rocsanna Namdar, PharmD, BCPS**
Assistant Professor
Department of Clinical Pharmacy
University of Colorado
Aurora, Colorado

**Lynn C. Nelson, PharmD, MBA**
Clinical Pharmacy Specialist, Infectious Diseases
University of Louisville Hospital
Louisville, Kentucky

**Melinda M. Neuhauser, PharmD, MPH, FCCP, FASHP**
Clinical Pharmacist, Infectious Diseases
Department of Veterans Affairs, Pharmacy Benefits
    Management Services
Hines, Illinois

**Tien M.H. Ng, PharmD, FCCP, BCPS (AQ-Cardiology)**
Associate Professor of Clinical Pharmacy and Medicine
University of Southern California
School of Pharmacy and Keck School of Medicine
Los Angeles, California

**David E. Nix, PharmD, BCPS (AQ-ID)**
Professor
University of Arizona College of Pharmacy
University of Arizona College of Medicine
University of Arizona Medical Center – University
    Campus
Tucson, Arizona

**Edith A. Nutescu, PharmD, FCCP**
Clinical Professor
University of Illinois at Chicago College of Pharmacy
Departments of Pharmacy Practice
Clinical Director, Antithrombosis Center
University of Illinois Hospital Health Sciences System
Chicago, Illinois

**Asad E. Patanwala, PharmD, BCPS**
Associate Professor
Department of Pharmacy Practice and Science
University of Arizona College of Pharmacy
Clinical Pharmacy Specialist, Emergency Medicine
University of Arizona Medical Center – University
    Campus
Tucson, Arizona

**Krina H. Patel, PharmD**
Adjunct Faculty
Department of Pharmacy Practice and Administration
Philadelphia College of Pharmacy
University of the Sciences
Philadelphia, Pennsylvania

**Susan L. Pendland, PharmD, MS**
Adjunct Associate Professor, University of Illinois at
    Chicago
Clinical Staff Pharmacist, St. Joseph Berea Hospital
Berea, Kentucky

**Hanna Phan, PharmD, BCPS**
Assistant Professor
Departments of Pharmacy Practice and Science, and
  Department of Pediatrics
Colleges of Pharmacy and Medicine
University of Arizona
Clinical Pharmacy Specialist, Pediatric Pulmonary Medicine
University of Arizona Medical Center – University Campus
Tucson, Arizona

**Beth Bryles Phillips, PharmD, FCCP, BCPS**
Clinical Professor
University of Georgia College of Pharmacy
Clinical Pharmacy Specialist
Charlie Norwood VA Medical Center
Athens, Georgia

**Melissa R. Pleva, PharmD, BCPS, BCNSP**
Adjunct Clinical Assistant Professor
Department of Clinical, Social, and Administrative Sciences
University of Michigan College of Pharmacy
Clinical Pharmacist Specialist, Department of Pharmacy
  Services
University of Michigan Hospital and Health Systems
Ann Arbor, Michigan

**April Miller Quidley, PharmD, BCPS, FCCM**
PGY2 Critical Care Residency Program Director
Critical Care Pharmacist
Vidant Medical Center
Greenville, North Carolina

**John J. Radosevich, PharmD, BCPS**
Clinical Pharmacist, Emergency Medicine
Maricopa Integrated Health System 2601 East Roosevelt
  Street
Phoenix, Arizona

**Évelyne Rey, MD, MSc, FRCPC**
Clinical Associate Professor
Department of Medicine and Obstetrics and Gynecology
University of Montreal (QC) Canada
Head, Division of Obstetrics and Gynecology
CHU Sainte-Justine, Montreal
Quebec, Canada

**Stephanie Reynolds, PharmD**
PGY2 Cardiology Pharmacy Practice Resident
West Palm Beach Veterans Affairs Medical Center
West Palm Beach, Florida

**Leigh Ann Ross, PharmD, FCCP, FASHP, BCPS**
Chair and Associate Professor
Department of Pharmacy Practice
Associate Dean for Clinical Affairs
University of Mississippi School of Pharmacy
Jackson, Mississippi

**Brendan S. Ross, MD**
Clinical Associate Professor
Department of Pharmacy Practice
University of Mississippi School of Pharmacy
Staff Physician
G.V. (Sonny) Montgomery Veterans Affairs Medical Center
Jackson, Mississippi

**Laurajo Ryan, PharmD, MSc, BCPS, CDE**
Clinical Associate Professor
University of Texas at Austin College of Pharmacy
University of Texas Health Science Center  School of
  Medicine
San Antonio, Texas

**Basma Sadaka, PharmD, BCPS**
Transplant Pharmacy Fellow
University of Cincinnati
University Hospital
Cincinnati, Ohio

**Lauren S. Schlesselman, M.A. Ed Psych, PharmD**
Associate Clinical Professor
University of Connecticut School of Pharmacy
Storrs, Connecticut

**Ramvinay S. Seddabattula, MD**
Infectious Diseases Fellow
University of Arizona College of Medicine
University of Arizona Medical Center – University Campus
Tucson, Arizona

**Roohollah Sharifi, MD, FACS**
Professor of Surgery/ Urology
University of Illinois at Chicago, College of Medicine
Chief of Urology
Jesse Brown VA Hospital
Chicago, Illinois

**Colin I. Sheffield, PharmD**
Coordinator, Cancer Center Specialty Pharmacy
Duke University Hospital
Durham, North Carolina

**Claire A. Simister, PharmD**
Clinical Pharmacy Specialist—Gynecology Oncology
The University of Texas MD Anderson Cancer Center
Houston, Texas

**Steven M. Smith, PharmD, MPH, BCPS**
Assistant Professor
Department of Clinical Pharmacy, Skaggs School of
  Pharmacy and Pharmaceutical Sciences
University of Colorado
Aurora, Colorado

**Sarah A. Spinler, PharmD, BCPS (AQ-Cardiology), FCCP, FAHA, FASHP, AACC**
Professor of Clinical Pharmacy
Philadelphia College of Pharmacy
University of the Sciences in Philadelphia
Philadelphia, Pennsylvania

**Sara A. Stahle, PharmD, BCPS**
Clinical Pharmacy Specialist – Critical Care
Pennsylvania Hospital
Philadelphia, Pennsylvania

**Robert J. Straka, BSc, PharmD, FCCP**
Professor
Department of Experimental and Clinical Pharmacology
University of Minnesota College of Pharmacy
Minneapolis, Minnesota

**Amy L. Stump, PharmD, BCPS**
Clinical Pharmacy Specialist, Ambulatory Care
Indiana University Health Methodist Family Medicine
    Residency Training Program
Indianapolis, Indiana

**Janice L. Stumpf, PharmD**
Clinical Associate Professor
University of Michigan College of Pharmacy
Clinical Pharmacist, Drug Information Service
University of Michigan Health System
Ann Arbor, Michigan

**Meghan K. Sullivan, PharmD**
Assistant Professor
University of New England College of Pharmacy
Portland, Maine

**Joseph M. Swanson, PharmD, BCPS**
Associate Professor of Clinical Pharmacy and Pharmacology
University of Tennessee
Colleges of Pharmacy and Medicine
Clinical Specialist
Regional Medical Center at Memphis
Memphis, Tennessee

**Eljim P. Tesoro, PharmD, BCPS**
Clinical Associate Professor
University of Illinois at Chicago
Clinical Pharmacist
University of Illinois Hospital & Health Sciences System
Chicago, Illinois

**Andrea N. Traina, PharmD, BCPS, BCACP**
Assistant Professor of Pharmacy Practice
St. John Fisher College
Wegmans School of Pharmacy
Clinical Pharmacy Specialist

Endocrine-Diabetes Care and Resource Center
Rochester General Health System
Rochester, New York

**Toby C. Trujillo, PharmD, BCPS (AQ-Cardiology)**
Associate Professor
University of Colorado Skaggs School of Pharmacy and
    Pharmaceutical Sciences
Clinical Specialist, Cardiology/Anticoagulation
University of Colorado Hospital
Aurora, Colorado

**Elena M. Umland, PharmD**
Professor of Pharmacy Practice
Associate Dean for Academic Affairs
Jefferson School of Pharmacy
Thomas Jefferson University
Philadelphia, Pennsylvania

**Sophia Vainrub, PharmD, BCPS**
Clinical Pharmacist, Internal Medicine
Froedtert Hospital
Milwaukee, Wisconsin

**Heather L. VandenBussche, PharmD**
Professor, Pharmacy Practice
Ferris State University College of Pharmacy
Bronson Methodist Hospital
Kalamazoo, Michigan

**Nicole D. Verkleeren, PharmD, BCPS**
Clinical Pharmacist, Critical Care
Forbes Regional Hospital
Monroeville, Pennsylvania

**Velliyur V. Viswesh, PharmD, BCPS**
Assistant Professor of Clinical and Administrative
    Sciences
California Northstate University College of Pharmacy
Rancho Cordova, California

**Geoffrey C. Wall, PharmD, FCCP, BCPS, CGP**
Professor of Clinical Sciences
Drake University College of Pharmacy and Health
    Sciences
Internal Medicine Clinical Pharmacist
Iowa Methodist Medical Center
Des Moines, Iowa

**Heidi J. Wehring, PharmD, BCPP**
Assistant Professor of Psychiatry, Maryland Psychiatric
    Research Center
University of Maryland Baltimore School of Medicine
Baltimore, Maryland

**Christy M. Weiland, PharmD, BCPS**
Clinical Faculty
University of Washington School of Pharmacy
University of Washington Medical Center
Clinical Pharmacist
Seattle, Washington

**Timothy E. Welty, PharmD, FCCP, BCPS**
Professor and Chair
Department of Clinical Sciences, College of Pharmacy and
    Health SciencesDrake University
Des Moines, Iowa

**Teri L. West, PharmD, BCPS**
Assistant Professor of Pharmacy Practice
Clinical Pharmacist
Lake Erie College of Osteopathic Medicine
School of Pharmacy
Bradenton, Florida

**Ann McMahon Wicker, PharmD, BCPS**
Medical Outcomes Specialist, Pfizer
Baton Rouge, Louisiana

**Jon P. Wietholter, PharmD, BCPS**
Clinical Assistant Professor
West Virginia University
Internal Medicine Clinical Pharmacist

Ruby Memorial Hospital
Morgantown, West Virginia

**Sheila M. Wilhelm, PharmD, BCPS**
Clinical Associate Professor
Wayne State University Eugene Applebaum College of
    Pharmacy and Health Sciences
Clinical Pharmacy Specialist
Harper University Hospital
Detroit, Michigan

**Susan R. Winkler, PharmD, BCPS, FCCP**
Professor and Chair
Department of Pharmacy Practice
Midwestern University Chicago College of Pharmacy
Downers Grove, Illinois

**Christopher G. Wood, PharmD, FCCP, FCCM, BCPS**
Associate Professor
University of Tennessee College of Pharmacy
Clinical Pharmacist
Regional Medical Center at Memphis
Memphis, Tennessee

# PREFACE

Determining and providing organized patient-specific pharmacotherapy recommendations involves a thorough evaluation of the patient's medical problems and medication issues. *Pharmacotherapy Principles and Practice Study Guide: A Case-Based Care Plan Approach,* 3rd edition, contains 103 patient cases that correspond to chapters published in the third edition of *Pharmacotherapy Principles and Practice.* Our goal for this companion textbook is to be a study guide for today's learners of the clinical application of pharmacotherapy through either self-study or during patient case discussion sessions with other health care professionals. The aim of this study guide is to help students navigate through the process of applying their knowledge of pharmacotherapy to a specific patient case by organizing patient data to logically assess a patient's medication issues and formulate a rational pharmacotherapy care plan.

Using a patient database form as an organized guide, students in the health care profession should learn how to apply their knowledge to evaluate the following key aspects of a patient case:

- *Medical Problem List:* Prioritize and organize each patient's medical problem list and corresponding medications

- *Laboratory Values:* Evaluate provided and missing laboratory values for issues related to each patient's medication and medical problem list

- *Drug Therapy Problem Worksheet:* Assess each patient for drug therapy problems and their causes by specifically focusing on drug dosing, missing medications, medications without an obvious indication, drug interactions, and the social and economical impact of certain pharmacotherapy recommendations

- *Pharmacotherapy Care Plan:* Formulate a comprehensive, rational, and practical patient care plan with pharmacotherapy recommendations that are organized by the prioritized medical problem list

- *Patient Education Summary:* Based on a patient's medical problem list and pharmacotherapy recommendations, summarize brief patient education points that are individualized to the patient case

A guide for reviewing and evaluating patient cases and preparing patient database forms is provided in greater detail in Chapter 1. The cases have been written in a realistic fashion, using terms and abbreviations that would be seen in a real patient's medical record. Definitions of abbreviations can be found in Appendix C. The Online Learning Center at www.PPPstudyguide.com has blank patient database forms that may be downloaded.

We, along with patient case authors, used published literature and our experiences as educators and clinicians to determine the focus of each patient case to be included in this textbook. If upon using this study guide, you feel that anything important has been left out, please let us know your thoughts for future editions.

We acknowledge the commitment of more than 150 patient case authors who dedicated their time and knowledge in the preparation of this third edition study guide. We also thank all of the editors and authors of *Pharmacotherapy Principles and Practice,* 3rd edition, who provided the pharmacotherapy background as reference material for this study guide's patient cases and question hints, and for their thoughts and suggestions as we developed the idea for this book.

We are grateful to everyone at McGraw-Hill who advised us and helped prepare this third edition study guide. We specifically thank Michael Weitz for all of his suggestions and insight in preparing this new textbook. In addition, we thank Peter Boyle, Harleen Chopra, and Laura Libretti for guiding us through the publication process and for the hard work related to the copyediting and formatting of each patient case.

At the University of Tennessee, we thank Dr. Christina Spivey for her suggestions to provide more consistency between this study guide and the companion *Pharmacotherapy Principles and Practice,* 3rd edition, textbook and LeeAnn Landphair for keeping all of the patient case chapter-related materials organized.

Lastly, we sincerely thank Dr. Edward W. Randell for conscientiously checking every laboratory value in each patient case for SI unit conversion.

Michael D. Katz, PharmD
Kathryn R. Matthias, PharmD, BCPS (AQ-ID)
Marie A. Chisholm-Burns, PharmD, MPH, FCCP, FASHP

# 1 Applying Pharmacotherapy Principles and Practice: How to Use This Study Guide

Michael D. Katz          Marie A. Chisholm-Burns
Kathryn R. Matthias

As health care becomes more and more complex in the 21st century, the health professional student is increasingly challenged to learn a rapidly expanding amount of information as well as necessary skills to apply that knowledge in a patient care setting. Students of pharmacotherapy quickly learn that the field is rapidly changing as our knowledge of human disease evolves and new drugs are developed to improve patient outcomes. Students also learn that while drug therapy can have tremendous beneficial effects on patient outcomes, such therapy also has the potential to cause harm. The "art" of pharmacotherapy is in applying knowledge and making therapeutic decisions that are most likely to have maximum positive benefit *for a specific patient*. As a companion book to *Pharmacotherapy Principles and Practice*, 3rd ed. (*PPP*), this Study Guide is designed to assist the student in learning to apply didactic knowledge to specific patient situations. Such application requires skills that cannot be learned in lectures or in other passive learning situations, but must be learned by practice and repetition. The more students practice applying their knowledge, using their patient assessment skills, and making therapeutic decisions in their preclinical courses, the more prepared they will be to apply these skills to real patients in their clinical rotations.

This Study Guide is more than a book of patient cases, but it uses patient cases to help students learn to apply pharmacotherapeutic knowledge and skills. Case-based learning is not a new concept in health sciences curricula. As a form of active learning, case-based learning allows the student to practice the skills necessary to provide patient care. The focus of the cases in this Study Guide is, of course, pharmacotherapeutics. A unique feature of this study guide is the expectation that the student will develop a pharmacotherapy care plan as the "output" for each case. What follows is a general discussion of the patient care process and then specific information regarding the use of the Study Guide and development of the pharmacotherapy care plan.

## PHARMACEUTICAL CARE AND THE PATIENT CARE PROCESS

Most pharmacy students are taught about pharmaceutical care early in their pharmacy curriculum. Pharmaceutical care, first described in the late 1980s and early 1990s,[1] can be summarized as "… patient-centered practice in which the practitioner assumes responsibility for a patient's drug-related needs and is held accountable for this commitment."[2] Although the definition of pharmaceutical care does not explicitly state that pharmacists are to perform these tasks, many feel that pharmaceutical care is the central mission of the pharmacy profession.

Although it may seem obvious that health professionals practice in a patient-centered way, all too often practitioners become distracted by technical or administrative tasks. Pharmacy students, after graduation, commit to patient-centered practice in the Oath of a Pharmacist[3]:

> I promise to devote myself to a lifetime of service to others through the profession of pharmacy. In fulfilling this vow:
> - I will consider the welfare of humanity and relief of suffering my primary concerns.
> - I will apply my knowledge, experience, and skills to the best of my ability to assure optimal outcomes for my patients.
> - I will respect and protect all personal and health information entrusted to me.
> - I will accept the lifelong obligation to improve my professional knowledge and competence.

- I will hold myself and my colleagues to the highest principles of our profession's moral, ethical, and legal conduct.
- I will embrace and advocate changes that improve patient care.
- I will utilize my knowledge, skills, experiences, and values to prepare the next generation of pharmacists. I voluntarily take these vows with the full realization of the responsibility with which I am entrusted by the public.

A central tenet underlying pharmaceutical care and our desire to improve drug therapy outcomes is the recognition that patients have drug therapy needs. Although sometimes these needs are obvious ("What can I take for my headache?"), in many cases the patient's drug therapy needs are unrecognized. For the practitioner committed to responsibility for a patient's drug-related needs, identifying such needs in an accurate and timely way is paramount. During any pharmaceutical care encounter, the patient must be assessed to determine whether the following drug therapy needs are being met[2]:

1. The medication is appropriate.
2. The medication is effective.
3. The medication is safe.
4. The patient is adherent.

The challenge for the beginning pharmacotherapeutic practitioner is in application. How does a student learn to take the scientific and factual information learned in the classroom and in readings and then apply it to patients so that drug therapy outcomes are maximized? The Study Guide is designed for this purpose, to teach the student the patient care process: how to organize patient information, assess patients in a systematic way, and develop a pharmacotherapy care plan.[4]

All clinicians need a structured rational thought process for making clinical decisions. What sets each profession and

professional apart is the application of a unique knowledge base and set of clinical skills to identify and solve problems and to prevent problems from occurring. In the context of drug therapy, Cipolle et al. have termed this structured process the "Pharmacotherapy Workup."[2]

There are three steps that comprise the patient care process and constitute the Pharmacotherapy Workup (see Figure 1-1): patient assessment, development of the pharmacotherapy care plan, and evaluation of the impact or results of the care plan. As Figure 1-1 indicates, each stage of the process is connected to the other stages, and the process is ongoing as the patient's situation changes.

## Assessment

The purpose of assessment is to gather patient-specific information and then determine if the patient's drug therapy needs are being met.[5] To develop the best possible pharmacotherapy plan for the patient, the information gathered must be as accurate and complete as possible. Inaccurate or incomplete information may result in bad therapeutic decisions. There are a variety of sources from which such information is gathered. Although the specific sources may differ on the basis of the patient's situation, the clinician must strive to obtain information from all available sources. The patient is a crucial source of information, as are family members, caregivers, and other health professionals. In a health-system setting (hospitals, ambulatory care clinics, etc.), the clinician also will have access to subjective and objective information recorded in the patient's medical record and other institutional databases. For the pharmacotherapy workup, particular attention must be given to obtaining a complete and accurate medication history. Remember that since the patient care process is continuous, the gathering of patient-specific information also must be ongoing. Such information must be documented in an organized and easily retrievable way that maintains patient confidentiality. Since there may be a large volume of

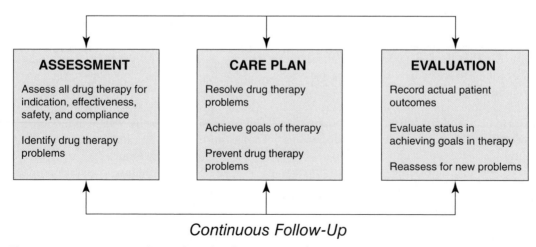

FIGURE 1-1.    The patient care process. (Reproduced with permission from Cipolle RJ, Strand LM, Morley PC. Pharmaceutical Care Practice. The Clinician's Guide, 2nd ed. New York, McGraw-Hill, 2004, p. 246.)

patient-specific information generated, particularly in a hospitalized patient, the use of a standardized patient data form facilitates the organization and retrievability of patient-specific information. Despite the clinician's best effort, in most cases there will be information that is inaccurate and/or incomplete. Never assume that you have all the information you need or that the information you have is correct. The clinician must be mindful of this and seek to "fill in the blanks" by asking appropriate follow-up questions or seeking additional information from other sources.

After all available information is collected, the next step is to develop a problem list.[6] The concept of problem list development is well established in the context of the problem-oriented medical record and the use of the SOAP (Subjective, Objective, Assessment, Plan) method of charting progress notes. The development of an accurate and complete problem list based on the patient's drug therapy needs is crucial in that the development of the pharmacotherapy care plan is derived from the patient's problem list. If a problem is not listed or is not accurate, then the plan will be incomplete or suboptimal. The problem list must be prioritized to ensure that the most important problems are addressed in a timely fashion. For the student learning pharmacotherapy, developing an accurate and complete list of problems is challenging since many pieces of subjective and objective information (findings) have to be interpreted before something can be labeled as a problem. In many cases, problems are medical diagnoses (hypertension, type 2 diabetes, etc.), and in some cases the problem may be a symptom (headache, nausea, pain, etc.). Keep in mind that the definition of a problem may change as more information is gathered. For example, a patient may present with fatigue and—in the absence of other information—that is how the patient's problem is defined at that specific time. However, if the patient is referred to a physician and is found to have hypothyroidism, then the patient's problem list is changed to hypothyroidism, with fatigue as a symptom of the patient's hypothyroidism. A common trap for the beginning student is listing every finding as a problem. With thought and—ultimately—experience, the student will begin to see that the patient's signs and symptoms may be "lumped" into broader problems. If the above-mentioned patient also has cold intolerance, cognitive impairment, weight gain, elevated TSH, and slightly elevated LDL cholesterol, the patient's problem is still hypothyroidism, since each of those findings is a common sign/symptom of hypothyroidism. Although the pharmacotherapy problem list may be very similar to the problem list generated by other clinicians or the problem list present in the patient's medical record, remember that the pharmacist, having a unique body of knowledge, should have a different way of looking at the patient, and the problem list may not be entirely the same. The pharmacotherapy workup must be focused on drug therapy issues, particularly on the presence or risk of drug therapy problems (DTPs). During the entire process, always ask yourself:

- Could the patient's problem(s) be caused by drug therapy?
- Could the patient's problem(s) be managed by a change in drug therapy?

## Drug Therapy Problems

The primary focus of the pharmacotherapy workup is the identification and management (treatment and prevention) of DTPs. A DTP is defined as any undesirable event or risk experienced by the patient that involves or is suspected to involve drug therapy and that actually or potentially interferes with a desired patient outcome.[7] Strand et al.'s original list of DTP categories has been expanded to 14 categories:

- Correlation between drug therapy and medical problems
- Need for additional drug therapy
- Unnecessary drug therapy
- Appropriate drug selection
- Wrong drug
- Drug regimen
- Dose too low
- Dose too high
- Therapeutic duplication
- Drug allergy/adverse drug event
- Interactions
- Failure to receive therapy
- Financial impact
- Patient knowledge of drug therapy

Since there are so many categories and specific types of DTPs, and since patients often receive multiple medications, it is important to use an organized, systematic approach to identify actual and potential DTPs. Once a DTP is identified and categorized, it is then necessary to identify the cause of the problem, thereby leading to potential solutions. When multiple DTPs are identified, they need to be prioritized to determine which problems should be addressed first. The patient's concerns must be considered in determining the problems that have the highest priority. Remember that the process of DTP identification is connected to the basic tenets of assessing the patient's drug therapy needs—appropriateness, effectiveness and safety of medications, and the patient's adherence.

## Pharmacotherapy Care Plan

The pharmacotherapy care plan[8,9] is the roadmap to achieving improved pharmacotherapy outcomes. It is the action plan developed on the basis of the assessment components described above. Care plans have been an integral component of nursing care, and other professionals or certain health care settings may utilize components of a care plan. However, there is no standard or widely accepted method of care plan development in Pharmacy. Guideline 12.1 of the accreditation standards for pharmacy education in the United States[10] states that "… the college or school must ensure that graduates are competent to provide patient-centered care, through the ability to design, implement, monitor, evaluate and adjust pharmacy care plans that are patient-specific…"

Ideally, the patient's care plan should be constructed with the patient's involvement and, in a multidisciplinary fashion, developed and altered in a cooperative way by all who are involved with the patient's care. Further, pharmacotherapy care planning should be a component of the patient's overall care plan. Care plans developed in isolation or not shared with the patient or other professionals are less likely to have the desired effect on patient outcomes. A pharmacotherapy care plan must be generated as part of the systematic patient care process and should be a dynamic document that reflects changes in the patient's conditions and drug therapy needs. The care plan is developed in a problem-oriented fashion. Each item in the patient's problem list must be addressed in the care plan, and the care plan should be prioritized in the same way as the problem list.

The pharmacotherapy care plan has several key components for each problem:

- Current drug regimen
- Drug therapy problems
- Therapy goals, desired endpoints
- Therapeutic recommendations
- Rationale
- Therapeutic alternatives
- Monitoring
- Patient education

In patients who have multiple problems, there likely will be some redundancy in the pharmacotherapy care plan in that some problems may be related, and some medications may be used for multiple indications. As the care plan is developed, it is important for the student to see and understand the connections among multiple problems and the pharmacotherapy plan. For example, a patient with hypertension, type 2 diabetes, and chronic kidney disease may be treated with an ACEI-I to lower BP, slow progression of renal disease, and reduce risk of cardiovascular events. The student must understand not only that the one drug may be used for several reasons but that the drug could affect the patient's problems in a variety of ways, such as improving BP control while causing an increase in serum potassium or an acute rise in serum creatinine. The risk and significance of these effects must be considered on the basis of the overall clinical picture. In some patients, unintended effects, at least to a defined point, may be acceptable.

Defining therapy goals and endpoints are crucial. You cannot determine whether the patient's desired outcomes are being achieved if you do not know what those desired outcomes are. Think of goals as broad or general outcomes, whereas endpoints are more specific parameters often used as indicators or surrogate markers to indicate that our goals are being achieved. The goals of therapy must be achievable and realistic for the patient. Drug therapy may aim to (1) cure a disease; (2) reduce or eliminate signs and/or symptoms; (3) slow or halt the progression of a disease; (4) prevent a disease; (5) normalize laboratory values; and/or (6) assist in the diagnostic process. Goals and endpoints must be observable, measurable, and describable using

specific parameters. Going back to our diabetic, hypertensive patient mentioned above, the goals of treating those disorders are to prevent cardiovascular disease (stroke, coronary artery disease, peripheral vascular disease), kidney disease, other microvascular complications of diabetes (retinopathy, neuropathy), etc. We also want the patient to feel better and have improved quality of life (QOL). An important goal of any pharmacotherapy care plan is the avoidance of adverse events. We do not want the patient to have side effects or a worsened QOL due to our recommended drug therapy. What would be endpoints for our patient? In our hypertensive diabetic patient, some endpoints would include BP <130/80 mm Hg, glycated hemoglobin <6.5–7% (0.065–0.07; 48–53 mmol/mol Hb), LDL cholesterol <130 mg/dL (<3.36 mmol/L), and weight loss of 22 lb (10 kg). Goals and endpoints should be associated with a time frame, describing, if possible and realistically, when the goal or endpoint is to be achieved (BP <130/80 mm Hg in 1 month; 22 lb (10 kg) weight loss in 6 months, etc.). The goals and endpoints part of the plan will be directly tied to the monitoring part of the plan, since monitoring is the way we will know if our goals and endpoints have been achieved.

Therapeutic recommendations are the interventions made to meet the patient's drug therapy needs. The recommendations must be specific and individualized to the patient's condition and drug therapy problems. For most problems, there are several ways to intervene to achieve the desired goals and endpoints. The clinician must consider all the possibilities and recommend a therapeutic course that is best for that patient, based on scientific evidence, patient history, cultural and health beliefs, psychosocial issues, health literacy, and cost. Remember that therapeutic recommendations for one problem may have an impact on other problems, so do not lose sight of the big picture.

Although it is important for the clinician to make appropriate therapeutic recommendations, providing a rationale for those recommendations is necessary. The rationale is *why* you are recommending what you are recommending. From an educational standpoint, providing a well-reasoned rationale shows that the student is thinking and understanding, rather than repeating what is in a book, guideline, or said by others. In the clinical practice setting, it is common for pharmacists to be asked to provide their rationale to physicians as part of a discussion about a patient's therapy. Pharmacists need to be adept at providing such a rationale in a succinct way. The rationale should be stated in a way that clearly describes why the recommendation was made for this patient, including why it was chosen over other alternatives, and any evidence available to support the recommendation should be provided.

In determining your therapeutic recommendations, several reasonable alternative regimens typically are available. Even after you have recommended your primary plan, the best alternatives must be kept in mind. The patient or prescriber may not agree with your primary recommendation and request an alternative. Your primary plan may not be effective, or an intolerable adverse event may occur, thereby requiring implementation of an alternative plan. As with your therapeutic recommendations, be specific with your alternative recommendations and base your alternative choices on relative effectiveness and safety based on the best evidence available.

Monitoring and follow-up are important components of the pharmacotherapy care plan and the overall patient care process.[11] Monitoring is how we determine whether our goals and endpoints (achieving positive goals and avoiding negative endpoints) are being reached. An effective monitoring plan must be realistic for the patient setting and include specific monitoring parameters (clinical and laboratory/diagnostic test), frequency of monitoring, and when the patient needs to be seen again for follow-up. Students often struggle with developing a monitoring plan since references often provide only general recommendations for what to monitor and how often. In most patients, the intensity and frequency of monitoring are dynamic. In a critically ill hospitalized patient, some pharmacotherapy monitoring parameters may be assessed multiple times daily. As the patient becomes more stable, leaves the ICU, and is, hopefully, discharged home, monitoring becomes less frequent. A patient initiated on warfarin in the hospital may have an INR measured daily. After discharge with a therapeutic INR, monitoring may be done weekly, and, as the patient's INR and clinical status remain stable, the frequency is slowly reduced until the INR is measured on a monthly basis. If the INR or the clinical picture changes, the frequency of INR monitoring likely will be increased temporarily. Regardless of the setting, the frequency of monitoring, particularly for those parameters involving blood collection or other invasive tests, must be realistic and based on how often the information truly is needed, what the patient can or is willing to allow, availability of vascular access, and, in the outpatient setting, the ability of the patient to travel to a laboratory or the availability of home care services. In the home setting, some of the monitoring may be done by the patient, such as assessing presence and severity of signs and symptoms, basic physical assessment parameters (e.g., weight, presence of edema), and certain diagnostic or laboratory tests (e.g., BP, blood glucose). The monitoring plan must be specific—what parameters, frequency of monitoring, who will monitor, and when and with whom the patient will follow-up. The results of monitoring naturally will influence the pharmacotherapy care plan, and, in many cases, there should be an upfront determination of what action will be taken based on the results of the monitoring plan (e.g., "If the patient's INR is <2, the warfarin dose will be increased from 4 to 5 mg daily").

Patient education is the final piece of the pharmacotherapy care plan. Patient adherence to drug therapy can be improved with effective and ongoing patient education, and, ideally, such education should be provided with verbal communication and written materials. Pharmacy students should utilize skills learned in their communications courses and information available in books[12,13] and begin applying those skills in case-based learning, small group discussions, and internship experience in preparation for their pharmacy practice experience rotations and, ultimately, pharmacy practice. The pharmacotherapy care plan must include a summary of what you will tell and provide the patient regarding their drug therapy.

Remember that our model for the patient care process involves continuous follow-up. As the pharmacotherapy care plan is implemented, the patient's response to therapy is monitored, and changes in therapy may be necessary. Changes in previous problems or the development of new signs and symptoms will require the assessment process and changes in the pharmacotherapy care plan. Although the patient care process and the application of your didactic knowledge to the patient care setting may seem daunting, by working through the cases in the Study Guide, your skills can only get better and better. Although this book can be used for self-study, ideally, some of the cases in this Study Guide will be used in a small group discussion setting under the guidance of a group facilitator, so you can see how other students think. Group settings also provide the opportunity to discuss and defend your therapeutic recommendations and practice your verbal communication skills. As you work through the patient cases, you will make mistakes and perhaps choose suboptimal therapy that even could cause harm. Beginners always make mistakes, and you should use the mistakes made by you and your fellow students as powerful learning opportunities. Here are some tips for success in patient care:

- CARE about the patient!
- Know your stuff—be prepared
- Realize that every patient is different
- Review and assess *all* available information
- Be organized and consistent in your approach
- Do not make snap judgments—is your assessment and approach supported by the evidence?
- NEVER make assumptions
- Be skeptical
- Think ahead, and think it through ("… then what?")

## HOW THE CASES ARE ORGANIZED

Each patient case in the Study Guide has been prepared in a standard format, similar to how you will see cases presented in a clinical setting. The use of an organized case format will assist you in learning where to find information about the patient and help you get accustomed to the format for when you will be presenting patients yourself in case discussions or rotations. The patient cases in the Study Guide are meant to be realistic. Patients usually will have multiple, sometimes related, problems, though each case will focus on one primary topic or problem. Patients will have DTPs requiring identification and management. The components of each case in the Study Guide will include:

1. *Patient Identification*—name, age, etc.
2. *Chief Complaint*—why the patient is seeking help, in the patient's own words

3. *History of Present Illness* (HPI)—the patient's story about why they are seeking help

4. *Past Medical History* (PMH)—including all significant illnesses, surgical procedures, injuries

5. *Family History*—age and health of immediate family (parents, siblings, children); for deceased relatives, the age and cause of death are included; any hereditary diseases should be noted

6. *Social History*—may include where the patient is from or lives, ethnicity/race, marital status, number of children, educational background, occupation, diet

7. *Tobacco/Alcohol/Substance Use*

8. *Allergy/Intolerances/Adverse Drug Events* (ADEs)—a common area where information from the patient is missing or incomplete

9. *Medication History*—should include current (or medications prior to admission if hospitalized) and previous medications; the list should include what the patient *actually* is taking, not just what is prescribed, and must include OTC drugs and dietary supplements (including herbal and complementary/alternative products).

10. *Review of Systems* (ROS)—systematic, head-to-toe questions asked to elicit symptoms and potential problems not noted by the patient in the HPI. Positive findings and pertinent negatives (significant absence of a symptom) are included.

11. *Physical Examination* (PE)—nature and completeness of the examination will depend on the patient's history and overall clinical picture. Rarely will a complete PE be done; rather, the examination will be targeted to the situation. Positive and pertinent negative findings will be included in the PE. If you are not familiar with the meaning or significance of some of the examination findings, make sure you look those up. Components of the PE may include:
   - General
   - Vital Signs (include pain as fifth vital sign)
   - Skin
   - HEENT
   - Neck and Lymph Nodes
   - Chest
   - Breasts (in women)
   - Cardiovascular
   - Abdomen
   - Neurology
   - Extremities
   - Genitourinary
   - Rectal

12. *Laboratory and Other Diagnostic Tests*—only data that are common and/or directly relevant to the case will be included. A list of normal laboratory values is included as Appendix B of this Study Guide. All laboratory results will be presented in conventional units typically used in the United States and in Systéme Internationale (SI) units for students using the book in other countries. If you are not familiar with the meaning or significance of some of the laboratory findings, make sure you look those up.

13. *Assessment*—the clinician's impression and/or diagnosis.

14. *Student Workup*—for each case, you will be asked if there is missing information and to evaluate and develop a Patient Database, Drug Therapy Problem Worksheet, and Pharmacotherapy Care Plan. When you are working with actual patients, you will find that the patient's history and information from other sources will be incomplete and/or inaccurate. Patient cases in the Study Guide will have missing information, and it is important that, as you evaluate each case, you recognize what needed information is missing so that you can make an accurate assessment of the patient. One way to remember to assess for missing information is to always create as one of your patient's problems "Inadequate Database," and then list the missing information elements under that problem in your Care Plan. A more detailed description of the Patient Database, Drug Therapy Problem Worksheet, and Pharmacotherapy Care Plan forms will follow.

15. *Targeted Questions*—each case will include a series of questions targeted toward helping you better understand the key elements of the case and the patient's primary problems. A unique feature of this Study Guide is that each question will be followed by a Hint, guiding you to the pages in *Pharmacotherapy Principles and Practice*, 3rd ed. (*PPP*) where you can find the information to answer the question.

16. *Follow-up*—some cases will provide a brief clinical follow-up that may include some outcomes of your initial Care Plan. The Follow-up section may include additional Targeted Questions, with Hints to further assist your studies.

17. *Global Perspective*—another unique feature of this Study Guide is the inclusion of a Global Perspective section that highlights an issue related to the case that is important to countries outside North America or involves different ethnic groups or races. Global Perspectives may highlight differences in disease incidence or manifestations, pharmacokinetics or pharmacodynamics, treatment standards, culturally based beliefs and/or treatments, and drug response.

18. *Case Summary*—a short summary of the key points addressed by the case.

19. *References*—will be included in the patient case only if a key reference has been published that is not included in *PPP*. For most cases, the references included in the relevant *PPP* chapters are excellent sources for you to obtain additional information.

## STUDENT CASE WORKUP

The desired student workup of each case in this Study Guide is the development of a Pharmacotherapy Care Plan. The principles of the pharmacotherapy workup, patient assessment, and development of a care plan were reviewed earlier in this chapter. Your workup of the Study Guide cases will apply these principles. To facilitate your accomplishing these tasks in a thoughtful, organized and systematic way, you are provided three forms—Patient Database, Drug Therapy Problem Worksheet (DTPW), and Pharmacotherapy Care Plan. The forms used in this Study Guide are adapted with permission from those originally developed by the American Society of Health-System Pharmacists (ASHP) in the early 1990s as part of its Clinical Skills program,[5,6,8,11] and these forms are currently used by participants in the ASHP Clinical Skills Competition (www.ashp.org/Import/ABOUTUS/Awards/ClinicalSkillsCompetition.aspx).

Different clinicians and institutions use many different types of patient-monitoring forms. Think of the forms used in this Study Guide as tools to help you learn to provide the best patient care. The forms are designed to help you organize information and to help you organize your thinking. Although you will find the use of such forms helpful, do not obsess about the forms or using them "right." Again, the forms are tools to help you achieve what you *should* obsess about—making the patient's drug therapy the best it can be.

To help you understand how to best utilize these forms as you workup the Study Guide cases, we have prepared a practice case presented in the same format as other cases in the Study Guide and a completed student workup. Before you embark on your first Study Guide patient case, look over the practice case and the completed forms. We have added some tips in certain places in the practice case forms to help you better understand their application. Learning to effectively assess patients and develop a care plan involves skills that require practice and repetition. As you begin learning pharmacotherapeutics, applying your didactic knowledge to patient situations may seem difficult, and it is likely you will make mistakes. That's okay! The point of this Study Guide is to help you learn and to develop your skills. Through your coursework, reading, and use of this Study Guide, you will see your knowledge and skills increase and you will become a great practitioner who will improve patient drug therapy outcomes.

## REFERENCES

1. Hepler CD, Strand LM. Opportunities and responsibilities in pharmaceutical care. Am J Hosp Pharm 1990 47: 533–543.
2. Cipolle RJ, Strand LM, Morley PC. Pharmaceutical Care Practice. The Clinician's Guide, 2nd ed. New York, McGraw-Hill, 2004.
3. American Association of Colleges of Pharmacy. www.aacp.org/resources/academicpolicies/studentaffairspolicies/Documents/OATHOFAPHARMACIST2008-09.pdf. Accessed October 1, 2012.
4. American Society of Health System Pharmacists. ASHP guidelines on a standardized method for pharmaceutical care. Am J Health Syst Pharm 1996 53:1713–1716.
5. Mason NA, Shimp LA. Module 2: Building a pharmacist's patient database. In: ASHP Clinical Skills Program—Advancing Pharmaceutical Care. Bethesda, MD, American Society of Health-System Pharmacists, 1993.
6. Shimp LA, Mason NA. Module 3: Constructing a patient's drug therapy problem list. In: ASHP Clinical Skills Program—Advancing Pharmaceutical Care. Bethesda, MD, American Society of Health-System Pharmacists, 1993.
7. Strand LM, Morley PC, Cipolle RJ, et al. Drug-related problems: Their structure and function. DICP 1990 24:1093–1097.
8. Jones W, Campbell S. Module 4: Designing and recommending a pharmacist's care plan. In: ASHP Clinical Skills Program—Advancing Pharmaceutical Care. Bethesda, MD, American Society of Health-System Pharmacists, 1993.
9. Galt K. Developing Clinical Practice Skills for Pharmacists. Bethesda, MD, American Society of Health-System Pharmacists, 2006.
10. American Council for Pharmacy Education. Accreditation Standards and Guidelines for the Professional Program in Pharmacy Leading to the Doctor of Pharmacy Degree, 2006. www.acpe-accredit.org/standards/default.asp. Accessed October 1, 2012.
11. Frye CB. Module 5: Monitoring the pharmacist's care plan. In: ASHP Clinical Skills Program—Advancing Pharmaceutical Care. Bethesda, MD, American Society of Health-System Pharmacists, 1993.
12. Beardsley RS, Kimberlin CL, Tindall WN. Communication Skills in Pharmacy Practice, 6th ed. Philadelphia, PA, Lippincott Williams & Wilkins, 2012.
13. Rantucci ML. Pharmacists Talking with Patients, 2nd ed. Philadelphia, PA, Lippincott Williams & Wilkins, 2007.

## PRACTICE CASE

### Case Learning Objectives

- Recognize the signs, symptoms, and risk factors for hypovolemia, hypokalemia, and metabolic alkalosis
- Develop an appropriate treatment and monitoring plan for hypovolemia, hypokalemia, and metabolic alkalosis
- Recognize the impact of pregnancy on medication choice and disease management

## PATIENT PRESENTATION

### Chief Complaint

"I feel so tired and dizzy, and I can't stop throwing up."

### History of Present Illness

Susan Jones is a 23-year-old woman brought to the urgent care center c/o severe weakness and dizziness. She states it started 3 days ago when she began to have frequent vomiting.

She thinks that "maybe I ate something bad." She also says that her bowel movements have been "a little looser than normal." She states that before she got sick 3 days ago, she felt fine.

## Past Medical History

Bulimia with two psychiatric hospitalizations

Depression, s/p suicide attempt × 1 (slashed wrists)

Pelvic inflammatory disease

## Family History

Mother died from drug overdose at age 34; she does not know her father.

## Social History

Single community college student; no children; works part time in restaurant.

## Tobacco/Alcohol/Substance Abuse

(+) cigarettes ½ ppd; admits to occasional marijuana use, denies current other illicit or unprescribed drug or alcohol use; used IV heroin until 1 year ago.

## Medications

Prozac 20 mg bid PO

Trazodone 50 mg q hs PO

K-DUR 40 mEq q AM PO

Methadone 120 mg q AM PO

Prilosec 20 mg q day PO

Lo-Estrin 1 q AM PO

## Review of Systems

(+) Weakness, dizziness, fatigue, nausea, and diarrhea; denies headache, chest pain, or abdominal pain; (+) dysuria; (−) vaginal pain or discharge.

## Physical Examination

▶ *General*

Very thin, chronically ill–appearing young woman who fainted when sitting up.

▶ *Vital signs*

BP 105/75 mm Hg lying, 70/0 mm Hg sitting; P 110 lying, 160 sitting; RR 12, T 37.1°C

Weight 47 kg (103.4 lb), height 5′4″ (163 cm)

▶ *Skin*

Dry, poor skin turgor; no rashes or lesions noted

▶ *HEENT*

PERRLA; mouth very dry; poor dentition

▶ *Neck and lymph nodes*

JVD 0 (neck veins flat); thyroid gland normal; no lymphadenopathy

▶ *Chest*

Clear to auscultation and percussion

▶ *Breasts*

Examination deferred

▶ *Cardiovascular*

Tachycardic; normal $S_1$, $S_2$; no murmurs, rubs, or gallops

▶ *Abdomen*

No tenderness or organomegaly; bowel sounds slightly hyperactive

▶ *Extremities*

Very thin; trace pedal edema; multiple "tracks" both arms

▶ *Genitourinary*

Normal vaginal discharge; uterus appears to contain approximately 12-week pregnancy

▶ *Rectal*

Mild hemorrhoids; Hemoccult (−)

## Laboratory Tests

### Fasting Obtained upon Admission

|           | Conventional Units | SI Units |
|-----------|--------------------|----------|
| Na        | 126 mEq/L          | 126 mmol/L |
| K         | 2.1 mEq/L          | 2.1 mmol/L |
| Cl        | 87 mEq/L           | 87 mmol/L |
| $CO_2$    | 32 mEq/L           | 32 mmol/L |
| BUN       | 8 mg/dL            | 2.9 mmol/L |
| SCr       | 0.5 mg/dL          | 44 μmol/L |
| Glu       | 110 mg/dL          | 6.1 mmol/L |
| Ca        | 8.7 mg/dL          | 2.18 mmol/L |
| Mg        | 1.8 mEq/L          | 0.90 mmol/L |
| Phosphate | 3.6 mg/dL          | 1.16 mmol/L |
| WBC       | $7.4 \times 10^3/mm^3$ | $7.4 \times 10^9/L$ |
| Hgb       | 11.6 g/dL          | 116 g/L; 7.2 mmol/L |
| Hct       | 34.6%              | 0.346 |
| Albumin   | 3.2 g/dL           | 32 g/L |
| PT        | 17 s               |  |
| INR       | 1.3                |  |

Urine pregnancy test (+)

ABG: pH 7.56, $pO_2$ 98 mm Hg (13.0 kPa), $O_2$ sat 99% (0.99), $pCO_2$ 44 mm Hg (5.9 kPa), $HCO_3$ 31 mEq/L (31 mmol/L)

Urine toxicology screen: (+) cocaine, THC, methamphetamine, nicotine, HCTZ

ECG: flat T waves; (+) U wave

## Assessment

Twenty-three-year-old pregnant woman with ECF volume depletion, vomiting and ? diarrhea, significant hypokalemia with ECG changes, hyponatremia, and metabolic alkalosis. Urine tox screen indicates active illicit drug use.

### Student Workup

**Missing Information?**

**Evaluate:**    Patient Database

Drug Therapy Problems

Care Plan (by Problem)

## TARGETED QUESTIONS

1. What signs and symptoms of ECF volume depletion, hypokalemia, and metabolic alkalosis does the patient have?

   *Hint: See pp. 506, 509, 524 in PPP*

2. What are the causes of this patient's alkalosis?

   *Hint: See p. 525 in PPP*

3. What are the risks of administering potassium intravenously?

   *Hint: See p. 510 in PPP*

4. What are the signs and symptoms of opioid withdrawal, and what drug interactions may occur with methadone?

   *Hint: See pp. 639, 641 in PPP*

5. What medications have proven to have teratogenic effects in humans?

   *Hint: See p. 851 in PPP*

## FOLLOW-UP

Three months later, the patient calls you after being discharged from an inpatient substance abuse program. She says she feels great, is staying clean, and her baby is doing well ("Look how fat I am!"). Her obstetrician recently told her that she has low thyroid and wants her to take levothyroxine. She is afraid that it will hurt her baby and she wants your advice. You look up her laboratory tests in the computer and note that her TSH is 10.1 µIU/mL (10.1 mIU/L). What is your advice to her?

*Hint: See pp. 794–796 in PPP*

## ⊙ GLOBAL PERSPECTIVE

Depression is a common mental disorder that presents with depressed mood, loss of interest or pleasure, feelings of guilt or low self-worth, disturbed sleep or appetite, low energy, and poor concentration. These problems can become chronic or recurrent and may lead to substantial impairments in an individual's ability to take care of his or her everyday responsibilities. At its worst, depression can lead to suicide, with the loss of about 850,000 lives every year.

In 2008, depression was the leading cause of disability worldwide as measured by years lived with disability (YLD) and the fourth-leading contributor to the global burden of disease based on disability-adjusted life-years (DALYs). By the year 2020, depression is projected to reach second place in the ranking of DALYs calculated for all ages and in both sexes. Today, depression already is the second cause of DALYs worldwide in the age category 15–44 years for both sexes combined. According to the World Health Organization, fewer than 25% of depressed patients have access to care, and, in some countries, fewer than 10% have access to care. Barriers to effective care include the lack of resources, lack of trained providers, and the social stigma associated with mental disorders, including depression.

## REFERENCE

World Health Organization. www.who.int/mental_health/management/depression/definition/en/index.html. Accessed October 1, 2012.

### CASE SUMMARY

- Young pregnant woman with history of depression, eating disorder, and substance abuse who presents with ECF volume depletion, hypokalemia, and metabolic alkalosis due to vomiting and diuretic use. Volume and potassium replacement must be initiated, and the underlying causes addressed to prevent recurrence.

- She is actively abusing drugs, placing her and the fetus at risk for multiple complications. Substance abuse treatment referral is warranted.

- The patient needs a referral to an obstetrician for assessment and prenatal care.

**For more information on the care plan and facilitator's guide please visit http://www.mhpharmacotherapy.com.**

## PATIENT DATABASE FORM

| | | | |
|---|---|---|---|
| **Patient Name:** Susan Jones | Real patient names are not used in this Study Guide. | **Patient ID:** | **Location:** Urgent Care |
| **Physician:** | | **Pharmacy:** | |
| **Age (or Date of Birth):** 23 yo | | **Race:** Caucasian | **Sex:** Female |
| **Height:** 5'4" (163 cm) | | **Weight:** 47 kg (103.4 lb) | |
| **Date of Admission/Initial Visit:** 6/1/2012 | | **Occupation:** Student, restaurant worker | |

### Allergies/Intolerances/ADRs

❏ No known drug allergies/ADRs

☒ Not known/inadequate information

| **Drug:** | **Reaction:** |
|---|---|

> A common area where information is missing or incomplete. No known drug allergies/ADRs is **NOT** the same as Not known. No known means the patients has been asked and/or chart reviewed, while Not known means there is missing information.

### HPI, PMH, FH, SH, etc…

Weakness, dizziness, vomiting,? diarrhea × 3 days

Hx eating disorder, depression (s/p suicide attempt), PID

Smokes ½ ppd, uses marijuana, Hx IVDU (+) dysuria on ROS

Appears dry—orthostatic, flat neck veins

Evidence of active IVDU

12 wk pregnant

> A summary of the key subjective and objective findings from the case.

| Prioritized Medical Problem List | Medication Profile |
|---|---|
| Hypovolemic hyponatremia, d/t vomiting,? diuretic use | |
| Hypokalemia with ECG changes | K-Dur 40 mEq q AM PO |
| Metabolic alkalosis due to #1 and #2 | |
| Active substance use with urine (+) cocaine, methamphetamine; no evidence for endocarditis | Methadone 120 mg q day PO |
| Tobacco use | |
| 12 wk pregnant by exam, (+) urine HCG | Lo-Estrin PO |
| Hx bulimia, appears to be malnourished | Fluoxetine 20 mg bid PO |
| ? Diarrhea | |
| Hx depression, s/p suicide attempt × 1 | |
| Dysuria, R/O UTI | |
| Inadequate database | ? Indications for trazodone, omeprazole |

> List of medications placed next to problem list to facilitate matching medications with indications. Note that some medications may have multiple indications.

> Get used to including Inadequate database or Missing Information on your problems list so you will remember to follow-up on all missing information.

The form is from *ASHP National Clinical Skills Competition Case Documents*, Copyright 2009, American Society of Health-System Pharmacists, Bethesda, MD (www.ashp.org). Adapted with permission.

| Vital Signs, Laboratory Data, and Diagnostic Test Results | | |
|---|---|---|
| Date | 6/1/2012 | |
| Weight (lb/kg) | 103.4 (47) | |
| Temperature (°C) | 37.1 | |
| Blood pressure (mm Hg) | 105/75 lying, 70/0 sitting | |
| Pulse | 110 lying, 160 sitting | |
| Respiratory rate | 12 | |
| Na<br>135–145 mEq/L (135–145 mmol/L) | 126 (126) | |
| K<br>3.3–4.9 mEq/L (3.3–4.9 mmol/L) | 2.1 (2.1) | |
| Cl<br>97–110 mEq/L (97–110 mmol/L) | 87 (87) | |
| $CO_2/HCO_3$<br>22–26 mEq/L (22–26 mmol/L) | 32 (32) | |
| BUN<br>8–25 mg/dL (2.9–8.9 mmol/L) | 8 (2.9) | |
| Creatinine (adult)<br>Male 0.7–1.3 mg/dL; female 0.6–1.1 mg/dL (male 62–115 µmol/L; female 53–97 µmol/L) | 0.5 (44) | |
| Creatinine clearance (adult)<br>85–135 mL/min (1.42–2.25 mL/s) | 129.9 (2.17) | |
| Glucose (fasting)<br>65–109 mg/dL (3.6–6.0 mmol/L) | 110 (6.1) | |
| Total Ca<br>8.6–10.3 mg/dL (2.15–2.58 mmol/L) | 8.7 (2.18) | |
| Mg<br>1.3–2.2 mEq/L (0.65–1.10 mmol/L) | 1.8 (0.9) | |
| $PO_4$<br>2.5–4.5 mg/dL (0.81–1.45 mmol/L) | 3.6 (1.16) | |
| Hemoglobin<br>Male 13.8–17.2 g/dL; female 12.1–15.1 g/dL (male 138–172 g/L; female 121–151 g/L) | 11.6 (116) | |
| Hematocrit<br>Male 40.7–50.3%; female 36.1–44.3% (male 0.407–0.503; female 0.361–0.443) | 34.6 (0.346); 7.2 mmol/L | |
| MCV<br>80.0–97.6 µm³ (80.0–97.6 fL) | | |
| WBC<br>4–10 × 10³/mm³ (4–10 × 10⁹/L) | 7.4 (7.4) | |
| Differential | | |
| Platelet<br>140–440 × 10³/mm³ (140–440 × 10⁹/L) | | |
| Albumin<br>3.5–5 g/dL (35–50 g/L) | 3.2 (32) | |
| Total bilirubin<br>0.3–1.1 mg/dL (5.13–18.8 µmol/L) | | |
| Direct bilirubin<br>0–0.3 mg/dL (0–5.1 µmol/L) | | |
| AST<br>11–47 IU/L (0.18–0.78 µkat/L) | | |

Having data in tabular form allows following trends over time (date as column heading).

| Vital Signs, Laboratory Data, and Diagnostic Test Results | | | |
|---|---|---|---|
| **ALT**<br>7–53 IU/L (0.12–0.88 µkat/L) | | | |
| **Alk phos (adult)**<br>38–126 IU/L (0.63–2.10 µkat/L) | | | |
| Urine HCG | Positive | | |
| **PH**<br>7.35–7.45 | 7.56 | | |
| **PO$_2$**<br>70–95 mm Hg (9.3–12.6 kPa) | 98 (13.0) | | |
| **O$_2$**<br>Saturation (90–110%) | 99 (0.99) | | |
| **PCO$_2$**<br>35–45 mm Hg (4.7–6.0 kPa) | 44 (5.9) | | |

Not every lab test is included on the blank forms, so you will need to add lab tests, normal values and normal values for tests not already on the form. Normal values may be found in Appendix B. Make sure you understand the significance of each lab test.

| Notes |
|---|
| Urine tox screen (+) for cocaine, THC, methamphetamine, HCTZ |
| ECG: NSR, rate 110, flattened T waves, (+) U wave |
| |
| |
| |
| |
| |

This is a free text area to add items that do not fit elsewhere or for quick notes to yourself or other clinicians who may be following the patient.

**DRUG THERAPY PROBLEM WORKSHEET**

This Worksheet will help you systematically assess the patient for the presence of and potential for all Drug Therapy Problems. After each problem is identified, you will then need to assess the significance of each problem, and integrate those problems with your overall Care Plan. Some medications may be associated with multiple problems. Make sure you are as specific as possible in identifying the problem so that appropriate action then can be taken.

| Type of Problem | Possible Causes | | |
|---|---|---|---|
| Correlation between drug therapy and medical problems | Drugs without obvious medical indications | Trazodone, omeprazole | |
| | Medications unidentified | | |
| | Untreated medical conditions | | |
| Need for additional drug therapy | New medical condition requiring new drug therapy | Pregnancy<br>If dysuria d/t UTI, needs nonteratogenic antimicrobial | Needs prenatal care |
| | Chronic disorder requiring continued drug therapy | | |
| | Condition best treated with combination drug therapy | | |
| | May develop new medical condition without prophylactic or preventative therapy or premedication | | |
| Unnecessary drug therapy | Medication with no valid indication | Lo-Estrin | Patient is pregnant |
| | Condition caused by accidental or intentional ingestion of toxic amount of drug or chemical | HCTZ contributed to fluid/electrolyte disorders | |
| | Medical problem(s) associated with use of or withdrawal from alcohol, drug, or tobacco | | |
| | Condition is better treated with nondrug therapy | | |
| | Taking multiple drugs when single agent as effective | | |
| | Taking drug(s) to treat an avoidable adverse reaction from another medication | | |
| Appropriate drug selection | Current regimen not usually as effective as other choices | | |
| | Current regimen not usually as safe as other choices | | |
| | Therapy not individualized to patient | | |
| Wrong drug | Medical problem for which drug is not effective | | |
| | Patient has risk factors that contraindicate use of drug | Need to assess teratogenic effects of all drugs; hormonal contraceptive in pregnancy | |
| | Patient has infection with organisms resistant to drug | | |
| | Patient refractory to current drug therapy | | |
| | Taking combination product when single agent appropriate | | |
| | Dosage form inappropriate | | |
| | Medication error | | |
| Drug regimen | PRN use not appropriate for condition | | |
| | Route of administration/dosage form/mode of administration not appropriate for current condition | | |
| | Length or course of therapy not appropriate | | |
| | Drug therapy altered without adequate therapeutic trial | | |
| | Dose or interval flexibility not appropriate | | |
| Dose too low | Dose or frequency too low to produce desired response in this patient | | |
| | Serum drug level below desired therapeutic range | | |
| | Timing of antimicrobial prophylaxis not appropriate | | |
| | Medication not stored properly | | |
| | Medication error | | |

Identified by comparing problem list and medication list.

Make sure all new problems are addressed (though all may not require drug therapy).

Even if a medication is indicated for the problem, it may not be the BEST therapy for that patient.

**DRUG THERAPY PROBLEM WORKSHEET**

| Type of Problem | Possible Causes | Problem List | Notes |
|---|---|---|---|
| Dose too high | Dose or frequency too high for this patient | Assess methadone dose with substance abuse provider | Make sure all drug doses have been adjusted for the patient's renal and liver function. |
| | Serum drug level above the desired therapeutic range | | |
| | Dose escalated too quickly | | |
| | Dose or interval flexibility not appropriate for this patient | Need for bid fluoxetine | |
| | Medication error | | |
| Therapeutic duplication | Receiving multiple agents without added benefit | | |
| Drug allergy/ adverse drug events | History of allergy or ADE to current (or chemically related) agents | | |
| | Allergy or ADE history not in medical records | Need allergy/ADE history | Allergy/ADE information commonly is missing or incomplete. |
| | Patient not using alert for severe allergy or ADE | | |
| | Symptoms or medical problems that may be drug induced | HCZT and fluid/ electrolyte disorders<br><br>Fluoxetine and insomnia | |
| | Drug administered too rapidly | | |
| | Medication error, actual or potential | | |
| Interactions (drug–drug, drug–disease, drug–nutrient, drug–laboratory test) | Effect of drug altered due to enzyme induction/ inhibition from another drug patient is taking | Fluoxetine and methadone | Slight reduction in methadone clearance; watch QTc |
| | Effect of drug altered due to protein-binding alterations from another drug patient is taking | | |
| | Effect of drug altered due to pharmacodynamic change from another drug patient is taking | Fluoxetine and trazodone | Both serotonin modulators |
| | Bioavailability of drug altered due to interaction with another drug or food | | Assessing for interactions is important, but make sure you assess for the clinical significance of the interaction in the patient. |
| | Effect of drug altered due to substance in food | | |
| | Patient's laboratory test altered due to interference from a drug the patient is taking | | |
| Failure to receive therapy | Patient did not adhere with the drug regimen | Unknown, but likely is nonadherent; likely not taking methadone since not in urine tox | ALWAYS assess adherence. If adherence problems are identified, find out the reasons for poor adherence and possible solutions. |
| | Drug not given due to medication error | | |
| | Patient did not take due to high drug cost/lack of insurance | Unknown | |
| | Patient unable to take oral medication | | |
| | Patient has no IV access for IV medication | | Financial or insurance problems are a common reason for poor adherence. |
| | Drug product not available | | |
| Financial impact | The current regimen is not the most cost-effective | | |
| | Patient unable to purchase medications/no insurance | Unknown | |
| Patient knowledge of drug therapy | Patient does not understand the purpose, directions, or potential side effects of the drug regimen | Unknown | Patients often have little understanding about their medications. Make sure you develop an educational plan appropriate for the patient. |
| | Current regimen not consistent with the patient's health beliefs | Unknown | |

# PHARMACOTHERAPY CARE PLAN

For acute problems, make sure your therapeutic recommendations are carried through to some resolution or stopping point and/or chronic therapy.

| Medical Problem List | Current Drug Regimen | Drug Therapy Problems | Therapy Goals, Desired Endpoints | Therapeutic Recommendations | Rationale | Therapeutic Alternatives | Monitoring |
|---|---|---|---|---|---|---|---|
| Hypovolemic hyponatremia | | HCTZ use may be contributing factor | Normal hemodynamics (BP, pulse, JVD), improved symptoms (weakness, dizziness); prevent recurrence by treating underlying cause | Normal saline IV 1 L now over 15 min, then 500 mL/h × 2. Repeat until no longer orthostatic; if able to take PO, add oral rehydration solution (ORS) 250 mL q 30 min; promethazine 25 mg PO/IM/PR q 4 h PRN N/V; pt needs to stop using HCTZ; if pt has diarrhea, order stool culture; R/O laxative abuse; stop using HCTZ | Severe signs and symptoms, presence of vomiting warrant IV fluid; normal saline best for treating ECF depletion, metabolic alkalosis; hyponatremia will correct with volume replacement | If able to take PO or IV access not available, ORS 500–1000mL/h as tolerated; metoclopramide 10 mg IV q 6 h PRN nausea | VS q 15 min × 2 h, then q 1 h while in urgent care. Recheck basic metabolic panel (BMP) in 4 h; pt to self-monitor symptoms, weight daily after discharge; repeat BMP in 2 d |
| Hypokalemia | K-Dur 40 mEq q AM PO | HCTZ | Normal serum K; normal ECG, no symptoms; prevent recurrence by treating underlying cause | KCl liquid 40 mEq PO now, repeat in 2 h; if serum K increasing, change to KCl SR 40 mEq bid × 2 d, then reassess; stop using HCTZ | Oral KCl safer than IV if pt able to take; pt has significant K deficit; need K replacement for correction of alkalosis; use liquid KCl for rapid absorption | If unable to take PO, IV KCl 10 mEq/ 100 mL with 10 mg lidocaine over 1 h × 4 doses | BMP in 2 h (recheck in 6 h if IV KCl given); ECG in 4 h |
| Metabolic alkalosis, due to decreased ECF, vomiting, ?diuretic use | | HCTZ | Normal ABG, electrolytes, ECF volume; prevent recurrence by treating underlying cause | Volume repletion, K replacement, treat vomiting as above; stop using HCTZ; if alkalosis slow to clear or serum Mg drops, provide Mg replacement as MgSO₄ 1 g IV in 100 mL NS over 1 h | Alkalosis will resolve with volume and K replacement and with removal of underlying causes; Mg deficiency can prevent resolution of hypokalemia, alkalosis, though serum Mg now normal | Alternatives to volume, K replacement as above; no indication for IV HCl administration; could give Mg replacement even though serum Mg in normal range | BMP, other monitoring as above; recheck serum Mg in 2 h |

*Callout notes:*

Drug therapy problems identified on DTPW listed in this column, tied to medical problem.

Goals and endpoints should be as specific as possible, and should include preventing adverse outcomes as well as seeking positive outcomes.

Therapeutic recommendations and alternatives must be specific (drug, route, dose, frequency, duration).

Make sure monitoring plan is specific (parameters, frequency) and realistic for the setting.

Your rationale should include why you chose your primary therapy (drug, route, etc.) versus the alternative(s); may include why you did not specifically address certain problems.

Note that some problems are connected to others, and their resolution may be connected to treatment of those related problems.

## PHARMACOTHERAPY CARE PLAN

| Medical Problem List | Current Drug Regimen | Drug Therapy Problems | Therapy Goals, Desired Endpoints | Therapeutic Recommendations | Rationale | Therapeutic Alternatives | Monitoring |
|---|---|---|---|---|---|---|---|
| Substance use | Methadone 120 mg q day PO | Urine tox (+) for cocaine, THC, methamphetamine | No use of illicit drugs; avoidance of medical complications of injection use such as skin abscesses endocarditis<br><br>Not all problems can be addressed or resolved. Some will require referral to other professionals or institutions. | Hold methadone since pt seems not to be taking and no evidence of narcotic withdrawal; if signs of withdrawal develop, begin methadone 20 mg q day inpatient; if methadone used, watch for potential interactions; blood cultures × 3 to R/O endocarditis; refer back to substance abuse provider after discharge; encourage enrollment in smoking cessation program; test for HIV, hepatitis B and C | Since urine tox was not positive for methadone, pt likely not taking; narcotic withdrawal not life-threatening, so best to wait to see if withdrawal signs develop and then treat with low-dose methadone; while no evidence of endocarditis (fever, murmur), best to R/O with blood cultures especially since she is pregnant | Begin methadone 20 mg q day if patient was taking methadone or other opioids chronically | Signs and symptoms of drug withdrawal; temperature q 6 h while in facility, then by pt daily; examine injection sites daily; CBC in 2 d; QTc if on methadone |
| Pregnancy | | Lo-Estrin, drugs of abuse, tobacco | Cessation of behavior that is high risk to the fetus; adequate prenatal care | DC Lo-Estrin; substance abuse program as per substance abuse provider; refer to OB for full assessment, prenatal care; prenatal vitamin 1 q day; nutrition consult; smoking cessation; need to review all current and future drugs for teratogenic effect | Substance abuse and malnutrition will severely compromise development and health of fetus | None | As per substance abuse provider, OB |

## PHARMACOTHERAPY CARE PLAN

| Medical Problem List | Current Drug Regimen | Drug Therapy Problems | Therapy Goals, Desired Endpoints | Therapeutic Recommendations | Rationale | Therapeutic Alternatives | Monitoring |
|---|---|---|---|---|---|---|---|
| Eating disorder, depression | Fluoxetine 20 mg bid PO | Drugs of abuse; fluoxetine bid ? causing insomnia; HCTZ use, ? laxative use | Normal eating patterns, no use of diuretics or laxatives; normal mood with no s/s depression | If patient has been taking fluoxetine, continue at 20 mg q day; psych consult; if insomnia, withhold hypnotics at this time since may be due to fluoxetine regimen and stimulant use; nutrition consult as above | Avoid SSRI withdrawal syndrome if she has been taking fluoxetine; if insomnia, may resolve with change in fluoxetine regimen, stimulant detox | Change antidepressant to less stimulating agent, i.e., sertraline 50 mg q day | As per psych |
| Dysuria | | | No symptoms; cure UTI if present | Urinalysis; if (+) for UTI, send for culture and start cephalexin 250 mg q 8 h × 7 d, start after all three blood cultures drawn | Cephalosporins safe in pregnancy, active against most common organism | Augmentin 500 mg q 8 h × 7 d | UTI s/s daily; repeat UA after antibiotic completed; stool frequency, consistency |
| Inadequate database | | | | Need allergy/ADE Hx; indications for trazodone, omeprazole; frequency of substance use; adherence with prescribed medications; use of diuretics, laxatives; screen for HIV, viral hepatitis; liver enzymes; previous pregnancies, deliveries | | | |

Therapy may be initiated or altered as missing information is obtained. In such cases make sure that you note when such therapy will be started based on obtaining certain information.

For the Study Guide cases, all you can do is list missing information. In a real-life setting, you must try to obtain the missing information from the appropriate sources (patient, family, medical record, other professionals or institutions).

<table>
<tr><td>**PATIENT EDUCATION SUMMARY**</td><td>Summarize your patient education in the type of language you would use with a real patient. Avoid use of medical terms or lingo, and keep in mind the patient's language skills, educational background, and culture.</td></tr>
</table>

**Notes**

- The problems you are having with your fluid and electrolytes are all related and are causing your weakness and dizziness. There are several reasons why these problems developed, including your vomiting and lack of food and fluid intake and your drug abuse. It appears that you are using an unprescribed diuretic, and that is causing or worsening these problems. Although we can easily treat these problems here, it is important that you take steps so that it does not happen again. You can help prevent this in the future by making sure you eat and drink fluids properly, do not use diuretics, and stop abusing drugs. After we give you some IV fluids, we will be giving you some oral fluids, as well as some oral potassium. It is very important that you take these as directed so that we can get your fluid and electrolyte levels back to normal. We have prescribed a medication, promethazine, for nausea and vomiting. Take it only if you need it and are unable to keep down oral fluids. Sometimes this medication can cause you to be a little drowsy or have a dry mouth. Let us know if that happens.

- From your urine screen and looking at your arms we can tell that you are actively abusing drugs. It will be crucial for you and your baby that you stop using immediately. We will refer you back to your substance abuse provider after you are discharged, and we strongly urge that you get involved with a program that will help you stay clean. Since it appears that you have not been using your methadone, we are going to withhold that for the time being. Since injecting drugs can put you (and your baby) at risk for infections like HIV and hepatitis, we are going to test you for those infections. Also, we are going to test you for a bacterial infection of the heart that happens sometimes in people who inject drugs. Smoking tobacco also is very harmful to you and your baby, and we strongly encourage you to stop smoking. Your substance abuse provider can help you with that also.

- We found that you are about 12 wk pregnant. We want to help you have a healthy baby, but the first thing you need to do is stop abusing drugs since they are so harmful to the development of your baby. Also, your nutrition does not appear to be very good, and you need to eat well enough so that your baby can get nutrients. We will refer you to an obstetrician, and we will start you on a prenatal vitamin to be taken every day. Since many medications can harm the baby during pregnancy, make sure all your providers know you are pregnant, and do not take any medication unless you check with your obstetrician or pharmacist. Do not start taking your birth control pills when you get home since you are pregnant.

- You had been prescribed fluoxetine (Prozac) for your depression and bulimia. If you have been taking it on a regular basis, we do not want to stop it suddenly. When you take this medication later in the day, sometimes it can cause problems sleeping, so we will give it to you just in the morning. We are going to have a psychiatrist consult with you so that we can determine the best way to manage these problems, with medications and with counseling.

- We noticed that you are complaining of some pain or burning when you urinate. This may be caused by a urinary tract infection, and we are going to test you for that. If you do have a urine infection, we will give you an antibiotic for that. Make sure you take every dose since a urine infection can harm your baby as well as you. The antibiotic we will give, cephalexin, will not harm your baby. Sometimes it can cause some diarrhea or skin rashes, so if that happens, please let us know.

# 2 Hypertension: Newly Diagnosed

Keri D. Hager          Stephanie Reynolds
Robert J. Straka

## CASE LEARNING OBJECTIVES

- Classify blood pressure levels
- Identify the goals of therapy for HTN
- Select appropriate HTN therapy based on patient's individual characteristics
- Develop an appropriate monitoring and follow-up plan
- Properly educate a patient about antihypertensive treatment

## PATIENT PRESENTATION

### Chief Complaint

"I need to get my meds renewed."

### History of Present Illness

Jose Vasquez is a 57-year-old Mexican American male who lost his job 6 months ago, and had not refilled any of his prescription medications for approximately 5 months because of cost (lost his insurance coverage). He has now started a new job and again has prescription drug coverage. He is concerned because his 52-year-old brother had a heart attack 2 years ago. Jose states his cholesterol was "where it was supposed to be" according to his previous physician while he was on simvastatin 40 mg in the past. Jose also mentions that his blood pressure has been in the 140s/90s at his gym, and he wonders if that is okay. He reports eating a low-fat diet, and exercises (walking, weightlifting) approximately 30 minutes three times/week.

### Past Medical History

Dyslipidemia 2006

Gout 2010

Seasonal allergic rhinitis since childhood

### Family History

Father died from MVA at the age of 35. Mother's age is 77 with HTN, osteoporosis, and a history of breast cancer. He has a brother (5 years younger) with dyslipidemia, HTN, type 2 DM; MI at age 50. He has two younger sisters, one has HTN, and both have dyslipidemia.

### Social History

Born in the United States after his parents emigrated from Mexico. Married and lives with his wife; has three sons aged 35, 32, and 26 (all healthy). Recently started working at the U.S. Post Office.

### Tobacco/Alcohol/Substance Use

Two to four drinks/week; tobacco use 1 ppd (41 pack-year history), "knows he should quit" but is unwilling to set a quit date given the stress of his new job; (–) illicit drug use.

### Allergies/Intolerances/Adverse Drug Events

NKDA

### Medications (Current)

Loratadine 10 mg PRN (Was taking allopurinol 200 mg and simvastatin 40 mg daily prior to losing insurance coverage.)

### Review of Systems

Constipation despite fiber-rich diet and at least 64 oz. (1.9 L) water daily. Otherwise unremarkable.

### Physical Examination

▸ *General*

Well-appearing, middle-aged, Hispanic male in no acute distress.

▶ **Vital Signs**

BP 146/94 mm Hg, repeat 144/92 mm Hg (right arm, regular cuff), P 56 bpm, RR 12, T 36°C.

Weight 168.4 lb (76.5 kg)

Height 66 in. (168 cm)

Denies pain

▶ **Skin**

Dry

▶ **HEENT**

PERRLA, EOMI intact; TMs appear normal

▶ **Neck and Lymph Nodes**

Thyroid gland smooth; (−) thyroid nodules; (−) lymphadenopathy; (−) carotid bruits

▶ **Chest**

Clear to auscultation

▶ **Cardiovascular**

RRR, normal $S_1$, $S_2$; (−) $S_3$ or $S_4$

▶ **Abdomen**

Not tender/not distended; (−) organomegaly

▶ **Neurology**

Grossly intact; deep tendon reflexes normal

▶ **Genitourinary**

Examination deferred

▶ **Rectal**

Examination deferred

## Laboratory Tests

### Fasting from Today

|  | Conventional Units | SI Units |
|---|---|---|
| Na | 143 mEq/L | 143 mmol/L |
| K | 4.2 mEq/L | 4.2 mmol/L |
| Cl | 99 mEq/L | 99 mmol/L |
| $CO_2$ | 25 mEq/L | 25 mEq/L |
| BUN | 13 mg/dL | 4.6 mmol/L |
| SCr | 1.2 mg/dL | 106 μmol/L |
| Glu | 111 mg/dL | 6.2 mmol/L |
| Total cholesterol | 240 mg/dL | 6.21 mmol/L |
| LDL cholesterol | 167 mg/dL | 4.32 mmol/L |
| HDL cholesterol | 38 mg/dL | 0.98 mmol/L |
| Triglycerides | 175 mg/dL | 1.98 mmol/L |
| TSH | 2.4 μIU/mL | 2.4 mIU/L |
| Uric acid | 9 mg/dL | 535 μmol/L |

## Laboratory Tests from 1 Year Ago

### Complete Metabolic Panel Within Normal Limits

|  | Conventional Units (mg/dL) | SI Units (mmol/L) |
|---|---|---|
| Total cholesterol | 170 | 4.40 |
| LDL cholesterol | 99 | 2.56 |
| HDL cholesterol | 42 | 1.09 |
| Triglycerides | 147 | 1.66 |

## Assessment

Fifty-seven-year-old male with untreated dyslipidemia and gout, impaired fasting glucose, as well as newly diagnosed HTN.

### Student Workup

**Missing Information?**

Evaluate:  Patient Database

Drug Therapy Problems

Care Plan (by Problem)

## TARGETED QUESTIONS

1. What is the patient's calculated Framingham 10-year coronary heart disease (CHD) risk?

   *Hint: See http://hp2010.nhlbihin.net/atpiii/calculator.asp*

2. What is the patient's target BP?

   *Hint: See p. 60 in PPP*

3. Which antihypertensive(s) would you consider initiating based on this patient's specific characteristics? Does he have any compelling indications for other options?

   *Hint: See pp. 62–70 in PPP*

4. How would you educate this patient about the medication(s) selected?

   *Hint: See p. 74 in PPP*

5. When and what would you monitor after initiating therapy?

   *Hint: See p. 73 in PPP*

## FOLLOW-UP

The patient returns for follow-up BP check 2 weeks later. BP 132/85 mm Hg, repeat 130/82 mm Hg (right arm, regular cuff). What actions, if any, would you take?

## ☼ GLOBAL PERSPECTIVE

HTN accounts for significant morbidity and mortality and has a worldwide prevalence estimated to include 1 billion individuals. Globally, 51% of all strokes and 45% of ischemic heart disease deaths are attributable to hypertension, and it is the leading risk factor for cause of death worldwide. The prevalence of HTN in the United States is among the highest in the world. Efforts to increase awareness, risk factor modification, control, and prevention are essential to reduce the global burden of cardiovascular disease. When designing an effective treatment plan for HTN, individual patient characteristics, comorbidities, the pharmacokinetic and pharmacodynamic properties of antihypertensive agents, and drug costs must be considered.

## CASE SUMMARY

- His current clinical picture is consistent with newly diagnosed HTN, and intervention is necessary.
- Lifestyle modification and pharmacotherapy are warranted to achieve target blood pressure and other risk factors for CVD.
- A variety of therapeutic options are available, and the advantages and disadvantages of each should be considered based on the patient's individual characteristics.

**For more information on the care plan and facilitator's guide please visit http://www.mhpharmacotherapy.com.**

# 3 Uncontrolled Hypertension

Keri D. Hager          Stephanie Reynolds
Robert J. Straka

## CASE LEARNING OBJECTIVES

- Classify blood pressure levels and treatment goals
- Recognize contributing factors in uncontrolled hypertension
- Recommend appropriate lifestyle modifications and pharmacotherapy for patients with uncontrolled hypertension on the basis of individual patient characteristics
- Construct an appropriate monitoring plan to assess hypertension treatment
- Properly educate a patient about antihypertensive treatment

## PATIENT PRESENTATION

### Chief Complaint

"My blood pressure at home is still high."

### History of Present Illness

Gusto Roubaix is a 66-year-old black male who presents with his wife to his health care provider complaining that his home BP readings continue to remain high. He was diagnosed with HTN 10 years ago, and it was well controlled until the past 18 months. He blames this on stress related to a poor real-estate market and a significant [>30 lb (>13.6 kg)] weight gain over the past 5 years (tries to practice portion control but dines out frequently; he does not have salt at the table or cook with salt). He is frustrated because his BP has not improved despite 1 hour of light aerobics (walking and water aerobics) daily, over the past 6 months. His home BP log, which he brought with him, reveals resting seated systolic BP levels ranging from 130 to 155 mm Hg and diastolic BP levels ranging from 70 to 90 mm Hg and a pulse of 50 to 58 bpm in the morning over the past 30 days. In addition, despite restricting his calories, he has not lost any weight. He complains of excessive fatigue, and his wife states she is always tired as well, as his snoring "keeps the whole house up all night long." He denies any dizziness or lightheadedness, edema, chest pain, or shortness of breath.

### Past Medical History

HTN (diagnosed 10 years ago)

Impaired fasting glucose

Metabolic syndrome

Dyslipidemia

Osteoarthritis of the knees (unresponsive to high-dose acetaminophen)

History of gout

GERD

Obstructive sleep apnea

BPH

Obesity

"Stress/fatigue"

### Family History

Mother deceased, stroke at age 82. Father is alive and well, aged 86. Sister diabetes and CKD, aged 59. Brother alive and well, aged 63.

### Social History

Lives in South Florida year round with his wife of 40 years.

### Tobacco/Alcohol/Substance Use

Social drinker, one to two glasses of wine nightly, (−) tobacco products, (−) illicit drugs.

### Allergies/Intolerances/Adverse Drug Events

Penicillin (angioedema)

## Medications (Current)

Aspirin 81 mg PO q AM

Verapamil SA 240 mg PO q 24 h

Metoprolol Succinate SA 200 mg PO q 24 h

Terazosin 5 mg PO q hs

Simvastatin 40 mg PO q hs

Omeprazole 20 mg PO q AM

Ibuprofen 400 mg PO 4 times daily PRN pain

OTC energy supplement PO daily

## Review of Systems

Frequent body aches that the patient attributes to exercise and arthritis; wakes up two to three times nightly to urinate with some hesitancy and dribbling; no chest pain at rest or with exercise; no SOB, dizziness, lightheadedness, or edema.

## Physical Examination

### ► General

Well-nourished, appears his age, overweight black male in no distress

### ► Vital Signs

BP 152/92 mm Hg, P 56 bpm (left-arm, regular-sized adult cuff), repeat 148/90 mm Hg, P 54 bpm

RR 16, T 37°C

Weight 184 lb (83.6 kg)

Height 68 in. (173 cm)

Currently denies pain

### ► Skin

Dry appearing skin; (–) rashes or lesions

### ► HEENT

PERRLA, EOMI; (–) sinus tenderness; TMs appear normal

### ► Neck and Lymph Nodes

(–) thyroid nodules; (–) lymphadenopathy; (–) carotid bruits

### ► Chest

Clear to auscultation

### ► Cardiovascular

RRR, normal $S_1$, $S_2$; (–) $S_3$ or $S_4$

### ► Abdomen

Not tender/not distended; (–) organomegaly

### ► Neurology

Grossly intact; DTRs normal

### ► Genitourinary

Examination deferred

### ► Rectal

Prostate is enlarged approximately 30 g, no areas of induration or nodularity

## Laboratory Tests

### Fasting Obtained 7 Days Ago

|  | Conventional Units | SI Units |
|---|---|---|
| Na | 142 mEq/L | 142 mmol/L |
| K | 4.2 mEq/L | 4.2 mmol/L |
| Cl | 98 mEq/L | 98 mmol/L |
| $CO_2$ | 24 mEq/L | 24 mmol/L |
| BUN | 12 mg/dL | 4.3 mmol/L |
| SCr | 1.2 mg/dL | 106 μmol/L |
| Glu | 104 mg/dL | 5.8 mmol/L |
| Total cholesterol | 146 mg/dL | 3.78 mmol/L |
| LDL cholesterol | 79 mg/dL | 2.04 mmol/L |
| HDL cholesterol | 36 mg/dL | 0.93 mmol/L |
| Triglycerides | 156 mg/dL | 1.76 mmol/L |

## Assessment

Sixty-six-year-old male with uncontrolled hypertension despite three antihypertensive agents.

### Student Workup

**Missing Information?**

Evaluate:     Patient Database

Drug Therapy Problems

Care Plan (by Problem)

## TARGETED QUESTIONS

1. What stage hypertension does this patient have and what is his target blood pressure?

   *Hint: See p. 54 in PPP*

2. What are some contributing factors in uncontrolled hypertension?

   *Hint: See p. 56 in PPP*

3. Based on this patient's individual characteristics, what are the advantages and disadvantages of different therapeutic options?

   *Hint: See Table 5-4 in PPP*

4. What risks and adverse effects of therapy would you discuss with the patient?

    *Hint: See Table 5-4 in PPP*

5. What are appropriate follow-up monitoring parameters?

    *Hint: See pp. 73–74 in PPP*

## FOLLOW-UP

Four weeks later, the patient returns for follow-up. He feels much better; his stress has actually improved because he is not nearly as fatigued, "maybe because I don't wake up to go to the bathroom three times per night anymore?" His wife adds, "That CPAP machine works wonders … he quit snoring … I am getting my usual 8 hours of sleep now." His pain is no better or worse on salsalate compared to when he was on ibuprofen; however he is satisfied with the current level of pain relief. He states that his body aches are "the same"; further questioning reveals these are not muscle weakness, cramping, or suggestive of statin myopathy. In addition, total CK was within normal limits. In the office, although improved, his seated blood pressure remains elevated and is consistent with his home blood pressure log (seated systolic BP levels ranging from 128 to 143 mm Hg and diastolic BP levels ranging from 68 to 84 mm Hg and a pulse of 60 to 74 bpm in the morning). The patient's BMP is within normal limits, and he reports no signs or symptoms of intolerance to his new therapeutic regimen. What additional interventions or modifications would you now make to improve the patient's blood pressure control?

## ⊙ GLOBAL PERSPECTIVE

Although the global burden of hypertension is growing substantially, it does not affect all groups or populations equally. It is estimated that 1 billion adults (333 million in economically developed and 639 million in economically developing countries) have hypertension, with those who reside in economically developing countries being increasingly affected. Eastern Europe and Latin American/Caribbean regions have the highest prevalence of hypertension, whereas prevalence of age-specific and age-adjusted hypertension continues to increase in China. Efforts to increase awareness, control, and prevention of hypertension are paramount in reducing the global burden of cardiovascular disease. Comprehensive risk-factor modifications (tobacco use, cholesterol, obesity, diabetes) are also essential, with special considerations given by region. In addition, the pharmacokinetic and pharmacodynamic properties of antihypertensive agents and adverse event profiles may differ among various populations. For example, African Americans are more likely to experience angioedema from ACE-Is while those of Chinese descent are more likely to experience cough. Finally, differences in drug cost, availability, and national resources may influence the approach to treating hypertension.

## CASE SUMMARY

- His current clinical picture is consistent with uncontrolled hypertension, and intervention is necessary.
- A thorough investigation of factors contributing to uncontrolled hypertension is warranted in addition to lifestyle and pharmacologic intensification.
- A variety of therapeutic options are available, and the advantages and disadvantages of each should be carefully considered based on the patient's individual characteristics.

For more information on the care plan and facilitator's guide please visit http://www.mhpharmacotherapy.com.

# 4 Heart Failure

Kimberly A. Ackerbauer    Tien M.H. Ng

## CASE LEARNING OBJECTIVES

- Differentiate among the common underlying etiologies of heart failure (HF), including ischemic, nonischemic, and idiopathic causes.
- Identify signs and symptoms of HF and classify a given patient by the New York Heart Association Functional Classification (NYHA FC) and American College of Cardiology/American Heart Association (AHA) HF Staging.
- Develop a specific evidence-based pharmacologic treatment plan for a patient with acute or chronic HF based on disease severity and symptoms.
- Properly educate a patient taking chronic HF medications.

## PATIENT PRESENTATION

### Chief Complaint

"I was so short of breath this morning I couldn't get out of bed. My legs have also been quite swollen, especially by the end of the day."

### History of Present Illness

DB is a 64-year-old Hispanic male who presents to the emergency department with a 3-day history of shortness of breath, lower extremity swelling, and an 18-lb (8-kg) weight gain. About 4 days ago, he ran out of medications and was unable to make it to the pharmacy to refill his medications. This morning, the shortness of breath persisted at rest to the point he could not get out of bed. This prompted him to come to the hospital. The patient also admits to waking up at night to catch his breath and needing at least three pillows to prop himself up while sleeping because he feels like he is drowning when laying flat. In the emergency room, he was placed on oxygen, given his home dose of amlodipine, given intravenous boluses of furosemide without much response, and then started on a furosemide intravenous infusion at 5 mg/h. After 3 hours, DB had no symptomatic relief and was transferred to the cardiac intensive care unit for further management.

### Past Medical History

HTN × 20 years
Bipolar disorder × 6 years

### Family History

Father had type 2 diabetes, HTN, and died at age 84 from an unknown cause. Mother is alive at age 87 with HTN and gout.

### Social History

Fluent in English and Spanish. Divorced and lives alone. He has a son who visits him about once a week for help around the house. Retired, used to work as a mechanic, now mainly sedentary. Eats mainly processed or premade foods.

### Tobacco/Alcohol/Substance Use

Denies alcohol use; (–) tobacco or illicit drug use

### Allergies/Intolerances/Adverse Drug Events

Benazepril (cough)

### Medications (Current)

HCTZ 25 mg PO q AM
Amlodipine 10 mg PO q 24 h
Lithium 300 mg PO q 8 h

### Review of Systems

Well-appearing male unable to lie flat in bed. No complaints of pain, headache, fever, or chills. Denies changes in mental status, nausea, or vomiting.

### Physical Examination

▶ *General*

Moderately distressed, obese, middle-aged Hispanic male.

▶ *Vital Signs*

BP 154/92 mm Hg, P 87, RR 27, T 37.3°C, $O_2$ saturation 92% (0.92) on 2 L via nasal cannula

Weight 211 lb (96 kg)

Height 68 in. (173 cm)

Denies pain

▶ **HEENT**

Unremarkable

▶ **Neck and Lymph Nodes**

Neck supple, (+) JVD

▶ **Chest**

Crackles bilaterally

▶ **Cardiovascular**

RRR, normal $S_1$, $S_2$, (+) $S_3$, (+) $S_4$ heart sounds, no murmurs, PMI displaced laterally

▶ **Abdomen**

(+) Bowel sounds, hepatomegaly

▶ **Neurology**

Alert and oriented × 3, no focal deficits

▶ **Extremities**

Warm, 2+ pulses (pedal/radial), 2+ bilateral lower extremity edema up to knees

▶ **Genitourinary**

Examination deferred

▶ **Rectal**

Examination deferred

## Laboratory Tests

### Fasting Obtained upon Admission

|  | Conventional Units | SI Units |
| --- | --- | --- |
| Na | 137 mEq/L | 137 mmol/L |
| K | 3.6 mEq/L | 3.6 mmol/L |
| Cl | 104 mEq/L | 104 mmol/L |
| $CO_2$ | 22 mEq/L | 22 mmol/L |
| BUN | 28 mg/dL | 10 mmol/L |
| SCr | 1.4 mg/dL | 124 μmol/L |
| Glu | 189 mg/dL | 10.5 mmol/L |
| Ca | 8.7 mg/dL | 2.18 mmol/L |
| Mg | 1.8 mEq/L | 0.90 mmol/L |
| Phosphate | 3.6 mg/dL | 1.16 mmol/L |
| WBC | $9.4 \times 10^3/mm^3$ | $9.4 \times 10^9/L$ |
| Hgb | 11.6 g/dL | 116 g/L; 7.2 mmol/L |
| Hct | 34.6% | 0.346 |
| MCV | 88.0 μm³ | 88.0 fL |

| Platelet | $213 \times 10^3/mm^3$ | $213 \times 10^9/L$ |
| --- | --- | --- |
| Albumin | 3.2 g/dL | 32 g/L |
| Total bilirubin | 1.5 mg/dL | 25.7 μmol/L |
| Direct bilirubin | 0.8 mg/dL | 13.7 μmol/L |
| AST | 89 IU/L | 1.48 μkat/L |
| ALT | 96 IU/L | 1.60 μkat/L |
| Alk phos | 180 IU/L | 3.00 μkat/L |
| PT | 17 s | |
| INR | 1.3 | |
| Total cholesterol | 164 mg/dL | 4.24 mmol/L |
| Triglycerides | 135 mg/dL | 1.53 mmol/L |
| LDL cholesterol | 96 mg/dL | 2.48 mmol/L |
| HDL cholesterol | 41 mg/dL | 1.06 mmol/L |
| Lithium | 0.8 mEq/L | 0.8 mmol/L |
| B-type natriuretic peptide | 9,022 pg/mL | 9,022 ng/L |

## Diagnostic Tests

▶ **Electrocardiogram**

Left ventricular hypertrophy, no acute ST-segment changes

▶ **Chest Radiograph**

Cardiomegaly, bilateral pleural effusions at the bases, no infiltrates (Figure 4-1)

**FIGURE 4-1.** Cardiomegaly with pulmonary venous congestion and bilateral pleural effusions. (Reproduced, with permission, from Usatine RP, Smith MA, Mayeaux Jr EJ, Chumley H, Tysinger J. The Color Atlas of Family Medicine. New York, McGraw-Hill, 2009, Fig 46-2.)

▶ *Echocardiogram*

Hypertrophied and dilated left ventricle, left ventricular EF 35% (0.35)

## Assessment

Sixty-four-year-old man presenting with new-onset HF.

### Student Workup

**Missing Information?**

Evaluate:     Patient Database
              Drug Therapy Problems
              Care Plan (by Problem)

## TARGETED QUESTIONS

1. What signs and symptoms of HF does this patient have?
   *Hint: See pp. 84–86 in PPP*

2. What NYHA functional class is this patient?
   *Hint: See p. 87 in PPP*

3. How do you determine when the addition of intravenous vasodilatory therapy is desirable in an acute HF patient?
   *Hint: See pp. 101–102 in PPP*

4. How do ACE-Is and β-blockers interfere with the pathophysiology of HF to improve patient survival?
   *Hint: See pp. 91–94 in PPP*

5. What education would you provide regarding lifestyle changes and self-monitoring for this patient?
   *Hint: See pp. 88, 106 in PPP*

## FOLLOW-UP

Six months later, DB returns to the clinic for a routine follow-up and medication refills. He states that he has no major complaints at this time. When prompted, he admits that over the past 3 months his exercise tolerance has decreased. He used to walk about six blocks to the grocery store and is now only able to walk two blocks. He denies any swelling in his legs but still needs three pillows while sleeping at night.

Furosemide 20 mg PO twice daily

Carvedilol 25 mg PO twice daily

Losartan 100 mg PO daily

Amlodipine 10 mg PO daily

Lithium 300 mg PO three times daily

▶ *Vital Signs*

BP 103/61 mm Hg, P 58, RR 18, T 37.4°C

Weight 204 lb (93 kg)

| | Conventional Units | SI Units |
|---|---|---|
| Na | 136 mEq/L | 136 mmol/L |
| K | 3.7 mEq/L | 3.7 mmol/L |
| Cl | 109 mEq/L | 109 mmol/L |
| $CO_2$ | 21 mEq/L | 21 mmol/L |
| BUN | 24 mg/dL | 8.6 mmol/L |
| SCr | 1.2 mg/dL | 106 µmol/L |
| Glu | 129 mg/dL | 7.2 mmol/L |

## TARGETED QUESTIONS

6. Are there any changes that could be made to his outpatient regimen to improve his symptoms and prognosis?
   *Hint: See pp. 91–96 in PPP*

### ⊙ GLOBAL PERSPECTIVE

Although the main etiologies of systolic HF are ischemic heart disease and hypertension in the United States, acquired etiologies can be more prevalent in developing countries. The availability of certain medications also varies from continent to continent. For example, in many countries in Europe and regions of Scandinavia, additional intravenous agents such as levosimendan are available for the treatment of acute HF. Finally, patterns of prescribing may differ among countries. This applies to both acute HF therapies such as inotropes and chronic medications such as β-blockers and ACE-Is.

### CASE SUMMARY

- His current clinical picture is consistent with being congested, necessitating aggressive diuresis and intravenous vasodilator therapy. It is appropriate to continue the furosemide infusion or give higher doses via intermittent boluses, and start an intravenous vasodilator.

- When clinically stable, this patient should be started on chronic disease-modifying agents that antagonize the renin-angiotensin-aldosterone system as well as the sympathetic nervous system.

- Prevention of future acute HF exacerbations with the use of diuretics, optimal management of the hypertension, and lifestyle modifications are necessary to improve this patient's long-term prognosis.

**For more information on the care plan and facilitator's guide please visit http://www.mhpharmacotherapy.com.**

# 5 Ischemic Heart Disease

Larisa H. Cavallari      Adam Bress

Robert J. DiDomenico

## CASE LEARNING OBJECTIVES

- Recognize the symptoms and diagnostic criteria of ischemic heart disease (IHD)
- Identify risk factors for the development of IHD
- Identify the treatment goals of IHD and appropriate lifestyle modifications and pharmacologic therapy to address each goal
- Design an appropriate therapeutic regimen for the management of IHD based on patient-specific information

## PATIENT PRESENTATION

### Chief Complaint

"I get pain in my chest and feel dizzy when I exercise. I have to stop exercising and rest for the pain and dizziness to go away."

### History of Present Illness

GP is a 61-year-old African American male who presents to his primary care physician complaining of chest pain radiating to his neck and left shoulder, excessive sweating, and dizziness (over the last month) when he attempts to exercise on a treadmill or stair stepper. He describes the pain as "feeling tight" and "pressure-like." The symptoms resolve after resting for a couple of minutes. He denies dyspnea, nausea, or vomiting. He also denies symptoms at rest, with change in body position, or in relation to meals. GP is concerned that he will not be able to exercise, which he is doing to lose weight. He is hoping that he can take something to prevent the chest pain and other symptoms that occur with exercise. He also reports swelling in his ankles that is worse after being on his feet all day and relieved with leg elevation.

### Past Medical History

HTN × 10 years

Depression × 6 months

Type 2 DM × 2 years

Bursitis in left hip × 6 months after slipping on the ice

### Family History

Mother died at age 45 from MI. Father is alive at age 78 S/P CABG at the age of 50. Son, aged 25, alive and well.

### Social History

He is a widower as of 6 months ago. GP currently lives at home with his 24-year-old son and cat. He is employed as a chef.

### Tobacco/Alcohol/Substance Use

(+) Tobacco; quit smoking 10 years ago, but restarted smoking about ½ ppd 6 months ago when his wife died. Denies illicit drug use; social drinker on the weekends.

### Allergies/Intolerances/Adverse Drug Events

Penicillin (develops hives)

### Medications (Current)

Fish oil 1,000 mg PO once daily

Sertraline 50 mg PO once daily

Lisinopril 40 mg PO once daily

HCTZ 25 mg PO once daily

Celecoxib 200 mg PO twice daily

Glipizide XL 10 mg PO once daily

## Review of Systems

Takes celecoxib twice daily for bursitis. Denies current dizziness, chest pain, diaphoresis, or dyspnea; (–) history of syncope, loss of consciousness, seizures, or visual changes. Reports that bursitis pain has largely resolved.

## Physical Examination

### ▶ General

Middle-aged, well-developed, African American male in no acute distress; conversant and pleasant

### ▶ Vital Signs

BP 144/92 mm Hg, P 82 bpm, RR 18, T 36.9°C

Weight 195 lb (88.6 kg)

Height 68 in. (173 cm)

(–) Pain

### ▶ Skin

Warm and dry; (–) pallor, rashes, or lesions

### ▶ HEENT

PERRLA, EOMI; oral mucosa moist; (–) pharyngeal erythema or exudate

### ▶ Neck and Lymph Nodes

Supple, no tenderness; (–) carotid bruits; (–) jugular vein distension; normal thyroid

### ▶ Chest

Clear to auscultation bilaterally

### ▶ Cardiovascular

RRR; normal $S_1$, $S_2$; (–) $S_3$ or $S_4$; (–) murmurs, rubs,

### ▶ Abdomen

Soft, nontender, nondistended; normal bowel sounds

### ▶ Neurology

Alert and oriented, cranial nerves II–XII intact

### ▶ Extremities

Bilateral lower extremity edema; warm; normal pulses

### ▶ Genitourinary

Examination deferred; per patient: (–) dysuria; (–) hematuria; (–) discharge

### ▶ Rectal

Examination deferred

## Laboratory Tests

### Fasting Obtained Prior to Clinic Visit

|  | Conventional Units | SI Units |
|---|---|---|
| Na | 141 mEq/L | 141 mmol/L |
| K | 4.4 mEq/L | 4.4 mmol/L |
| Cl | 101 mEq/L | 101 mmol/L |
| $CO_2$ | 24 mEq/L | 24 mmol/L |
| BUN | 10 mg/dL | 3.6 mmol/L |
| SCr | 1.1 mg/dL | 97 μmol/L |
| Glu | 130 mg/dL | 7.2 mmol/L |
| Ca | 10.0 mg/dL | 2.50 mmol/L |
| Mg | 1.7 mEq/L | 0.85 mmol/L |
| Phosphate | 4.1 mg/dL | 1.32 mmol/L |
| Hgb | 15.1 g/dL | 151 g/L; 9.38 mmol/L |
| Hct | 45.3% | 0.453 |
| WBC | $8.0 \times 10^3/mm^3$ | $8.0 \times 10^9/L$ |
| Platelets | $313 \times 10^3/mm^3$ | $313 \times 10^9/L$ |

## Assessment

Sixty-one-year-old man with symptoms consistent with chronic stable angina. GP's primary care physician has scheduled a treadmill stress echocardiogram (echo stress test) to evaluate him for IHD and assess his left ventricular systolic function.

### Student Workup

**Missing Information?**

Evaluate: Patient Database

Drug Therapy Problems

Care Plan (by Problem)

## TARGETED QUESTIONS

1. What symptoms of chronic stable angina does the patient have?

   *Hint: See p. 114 in PPP*

2. What are the patient's risk factors for IHD?

   *Hint: See p. 111 in PPP*

3. What is your assessment of GP's current antihypertensive regimen?

   *Hint: See p. 120 in PPP and Hypertension chapter*

## FOLLOW-UP

One week later, the patient's echo stress test comes back positive for inducible myocardial ischemia (i.e., positive for CAD), and shows normal left ventricular systolic function (i.e., no evidence of left ventricular dysfunction). He is diagnosed with chronic stable angina.

4. A coronary angiogram is scheduled in 1 week with possible PCI. What antiplatelet therapy would you recommend if the patient does undergo coronary stenting for management of his chronic stable angina?

   *Hint: See pp. 156–157 in PPP*

5. What therapy do you recommend to manage the patient's current symptoms of angina?

   *Hint: See pp. 122–126 in PPP*

6. Now that you have addressed the patient's antianginal medications, what additional medications (other than those addressed in question 4) would you consider now that he has been diagnosed with IHD?

   *Hint: See pp. 120–122 in PPP*

7. What lifestyle modifications are appropriate for this patient?

   *Hint: See pp. 118–119 in PPP*

## GLOBAL PERSPECTIVE

In general, persons of African descent may have lesser antihypertensive response to β-blockers or ACE-I monotherapy than those of other racial groups. However, this is not a reason to avoid these drugs in an African American patient when a compelling indication (e.g., IHD, diabetes) exists for their use. These drugs may still have cardio- and reno-protective effects despite less blood pressure lowering effect. Concomitant use of these drugs with a thiazide diuretic may significantly enhance blood pressure response.

## CASE SUMMARY

- His current clinical picture is consistent with chronic stable angina.
- Therapy to relieve acute symptoms of ischemia and prevent recurrent angina should be initiated.
- Additional drug therapy and lifestyle modifications to address the patient's risk factors for IHD to reduce the risk for an acute coronary syndrome is warranted.

**For more information on the care plan and facilitator's guide please visit http://www.mhpharmacotherapy.com.**

# 6 Acute Coronary Syndromes

Sarah A. Spinler

## CASE LEARNING OBJECTIVES

- List key electrocardiographic and clinical features identifying a patient with non–ST-segment elevation (NSTE) acute coronary syndrome (ACS) who is at high risk of myocardial infarction (MI) or death
- Devise a pharmacotherapy treatment plan for a patient with ST-segment elevation myocardial infarction (STEMI) given patient-specific data
- Devise a pharmacotherapy treatment and monitoring plan for a patient with NSTE ACS given patient-specific data
- Formulate a monitoring plan for a patient with NSTE ACS receiving aspirin, clopidogrel, β-blocker, anticoagulant, and glycoprotein IIb/IIIa receptor inhibitor
- Devise a pharmacotherapy and risk-factor modification treatment plan for secondary prevention of coronary heart disease (CHD) events in a patient following MI
- List the quality performance measures of care for MI

## PATIENT PRESENTATION

### Chief Complaint

"My chest discomfort is gone now that they put a stent in my coronary artery."

### History of Present Illness

Jonathan Wright is a 66-year-old male who presented to the emergency department (ED) by ambulance at 14:00 complaining of 4 hours of continuous chest pressure that started while raking leaves. JW developed substernal chest pressure at 10:00 about 30 minutes after starting to rake leaves at his home. He stopped and rested but the chest pressure did not resolve. Local paramedics were summoned, and he was given three 0.4 mg SL NTG tablets by mouth, 325 mg aspirin by mouth, and morphine 2 mg IV push at 13:30 without relief of chest discomfort. He was brought to the ED by ambulance. A 12-lead ECG was performed, and NTG 10 mcg/min IV infusion was initiated at 14:15. The cardiology attending consulted with the interventional cardiologist and the decision was made to bring JW to the cardiac catheterization laboratory for coronary angiography (see Figure 6-1). Bivalirudin was initiated at the time of percutaneous coronary intervention (PCI) and was discontinued in the cardiac catheterization laboratory following successful PCI. The patient is now in the CCU s/p PCI with placement of a bare metal stent in the LAD coronary artery.

### Past Medical History

HTN × 5 years

### Family History

Father with MI at age 75; mother and sister alive with type 2 DM

### Social History

Retired former newspaper reporter

### Tobacco/Alcohol/Substance Use

Nonsmoker. Denies use of alcohol or illicit drugs

### Allergies/Intolerances/Adverse Drug Events

None

### Medications (Current)

NTG 10 mcg/min IV

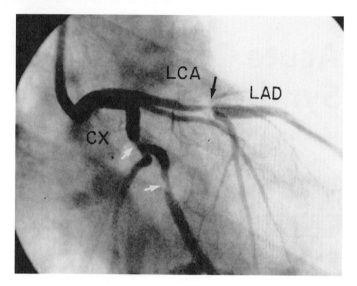

**FIGURE 6-1.** Coronary angiogram of the left coronary artery (LCA) with a tight stenosis in the proximal left anterior descending (LAD) artery (black arrow). The circumflex artery (CX) has two moderately severe stenoses (white arrows). (Reproduced, with permission from Usatine RP, Smith MA, Mayeaux Jr EJ, Chumley H, Tysinger J The Color Atlas of Family Medicine. New York, McGraw-Hill, 2009, Fig 45-1.)

## Medications Taken Prior to Admission

Amlodipine 10 mg PO once daily

ASA 325 mg PO once daily

## Review of Systems

Previous 10/10 chest pressure now 1/10; (−) nausea, abdominal pain, or headache

## Physical Examination

### ▸ General

Elderly male in less distress

### ▸ Vital Signs

BP 140/90 mm Hg, P 88 bpm, RR 17, T 37°C

Weight 198 lb (90 kg)

Height 71 in. (180 cm)

Denies pain, but 1/10 chest pressure

### ▸ HEENT

Normal; (−) AV nicking, (−) papilledema

### ▸ Chest

Clear to A&P, JVD 4 cm, PMI left midclavicular line 4th intercostal space

### ▸ Cardiovascular

RRR, normal $S_1$, $S_2$, (−) $S_3$ or $S_4$, (−) M/R/G

### ▸ Abdomen

Not tender/not distended, normal bowel sounds

### ▸ Neurologic

A&O × 3, cranial nerves II–XII intact

### ▸ Genitourinary

Deferred

### ▸ Rectal

(−) Occult blood

### ▸ Extremities

No bruits, pulses 2+, (−) edema

## Laboratory Tests

### Nonfasting Obtained in the ED

ECG: In ED showed sinus tachycardia with 2 mm ST depression in leads $V_2$–$V_4$; normal PR, QRS, and QTc intervals; post-PCI ECG shows NSR with resolution of ST depression, no Q waves.

|  | Conventional Units | SI Units |
|---|---|---|
| Sodium | 140 mEq/L | 140 mmol/L |
| Potassium | 4.2 mEq/L | 4.2 mmol/L |
| Chloride | 105 mEq/L | 105 mmol/L |
| $CO_2$ | 24 mEq/L | 24 mmol/L |
| BUN | 16 mg/dL | 5.7 mmol/L |
| SCr | 1.0 mg/dL | 88 mmol/L |
| Glucose | 99 mg/dL | 5.5 mmol/L |
| Hgb | 14.7 g/dL | 147 g/L; 9.12 mmol/L |
| Hct | 44.0% | 0.440 |
| Plt | $220 \times 10^3/mm^3$ | $220 \times 10^9/L$ |
| WBC | $4.3 \times 10^3/mm^3$ | $4.3 \times 10^9/L$ |
| Troponin I | 7.5 ng/mL | 7.5 mcg/L |
| LDL cholesterol | 110 mg/dL | 2.84 mmol/L |
| Triglycerides | 240 mg/dL | 2.71 mmol/L |
| HDL cholesterol | 35 mg/dL | 0.91 mmol/L |
| Magnesium | 2.0 mEq/L | 1.00 mmol/L |
| AST | 30 U/L | 0.50 μkat/L |
| ALT | 30 U/L | 0.50 μkat/L |
| aPTT | 30 s |  |
| INR | 1.0 |  |

$O_2$ sat = 99% (0.99) on RA

## Assessment

Sixty-six-year-old male with signs, symptoms, and laboratory tests consistent with ACS.

### Student Workup

**Missing Information?**

**Evaluate:** Patient Database
Drug Therapy Problems
Care Plan (by Problem)

## TARGETED QUESTIONS

1. What type of ACS is this?
   *Hint: See pp. 135–136 in PPP*

2. What signs and symptoms of ACS does this patient have?
   *Hint: See pp. 136–137 in PPP*

3. What are this patient's risk factors for developing CHD?
   *Hint: See Tables 7-2, 8-1 in PPP*

4. How is the diagnosis of MI made?
   *Hint: See pp. 136–138 in PPP*

5. What high risk of death or MI characteristics does this patient have?
   *Hint: See Table 8-1 in PPP*

6. How does timing of PCI influence the choice and timing of antiplatelet therapy (in addition to aspirin administered at the time of patient presentation or prior to hospital presentation)?
   *Hint: See pp. 150–154 in PPP*

7. In which patient subgroups is the benefit of reduction in cardiovascular death, MI, or stroke not greater than the risk of major bleeding in patients treated with prasugrel versus clopidogrel following PCI?
   *Hint: See Wiviott SD, Braunwald E, McCabe CH, et al. TRITON-TIMI 38 Investigators. Prasugrel versus clopidogrel in patients with acute coronary syndromes. N Engl J Med 2007 357: 2001–2015, and Wiviott SD, Desai N, Murphy SA, et al. Efficacy and safety of intensive antiplatelet therapy with prasugrel from TRITON-TIMI 38 in a core clinical cohort defined by worldwide regulatory agencies. Am J Cardiol 2011 108: 905–911.*

8. What is the minimal duration of time that dual antiplatelet therapy should be continued?

*Hint: See Levine GN, Bates ER, Blankenship JC, et al; American College of Cardiology Foundation; American Heart Association Task Force on Practice Guidelines; Society for Cardiovascular Angiography and Interventions. 2011 ACCF/AHA/SCAI Guideline for Percutaneous Coronary Intervention. A report of the American College of Cardiology Foundation/ American Heart Association Task Force on Practice Guidelines and the Society for Cardiovascular Angiography and Interventions. J Am Coll Cardiol 2011 58:44–122.*

9. How is the dose of the β-blocker titrated?
   *Hint: See p. 155 and Table 8-2 in PPP*

10. How would your selection of pharmacotherapy differ if this patient presented with signs and symptoms of acute heart failure (HF)?
    *Hint: See Table 8-2 in PPP*

11. What is the single best predictor of mortality in this patient?
    *Hint: See Table 8-1 in PPP*

## FOLLOW-UP

12. The patient presents to his cardiologist 2 weeks following discharge. His BP is 142/90 mm Hg, pulse 55 bpm, and he is afebrile. His chemistry panel includes potassium of 4.2 mEq/L (4.2 mmol/L) and SCr 1.07 mg/dL (95 μmol/L). What recommendations would you make to the physician regarding his pharmacotherapy regimen?
    *Hint: See Table 8-2 in PPP*

13. The patient presents to his cardiologist 6 weeks following discharge. The patient's LDL cholesterol is 68 mg/dL (1.76 mmol/L), but his fasting triglycerides are still elevated at 185 mg/dL (2.09 mmol/L) and HDL cholesterol still low at 36 mg/dL (0.93 mmol/L). What recommendations would you make to the physician regarding his pharmacotherapy regimen?
    *Hint: See p. 256 in PPP*

## ⟳ GLOBAL PERSPECTIVE

According to the World Health Organization, cardiovascular diseases (CVDs) are the leading cause of death globally. MI is the most common type of CVD. Almost 30% of deaths worldwide are caused by CVD. Almost 80% of CVD deaths occur in low- and middle-income countries. More than 20 million people survive MIs and require secondary preventative care.

## CASE SUMMARY

- His current clinical picture is NSTE ACS, and early PCI restored blood flow through the LAD to myocardium.
- He was diagnosed with MI due to his symptoms, ECG findings, and an elevation in serum or plasma cardiac biomarker troponin.
- Acute pharmacotherapy should be initiated for in-hospital management.
- Secondary prevention pharmacotherapy should be started prior to hospital discharge.

- Key clinical practice guidelines and performance measures guide pharmacotherapy selection.
- Patients should be monitored for resolution of MI signs and symptoms, development of MI complications, and pharmacotherapy adverse effects.

**For more information on the care plan and facilitator's guide please visit http://www.mhpharmacotherapy.com.**

# 7 Atrial Fibrillation

Toby C. Trujillo

## CASE LEARNING OBJECTIVES

- Compare and contrast the risk factors for and the features, mechanisms, etiologies, symptoms, and goals of therapy of atrial fibrillation (AF)
- Compare and contrast the mechanisms of action of drugs used for ventricular rate control, conversion to sinus rhythm, and maintenance of sinus rhythm in patients with AF, and explain the importance of anticoagulation for patients with AF
- Design individualized drug therapy treatment plans for patients with AF

## PATIENT PRESENTATION

### Chief Complaint

"I was supposed to come back if I didn't feel right."

### History of Present Illness

Linda Leong is an 81-year-old Asian female who approximately 1 month ago presented to the emergency department with complaints of SOB, palpitations, fatigue, lightheadedness, and weakness of unspecified duration. She was found to be in AF with a ventricular rate of 130 bpm. At the time of admission, no atrial thrombus was present via transesophageal echocardiography (TEE). Diltiazem was initiated to control her ventricular rate with good response, and IV heparin for bridging plus long-term warfarin was initiated for stroke prevention. The decision for cardioversion was deferred at that time, and she was discharged on diltiazem, warfarin, and her other chronic medications. During the hospitalization, LL was also noted to have lower extremity edema and an elevated JVD, and she was treated with furosemide. She presents today in the cardiology clinic for follow-up. She states she has been compliant with her medications, still feels tired, and occasionally notices she has a fast heart rate.

### Past Medical History

AF

HTN

Heart failure (HF) (EF 50% [0.50] 1 mo ago)

Glaucoma

Dementia

Heartburn

### Family History

Mother had CAD and died of an MI at age 66. Father died of lung cancer at age 81. She has one younger brother and sister who are healthy.

### Social History

Married and lives with her husband of 47 years.

### Tobacco/Alcohol/Substance Use

Occasional glass of wine with dinner; (−) tobacco or illicit drug use

### Allergies/Intolerances/Adverse Drug Events

No known drug allergies

### Medications (Current)

Diltiazem XR 240 mg PO once daily

Warfarin 2.5 mg PO once daily

Lisinopril 40 mg PO once daily

Furosemide 20 mg PO once daily

Donepezil 10 mg PO once daily

Ranitidine 150 mg PO once daily

Travoprost Z 0.004% one drop each eye once daily

Multivitamin PO once daily

### Review of Systems

Still reports fatigue over the last month since discharge from the hospital, difficulty in completing chores in the yard; occasional headaches relieved with nonaspirin pain reliever,

(–) changes in vision; occasional palpitations, SOB, and DOE; (–) heartburn or change in appetite; (–) recent changes in memory or cognition.

## Physical Examination

### ▸ General

Well-appearing, elderly Asian woman in no acute distress

### ▸ Vital Signs

BP 135/85 mm Hg, P 90 bpm, RR 14, T 37.1°C

Weight 143.0 lb (65.0 kg)

Height 68 in. (173 cm)

### ▸ Skin

(–) Rashes or lesions

### ▸ HEENT

PERRLA, mucosal membranes dry

### ▸ Neck and Lymph Nodes

(–) JVD; (–) carotid bruits

### ▸ Chest

Clear to auscultation

### ▸ Breasts

Examination deferred

### ▸ Cardiovascular

Irregularly irregular rhythm; slightly tachycardic; no murmurs, rubs, or gallops

### ▸ Abdomen

Not tender, not distended; (–) hepatomegaly

### ▸ Neurology

Alert and oriented × 3

### ▸ Genitourinary

Examination deferred

### ▸ Rectal

Examination deferred

## Laboratory Tests

### Fasting Drawn Today

| | Conventional Units | SI Units |
| --- | --- | --- |
| Na | 140 mEq/L | 140 mmol/L |
| K | 4.3 mEq/L | 4.3 mmol/L |
| Cl | 104 mEq/L | 104 mmol/L |
| $CO_2$ | 22 mEq/L | 22 mmol/L |
| BUN | 22 mg/dL | 7.9 mmol/L |
| SCr | 1.6 mg/dL | 141 μmol/L |
| Glu | 84 mg/dL | 4.7 mmol/L |
| Ca | 8.9 mg/dL | 2.23 mmol/L |
| Mg | 1.8 mEq/L | 0.90 mmol/L |
| Phosphate | 3.8 mg/dL | 1.23 mmol/L |
| Triglycerides | 175 mg/dL | 1.98 mmol/L |
| Hgb | 13.5 g/dL | 135 g/L; 8.38 mmol/L |
| Hct | 39.7% | 0.397 |
| WBC | $7.6 \times 10^3/mm^3$ | $7.6 \times 10^9/L$ |
| Albumin | 3.8 g/dL | 38 g/L |
| AST | 26 U/L | 0.43 μkat/L |
| ALT | 24 U/L | 0.40 μkat/L |
| Prothrombin | 20 s | |
| INR | 1.5 | |
| Total cholesterol | 238 mg/dL | 6.15 mmol/L |
| LDL cholesterol | 158 mg/dL | 4.09 mmol/L |
| HDL cholesterol | 45 mg/dL | 1.16 mmol/L |

## Assessment

Seventy-seven-year-old Asian female who presents with continuing symptoms of AF, now here for follow-up in the cardiology clinic 1 month after being hospitalized for new-onset AF.

### Student Workup

**Missing Information?**

**Evaluate:**    Patient Database

Drug Therapy Problems

Care Plan (by Problem)

## TARGETED QUESTIONS

1. What underlying etiologies are present in this patient for the development of AF?

   *Hint: See pp. 177–178 in PPP*

2. How should this patient's AF be classified?

   *Hint: See pp. 178–179 in PPP*

3. Should this patient undergo emergent electrical cardioversion at this time?

   *Hint: See pp. 179–180 in PPP*

4. Should the patient receive aspirin for the prevention of stroke?

   *Hint: See pp. 184–185 in PPP*

5. Should the patient receive anti-arrhythmic drug therapy at this time?

   *Hint: See pp. 182–184 in PPP*

## FOLLOW-UP

6. Five weeks later, the patient returns for follow-up. She continues to experience SOB, DOE, and occasional palpitations. Her current vitals reveal a BP of 125/80 mm Hg and a HR of 78 bpm. Today her INR is 2.7 (3 weeks ago, it was 2.2). What antiarrhythmic agent would be recommended for LL at this time to restore and maintain normal sinus rhythm?

   *Hint: See pp. 182–184 in PPP*

## ○ GLOBAL PERSPECTIVE

In a majority of patients, therapeutic anticoagulation with warfarin is the preferred treatment strategy to prevent stroke in patients with AF. Although warfarin has been used in the United States for many years, it is important to note that different vitamin K antagonists are used in other countries worldwide, including acenocoumarol and phenprocoumon. Although the mechanism of action for these agents is similar to that of warfarin, there are major differences in the pharmacokinetics of the compounds, and, hence, differences in how health care professionals may perform routine dose titration and management of therapy. It is important to clarify which specific coumarin derivative the patient is taking to optimally manage their anticoagulation. In 2010, alternatives to oral vitamin K antagonists began to appear in both the U.S. and European markets. At the time of publication, these options include the oral direct thrombin inhibitor dabigatran, and the oral direct factor Xa inhibitor rivaroxaban. Both agents are also available for venous thromboembolism (VTE) prevention outside the United States, but only rivaroxaban has a U.S. FDA-approved indication for VTE prevention. As experience with these new drugs is observed and study results published around the world, a better understanding of where these new oral anticoagulants fit into clinical practice will develop. Additional agents, such as apixaban, are also likely to enter the marketplace in the near future based on the results from randomized controlled trials.[1]

## REFERENCE

1. Connolly SJ, Ezekowitz MD, Yusuf S, et al. Dabigatran versus warfarin in patients with atrial fibrillation. N Engl J Med 2009 361:1139–1151.

## CASE SUMMARY

- LL's current clinical picture is consistent with AF diagnosed 1 month earlier.
- Current rate-control therapy is successful at reducing HR to <110 bpm. However, patient still experiencing symptoms attributable to the disease and may need to consider restoration of normal sinus rhythm.
- Patient is currently receiving therapy for stroke prevention, but there is a need to question whether current therapy is appropriate.
- Patient has elevated total and LDL cholesterol and there is a need to assess whether treatment is needed.

**For more information on the care plan and facilitator's guide please visit http://www.mhpharmacotherapy.com**

# 8 Deep Venous Thrombosis

Michelle T. Martin          Edith A. Nutescu

## CASE LEARNING OBJECTIVES

- Recognize the signs and symptoms of venous thromboembolism (VTE)
- Identify elements needed for a proper diagnosis of deep venous thrombosis (DVT)
- Develop a treatment and monitoring plan for patients with DVT
- Select an appropriate bridging plan to oral anticoagulation
- Educate a patient on anticoagulation therapy

## PATIENT PRESENTATION

### Chief Complaint
"My left leg hurts so bad I can't handle it anymore."

### History of Present Illness
Melinda Smith is a 38-year-old white female who presents to the emergency department with a 2-day H/O edema, severe pain, and warmth in her LLE. She returned home to Chicago, Illinois, 2 days ago from London, England, where she traveled for a long weekend (a gift from her husband). She reports that these symptoms developed after the flight. She had tried massaging her leg, but it is tender and painful to touch. She tried placing a warm towel on it to alleviate the pain, but she states that her leg has become increasingly warm since the symptoms appeared. She states she hates going to the doctor, so she did not want to have her symptoms evaluated initially 2 days ago.

### Past Medical History
Tobacco use × 18 years
Use of hormonal contraceptive × 5 years
Obesity
HTN × 2 years
GERD × 10 years
Occasional aches and pains

### Family History
Mother: DVT age 63; per patient, she "took blood thinners"
Sister: varicose veins

### Social History
Patient works as a receptionist at a law office. She is married and lives with her husband of 10 years. They have two children aged 8 and 5 years.

### Tobacco/Alcohol/Substance Use
(+) 1.5 ppd × 18 yr
(+) Social drinker 2–3 drinks/wk
(−) Denies illicit drug use

### Allergies/Intolerances/Adverse Drug Events
Amoxicillin (rash at age 3)

### Medications (Current)
HCTZ 25 mg PO daily
Omeprazole 20 mg PO (she states she takes it PRN)
Norgestimate/ethinyl estradiol PO daily
Ibuprofen 200 mg PO PRN headache or pain
Multivitamin PO daily

### Review of Systems
Occasional headaches and back pain relieved by ibuprofen

### Physical Examination
▶ *General*
Obese, Caucasian woman in pain

▶ *Vital Signs*

BP 132/78 mm Hg, P 68 bpm, RR 16, T 36.4°C

Weight 220 lb (100 kg)

Height 64 in. (163 cm)

Pain 9/10 in LLE

▶ *Skin*

(−) Rashes or lesions; (−) trauma of LLE; (+) erythema in LLE

▶ *HEENT*

PERRLA, EOMI

▶ *Neck and Lymph Nodes*

(−) Thyroid nodules; (−) lymphadenopathy; (−) carotid bruits

▶ *Chest*

Clear to auscultation; no wheezes or crackles

▶ *Breasts*

Examination deferred

▶ *Cardiovascular*

RRR, normal $S_1$, $S_2$; (−) $S_3$ or $S_4$

▶ *Abdomen*

Obese, not tender; not distended; (−) organomegaly; (+) bowel sounds

▶ *Extremities*

1+ pitting edema; tenderness to palpation in LLE; (+) pedal pulses

▶ *Neurology*

Grossly intact; deep tendon reflexes normal

▶ *Genitourinary*

Examination deferred

▶ *Rectal*

Examination deferred

## Laboratory Tests/Imaging

### Venous Duplex Exam Results

LLE: Evidence of acute nonoccluding thrombus in the popliteal vein

RLE: No evidence of thrombus

|  | Conventional Units | SI Units |
|---|---|---|
| Na | 137 mEq/L | 137 mmol/L |
| K | 4.4 mEq/L | 4.4 mmol/L |
| Cl | 103 mEq/L | 103 mmol/L |
| $CO_2$ | 25 mEq/L | 25 mmol/L |
| BUN | 13 mg/dL | 4.6 mmol/L |
| SCr | 0.7 mg/dL | 62 μmol/L |
| Glu | 108 mg/dL | 6.0 mmol/L |
| Ca | 10.1 mg/dL | 2.53 mmol/L |
| Mg | 2.1 mg/dL | 0.86 mmol/L |
| Phosphate | 4.1 mg/dL | 1.32 mmol/L |
| Hgb | 12.3 g/dL | 123 g/L; 7.63 mmol/L |
| Hct | 37.4% | 0.374 |
| WBC | $8.8 \times 10^3/mm^3$ | $8.8 \times 10^9/L$ |
| MCV | 75 μm³ | 75 fL |
| Albumin | 3.6 g/dL | 36 g/L |

## Assessment

MS is a 38-year-old obese woman with symptoms and imaging consistent with LLE DVT.

### Student Workup

**Missing Information?**

Evaluate:    Patient Database

Drug Therapy Problems

Care Plan (by Problem)

## TARGETED QUESTIONS

1. What signs and symptoms of DVT does the patient have?

   *Hint: See pp. 201–203*

2. What are the patient's risk factors for developing a DVT? What are other acquired and inherent risk factors for DVT?

   *Hint: See pp. 199–200 in PPP*

3. What clinical and objective criteria should be used to diagnose this patient's DVT?

   *Hint: See pp. 202–203 in PPP*

4. What is your plan for managing this patient's recent DVT? What initial treatment should the patient start? What needs to be monitored? How would you transition this patient to an oral anticoagulant?

   *Hint: See pp. 206–220 in PPP*

5. For how long should this patient be treated with an oral anticoagulant? What laboratory values should be monitored, and what is her goal INR?

   *Hint: See Table 10-13 and pp. 206–220 in PPP*

6. What risks and adverse effects of therapy would you discuss with the patient?

   *Hint: See Tables 10-8, 10-9 and pp. 215–220 in PPP*

7. What can be done to reduce this patient's risk of recurrent DVT?

   *Hint: See Table 10-1 in PPP*

## FOLLOW-UP

8. The patient was hospitalized for three nights. Because of her family history (her mother had a history of DVT), a hypercoagulability panel was ordered, which included laboratory values for factor V Leiden, prothrombin G20210A mutation, proteins C and S activity, anticardiolipin antibodies, antithrombin, and lupus anticoagulant. All results came back negative.

   The patient was given warfarin 10 mg nightly for 2 days, then warfarin 5 mg nightly. She was started on enoxaparin 100 mg SC q 12 h upon discharge. Two days after the patient was discharged, she presents to the Antithrombosis Clinic for monitoring of her INR. Her INR is 1.73 (after five doses of warfarin). What changes in her therapy, if any, would you recommend?

   *Hint: See Figure 10-9 and pp. 217–218 in PPP*

## GLOBAL PERSPECTIVE

Hepatic metabolism of warfarin varies greatly among patients, leading to very large interpatient differences in dose requirements. Genetic variations in these isoenzymes, specifically polymorphisms in CYP2C9*2, CYP2C9*3, and VCORC1 genotypes result in a significantly lower warfarin dose requirement to achieve a therapeutic response. Ethnic differences exist in the expression of these phenotypes, but the expression is not adequately uniform to allow consistent dose predictions in various ethnic populations. Genetic polymorphism can be identified by pharmacogenetic testing; however, the utility and cost effectiveness of such testing is controversial.

## CASE SUMMARY

- The patient's clinical picture is consistent with DVT.
- After initial acute therapy with a short-acting parenteral anticoagulant, the patient should be transitioned to and complete a 3-month course of oral anticoagulation therapy.
- Anticoagulation prophylaxis needs to be considered in the future if patient will be exposed to risk of VTE (i.e., surgical procedures, long flights, pregnancy).
- The patient can make lifestyle adjustments to decrease her risk for future events.

For more information on the care plan and facilitator's guide please visit http://www.mhpharmacotherapy.com.

# 9 Ischemic Stroke

Susan R. Winkler

## CASE LEARNING OBJECTIVES

- Recognize the signs and symptoms of acute ischemic stroke
- Identify risk factors for ischemic stroke in a patient and provide appropriate patient education
- Determine whether thrombolytic therapy is indicated in a patient with acute ischemic stroke
- Develop an appropriate patient-specific therapeutic plan for acute ischemic stroke
- Develop an appropriate therapeutic plan for outpatient management of a patient with ischemic stroke, including an appropriate agent to prevent stroke recurrence

## PATIENT PRESENTATION

### Chief Complaint

"I just could not get the words out. I tried to speak, but nothing would come out."

### History of Present Illness

Catherine Smith is an 81-year-old Caucasian woman who was taken by the paramedics to the local hospital after experiencing weakness in her right hand and difficulty speaking during dinner with her neighbors. Her neighbors noted that she was having difficulty holding her fork and her speech seemed jumbled, so they immediately called the paramedics. She arrived in the emergency department within 90 minutes of the onset of her symptoms. She has been feeling tired and anxious since the death of her husband 4 months ago. Her appetite has been poor and she has lost 11 lb (5 kg) during this time. In the past 2 weeks, she has had several episodes where she experienced tingling in the fingers of her right hand and difficulty speaking; however, these episodes resolved within 15–20 minutes. She previously experienced these symptoms in 2007.

### Past Medical History

HTN for 18 years

PVD diagnosed in 2003

Anemia diagnosed 6 months ago

Anxiety diagnosed 2 months ago

### Family History

Both parents are deceased. She has no siblings. She has two adult sons who are healthy.

### Social History

She worked as an administrative assistant, and is retired for 22 years. She has two children aged 51 and 45 years.

### Tobacco/Alcohol/Substance Use

Social drinker; (–) tobacco or illicit drug use

### Allergies/Intolerances/Adverse Drug Events

NKDA

### Medications (Current)

Lisinopril/HCTZ 10/12.5 mg, 1 tablet PO every morning

Atenolol 25 mg, 1 tablet PO every evening

Aspirin 325 mg, 1 tablet PO every morning

Ferrous gluconate 300 mg, 1 tablet PO every morning with food

Citrucel fiber shake, 1 shake PO daily

Alprazolam 0.25 mg, 1 tablet PO 3 times daily PRN anxiety

### Medications (Prior)

Cilostazol 50 mg, 1 tablet PO twice daily, discontinued due to diarrhea

### Review of Systems

Denies headache; (–) blurred vision; (–) dizziness; has had difficulty ambulating in recent months due to generalized weakness; no history of migraine headaches or seizures

## Physical Examination

▶ **General**

Elderly, Caucasian woman, appearing weak and slightly anxious

▶ **Vital Signs**

BP 158/94 mm Hg, P 84, RR 14, T 36.9°C

Weight 147.4 lb (67.0 kg)

Height 64 in. (163 cm)

Denies headache or pain

▶ **Skin**

Warm and dry to touch

▶ **HEENT**

PERRLA, EOMI; no nystagmus; slight right-sided facial droop

▶ **Neck and Lymph Nodes**

(+) Carotid bruits on the left side; (−) lymphadenopathy

▶ **Chest**

Clear to auscultation

▶ **Breasts**

Examination deferred

▶ **Cardiovascular**

RRR, normal $S_1$, $S_2$; (−) $S_3$; (+) $S_4$

▶ **Abdomen**

Soft, nontender, nondistended; (+) BS; (−) organomegaly

▶ **Neurology**

A&O × 3; (+) dysarthria; slight right-sided facial droop; strength RUE 2/5; RLE 3/5; LUE 5/5; LLE 4/5 DTRs 2+ throughout; normal Babinski reflex

▶ **Extremities**

No cyanosis, clubbing, or edema; pulses 1+ bilaterally

▶ **Genitourinary**

Examination deferred

▶ **Rectal**

Examination deferred

## Laboratory Tests

|  | Conventional Units | SI Units |
|---|---|---|
| Na | 145 mEq/L | 145 mmol/L |
| K | 4.3 mEq/L | 4.3 mmol/L |
| Cl | 100 mEq/L | 100 mmol/L |
| $CO_2$ | 28 mEq/L | 28 mmol/L |
| BUN | 16 mg/dL | 5.7 mmol/L |
| SCr | 1.2 mg/dL | 106 μmol/L |
| Glu | 115 mg/dL | 6.4 mmol/L |
| Ca | 8.7 mg/dL | 2.18 mmol/L |
| Mg | 1.7 mEq/L | 0.85 mmol/L |
| Phosphate | 3.2 mg/dL | 1.03 mmol/L |
| Hgb | 11.6 g/dL | 116 g/L; 7.19 mmol/L |
| Hct | 35.2% | 0.352 |
| WBC | $5.6 \times 10^3/mm^3$ | $5.6 \times 10^9/L$ |
| Platelets | $264 \times 10^3/mm^3$ | $264 \times 10^9/L$ |
| aPTT | 24.6 s |  |
| Total cholesterol | 223 mg/dL | 5.77 mmol/L |
| LDL cholesterol | 121 mg/dL | 3.13 mmol/L |
| HDL cholesterol | 46 mg/dL | 1.19 mmol/L |
| Triglycerides | 184 mg/dL | 2.08 mmol/L |

## Diagnostic Tests

ECG: NSR

Head CT scan: (−) Hemorrhage; evidence of left-sided infarct (see Fig. 9-1)

Carotid Doppler: Decreased flow left carotid; 48% stenosis in left carotid

## Assessment

Eighty-one-year-old woman who presents to the emergency department with signs and symptoms consistent with a left-sided ischemic stroke. Diagnostic tests completed in the emergency department confirm the diagnosis of ischemic stroke.

### Student Workup

**Missing Information?**

**Evaluate:**   Patient Database

Drug Therapy Problems

Care Plan (by Problem)

**FIGURE 9-1.** CT scan of left-sided stroke. Reproduced, with permission, from Ropper AH, Samuels MA (eds). Adams and Victor's Principles of Neurology, 9th ed. New York, McGraw-Hill, Inc., 2009.

## TARGETED QUESTIONS

1. What signs, symptoms, and diagnostic tests are consistent with an ischemic stroke in this patient?

    *Hint: See p. 232 in PPP*

2. What risk factors for ischemic stroke are evident in this patient?

    *Hint: See p. 232 in PPP*

3. Would this patient be a candidate for thrombolytic therapy with alteplase or for carotid endarterectomy?

    *Hint: See pp. 234–238 in PPP*

4. How is alteplase administered and monitored acutely in the clinical setting?

    *Hint: See pp. 235–236 and Table 11-4 in PPP*

5. What long-term therapy would be appropriate in this patient for secondary stroke prevention, including the management of risk factors?

    *Hint: See pp. 235–236 and Table 11-3 in PPP*

## FOLLOW-UP

6. The patient returns for follow-up 3 weeks after her acute ischemic stroke. Her BP at this visit is 146/84 mm Hg, which is more than the goal of <120/80 mm Hg. How would you manage her BP at this point? Should she continue long-term statin therapy?

    *Hint: See p. 239 in PPP*

## ☉ GLOBAL PERSPECTIVE

Stroke has decreased to the fourth leading cause of death in the United States; however, it remains a major cause of long-term disability. Strokes occur more commonly in people 65 years and older, with the stroke risk doubling every decade after age 55 years. Stroke mortality has declined; however, hypertension, atrial fibrillation, and cigarette smoking continue to be important risk factors for stroke. Worldwide, stroke is the second most common cause of death. Approximately 20 million strokes occur globally each year, resulting in 5.7 million deaths annually. In developing countries, stroke mortality has declined due to global efforts to decrease cigarette smoking and manage hypertension. The incidence of stroke is expected to increase over the next decade due to the aging of the population.

## CASE SUMMARY

• The patient has experienced an acute left-sided ischemic stroke, so thrombolytic therapy is indicated in this case.

• She has risk factors for stroke, including hypertension, hyperlipidemia, previous transient ischemic attacks (TIAs), and PVD that require aggressive management to achieve target endpoints.

For more information on the care plan and facilitator's guide please visit http://www.mhpharmacotherapy.com.

# 10 Dyslipidemia

Jeannie Kim Lee        Kristina De Los Santos

## CASE LEARNING OBJECTIVES

- Determine a patient's coronary heart disease (CHD) risk and corresponding treatment goal according to the National Cholesterol Education Program Adult Treatment Panel (NCEP ATP) III guidelines
- Recommend appropriate therapeutic lifestyle changes and pharmacotherapy interventions for patients with dyslipidemia
- Describe the components of a monitoring plan to assess the effectiveness and adverse effects of pharmacotherapy for patients with dyslipidemia

## PATIENT PRESENTATION

### Chief Complaint

"My doctor sent me here for you to check my cholesterol."

### History of Present Illness

Joe Sanchez is a 68-year-old Hispanic male who is referred to the pharmacy clinic for lipid evaluation and management. He is new to this clinic, having recently been seen by one of the clinic's primary care physicians. He is feeling well with no complaints today. His last appointment with his primary care provider was 2 months ago when the dose of his BP medication was increased, so laboratory tests were drawn. That provider felt he would benefit from a pharmacist evaluation of his cholesterol, so he consulted a clinic pharmacist to assess JS's lipid panel and other pertinent laboratory results, initiate treatment for his lipid management, and follow-up to monitor for the efficacy and safety of the therapy. JS has long-standing HTN and was started on prescription medications several years ago, in addition to aspirin. He questions the safety of prescription medications as "they are not natural," and is resistant to taking prescription medications. He drinks four 8 oz (240 mL) glasses of grapefruit juice every day, stating that "it keeps me healthy."

### Past Medical History

HTN

Osteoarthritis

BPH

Obesity

### Family History

Father died from complications of CAD at age 52. Mother is alive at 91 with advanced dementia and diabetes.

### Social History

JS is a devout Catholic born in Tucson, Arizona. He speaks Spanish and English. He is married and lives with his wife of 43 years, and they have four children, aged 41, 38, 36, and 35. He is retired from his job at the U.S. Postal Service, and he now works part-time as a handyman.

### Tobacco/Alcohol/Substance Use

Current smoker, ½ ppd; drinks six beers each weekend; has never used illicit drugs

### Allergies/Intolerances/Adverse Drug Events

Penicillin (unknown reaction)

### Medications (Current)

HCTZ 25 mg daily PO, last refill June 26, 2012 (30-d supply)

Lisinopril 20 mg daily PO, last refill June 26, 2012 (30-d supply)

Doxazosin 4 mg at bedtime PO, last refill July 31, 2012 (30-d supply)

Ibuprofen 200 mg PRN PO for knee and low back pain

Aspirin 81 mg daily PO

### Review of Systems

(−) Headache, dizziness, light-headedness; (−) chest pain, palpitations; (−) infection; (−) urinary frequency; (+) nocturia one time per night (down from five times since starting doxazosin); (−) constipation, diarrhea, nausea; occasional knee and back pain relieved with ibuprofen.

## Physical Examination [from Last Primary Care Provider (PCP) Visit 2 Weeks Ago]

▶ *General*

Well-appearing, elderly, Hispanic male in no acute distress

▶ *Vital Signs*

BP 142/90 mm Hg, P 78, RR 14, T 36.2°C

Weight 245 lb (111 kg)

Height 66 in. (168 cm)

Pain 2/10 today

▶ *Skin*

Dry-appearing skin and scalp; (–) rashes or lesions

▶ *HEENT*

PERRLA, EOMI; trace periorbital edema; (–) sinus tenderness; TMs appear normal

▶ *Neck and Lymph Nodes*

Thyroid gland normal; (–) thyroid nodules; (–) lymphadenopathy; (–) carotid bruits

▶ *Chest*

Clear to auscultation

▶ *Cardiovascular*

RRR, normal $S_1$, $S_2$; (–) $S_3$ or $S_4$

▶ *Abdomen*

Not tender/not distended; (–) organomegaly

▶ *Neurology*

Grossly intact; deep tendon reflexes normal

▶ *Genitourinary*

Examination deferred

▶ *Rectal*

Examination deferred

### Laboratory Tests

#### Fasting Obtained 2 Weeks Ago

|  | Conventional Units | SI Units |
|---|---|---|
| Na | 137 mEq/L | 137 mmol/L |
| K | 3.9 mEq/L | 3.9 mmol/L |
| Cl | 102 mEq/L | 102 mmol/L |
| $CO_2$ | 25 mEq/L | 25 mmol/L |
| BUN | 19 mg/dL | 6.8 mmol/L |
| SCr | 1.1 mg/dL | 97 μmol/L |

| Total cholesterol | 263 mg/dL | 6.80 mmol/L |
|---|---|---|
| LDL cholesterol | 168 mg/dL | 4.34 mmol/L |
| HDL cholesterol | 51 mg/dL | 1.32 mmol/L |
| Triglycerides | 274 mg/dL | 3.10 mmol/L |
| AST | 16 IU/L | 0.27 μkat/L |
| ALT | 14 IU/L | 0.23 μkat/L |

### Assessment

Sixty-eight-year-old man with recently diagnosed dyslipidemia as well as HTN, BPH, and obesity.

---

### Student Workup

**Missing Information?**

**Evaluate:**    Patient Database

Drug Therapy Problems

Care Plan (by Problem)

---

## TARGETED QUESTIONS

1. What risk factors for CAD does JS have?

   *Hint: See Table 12-4 in PPP*

2. What are JS's 10-year CAD risk, his risk category, and his LDL goal?

   *Hint: See Tables 12-6 and Figure 12-6 in PPP*

3. Would JS benefit from any lifestyle modifications? If yes, specify.

   *Hint: See Table 12-7 in PPP*

4. If pharmacologic treatment is appropriate for JS, what medication would you choose and how would you plan his monitoring and follow-up?

   *Hint: See Tables 12-8 and 12-9 in PPP*

5. What education does JS require to be successful with his treatment plan?

   *Hint: See Tables 12-7 and 12-9, and p. 265 in PPP*

## FOLLOW-UP

6. Five years later, JS returns for follow-up. He now has diabetes, has experienced a silent MI, and is developing early signs of Alzheimer disease. He successfully quit smoking 1 year after this silent MI was discovered.

   His fasting laboratory tests include:

   Total cholesterol 270 mg/dL (6.98 mmol/L)

   LDL cholesterol 122 mg/dL (3.15 mmol/L)

   HDL cholesterol 41 mg/dL (1.06 mmol/L)

   Triglycerides 410 mg/dL (4.63 mmol/L)

What is JS's LDL goal now? How would the treatment plan change? How should the view of JS's triglycerides be altered given his new diagnoses? How should his cholesterol be managed as his age and Alzheimer disease progress?

*Hint: See Tables 12-3 and 12-9 in PPP*

## ☽ GLOBAL PERSPECTIVE

Dyslipidemia is a global issue. A clinician must be aware that various ethnic groups may vary in their risk and presentation for CHD. For instance, South Asians, who make up 25% of the global population, have a three- to five-fold increased risk of cardiovascular morbidity and mortality as compared with other ethnic groups. Despite their significantly higher risk of CHD due to a high prevalence of risk factors, they are less likely to receive preventative statin treatment due to their low baseline serum cholesterol levels compared with Caucasian patients. In addition, there is a paucity of data for statin treatment in South Asian patients. For South Asians living in the United States, the U.S. Food and Drug Administration (US FDA) recommends that the starting dose of rosuvastatin be 5 mg (instead of 10 mg) due to a pharmacokinetic study that showed South Asians had a 1.6- to 2.3-fold increased exposure to rosuvastatin compared with Caucasian patients.

## CASE SUMMARY

- JS's current clinical picture is consistent with newly diagnosed dyslipidemia.

- Initial goals and treatment vary widely on the basis of risk factors. All patients may benefit from lifestyle modifications. Medication therapy is indicated as determined by the NCEP ATP III guidelines.

- Statins are usually first-line therapy for lowering LDL cholesterol.

**For more information on the care plan and facilitator's guide please visit http://www.mhpharmacotherapy.com.**

# 11 Hypovolemic Shock

Christopher G. Wood    Joseph M. Swanson

## CASE LEARNING OBJECTIVES

- Describe the clinical presentation, including signs, symptoms, and laboratory test measurements for the typical hypovolemic shock patient
- Prepare a treatment plan with clearly defined outcome criteria for a hypovolemic shock patient that includes both fluid management and pharmacologic therapy
- Compare and contrast relative advantages and disadvantages of crystalloids, colloids, and blood products in the treatment of hypovolemic shock
- Formulate a stepwise monitoring strategy for a hypovolemic shock patient

## PATIENT PRESENTATION

### Chief Complaint

"Some guy shot me in the stomach! It hurts really bad!"

### History of Present Illness

EM is a 25-year-old male who was at a nightclub and got into an argument with other patrons. During the argument he was shot in the abdomen with a handgun. He was transported to the trauma center by ambulance within approximately 30 minutes of his injury. In the ambulance, he was alert and oriented, and his vital signs were BP 140/95 mm Hg, HR 90, and RR 14. The paramedics reported that the patient had "moderate" blood loss from the bullet entry site. On arrival to the trauma center, he became restless and confused during his interview by the trauma team. His admission BP was 110/70 mm Hg, HR 110, RR 24, and SaO$_2$ 85% (0.85) and dropping. Subsequently, he was endotracheally intubated and placed on mechanical ventilation. He had two large-bore venous catheters and a urinary catheter placed.

### Past Medical History

Noncontributory

### Family History

Noncontributory

### Social History

Single, employed at a local factory

### Tobacco/Alcohol/Substance Use

Social drinker; (–) tobacco; (+) marijuana use

### Allergies/Intolerances/Adverse Drug Events

Penicillin (unknown type)

### Medications (Current)

Unable to be determined prior to intubation

### Review of Systems

Before intubation, the patient complained of generalized weakness. His urine output in the catheter collection system was noted to be very dark yellow.

### Physical Examination

▸ *General*

Well-nourished, young, African American male with increasing confusion and restlessness in some distress.

▸ *Vital Signs (10 Minutes after Admission)*

BP 80/45 mm Hg, HR 120, RR 20 (mechanically ventilated), T 36°C

Weight 198 lb (90 kg)

Height 70 in. (178 cm)

▸ *Skin*

Cool

▸ *HEENT*

PERRLA, EOMI, otherwise normal; oral endotracheal tube in place

▸ *Neck and Lymph Nodes*

Normal

▸ *Chest*

(+) Breath sounds and clear to auscultation bilaterally

▸ *Cardiovascular*

Tachycardic and hypotensive; normal heart sounds

▸ *Abdomen*

Bullet entry wound (1 cm) in left lower quadrant with active bleeding from the wound; very tender around entry wound.

▸ *Neurology*

Grossly intact; increasing confusion

▸ *Genitourinary*

Urinary catheter in place

▸ *Rectal*

Grossly heme positive

## Laboratory Tests (on Admission)

### Arterial Blood Gas

|         | Conventional Units | SI Units  |
|---------|--------------------|-----------|
| pH      | 7.28               | —         |
| $PCO_2$ | 50 mm Hg           | 6.65 kPa  |
| $PO_2$  | 82 mm Hg           | 109 kPa   |
| $HCO_3$ | 21 mEq/L           | 21 mmol/L |
| $SaO_2$ | 84%                | 0.84      |

### Metabolic Panel

|        | Conventional Units | SI Units   |
|--------|--------------------|------------|
| Na     | 144 mEq/L          | 144 mmol/L |
| K      | 3.9 mEq/L          | 3.9 mmol/L |
| Cl     | 105 mEq/L          | 105 mmol/L |
| $HCO_2$| 20 mEq/L           | 20 mEq/L   |
| BUN    | 22 mg/dL           | 7.9 mmol/L |
| Cr     | 1.7 mg/dL          | 150 μmol/L |
| Glu    | 175 mg/dL          | 9.7 mmol/L |

## Assessment

Twenty-five-year-old male with emerging hemorrhagic hypovolemic shock

**Student Workup**

**Missing Information?**

Evaluate:    Patient Database

Drug Therapy Problems

Care Plan (by Problem)

## TARGETED QUESTIONS

1. What signs and symptoms of hypovolemic shock does the patient have?

   *Hint: See Table 13-2 and pp. 272–273 in PPP*

2. What alterations of key hemodynamic parameters are occurring in this patient?

   *Hint: See Figure 13-1 in PPP*

3. What are the immediate treatment goals in the first hour of hypovolemic shock?

   *Hint: See Figure 13-3 and p. 273 in PPP*

4. What should be administered for initial therapy of hypovolemic shock? Compare the advantages and disadvantages of colloids and crystalloids for fluid resuscitation.

   *Hint: See Figure 13-3 and pp. 275–277 in PPP*

5. One hour after the initial therapy for hypovolemic shock, what additional therapy is needed?

   *Hint: See Figure 13-3, Table 13-4, and pp. 277–278 in PPP*

## FOLLOW-UP

After the initial resuscitation period, an exploratory laparotomy was performed in the operating room. The patient had a penetrating injury to the colon with heavy contamination of colonic contents into the peritoneal space. The sites of acute bleeding were surgically repaired. The following morning, the patient is in the ICU on mechanical ventilation and a pulmonary artery catheter has been placed. The patient's vital signs are BP 85/64 mm Hg, HR 110, pulmonary artery wedge (occlusion) pressure 17 mm Hg, cardiac index 5 L/min/m², and RR 18 (ventilated). Pertinent labs/findings include Hgb 8.4 g/dL (84 g/L; 5.21 mmol/L), lactate 55.9 mg/dL (6.20 mmol/L), and SCr 1.9 mg/dL (168 μmol/L). Within the last hour, the patient's mental status has deteriorated and is now obtunded.

6. What therapy should be administered now for his ongoing shock?

   *Hint: See Figure 13-3 and pp. 277–278 in PPP*

7. What are the treatment goals for EM's shock within the first 24 hours of onset?

   *Hint: See p. 273 in PPP*

8. What supportive care pharmacotherapy should be started?

   *Hint: See pp. 278–279 in PPP*

9. What antimicrobial surgical prophylaxis, if any, should be started?

   *Hint: See antimicrobial prophylaxis chapter in PPP*

## ☉ GLOBAL PERSPECTIVE

Hypovolemic shock, especially related to trauma, is a leading cause of morbidity and mortality for younger populations regardless of country or ethnic group. The incidence of violence-related trauma (e.g., gunshot wounds) varies based on multiple sociopolitical factors. Treatment of hemorrhagic shock as presented in this case will vary somewhat worldwide depending on the health care infrastructure. For example, the ability to transfer patients quickly to a trauma center, familiarity with assessment and rapid management of bleeding, and rapid fluid resuscitation may all vary widely. In addition, the use of tranexamic acid varies among countries. This therapy was studied in Europe and developing countries but has not been widely adopted in the United States. A cultural factor in some patients will be a social and/or religious prohibition against receiving blood products.

## CASE SUMMARY

- Rapid assessment of the type and severity of hypovolemic shock, and rapid restoration of systolic blood pressure are key components of initial therapy.
- Ongoing therapy (i.e., first 24 hours) focuses on continued volume resuscitation and reversal of organ dysfunction.

For more information on the care plan and facilitator's guide please visit http://www.mhpharmacotherapy.com.

# 12 Chronic Asthma

Brice Labruzzo Mohundro   Wallace G. Leader

- Classify asthma severity
- Assess the existing treatment regimen and proper inhalation technique
- Develop a therapeutic plan (including treatment and monitoring) using patient-specific data that maximize patient response while minimizing adverse drug events and other drug-related problems
- Discuss proper instructions that are to be provided to a patient prescribed asthma medications

## PATIENT PRESENTATION

### Chief Complaint

Desiree Adams is a 36-year-old African American female who presents to a family medicine clinic for follow-up after a recent emergency department (ED) visit for an "asthma attack."

### History of Present Illness

DA reports having asthma as a child but was told by her mother that she grew out of it. She believes it was around the seventh grade when she stopped using an inhaler. She does not recall the name of the medication she used. On discharge from the ED, the patient was provided with a prescription for prednisone 20 mg daily for 1 week and an albuterol inhaler, but she is not sure if she is using the inhaler correctly. DA reports she finished the 7 days of prednisone a few days ago and is having less difficulty breathing than when she presented to the ED; however, she complains of a cough that she thinks appeared when she began working a second job (about 6 months ago). The patient experiences SOB most days of the week, which is sometimes accompanied by wheezing and a funny feeling in her chest. DA denies any nighttime symptoms. She is concerned because she is not able to run around with her kids when she gets home from work like she used to. She notices on her days off from the dry cleaning business, she is usually symptom free unless she is around cats or mowing the yard. In addition to her respiratory complaints, the patient tells you she is experiencing heartburn several times per week, which she has been self-treating with Tums.

### Past Medical History

Allergic rhinitis (allergic to cat dander and pollen per intradermal allergy testing) × 20 yr

Asthma (diagnosed at age 5 years, no treatment since approximately the age of 12 yr)

HTN × 3 yr

### Family History

Both parents have HTN; father and younger sister have asthma and allergic rhinitis.

### Social/Work History

Single mother of three living in a house with no pets. Her primary job is working as a cashier at a grocery store, but she also works a second job at a family-owned dry cleaning business.

### Tobacco/Alcohol/Substance use

She denies current tobacco and alcohol use.

### Allergy/Intolerance/Adverse Event History

Sulfamethoxazole/trimethoprim—rash

### Medication History

Albuterol HFA 90 mcg one to two puffs every 4–6 hr as needed for shortness of breath

Loratadine 10 mg by mouth daily as needed for allergies

Extended-release propranolol 120 mg by mouth daily for hypertension

Norgestimate/ethinyl estradiol one tablet by mouth daily

### Review of Systems

Unremarkable except for what is noted above

## Physical Examination

▶ *General*

Well-developed, well-nourished black female in no acute distress

▶ *Vital Signs*

BP 142/90 mm Hg, P 65, RR 20, T 37°C

Weight 180 lb (82 kg)

Height 65 in. (165 cm)

Denies pain

▶ *Skin*

Red and flaky inside elbows and behind knees

▶ *HEENT*

WNL except for nasal polyps

▶ *Chest*

Clear to auscultation bilaterally

▶ *Cardiovascular*

RRR; $S_1$ and $S_2$ normal; no rubs, gallops, or murmurs

## Laboratory and Other Diagnostic Tests

### Spirometry

|  | Prealbuterol (% Predicted) | Postalbuterol (% Predicted) |
|---|---|---|
| $FEV_1$ | 82 [0.82] | 96 [0.96] |
| FVC | 98 [0.98] | 109 [1.09] |
| $FEV_1/FVC$ | 0.84 | 0.88 |

### Assessment

Thirty-six-year-old female with signs, symptoms, and diagnostic tests consistent with asthma

### Student Workup

**Missing Information/Inadequate Data?**

Evaluate:    Patient Database

Drug Therapy Problems

Care Plan (by Problem)

## TARGETED QUESTIONS

1. How would you classify the patient's asthma severity?

   Hint: See http://www.nhlbi.nih.gov/guidelines/asthma

2. Why are inhaled corticosteroids a preferred therapy for all severities of persistent asthma?

   Hint: See pp. 290–293 in PPP

3. What disease states and medications can potentially worsen asthma?

   Hint: See p. 287 in PPP

4. What adverse effects of inhaled corticosteroids would you discuss with the patient?

   Hint: See p. 291 in PPP

5. Explain the steps involved with a properly metered dose inhaler technique.

   Hint: See Figure 14-1 in PPP

## FOLLOW-UP

6. Four weeks later, the patient returns for follow-up. The coughing has resolved; however, she is using albuterol three to four times per week for SOB. What level of control is the patient currently experiencing? What changes, if any, would you make to her asthma treatment?

   Hint: See Figure 14-2 in PPP

## ☺ GLOBAL PERSPECTIVE

Asthma is a significant global public health problem, affecting patients in both developed and undeveloped countries. Using conservative criteria, it is estimated that approximately 300 million people worldwide have asthma. International asthma prevalence patterns cannot be explained using current knowledge of asthma pathogenesis; however, asthma prevalence appears to increase in areas that become more urbanized and adopt Western lifestyles. These increases are associated with increases in atopic sensitization and correspond with increases in other atopic disorders, such as allergic rhinitis and eczema. Globally, asthma is responsible for approximately 15 million disability-adjusted life years, a measurement of years of healthy life lost because of the disease, which is similar to that of diabetes mellitus and schizophrenia. Despite the existence of evidence-based guidelines for asthma care, wide variations in the clinical management of asthma exist worldwide.

Major barriers to effective asthma therapy include access to care and cost of therapy. In many areas, patients do not have access to basic asthma medications or medical care, leading to suboptimal long-term therapy and increased risk of death from an acute asthma. One of the primary barriers to appropriate asthma control is the cost of medications, and many patients in countries located in Central America, Africa, South Asia, and the Middle East do not have access to essential asthma medications.

### CASE SUMMARY

- Her presentation is consistent with mild persistent asthma.
- A daily controller medication should be initiated to improve asthma control.
- Comorbid conditions that may interfere with asthma control should be managed.

For more information on the care plan and facilitator's guide please visit http://www.mhpharmacotherapy.com.

# 13 Acute Asthma Exacerbation

Ann McMahon Wicker    Wallace G. Leader

## CASE LEARNING OBJECTIVES

- Classify current asthma severity
- Recognize the clinical signs and symptoms of asthma
- Develop an appropriate treatment and monitoring plan for acute asthma therapy
- List the factors that may affect a patient's adherence to asthma therapy
- Educate a patient who is on asthma medication about the use of inhaled delivery devices, peak flow meters, and asthma education plans

## PATIENT PRESENTATION

### Chief Complaint

"I am having trouble catching my breath."

### History of Present Illness

Jeremy Weber is an 11-year-old African American male who presents to the emergency department (ED) complaining of shortness of breath, which has been getting progressively worse over the past 12 hours. His shortness of breath started on the playground at school after a kickball game with his classmates. After the game, in addition to shortness of breath, JW experienced wheezing, coughing, and chest tightness. At this time, he self-treated his breathing difficulty with an old Primatene Mist inhaler that he carries in his pocket wherever he goes. Initially, he was having difficulty breathing, but now he is in acute distress. On arrival to the ED, his oxygen saturation ($SAO_2$) was 85% (0.85) and he was able to answer questions only with single words. He was treated with three nebulized albuterol treatments with some relief; repeat $SAO_2$ was 90% (0.90). JW has had a runny nose and watery eyes for the past 2 weeks, which is not unusual for him.

### Past Medical History

Asthma × 8 years with five hospitalizations since diagnosis, but no history of intubation

Perennial allergic rhinitis × 5 years

ADHD × 3 years

### Family History

Positive for allergic rhinitis (mother and sister)

### Social History/Work History

Currently enrolled in the fifth grade and lives with his mother, father, and sister. There are no animals at home.

### Tobacco/Alcohol/Substance Abuse

Denies any tobacco use, but does have exposure to second-hand smoke at home. Also denies any alcohol or drug use.

### Allergies/Intolerances/Adverse Drug Events

No known drug allergies

### Medications (Prior to Admission)

Primatene Mist inhaler one to two puffs PRN

Albuterol 90 mcg one to two puffs every 4 to 6 hours PRN shortness of breath (has not been filled in over 6 months)

Cetirizine 10 mg PO daily PRN allergies

Methylphenidate 10 mg PO q 9 AM and 3 PM

### Review of Systems

Negative, except for above

### Physical Examination

▶ *General*

The patient appears slightly anxious, is in respiratory distress, and looks sick. He is having trouble speaking.

▶ *Vital Signs*

BP 99/51 mm Hg, P 108, RR 26, T 36.7°C, and $O_2$ saturation
   90% (0.90) on 2L nasal cannula

Weight 78.3 lb (35.6 kg)

Height 58 in. (147 cm)

Denies pain

▶ *HEENT*

Has boggy, indurated, and edematous nasal mucosa. Red,
watery eyes and clear mucoid nasal discharge are noted.

▶ *Chest*

The patient has significant respiratory distress with marked
respiratory effort and use of accessory muscles; diffuse expiratory wheezes bilaterally; no crackles or rhonchi noted.

▶ *Cardiovascular*

Tachycardic, RRR. No murmurs appreciated

▶ *Abdomen*

Soft, nontender, and nondistended. Positive bowel sounds

▶ *Neurology*

Alert and oriented × 3

## Laboratory Tests

$SAO_2$ prenebulizer 85% (0.85)

$SAO_2$ postnebulizer 90% (0.90)

|  | Prealbuterol (% Predicted) | Postalbuterol (% Predicted) |
|---|---|---|
| $FEV_1$ | 82 [0.82] | 96 [0.96] |
| FVC | 98 [0.98] | 109 [1.09] |
| $FEV_1$/FVC | 0.84 | 0.88 |

## Diagnostic Studies

CXR shows normal cardiac shadow and clear lung fields. ECG
shows sinus tachycardia.

## Assessment

This is an 11-year-old African American male with an acute
asthma exacerbation.

### Student Workup

#### Missing Information/Inadequate Data?

**Evaluate:**   Patient Database

Drug Therapy Problems

Care Plan (by Problem)

## TARGETED QUESTIONS

1. What is this patient's acute asthma exacerbation severity?
   *Hint: See http://www.nhlbi.nih.gov/guidelines/asthma*

2. Describe signs and symptoms this patient has that are
   consistent with an acute asthma exacerbation.
   *Hint: See pp. 285–286 in PPP*

3. What medications would be most appropriate in an acute
   asthma exacerbation?
   *Hint: See Figures 14-3 and 14-4 in PPP*

4. When should this patient perform peak flow
   measurements to determine his personal best?
   *Hint: See p. 300 in PPP*

5. This patient's mother is concerned about the adverse
   effects associated with corticosteroid use in children. How
   would you counsel her regarding her concern?
   *Hint: See p. 291 in PPP*

## FOLLOW-UP

6. JW is admitted to the hospital. On further questioning,
   he reports awakening about three times per month. He
   also admits to taking breaks during activity to catch his
   breath, using his Primatene Mist inhaler about five times
   per week. What medications should JW be discharged
   home on? What counseling advice, if any, would you give
   to him? If he did not respond to the initial therapy, what
   adjunctive therapies could have been considered?

## ↻ GLOBAL PERSPECTIVE

Asthma is a significant public health problem globally,
affecting patients in both developed and undeveloped
countries. It is estimated that asthma accounts for one
in 250 deaths worldwide. The majority of asthma deaths
worldwide are preventable. Most acute asthma-related
deaths are due to the lack of appropriate intensification of
therapy because of inappropriate assessment of the severity
of the exacerbation causing delays in obtaining medical
assistance or lack of access to medical care. The number
of hospitalizations due to asthma are higher and length
of asthma-related hospital stays is longer in developing
countries than in more affluent countries.

### CASE SUMMARY

- His current clinical picture is consistent with a severe acute
  asthma exacerbation, and medications to manage this
  exacerbation should be initiated.

- All patients with a diagnosis of asthma, regardless of severity,
  should have an appropriate rescue inhaler available.

For more information on the care plan and facilitator's
guide please visit http://www.mhpharmacotherapy.com.

# 14 Chronic Obstructive Pulmonary Disease

Nicole D. Verkleeren

## CASE LEARNING OBJECTIVES

- Identify the signs and symptoms of a COPD exacerbation
- List the treatment goals for a patient with COPD
- Design an appropriate treatment regimen for a patient with a COPD exacerbation
- Develop a monitoring plan to assess the effectiveness and adverse effects of pharmacotherapy for COPD
- Formulate an appropriate education plan for a patient with COPD

## PATIENT PRESENTATION

### Chief Complaint

"My breathing just isn't getting better. I'm so tired and out of breath, I couldn't even read a book to my grandson yesterday."

### History of Present Illness

Samuel Smarthe is a 67-year-old male who presents to the emergency department with complaints of increasing SOB over the past 4–5 days. He was seen by his primary care physician 3 days ago and was given a prescription for prednisone and told to increase his rescue inhaler use as needed. He comes to the ED this evening because his SOB has continued to worsen and he is increasingly tired and weak. In the last year, he has been hospitalized five times for similar symptoms, most recently 5 weeks ago. He has been using inhalers for his COPD for the past 11 years. About 6 months ago, his ICS dose was increased. He is supposed to use O$_2$ at home, but he admits to being nonadherent with this.

### Past Medical History

COPD diagnosed 12 years ago

HTN diagnosed at age 35

Chronic atrial fibrillation × 5 years

Hyperlipidemia diagnosed at age 45

GERD × 2 years

Osteoarthritis (OA) × 10 years

### Family History

Father died at age 70 of lung cancer. Mother died at age 35 in a motor vehicle accident. He has one brother with CAD and an "irregular heartbeat," who is alive.

### Social History

The patient is married and lives with his wife of 45 years, his youngest daughter, and his 3-year-old grandson. He has two other children who live out of state. He is a retired steel-mill worker, and he and his wife care for their grandson during the day while his daughter is at work.

### Tobacco/Alcohol/Substance Use

Smokes ½ ppd of cigarettes; he cut back about 6 months ago from 1½ ppd for 47 years. No alcohol or illicit drug use.

### Allergies/Intolerances/Adverse Drug Events

None

### Medications (Prior to Admission)

Simvastatin 20 mg PO q h

Atenolol 50 mg PO daily

Warfarin 7.5 mg PO on Mondays and Fridays, 5 mg PO on all other days

Prednisone 30 mg PO daily × 10 d (started 3 d ago)

Fluticasone/salmeterol 500 mcg/50 mcg one inhalation q 12 h

Tiotropium 18 mcg one inhalation q 24 h

Albuterol MDI one to two puffs q 4–6 h PRN SOB (used as often as q 20 min in the hours before presentation)

Famotidine 20 mg PO twice daily

Acetaminophen 500 mg PO q 6 h PRN arthritis pain

## Review of Systems

Increasing fatigue over the past week; (−) nasal congestion or drainage; (+) SOB, cough with increased thick, tan, sputum production; (−) fever; (−) chest pain; (−) muscle pain/weakness; (+) moderate arthritis pain in the knees usually relieved by acetaminophen; (−) unusual bleeding/bruising; (−) constipation; (−) sick contacts; (−) recent travel

## Physical Examination

### ▶ General

Slightly frail, elderly white man who appears older than his stated age, in moderate respiratory distress since receiving treatment in the ED

### ▶ Vital Signs

BP 115/68 mm Hg, P 92, RR 26, T 36.9°C

Weight 134 lb (60.9 kg)

Height 70 in. (178 cm)

2/10 arthritic pain in both knees

### ▶ Skin

Warm, dry, and intact

### ▶ HEENT

PERRLA, EOMI; TMs appear normal; white patches cover tongue and inside of mouth

### ▶ Neck and Lymph Nodes

(−) Lymphadenopathy; (−) thyromegaly; (−) carotid bruits; (+) mild bilateral JVD; use of accessory muscles for breathing noted

### ▶ Chest

Barrel-shaped chest; lung sounds distant; (+) rhonchi; (−) rales and crackles; bilateral wheezes on inspiration and expiration

### ▶ Cardiovascular

Irregularly irregular rhythm, normal $S_1$, $S_2$; (−) $S_3$ or $S_4$; no murmurs or rubs

### ▶ Abdomen

Nontender, nondistended; (−) organomegaly; paradoxical abdominal motion observed

### ▶ Neurology

Alert and oriented × 3; cranial nerves II–XII intact

### ▶ Extremities

Cool, slightly cyanotic, no clubbing, 1+ edema of lower extremities; radial and pedal pulses 2+ bilaterally; slightly decreased range of motion in both knees; (−) joint swelling or tenderness

## Laboratory Tests

|  | Conventional Units | SI Units |
|---|---|---|
| Na | 139 mEq/L | 139 mmol/L |
| K | 3.1 mEq/L | 3.1 mmol/L |
| Cl | 107 mEq/L | 107 mmol/L |
| BUN | 22 mg/dL | 7.9 mmol/L |
| SCr | 1.3 mg/dL | 115 μmol/L |
| Glucose | 117 mg/dL | 6.5 mmol/L |
| Hemoglobin | 14.1 g/dL | 141 g/L; 8.75 mmol/L |
| Hematocrit | 41.1% | 0.411 |
| WBC | $9.8 \times 10^3/mm^3$ | $9.8 \times 10^9/L$ |
| Platelets | $257 \times 10^3/mm^3$ | $257 \times 10^9/L$ |
| PT | 28.5 s | |
| INR | 2.6 | |
| ABG | | |
| pH | 7.27 | |
| $PCO_2$ | 59.1 mm Hg | 7.9 kPa |
| $PO_2$ | 58.5 mm Hg | 7.8 kPa |
| $HCO_3$ | 28 mEq/L | 28 mmol/L |
| $SaO_2$ | 86% | 0.86 |

## Diagnostic Tests

CXR (see Figure 14-1) shows hyperinflation of the lungs; flattened diaphragm; (−) infiltrates, effusion.

ECG reveals atrial fibrillation with controlled ventricular rate; (−) U-waves, T-waves normal.

## Assessment

Sixty-seven-year-old man with signs, symptoms, and laboratory tests consistent with a COPD exacerbation requiring hospitalization and noninvasive mechanical ventilation.

### Student Workup

#### Missing Information?

| Evaluate: | Patient Database |
|---|---|
| | Drug Therapy Problems |
| | Care Plan (by Problem) |

**FIGURE 14-1.**  PA radiograph showing flattened hemidiaphragms and decreased vascular markings. (Reproduced, with permission, from Usatine RP, Smith MA, Mayeaux Jr EJ, Chumley H, Tysinger J. The Color Atlas of Family Medicine. New York, McGraw-Hill, 2009, Fig 54-2.)

## TARGETED QUESTIONS

1.  What signs and symptoms of a COPD exacerbation does the patient have?

    *Hint: See p. 314 in PPP*

2.  What are the indications for antibiotic use in the treatment of a COPD exacerbation, and what should be taken into consideration when choosing an antibiotic for this patient?

    *Hint: See pp. 315–316 in PPP*

3.  Why might theophylline be avoided in this patient?

    *Hint: What side effect(s) of theophylline might worsen an underlying condition in this patient? See p. 313 in PPP*

4.  What indications for mechanical ventilation does this patient display?

    *Hint: See pp. 316–317 in PPP*

## FOLLOW-UP

5.  Three days later, the patient's blood gases have improved, he remains afebrile, culture results are negative, and he is no longer requiring mechanical ventilation.

What changes, if any, would you make to his drug therapy regimen? What considerations regarding his pharmacotherapy regimen should be considered as this patient is being discharged?

*Hint: See p. 315 in PPP for antibiotic duration and the section on immunizations on p. 314 in PPP*

## ⟳ GLOBAL PERSPECTIVE

According to U.S. epidemiologic data, Caucasians are more likely than other races and ethnic groups to have COPD; this trend differs from most other lung diseases. Not only are white Americans more prone to COPD, but they are also more likely to die from the disease than are African Americans or Hispanics. Although epidemiologic data can be difficult to interpret, particularly when discussing a disease that is underdiagnosed such as COPD, with prevalence rates in whites and African Americans nearly double those seen in Hispanics, a genetic component that is specific to certain ethnicities seems likely. This theory is supported in Asians and Pacific Islanders, in whom some research suggests that they may possess a genetic component that reduces their risk of COPD. In many countries, the prevalence of COPD is increasing, reflecting increased rates of smoking over the past 20 years.

## CASE SUMMARY

-   His clinical presentation indicates the need for hospitalization, mechanical ventilation, and antibiotics in addition to standard treatment for a COPD exacerbation.

-   His underlying medical conditions (e.g., atrial fibrillation) and existing medications (warfarin) must be taken into consideration when designing a drug therapy regimen and establishing therapeutic goals and monitoring.

-   Unnecessary use of antibiotics should be avoided; therefore, when they are used, they should be discontinued as soon as it is appropriate.

For more information on the care plan and facilitator's guide please visit http://www.mhpharmacotherapy.com.

# 15 Cystic Fibrosis

Hanna Phan                    Nicole M. Even

## CASE LEARNING OBJECTIVES

- Describe the signs and symptoms of a respiratory exacerbation of cystic fibrosis (CF)
- Determine appropriate pharmacotherapy, including antimicrobial choice and patient monitoring for a patient with an acute CF exacerbation
- Describe appropriate nutritional assessment and management of a patient with CF

## PATIENT PRESENTATION

### Chief Complaint

"Increased work of breathing and worsening respiratory symptoms" per stepmother

### History of Present Illness

JM is a 12-year-old Caucasian female brought to the emergency department for worsening respiratory symptoms. The patient's stepmother states that JM was treated with ciprofloxacin 750 mg PO BID at home for the past 2 weeks without resolution of symptoms. JM has had increased cough with very dark-green colored sputum, SOB, and lethargy. She has lost 8 pounds (3.6 kg) over the last month and is having abnormal stools (4–6 stools/d) that are foul smelling and greasy.

### Past Medical History

JM was diagnosed with cystic fibrosis (CF) at the age of 6 months. Her CF genotype is ΔF508 homozygous. Previous hospitalizations: she is frequently hospitalized ~ every 2–3 months for acute pulmonary CF exacerbations. She has pancreatic insufficiency requiring supplementation. History of iron deficiency anemia, GERD, allergic rhinitis. Her baseline FEV1 is 80% (0.80) of predicted.

### Family History

JM has one 19-year-old brother who no longer lives with the family who also has CF (same genetic mutations) and has frequent hospitalizations for acute CF exacerbations.

### Social History

JM is a sophomore at a local high school. She lives with her father and stepmother. She is nonadherent to her nebulized medications and airway clearance (misses at least once daily) and occasionally forgets to take her pancreatic enzymes (about 1–2 times/wk). Her stepmother works full time and JM does not participate in any sports or extracurricular activities outside of school.

### Allergies/Intolerances/Adverse Drug Events

NKDA

### Medications

▶ **Home Therapy**

Vitamin A-D-E-K supplement (Source CF) 1 gel cap PO BID

Albuterol 2.5 mg nebulized BID

Dornase alfa 2.5 mg nebulized daily

Pancreatic enzyme (Creon) eight 12,000 capsules PO with meals and 4 capsules with snacks

Vitamin E 400 IU PO BID

Tobramycin inhalation solution (TOBI) 300 mg nebulized bid, 28 days on/off alternating with aztreonam, currently "on" month

Airway clearance via high frequency chest wall oscillation vest bid (patient does only once daily)

Ferrous sulfate 325 mg PO BID

Loratadine 10 mg PO daily

▶ **Current Inpatient Therapy**

Meropenem 850 g IV q 8 h

Ciprofloxacin 750 mg PO q 12 h

Albuterol 2.5 mg nebulized q 4–6 h PRN

Airway clearance via percussion and postural drainage (P + PD) BID

Source CF 1 gel cap PO BID

Creon eight 12,000 capsules PO with meals and 4 capsules with snacks

Dornase alfa 2.5 mg nebulized daily

Ferrous sulfate 325 mg PO bid

Loratadine 10 mg PO daily

Vitamin E 400 IU PO BID

## Immunizations

Up to date

## Review of Systems

▶ *General*

Fatigue and weakness with increased productive cough; increased stool (noted that it floats versus well-formed, sinking).

## Physical Examination

▶ *Vital Signs*

HR 97, BP 113/70 mm, RR 19, T 36.6°C

Height 67 in. (171 cm)

Weight 95 lb (43 kg)

$O_2$ saturation 87% (0.87) on RA, 96% (0.96) with 1L nasal cannula

Spirometry (% predicted) $FEV_1$ 68 (0.68); FVC 76 (0.76); $FEV_1$/FVC 90 (0.90); PEF 74 (0.74)

▶ *Skin/Extremities*

Clubbing noted with no cyanosis; capillary refill <2 s

▶ *HEENT*

EOMI, PERRLA

▶ *Neck and Lymph Nodes*

(−) Lymphadenopathy

▶ *Chest*

Crackles bilaterally in the upper lobes greater than lower lobes, poor air entry

▶ *Cardiovascular*

RRR, no murmurs, rubs, or gallops

▶ *Abdomen*

Nondistended, nontender, normal bowel sounds. Complains of heartburn symptoms 2–3/wk. Normal diet but not very hungry and doesn't feel like eating anything some days.

▶ *Neurology*

Grossly intact; DTRs normal; A&O × 4

▶ *Genitourinary*

Examination deferred. Urine output: good, ~ 2 mL/kg/h

▶ *Rectal*

Examination deferred

## Laboratory Tests

### Nonfasting (8/20)

|  | Conventional Units | SI Units |
|---|---|---|
| Na | 139 | 139 mmol/L |
| K | 3.5 | 3.5 mmol/L |
| Cl | 106 | 106 mmol/L |
| $HCO_3$ | 25 | 25 mmol/L |
| BUN | 12 mg/dL | 4.3 mmol/L |
| SCr | 0.7 mg/dL | 62 μmol/L |
| Glucose | 120 mg/dL | 6.7 mmol/L |
| Ca | 8.7 mg/dL | 2.18 mmol/L |
| Mg | 1.5 mEq/L | 0.75 mmol/L |
| $PO_4$ | 3 mEq/L | 0.97 mmol/L |
| Albumin | 2.5 g/dL | 25 g/L |
| WBC | $8.2 \times 10^3/mm^3$ | $8.2 \times 10^9/L$ |
| MCV | 79 μm³ | 79 fL |
| Segs | 57% | 0.57 |
| Bands | 13% | 0.13 |
| Lymphs | 25% | 0.25 |
| Monos | 5% | 0.05 |
| Eos | 3% | 0.03 |
| Baso | 1% | 0.01 |
| Hemoglobin | 12 g/dL | 120 g/L; 7.45 mmol/L |
| Hematocrit | 36.5% | 0.365 |
| Platelets | $350 \times 10^3/mm^3$ | $350 \times 10^9/L$ |
| PT | 14.6 s | |
| INR | 1.2 | |
| AST | 21 IU/L | 0.35 μkat/L |
| ALT | 23 IU/L | 0.38 μkat/L |
| Alk phos | 148 IU/L | 2.47 μkat/L |
| Tbili | 0.1 mg/dL | 1.7 μmol/L |
| Vitamin A (retinol) | 3 mcg/dL | 0.105 μmol/L |
| Vitamin E (alpha tocopherol) | 1.1 mg/dL | 25.54 μmol/L |
| Vitamin D (25-OH total) | 5.1 ng/mL | 12.73 nmol/L |

## Cultures

### 6/16 respiratory sputum

**3+ *Pseudomonas aeruginosa*, mucoid**

Susceptible:

| | |
|---|---|
| tobramycin | MIC 4 mcg/mL or mg/L |
| amikacin | MIC ≤ 1 mcg/mL or mg/L |
| meropenem | MIC 4 mcg/mL or mg/L |
| aztreonam | MIC 4 mcg/mL or mg/L |

Intermediate:

| | |
|---|---|
| cefepime | MIC 16 mcg/mL or mg/L |
| piperacillin/tazobactam | MIC 32 mcg/mL or mg/L |
| ciprofloxacin | MIC 4 mcg/mL or mg/L |

Resistant:

| | |
|---|---|
| gentamicin | MIC 8 mcg/mL or mg/L |

**3+ *Pseudomonas aeruginosa*, non-mucoid**

Susceptible:

| | |
|---|---|
| tobramycin | MIC 2 mcg/mL or mg/L |
| amikacin | MIC ≤ 1 mcg/mL or mg/L |
| meropenem | MIC 4 mcg/mL or mg/L |
| aztreonam | MIC 4 mcg/mL or mg/L |

Intermediate:

| | |
|---|---|
| cefepime | MIC 16 mcg/mL or mg/L |
| ciprofloxacin | MIC 4 mcg/mL or mg/L |

Resistant:

| | |
|---|---|
| gentamicin | MIC 8 mcg/mL or mg/L |
| piperacillin/tazobactam | MIC 64 mcg/mL or mg/L |

### 8/20 respiratory sputum
**FINAL Pending**

Gram stain: negative

3+ Gram-negative rods, nonlactose fermenting

## Assessment

After reviewing the JM's lab values and clinical examination results, she is diagnosed with a CF exacerbation.

## TARGETED QUESTIONS

1. What signs and symptoms of JM's presentation are indicative of a CF pulmonary exacerbation?

   *Hint: See p. 324 in PPP*

2. Is JMs current antimicrobial regimen the most appropriate for her CF exacerbation? If not, what changes would you make? Why? What laboratory values and clinical parameters need to be monitored while JM's is on the antibiotic regimen you have recommended?

   *Hint: See pp. 326–328 in PPP*

3. What pulmonary-related recommendations would you make for JM's treatment?

   *Hint: See pp. 325–326 in PPP*

4. What factors may have contributed to JM's continued nutritional problems?

   *Hint: See p. 325 in PPP*

5. What dietary goals and recommendations can you make for JM to follow when she is discharged?

   *Hint: See pp. 325, 329 in PPP*

## FOLLOW-UP

JM returns to clinic 1 month after her being discharged for her CF exacerbation. You interview her and find out that she is still not adhering to her home medication regimen. On further questioning, you find out that she frequently over-sleeps and almost misses her bus to school on a daily basis, forgets to take her medications when she comes home from school, and doesn't bother counting her enzymes so she just "takes a handful" if she remembers before she eats.

6. How can you reinforce the importance of adherence to JM? What strategies can you recommend to help her become more adherent to her therapy?

   *Hint: See p. 331 in PPP*

## ⟳ GLOBAL PERSPECTIVE

Cystic fibrosis is one of the most common genetic disorders in the white population (e.g., 90% of CF patients in the United States are white); however, it affects a wide variety of races and ethnicities, including African American (1 in 15,000), Hispanic (1 in 1,900), and Asian (1 in 32,000).[1,2] CF affects approximately 70,000 individuals worldwide.[2] A cure for CF has yet to be discovered. Due to the known disease-related complications throughout life, complex treatment regimens, and need for life-long disease education for patients and families, specialized patient care resources are necessary.[3] Currently, interdisciplinary CF care teams are predominantly found in North America and Europe, given the greater geographic density of patients diagnosed with CF. Interdisciplinary CF patient care teams often include medicine, nursing, respiratory therapy, nutrition, pharmacy, and social work disciplines. CF and CF-related diseases (e.g., CF-related diabetes) are often underrecognized and underdiagnosed in Latin America, Africa, and areas of Asia. As a result, patients may be diagnosed later in life after complications have developed, some of which are not reversible, such as loss of lung function due to frequent pulmonary exacerbations. Providers in developing countries may miss the diagnosis of CF due to the commonality of respiratory and gastrointestinal disorders as a result of malnutrition. Lack of knowledge about the disease and poor access to health care limit the availability of CF care in developing counties.[3] International foundations and organizations including the CF Foundation, World Health Organization, European CF Society, and CF Worldwide continue to increase awareness of the disease, provide education and resources to patients and families, and facilitate advances in patient care and outcomes.

## REFERENCES

1. Cystic Fibrosis Foundation. Cystic Fibrosis Patient Registry, 2011. Annual Data Report to the Center Directors. Bethesda, MD: The Foundation, 2012.
2. Gibson RL, Burns JL, Ramsey BW. Pathophysiology and management of pulmonary infections in cystic fibrosis. Am J Respir Crit Care Med 2003 168:918–51.
3. World Health Organization and Cystic Fibrosis Worldwide. The molecular genetic epidemiology of cystic fibrosis (2004). Available at: http://www.cfww.org/who/. Accessed February 10, 2013.

## CASE SUMMARY

- The patient's current clinical picture is consistent with a pulmonary exacerbation secondary to CF. Patient also presents with poor nutritional status due to pancreatic insufficiency possibly due to poor adherence to pancreatic enzyme replacement therapy.

- Care should be taken in selection, dosing, and monitoring of antimicrobial therapy used as part of pulmonary exacerbation treatment as there are pharmacokinetic differences that should be accounted for and the risk of adverse effects should be considered.

- The patient will require education regarding cystic fibrosis, including correct use of medications (e.g., timing of pancreatic enzymes, order of aerosolized therapies) and the importance of adherence to airway clearance and drug therapies.

For more information on the care plan and facilitator's guide please visit http://www.mhpharmacotherapy.com.

# 16 Gastroesophageal Reflux Disease

Jeannie Kim Lee          Stephanie J. Davis

## CASE LEARNING OBJECTIVES

- Differentiate between typical, atypical, and complicated symptoms of GERD
- Recommend appropriate lifestyle modifications and pharmacotherapy interventions for patients with GERD
- Formulate a monitoring plan to assess the effectiveness and safety of pharmacotherapy for GERD
- Educate patients on appropriate lifestyle modifications and drug therapy issues, including adherence, adverse effects, and drug interactions

## PATIENT PRESENTATION

### Chief Complaint

"I have burning in my chest when I am in my recliner after supper watching the evening news."

### History of Present Illness

Gertie Burns is a 67-year-old woman who presents to her primary care provider complaining of burning sensation in chest every morning before breakfast and evening after supper. She has also noticed persistent cough and hoarseness develop in the last 2 years. She has had similar symptoms in the distant past but did not pay close attention while busy working multiple shifts as a registered nurse (RN). The burning pain had improved with weight loss, resulting from diet and exercise, when Gertie was in her fifties. However, after retirement, she gained her weight back with her new sedentary lifestyle and diet consisting of deep-fried Cajun meals. She has been self-treating her symptoms with Tums and drinking more milk to relieve the burning. The Tums has been working some but not to her satisfaction. She eats dinner around 5:30 pm, so it can be finished by the time the news comes on every evening at 6 pm. She is inquiring if she should purchase Tagamet since she saw a commercial on television about it treating stomach acid.

### Past Medical History

HTN × 16 years

Osteoarthritis × 9 years

Osteoporosis × 3 months

Onychomycosis of the left big toe × 4 weeks

Impaired renal function

Constipation

Seasonal allergies

### Family History

Father had stroke and died at age 74. Mother died of cancer at age 83. Patient has one sister who is 71 and has osteoporosis.

### Social History

GB is an African American woman originally from Louisiana. She is married and lives with her husband of 47 years who is a smoker (smoked 1 ppd × 40 years). She and her husband have three daughters, aged 47, 45, and 40. She is a retired RN and works as a volunteer at a local hospital.

### Tobacco/Alcohol/Substance Use

Social drinker; (−) tobacco or illicit drug use

### Allergies/Intolerances/Adverse Drug Events

NKDA

### Medications (Current)

MOM 30 mL PO q 24 h PRN constipation

Alendronate 70 mg PO weekly

Nifedipine XL 30 mg PO q 24 h

Calcium carbonate 1,000 mg PO q 12 h

Terbinafine 250 mg PO q 24 h × 12 weeks

Tums 1–2 tablets PRN heartburn

Ibuprofen 400 mg PO q 8 h and PRN joint pain and headache

Loratadine 10 mg PO q 24 h PRN allergies

## Review of Systems

Occasional sinus headache relieved with ibuprofen and loratadine; (–) eye itching, runny nose, congestion, tinnitus, vertigo, or infections; occasional cough and hoarseness; burning in the chest nonradiating and no pressure; (–) history cardiac disease; frequent bilateral knee pain; (–) change in urinary frequency; occasional constipation; (–) PUD or IBD; (+) dry skin; (+) toenail fungal infection.

## Physical Examination

### ▶ General

Well-appearing, older, and slightly overweight African American woman in no acute distress

### ▶ Vital Signs

BP 137/76 mm Hg, P 72, RR 14, T 36.2°C

Weight 142.4 lb (64.7 kg); BMI 26.1 kg/m$^2$

Height 62 in. (157 cm)

No pain

### ▶ Skin

Dry-appearing skin and scalp; (–) rashes or lesions

### ▶ HEENT

PERRLA, EOMI; trace periorbital edema; (–) sinus tenderness; TMs appear normal

### ▶ Neck and Lymph Nodes

Thyroid gland normal; (–) thyroid nodules; (–) lymphadenopathy; (–) carotid bruits

### ▶ Chest

Clear to auscultation

### ▶ Breasts

Examination deferred

### ▶ Cardiovascular

RRR, normal S$_1$, S$_2$; (–) S$_3$ or S$_4$

### ▶ Abdomen

Not tender/not distended; (–) organomegaly

### ▶ Neurology

Grossly intact; DTRs normal

### ▶ Genitourinary

Examination deferred

### ▶ Rectal

Examination deferred

## Laboratory Tests

### Fasting Obtained 6 Days Ago

|  | Conventional Units | SI Units |
|---|---|---|
| Na | 140 mEq/L | 140 mmol/L |
| K | 4.2 mEq/L | 4.2 mmol/L |
| Cl | 101 mEq/L | 101 mmol/L |
| CO$_2$ | 22 mEq/L | 22 mmol/L |
| BUN | 8.2 mg/dL | 2.9 mmol/L |
| SCr | 0.9 mg/dL | 80 μmol/L |
| Glucose | 109 mg/dL | 6.0 mmol/L |
| Ca | 8.2 mg/dL | 2.05 mmol/L |
| Mg | 1.6 mEq/L | 0.80 mmol/L |
| Phosphate | 4.0 mg/dL | 1.29 mmol/L |
| Hemoglobin | 13.9 g/dL | 139 g/L; 8.63 mmol/L |
| Hematocrit | 40.1% | 0.401 |
| WBC | 7.9 × 10$^3$/mm$^3$ | 7.9 × 10$^9$/L |
| MCV | 81 μm$^3$ | 81 fL |
| Albumin | 4.2 g/dL | 42 g/L |
| AST | 18 IU/L | 0.30 μkat/L |
| ALT | 18 U/L | 0.30 μkat/L |

## Assessment

Sixty-seven-year-old woman with symptoms consistent with GERD

## Student Workup

### Missing Information?

**Evaluate:**  Patient Database

Drug Therapy Problems

Care Plan (by Problem)

## TARGETED QUESTIONS

1.  What typical and atypical symptoms of GERD does the patient have?

    *Hint: See p. 326 in PPP*

2.  Which of the patient's lifestyle and medications may make the GERD symptoms worse?

    *Hint: See Table 17-1 in PPP*

3.  What medications decrease lower esophageal sphincter pressure?

    *Hint: See Table 17-1 in PPP*

4. How would you answer the patient's question about taking cimetidine (Tegment) for her GERD?

   *Hint: See p. 339 in PPP. Cytochrome p-450 interactions should be explored*

5. What would be the drug of choice for the patient's acid suppression therapy, and how long should the patient be treated?

   *Hint: See pp. 338–341 and Table 17-2 in PPP*

6. What risks and adverse effects of therapy would you discuss with the patient?

   *Hint: See pp. 338–341 and Table 17-2 in PPP*

## FOLLOW-UP

7. Twelve weeks later, Gertie returns for her second follow-up. She has lost 6 lb (2.7 kg) and is adhering to most of the lifestyle modification recommendations provided during the last visit. She is now taking the alendronate correctly every Sunday morning. She is no longer having GERD symptoms, except when she goes out to the local barbecue restaurant and eats fried pickles. Would you consider a change in her current acid suppression therapy? If yes, what change would you recommend? What are the potential risks of taking PPIs for the long term? What actions, if any, would you take?

   *Hint: See pp. 339–340 in PPP*

## ⟳ GLOBAL PERSPECTIVE

Genetic variations among patients may change PPI effectiveness because of an alteration in their ability to metabolize drugs through the cytochrome p-450 (CYP450) enzyme system. It is unclear which patients have a polymorphic gene variation that makes them slow or fast metabolizers. Drug interactions with omeprazole are associated more often with those who are considered "slow metabolizers." Asian populations have a greater number of PPI rapid metabolizers compared to Caucasian populations. Rapid metabolizers may not receive optimal therapeutic effect from PPI therapy. PPIs may differ in the extent of drug–drug interaction related to the CYP450 enzyme system. For example, esomeprazole is metabolized more readily by CYP3A4 enzymes and may be affected less by the patient's genotype. Therefore, patients on PPI therapy should be monitored routinely for drug interactions and associated drug-related problems.

## CASE SUMMARY

- Patient's current clinical picture is consistent with GERD, presenting with typical as well as atypical symptoms warranting acid suppression therapy.
- An initial PPI trial (e.g., omeprazole 20 mg daily is reasonable) of 8 weeks, along with lifestyle modification, can determine the diagnosis of GERD.
- Overuse of PPI agents should be avoided, especially in the elderly, with serious complications related to prolonged and high-dose PPI use.

**For more information on the care plan and facilitator's guide please visit http://www.mhpharmacotherapy.com.**

# 17 Peptic Ulcer Disease

Geoffrey C. Wall

## CASE LEARNING OBJECTIVES

- Recognize the signs and symptoms of peptic ulcer disease (PUD)
- Identify the desired therapeutic outcomes for patients with PUD
- Identify factors that guide selection of an appropriate *Helicobacter pylori* eradication regimen
- Formulate a monitoring plan for patients with PUD on follow-up

## PATIENT PRESENTATION

### Chief Complaint

"I'm been very nauseated lately. My stomach burns after I eat anything."

### History of Present Illness

Robert Benton is a 51-year-old man who presents to his local hospital's emergency department complaining of feeling dizzy, with nausea (no vomiting), lethargy, and epigastric pain—described as "burning" off and on during the day, but especially after eating. He has recently moved to this area from another state and has yet to establish a primary care provider. He has never experienced the symptoms described before. He rarely saw his prior primary care physician in the past, although he had visited her for increasing left-knee pain that she ascribed to osteoarthritis. The patient does not like to take "artificial" medications and refused any treatment for his osteoarthritis. He denies any melena, frank blood in stool, throwing up blood, chest pain, or any other symptoms. Because of the nausea he has not eaten or drunk much in the last 3 days.

### Past Medical History

Osteoarthritis of left knee.

"High cholesterol" "diagnosed" at a health fair 1 year ago. He had not told his former primary care physician about this.

### Family History

His father had a history of HTN and hyperlipidemia, but died of colon cancer at age 72. Mother is alive and well at age 74. He has no siblings.

### Social History

The patient is married and lives with his second wife. He has one son from a prior marriage, aged 18. He works as a certified public accountant. He is generally uncomfortable with taking medications, and feels that "natural" medicines are preferable to "artificial pills" (his words).

### Tobacco/Alcohol/Substance Use

Social drinker; (–) tobacco or illicit drug use

### Allergies/Intolerances/Adverse Drug Events

Penicillin (unknown reaction)

### Medications (Current)

A herbal preparation, "some sort of yeast product," for his "high cholesterol"

### Review of Systems

Nausea and epigastric pain as listed above; (–) changes in bowel habit or change in color/consistency of stool; dizzy and tired × 2 days, as listed above; anorexia, as listed above; (–) tinnitus, vertigo, or infections; (+) left-knee pain, especially when kneeling or first thing in the morning.

### Physical Examination

▶ *General*

Well-appearing white man, with minimal distress

▶ **Vital Signs**

BP 122/79 mm Hg, P 64 (sitting), BP 99/69 mm Hg, P 82 (standing), RR 11, T 37.2°C

Weight 165 lb (75 kg)

Height 70 in. (178 cm)

Pain was 2/10 in knees this morning

Epigastric pain 4/10

▶ **HEENT**

PERRLA, EOMI; (−) sinus tenderness; TMs appear normal

▶ **Skin**

Decreased skin turgor

▶ **Neck and Lymph Nodes**

Thyroid gland smooth; (−) thyroid nodules; (−) lymphadenopathy; (−) carotid bruits; flat neck veins

▶ **Chest**

Clear to auscultation

▶ **Cardiovascular**

RRR, normal $S_1$, $S_2$; (−) $S_3$ or $S_4$

▶ **Abdomen**

Not tender/not distended; (+) epigastric pain, not worse on palpation

▶ **Neurology**

Grossly intact; DTRs normal

▶ **Genitourinary**

Examination deferred

▶ **Rectal**

Normal rectal tone; smooth prostate with no nodules; minimal stool in rectal vault that is occult blood (−)

## Laboratory Tests

### Obtained While in ED

|  | Conventional Units | SI Units |
| --- | --- | --- |
| Na | 140 mEq/L | 140 mmol/L |
| K | 3.9 mEq/L | 3.9 mmol/L |
| Cl | 100 mEq/L | 100 mmol/L |
| $CO_2$ | 22 mEq/L | 22 mmol/L |
| BUN | 40 mg/dL | 14.3 mmol/L |
| SCr | 0.7 mg/dL | 62 μmol/L |
| Glucose | 89 mg/dL | 4.9 mmol/L |
| Ca | 9.4 mg/dL | 2.35 mmol/L |
| Mg | 1.8 mEq/L | 0.90 mmol/L |
| Phosphate | 3.8 mg/dL | 1.23 mmol/L |
| Hemoglobin | 14.1 g/dL | 8.75 mmol/L (141 g/L) |
| Hematocrit | 40.1% | 0.401 |
| WBC | $8.2 \times 10^3/mm^3$ | $8.2 \times 10^9/L$ |
| MCV | 88 μm³ | 88 fL |
| Platelets | $247 \times 10^3/mm^3$ | $247 \times 10^9/L$ |
| *H. pylori* serology | (+) | |
| TSH | 4.2 μIU/mL | 4.2 mIU/L |
| Stool for occult blood | (−) | |
| Total cholesterol | 220 mg/dL | 5.69 mmol/L |
| LDL cholesterol | 122 mg/dL | 3.15 mmol/L |
| HDL cholesterol | 46 mg/dL | 1.19 mmol/L |

## Assessment

Fifty-one-year-old man with history, signs, symptoms, and laboratory tests consistent with the following:

Probable PUD, without acute GI bleeding

Probable *H. pylori* infection

Fluid depletion secondary to nausea and decreased intake

Osteoarthritis currently untreated

Dyslipidemia currently on herbal treatment

Health maintenance: colon cancer screening

### Student Workup

**Missing information?**

**Evaluate:**    Patient Database

Drug Therapy Problems

Care Plan (by Problem)

## TARGETED QUESTIONS

1. What signs and symptoms of PUD does this patient have?

   *Hint: See p. 350 in PPP*

2. What treatment regimen for *H. pylori* infection would you select in this patient? What specific parts of the patient database would guide your decision?

   *Hint: See pp. 351–353 in PPP*

3. What medications should be *avoided* in this patient to treat his osteoarthritis?

   *Hint: See pp. 354–355 in PPP*

4. What risks and adverse effects of therapy would you discuss with this patient?

   *Hint: See pp. 351–354 in PPP*

5. How would you initially treat the patient's dehydration?

*Hint: The patient is mildly volume depleted, probably owing to the decreased oral intake he has had over the last several days. He is orthostatic and has a high BUN:Cr ratio (although a significant GI bleeding can often cause the BUN to rise secondary to partially digested blood). See Chapter 27, Fluids and Electrolytes in PPP for more details on managing fluid status.*

## FOLLOW-UP

6. The patient is referred to a new primary care physician to establish care and for follow-up. The patient is seen 5 days after completing *H. pylori* eradication therapy. Although he feels somewhat better, he still complains of epigastric pain after meals. However, this pain is diminished and the nausea he felt before has abated. He is eating and drinking normally at this time. The patient is then referred to a gastroenterologist who performs an upper GI endoscopic procedure on him. The endoscopy reveals several shallow duodenal ulcers that are partially healed with no blood or visible blood vessels. Biopsy of one of these ulcers is subjected to a tissue CLO test that reveals *H. pylori* infection. The patient confirms that he was adherent to the original *H. pylori* eradication regimen. What actions, if any, would you take?

*Hint: See p. 353 in PPP*

## ⟳ GLOBAL PERSPECTIVE

*H. pylori* infection is one of the most common causes of duodenal ulcers worldwide. The organism is a microaerophilic Gram-negative rod that thrives within the low-pH environment of the stomach. Although the host and organism factors that lead to development of peptic ulcers in *H. pylori* infection are becoming better understood, what actually triggers symptomatic disease is still a mystery. Roughly 50% of the world's population is infected with the organism, yet only a small percentage of patients ever develop clinical PUD. Further, *H. pylori* is an inherently resistant organism requiring multiple antimicrobials and antisecretory agents for treatment. Resistance patterns for the organism vary significantly, depending on country with high percentages of metronidazole resistance in Asia and moderate resistance rates to clarithromycin in Europe. As it is not clinically feasible to perform traditional culture and sensitivities on this organism, the results of surveillance programs that outline general resistance patterns by geographic location should be known by the clinicians practicing in that region.

## CASE SUMMARY

- This patient has probable *H. pylori* PUD. As he is demonstrating no signs and symptoms of acute GI bleeding, has no alarm symptoms concerning for cancer (i.e., weight loss, night sweats), and is relatively young, he may be treated empirically.

- Normally a standard regimen consisting of amoxicillin, clarithromycin, and a PPI would be initiated. Unfortunately, the patient has a listed allergy to penicillin. Clarification of the reaction would be helpful. In addition, the patient may be taking Chinese red yeast rice for his dyslipidemia. As this compound is essentially a less refined version of HMG CoA reductase inhibitors, the possibility that the clarithromycin may interact with the compound increasing the risk for rhabdomyolysis also exists. Thus, a secondary regimen should be selected.

- The patients' dyslipidemia should be evaluated appropriately by his primary care physician, and if necessary, appropriate nonpharmacologic and/or pharmacologic treatment should be initiated.

- For the patient's osteoarthritis, aspirin or NSAID should be avoided, especially in the immediate post-PUD treatment phase. Scheduled acetaminophen would be a reasonable alternative. If in the future the patient requires chronic use of either aspirin or an NSAID, appropriate gastroprotection could be considered as could a low-potency opioid or a local corticosteroid injection.

- During follow-up, it appears that the *H. pylori* infection was not eradicated. New guidelines suggest that patients who have received an *H. pylori* eradication regimen should be tested to insure the regimen was successful. Given the patient's allergy and medication history outlined above, the number of salvage regimens that can be used for the patient is limited. A furazolidone, tetracycline, bismuth, and PPI regimen would be one of the few choices left in this situation.

**For more information on the care plan and facilitator's guide please visit http://www.mhpharmacotherapy.com.**

# 18 Ulcerative Colitis

Brian A. Hemstreet

## CASE LEARNING OBJECTIVES

- Recognize the signs and symptoms of ulcerative colitis (UC)
- Identify the goals of therapy for patients with UC
- Develop an appropriate treatment and monitoring plan for UC
- Select appropriate drug therapy for a patient with active UC
- Properly educate a patient regarding proper use and potential adverse effects associated with drug treatments for UC

## PATIENT PRESENTATION

### Chief Complaint

"I'm still having abdominal pain and diarrhea when I lower my dose of prednisone."

### History of Present Illness

Allison Gentry is a 29-year-old woman who presents to her gastroenterologist complaining of 2–4 bloody bowel movements per day, intermittent crampy abdominal pain, low-grade fever, and feeling fatigued. She was initially diagnosed with UC 15 months ago. At that time she was placed on Asacol 4.8 g/d, which initially induced remission of her UC. Five months ago she experienced a flare of her UC, for which she received a course of prednisone 60 mg daily. Since that time she has been unable to taper off the prednisone. Her typical UC symptoms, particularly sharp abdominal pain, bloody diarrhea, and low-grade fever reappear once her daily prednisone dose is lowered below 30 mg daily. She still takes her Asacol and reports adherence to this therapy. Over the last 2 months she has noticed an increase in fatigue as well. She feels like she wants to rest all the time and she is unable to jog as far as she used to when her symptoms were under better control. She has also had a 15 lb (6.8 kg) weight gain over the last 5 months and is experiencing intermittent outbreaks of acne, which she views as very embarrassing. She is frustrated with the fact that her UC was initially under control, but now seems to be less responsive to her Asacol. Since she has recently gotten engaged and is planning her wedding for next year, she would like to be tapered off the prednisone as soon as

possible. Likewise, she and her fiancé have also discussed the desire to have children once they are married.

### Past Medical History

UC (classified as pancolitis by colonoscopy 15 months ago)

UTI (3 years ago)

GERD

### Family History

Father had colon cancer at the age of 54, and is still alive following resection and chemotherapy. Mother is alive at the age of 70 with hypothyroidism. She has two younger sisters, both healthy.

### Social History

Engaged and lives with her fiancé. No children. Works as a physical therapist at a local hospital. Sexually active.

### Tobacco/Alcohol/Substance Use

Occasional alcohol use; (+) tobacco use 1 ppd for 10 years, (−) illicit drug use.

### Allergies/Intolerances/Adverse Drug Events

Sulfa (rash after receiving Bactrim DS)

### Medications (Current)

Loperamide 2 mg PO as needed for diarrhea

Asacol 400 mg, four tablets PO three times daily

Prednisone 40 mg q day

Omeprazole OTC 20 mg PO as needed

Magnesium/aluminum hydroxine antacid liquid one to two teaspoons PO as needed

Ibuprofen 200 mg tablets, three to four tablets PO as needed for pain and headaches

## Review of Systems

Occasional H/A and muscle aches relieved with ibuprofen, (+) fatigue, (−) SOB, (+) bloody bowel movements with crampy abdominal pain, (+) acne, (+) weight gain, (−) rash or yellowing of skin, (+) subjective low-grade fever, (+) GERD, partially relieved with omeprazole or antacid.

## Physical Examination

### ▸ General

Well-appearing, young white woman in no acute distress

### ▸ Vital Signs

BP 130/76 mm Hg, P 85, RR 17, T 37.6°C

Weight 138.6 lb (63.0 kg)

Height 68 in. (173 cm)

Denies pain

### ▸ Skin

Face appears oily, with acne on upper back and forehead; (+) pallor

### ▸ HEENT

PERRLA, EOMI; (−) sinus tenderness; TMs appear normal.

### ▸ Neck and Lymph Nodes

Thyroid gland smooth, no thyromegaly (−) thyroid nodules; (−) lymphadenopathy; (−) carotid bruits.

### ▸ Chest

Clear to auscultation

### ▸ Breasts

Examination deferred

### ▸ Cardiovascular

RRR, normal $S_1$, $S_2$; (−) $S_3$ or $S_4$

### ▸ Abdomen

Tender to deep palpation in LLQ/not distended; (−) organomegaly, (−) rebound

### ▸ Neurology

Grossly intact; DTRs normal

### ▸ Genitourinary

Examination deferred

### ▸ Rectal

(−) Hemorrhoids

## Laboratory Tests

### Fasting Obtained 2 Days Ago

|  | Conventional Units | SI Units |
|---|---|---|
| Na | 138 mEq/L | 138 mmol/L |
| K | 3.1 mEq/L | 3.1 mmol/L |
| Cl | 98 mEq/L | 98 mmol/L |
| $CO_2$ | 27 mEq/L | 27 mmol/L |
| BUN | 15 mg/dL | 5.4 mmol/L |
| SCr | 1.0 mg/dL | 88 μmol/L |
| Glu | 119 mg/dL | 6.6 mmol/L |
| Ca | 9.0 mg/dL | 2.25 mmol/L |
| Mg | 1.8 mEq/L | 0.90 mmol/L |
| Phosphate | 3.8 mg/dL | 1.23 mmol/L |
| Hgb | 10.0 g/dL | 100 g/L; 6.21 mmol/L |
| Hct | 30.7% | 0.307 |
| WBC | $8.6 \times 10^3/mm^3$ | $8.6 \times 10^9/L$ |
| MCV | 74 μm³ | 74 fL |
| Platelets | $230 \times 10^3/L$ | $230 \times 10^9/L$ |
| ALT | 25 U/L | 0.42 μkat/L |
| AST | 20 U/L | 0.33 μkat/L |
| Bilirubin total | 0.9 mg/dL | 15.4 μmol/L |
| TSH | 3.8 mIU/L | 3.8 μIU/L |
| Albumin | 3.9 g/dL | 39 g/L |
| C-reactive protein (CRP) | 5 mg/dL | 50 mg/L |

## Assessment

Twenty-nine-year-old woman with signs, symptoms, and laboratory tests consistent with active UC.

### Student Workup

**Missing Information?**

| Evaluate: | Patient Database |
|---|---|
| | Drug Therapy Problems |
| | Care Plan (by Problem) |

## TARGETED QUESTIONS

1. What signs and symptoms of UC does the patient have?
   *Hint: See p. 362 in PPP*

2. How would you assess the appropriateness of her drug therapy for UC when she was initially diagnosed 15 months ago?

    *Hint: See pp. 363–367 in PPP*

3. How would you assess and classify this patient's UC at this point in time?

    *Hint: See p. 362 in PPP*

4. What are potential risks of long-term oral corticosteroid use in this patient?

    *Hint: See p. 365 in PPP*

5. What are potential pharmacotherapeutic intervention(s) that could be made at this time to manage this patient's UC?

    *Hint: See pp. 363–367 in PPP*

## FOLLOW-UP

6. The patient is seen again in clinic 8 months later. Her symptoms have improved and she has been able to reduce her dose of prednisone to 10 mg daily. She has lost 7 lb (3.2 kg) and her acne is much improved. She inquires about smoking cessation, stating that she wishes to quit in anticipation of beginning to try to conceive within the next year. She knows it is difficult to quit and is willing to try. How will reductions in tobacco use affect her UC? What recommendations would you make regarding smoking cessation therapy for this patient?

## GLOBAL PERSPECTIVE

Treatment of UC may involve many different therapies aimed at suppressing the inflammatory response. Among these therapies are azathioprine and 6-mercaptopurine, which possess potent immunosuppressive properties. Although effective for treatment of UC, thiopurine drugs may be associated with serious toxicities, such as bone marrow suppression and hepatotoxicity. Azathioprine is metabolized to its active form largely by the enzyme thiopurine methyltransferase (TPMT). Genetic polymorphisms in the TPMT enzymes among various ethnic groups may lead to some patients having low enzyme activity. These patients would be at risk for accumulation of azathioprine at standard doses typically used in UC, resulting in severe and prolonged leucopenia and increased risk of hepatotoxicity. TPMT mutations resulting in slower metabolism are more prevalent in Asian and African populations. For this reason, the FDA recommends that patients should be tested for TPMT activity prior to initiating therapy to decide if the drug should be avoided or given in a reduced dose.

## CASE SUMMARY

- Her current clinical picture is consistent with UC.
- Initiation of therapy to induce and maintain remission as well as to provide long-term steroid-sparing effects is preferable.
- Appropriate baseline monitoring should be performed prior to initiating therapy with the selected agent(s).

For more information on the care plan and facilitator's guide please visit http://www.mhpharmacotherapy.com.

# 19 Nausea and Vomiting

Sheila M. Wilhelm          Jamie Hwang
Holly Chiu

## CASE LEARNING OBJECTIVES

- Recognize the causes and risk factors for nausea and vomiting
- Identify the goals of therapy for nausea and vomiting
- Develop and recommend an appropriate treatment for patients with nausea and vomiting associated with cancer chemotherapy and surgery
- Implement a monitoring plan for nausea and vomiting
- Properly educate a patient taking antiemetics

## PATIENT PRESENTATION

### Chief Complaint

"I feel nauseated and it feels like I need to vomit."

### History of Present Illness

JM is a 60-year-old Caucasian woman with complaints of nausea and vomiting after a laparotomy with total abdominal hysterectomy and bilateral salpingo-oophorectomy for staging and initial treatment of ovarian cancer.

Prior to her procedure, JM had been given dexamethasone 4 mg IV for prophylaxis of nausea and vomiting (N/V) and received the institution's standard anesthesia protocol with thiopental 4.5 mg/kg, atracurium 0.5 mg/kg, and fentanyl 0.05 mg followed by tracheal intubation along with 75% nitrous oxide, 0.5–2% isoflurane, and oxygen therapy.

The procedure results indicated stage III ovarian cancer. JM seemed to have tolerated the procedure well except that she felt nauseated and vomited once despite antiemetic prophylaxis. She has been given hydrocodone/acetaminophen 7.5/750 mg four times a day, which is adequately controlling her pain associated with the procedure. For N/V, she received dexamethasone again postoperatively that failed to control her symptoms. For the new diagnosis of stage III ovarian cancer, she will be started on cisplatin and paclitaxel in the oncology clinic 1 week following surgery.

### Past Medical History

HTN × 8 years
DM × 5 years
GERD × 3 years

### Family History

Mother died of breast cancer at the age of 65. Father is alive at age 70 with HTN and diabetes. She has one sister who also has diabetes.

### Social History

Lives at home with husband. Works as a paralegal.

### Tobacco/Alcohol/Substance Use

Drinks one glass of wine every night; occasionally smokes tobacco, negative for illicit drug use

### Allergies/Intolerances/Adverse Drug Events

No known drug allergies (NKDA)

### Medications Prior to Admission (PTA)

HCTZ 25 mg PO daily
Glyburide 5 mg PO twice daily
Metformin 500 mg PO twice daily

Omeprazole 20 mg PO daily

Acetaminophen 650 mg PO PRN for HA

## Medications (Current)

HCTZ 25 mg PO daily

Glyburide 5 mg PO twice daily

Metformin 500 mg PO twice daily

Pantoprazole 40 mg PO daily

## Review of Systems

Occasional headaches relieved with non-aspirin pain reliever; (–) tinnitus, vertigo, or infections; frequent body aches that she attributes to lack of exercise; (–) change in urinary frequency, but she has noticed an increase in the number of episodes of constipation in the past year; reports cold extremities; (–) history of seizures, syncope, or loss of consciousness; (+) dry skin.

## Physical Examination

▶ *General*

Well-appearing, middle-aged, Caucasian woman in no acute distress

▶ *Vital Signs*

BP 149/85 mm Hg, P 65, RR 19, T 36.1°C

Weight 134 lb (61 kg)

Height 67 in. (170 cm)

Denies pain

▶ *Skin*

Dry appearing skin and scalp; (–) rashes or lesions

▶ *HEENT*

PERRLA, EOMI; trace periorbital edema; (–) sinus tenderness; TMs appear normal

▶ *Chest*

Clear to auscultation

▶ *Breasts*

Examination deferred

▶ *Cardiovascular*

RRR, normal $S_1$, $S_2$; (–) $S_3$ or $S_4$

▶ *Abdomen*

Not tender/not distended; (–) organomegaly

▶ *Neurology*

Grossly intact; deep tendon reflexes normal

▶ *Genitourinary*

Examination deferred

▶ *Rectal*

Examination deferred

## Laboratory Tests

### Fasting Obtained 2 Days Ago

|  | Conventional Units | SI Units |
|---|---|---|
| Na | 143 mEq/L | 143 mmol/L |
| K | 4.1 mEq/L | 4.1 mmol/L |
| Cl | 100 mEq/L | 100 mmol/L |
| $CO_2$ | 24 mEq/L | 24 mmol/L |
| BUN | 8 mg/dL | 2.9 mmol/L |
| SCr | 0.7 mg/dL | 62 µmol/L |
| Glu | 130 mg/dL | 7.2 mmol/L |
| Ca | 9.4 mg/dL | 2.35 mmol/L |
| Mg | 1.8 mEq/L | 0.90 mmol/L |
| Phosphate | 3.8 mg/dL | 1.23 mmol/L |
| Hgb | 13.0 g/dL | 130 g/L; 8.07 mmol/L |
| Hct | 40% | 0.40 |
| WBC | $6 \times 10^3/mm^3$ | $6 \times 10^9/L$ |
| MCV | 83 µm³ | 83 fL |
| Platelets | $230 \times 10^3/mm^3$ | $230 \times 10^9/L$ |
| Albumin | 3.8 g/dL | 38 g/L |
| CA-125 | 90 U/mL | 90 kU/L |
| Total cholesterol | 159 mg/dL | 4.11 mmol/L |
| LDL cholesterol | 85 mg/dL | 2.20 mmol/L |
| HDL cholesterol | 30 mg/dL | 0.78 mmol/L |
| Triglycerides | 90 mg/dL | 1.02 mmol/L |

## Assessment

Sixty-year-old woman with signs, symptoms, and risk factors consistent with postoperative nausea and vomiting (PONV); at risk in future for chemotherapy-induced nausea and vomiting (CINV)

### Student Workup

**Missing Information?**

| **Evaluate:** | Patient Database |
|---|---|
| | Drug Therapy Problems |
| | Care Plan (by Problem) |

## TARGETED QUESTIONS

1. What risk factors does this patient have that contribute to development of PONV?

   *Hint: See p. 383 in PPP*

2. Why did the patient develop N/V despite the prophylaxis for PONV?

   *Hint: See p. 384 in PPP*

3. What therapy would be most appropriate to treat the patient's PONV that developed despite prophylaxis?

   *Hint: See p. 384 and Table 20-2 in PPP*

4. What risks and adverse effects of PONV therapy would you discuss with the patient?

   *Hint: See Table 20-2 in PPP*

## FOLLOW-UP

One week later, patient presents to the oncology clinic. She is to be started on cisplatin and paclitaxel for the management of stage III ovarian cancer.

5. What risk factors does this patient have that contribute to development of CINV?

   *Hint: See pp. 382–383 in PPP*

6. What prevention regimen is recommended for acute CINV?

   *Hint: See Table 20-4 in PPP*

7. What prevention regimen is recommended for delayed CINV?

   *Hint: See Table 20-4 in PPP*

8. What breakthrough treatment is recommended for this patient's CINV?

   *Hint: See pp. 382–383 in PPP*

9. What risks and adverse effects of CINV therapy would you discuss with the patient?

   *Hint: See Table 20-2 in PPP*

## ☺ GLOBAL PERSPECTIVE

Domperidone, which is widely available in many countries (including Mexico) but is not FDA approved in the United States, is pharmacologically similar to metoclopramide but has minimal passage across the blood–brain barrier. It has similar CTZ-mediated antiemetic efficacy to metoclopramide but is less likely to cause centrally mediated adverse effects (e.g., extrapyramidal reactions, tardive dyskinesia). Patients from other countries or Americans who travel to other countries may receive domperidone for N/V, GERD, or gastroparesis. Domperidone can prolong the QT interval and it should not be used in patients who have QT prolongation or are receiving other medications that may cause QT prolongation.

## CASE SUMMARY

- Patient has multiple risk factors for N/V, and prophylactic therapy for PONV and CINV should be initiated.
- Combinations of antiemetics are recommended for preventing PONV for high-risk patients.
- Cisplatin is a highly emetogenic chemotherapy. A combination of antiemetics with different mechanisms of action is recommended for prevention of acute and delayed CINV.

For more information on the care plan and facilitator's guide please visit http://www.mhpharmacotherapy.com.

# 20 Diarrhea

Yolanda B. McKoy-Beach     Clarence E. Curry, Jr

## CASE LEARNING OBJECTIVES

- Recognize the signs and symptoms of diarrhea
- Distinguish between acute and chronic diarrhea
- Explain how medication use can lead to diarrhea
- Identify the goals of therapy for diarrhea
- Develop an appropriate treatment plan for a patient with diarrhea

## PATIENT PRESENTATION

### Chief Complaint

"I have diarrhea, I think. I have also been throwing up and I have watery stools at different times."

### History of Present Illness

Jose Zapata is a 40-year-old Latino male who is a native of Mexico. The patient complains of symptoms described as abdominal pain, vomiting, and loose watery stools occurring at different times. These symptoms have been occurring for a couple of weeks. He reports that he recently went home to Mexico and "ate a lot of vegetables and fruits" that were grown on his parents' land. He also reports feeling a bit sluggish after being home a couple of days, and his mother suggested he drink some aloe vera juice, which he consumed for the first couple of days. He says that he returned to the United States about 2 weeks ago and that he really hasn't noticed a change in the frequency of the bouts of diarrhea.

JZ became a patient at the community clinic approximately 2 months ago. On his initial visit, he described symptoms of polyuria, polydipsia, and weight loss of 10 lb (4.5 kg) over the previous couple of months without trying to lose weight. At that time, a fingerstick was performed in the clinic and the result showed a blood glucose level of 190 mg/dL (10.5 mmol/L). He reports that afterward he came to the clinic on two different occasions to have fingersticks done. The results were 154 mg/dL (8.5 mmol/L) and 172 mg/dL (9.5 mmol/L), respectively. Based on those results, he was started on metformin 500 mg once daily for 7 days, then 500 mg twice daily. He thinks the episodes of diarrhea and vomiting began after the metformin was increased to 1,000 mg twice daily at his last clinic visit. Today he is also feeling "very down" and misses his wife and children.

### Past Medical History

Type 2 DM diagnosed 6 weeks ago

HTN diagnosed 1 year ago in Mexico

Dyslipidemia diagnosed at the last clinic visit

### Family History

Father (+) type 2 DM; mother (+) HTN and type 2 DM. His wife and children are all in good health.

### Social History

Originally a native of Mexico; has been in the United States for 4 years.

The patient has a seventh-grade education; nonsmoker; patient has no health insurance and receives prescription medications through a national chain pharmacy's $4.00 generic drugs.

### Tobacco/Alcohol/Substance Use

Denies alcohol use

### Medication History (Current)

Metformin 1,000 mg PO twice daily

Lisinopril 10 mg PO daily

Aspirin 81 mg PO daily

Pravastatin 10 mg PO nightly

Preparation-H PRN

## Allergies

NKDA

## Physical Examination

▶ *General*

Well-nourished male in no acute distress; appears depressed.

▶ *Vital Signs*

BP 146/90 mm Hg, HR 80 bpm, RR 18, T 36.2°C

Weight 220 lb (100 kg)

Height 69 in. (175 cm)

BMI 31 kg/m$^2$

Denies pain

▶ *HEENT*

PERRLA, EOMI

▶ *Cardiovascular*

RRR; $S_1$ and $S_2$ normal; no $S_3$ or $S_4$

▶ *Chest*

Clear to auscultation and percussion

▶ *Abdomen*

No hepatomegaly or splenomegaly; nontender, distended; normoactive bowel sounds

▶ *Genitourinary*

Within normal limits

▶ *Rectal*

No fissures or hemorrhoids; palpable stool; heme (−)

▶ *Neurology*

Alert and oriented × 3; cranial nerves intact; (−) Babinski

## Laboratory and Diagnostic Tests

|         | Conventional Units          | SI Units                    |
|---------|-----------------------------|-----------------------------|
| Na      | 134 mEq/L                   | 134 mmol/L                  |
| K       | 4.1 mEq/L                   | 4.1 mmol/L                  |
| Cl      | 101 mEq/L                   | 101 mmol/L                  |
| HCO$_3$ | 30.7 mEq/L                  | 30.7 mmol/L                 |
| BUN     | 23 mg/dL                    | 8.2 mmol/L                  |
| Scr     | 0.9 mg/dL                   | 80 μmol/L                   |
| Glu     | 150 mg/dL                   | 8.3 mmol/L                  |
| AST     | 18 IU/L                     | 0.30 μkat/L                 |
| ALT     | 22 IU/L                     | 0.37 μkat/L                 |
| Alk phos | 80 IU/L                    | 1.33 μkat/L                 |
| Ca      | 9.3 mg/dL                   | 2.33 mmol/L                 |
| PO$_4$  | 4.6 mg/dL                   | 1.49 mmol/L                 |
| Hgb     | 14.4 g/dL                   | 144 g/L; 8.94 mmol/L        |
| Hct     | 41%                         | 0.41                        |
| WBC     | $5.98 × 10^3$ mm            | $5.98 × 10^9$/L             |
| Total cholesterol | 213 mg/dL         | 5.51 mmol/L                 |
| HDL cholesterol | 39 mg/dL            | 1.01 mmol/L                 |
| LDL cholesterol | 124 mg/dL           | 3.21 mmol/L                 |
| Triglyceride | 241 mg/dL              | 2.72 mmol/L                 |
| HbA$_{1c}$ | 8.2%                     | 0.082; 66 mmol/mol Hgb      |

## Urinalysis

Clear and colorless

## Stool

(−) blood; (−) ova and parasites

Stool culture is pending

## Assessment

Forty-year-old man with signs and symptoms of diarrhea.

### Student Workup

**Missing Information/Inadequate Data?**

| Evaluate: | Patient Database |
|-----------|------------------|
|           | Drug Therapy Problems |
|           | Care Plan (by Problem) |

## TARGETED QUESTIONS

1. What signs and symptoms of diarrhea does the patient have?

   *Hint: See p. 396 in PPP*

2. What medications can cause diarrhea?

   *Hint: See Table 21-3 in PPP*

3. When should a colonoscopy be performed in a person with chronic diarrhea?

   *Hint: See p. 396 in PPP*

4. What is the primary management for diarrhea?

   *Hint: See pp. 396–397 in PPP*

5. Should this patient be treated for dehydration? Why or why not?

   *Hint: See p. 397 in PPP*

## FOLLOW-UP

Two weeks later, the patient returns for follow-up. He reports that the diarrhea has resolved. The metformin dose, which was lowered to 500 mg twice daily, will now be gradually increased over the next 4–6 weeks to achieve the target dose of 2,000 mg/d.

## ⟳ GLOBAL PERSPECTIVE

Diarrhea is not a disease but rather a symptom of another problem. Dehydration is frequently a consequence of diarrhea, and its effect in the very young or the elderly can be significant. Diarrhea is classified as acute or chronic and can be brought on by infectious microorganisms or by noninfectious causes, including medications. In developing countries, diarrhea, often resulting from infectious causes, is a major cause of morbidity and mortality. Lactose intolerance, the result of a deficiency of lactase, is a common cause of diarrhea. It occurs widely throughout the world, affecting virtually all racial and ethnic groups, although it is seen less often in northern Europe. Irritable bowel syndrome (IBS) is another condition seen worldwide that is frequently characterized by diarrhea. The availability of clean water is perhaps the single most important way to curb infectious diarrheal illnesses seen in developing countries. Treatment for diarrhea in the developing world is most often accomplished through the use of oral rehydration therapy. In any part of the world, significantly dehydrated patients and those whose diarrhea is caused by an invasive microorganism, as well as the very young or the elderly and those with comorbidities, may require more extensive evaluation, treatment, and monitoring.

## CASE SUMMARY

- Current clinical picture is consistent with acute or persistent diarrhea that could have been caused by an infectious agent (traveler's diarrhea) or is drug-induced.
- The treatment of suspected traveler's diarrhea is bismuth subsalicylate regular strength. The recommended adult dose is 30 mL or 2 tablets, repeated every 30–60 min as needed, not to exceed eight doses.
- The treatment of suspected drug-induced diarrhea is to decrease or discontinue the causative agent.

For more information on the care plan and facilitator's guide please visit http://www.mhpharmacotherapy.com.

# 21 Constipation

Beverly C. Mims    Clarence E. Curry, Jr

## CASE LEARNING OBJECTIVES

- Identify the causes of constipation
- Recognize the symptoms of functional constipation
- Identify the goals of therapy for functional constipation
- Recommend lifestyle modifications and therapeutic interventions for the treatment of functional constipation

## PATIENT PRESENTATION

### Chief Complaint

"I'm constipated. I haven't had a bowel movement in 4 days, and this isn't the first time it has happened."

### History of Present Illness

Quoba Nestor is a 48-year-old female who presents to her physician's office complaining of constipation. QN is evaluated every 6 months by her primary-care physician and was last seen 5 months prior to presentation. Upon further questioning by her physician, QN reported that she often has to strain when attempting to have a bowel movement. When she does have a movement, her stools are small, dry, and hard. She had used docusate in the past with some benefit, but recently it seemed to stop working. She has tried psyllium in the past, but she didn't like mixing it with so much water and it made her constipation worse. QN denied abdominal pain. QN has a history of HTN and neuropathic, joint, and muscle pain.

### Past Medical History

Essential HTN

Neuropathic pain—radiculopathy caused by traumatic injury

### Family History

Father is alive at age 72 and has CAD, HTN, osteoarthritis, and type 2 DM. Mother is alive at age 67 with type 2 DM, HTN, osteoarthritis, and hypercholesterolemia. QN has three siblings; all are living. Two siblings are known to have migraine headaches and HTN, and one sibling has type 1 DM.

### Social History

QN is a divorced mother of two children aged 19 and 15. She works as a paralegal for the county government.

### Tobacco/Alcohol/Substance Use

(−) Alcohol, tobacco, or illicit drug use

### Allergies/Intolerances/Adverse Drug Events (ADEs)

Gabapentin (pruritus)

### Medications (current)

Lisinopril 40 mg PO q day

HCTZ 25 mg PO q day

Amitriptyline 50 mg PO at bedtime

Multivitamin 1 tablet PO every 24 hours

Ibuprofen 200 mg PO every 8 hours as needed for headaches and joint and muscle pain

### Review of Systems

Occasional headaches and joint and muscle aches and pains are relieved with ibuprofen; noticed a change in bowel habits when she started taking amitriptyline for neuropathic pain caused by traumatic injury; feels full

### Physical Examination

▶ *General*

Well-developed, well-nourished middle-aged female in no acute distress

▶ *Vital Signs*

BP 120/80 mm Hg, P 70, RR 20, T 37.0°C

Weight 146 lb (66.4 kg)

Height 60 in. (152 cm)

Denies pain

▶ *Skin*

Dry-appearing skin; skin intact; (−) rashes or lesions

▶ *HEENT*

PERRLA, EOMI, (−) sinus tenderness

▶ *Neck and Lymph Nodes*

Supple w/o JVD, bruits, or thyromegaly

▶ *Chest*

Clear to auscultation

▶ *Cardiovascular*

Within normal limits w/o gallop, murmur, rub, click, or irregularity

▶ *Abdomen*

No scars, lesions, or rashes; round, soft, nontender, symmetrical abdomen; hypoactive bowel sounds; no visible pulsations; no bruits; no guarding

▶ *Neurology*

Grossly intact; DTRs normal

▶ *Genitourinary*

Deferred

▶ *Rectal*

Anal sphincter pressure normal; (+) small pieces of hard stool in rectal vault; (−) external hemorrhoids

## Laboratory Tests

|      | Conventional Units | SI Units |
|------|--------------------|----------|
| Na   | 139 mEq/L          | 139 mmol/L |
| K    | 4.0 mEq/L          | 4.0 mmol/L |
| Cl   | 100 mEq/L          | 100 mmol/L |
| $CO_2$ | 24 mEq/L         | 24 mmol/L |
| BUN  | 11 mg/dL           | 3.9 mmol/L |
| SCr  | 0.6 mg/dL          | 53 μmol/L |
| Glu  | 160 mg/dL          | 8.9 mmol/L |
| Ca   | 9.7 mg/dL          | 2.43 mmol/L |
| Mg   | 1.8 mEq/L          | 0.90 mmol/L |
| Phosphate | 3.2 mg/dL     | 1.03 mmol/L |
| Hgb  | 14.7 g/dL          | 147 g/L; 9.13 mmol/L |
| Hct  | 38.6%              | 0.386 |
| WBC  | $7 \times 10^3/mm^3$ | $7 \times 10^9/L$ |
| Albumin | 3.9 g/dL        | 39 g/L |
| Stool occult blood | (−)   | |

## Assessment

Forty-eight-year-old woman with complaints consistent with constipation.

---

**Student Workup**

**Missing Information/Inadequate Data?**

**Evaluate:**    Patient Database

Drug Therapy Problems

Care Plan (by Problem)

---

## TARGETED QUESTIONS

1. What symptoms of constipation does the patient have?

   *Hint: See p. 390 in PPP*

2. What medications and other products can cause or worsen constipation?

   *Hint: See Table 21-1 in PPP*

3. What risks and/or adverse effects associated with laxative products should be considered as you prepare to recommend a product and discuss its use with the patient?

   *Hint: See pp. 391–394 in PPP*

## FOLLOW-UP

Two weeks later, the patient returns for follow-up. She feels better and reports the absence of small hard stools and the need to strain when defecating. She regularly sets aside time to have a bowel movement and reports a symptom-free experience at least three to four times weekly since being on medication.

4. How long should this patient continue to take medication to sustain a symptom-free bowel movement?

5. Should sugar-containing products be excluded from consideration now or in the future for this patient?

## ⊙ GLOBAL PERSPECTIVE

Constipation occurs all over the world. Perhaps as much as 12% or more of the world's population has constipation at one time or another. It appears that inhabitants of developed countries have a higher incidence than those living in developing countries, perhaps because the diet in developed countries contains less fiber. Around the world, many people choose to treat constipation without the aid of commercially available laxatives. Some people attempt to self-treat constipation by altering their diet, and herbal remedies are popular in many parts of the world. Among those herbs used are buckthorn, flaxseed, aloe, fenugreek, and beetroot. In many cultures, fruit is favored for constipation relief. These may include pears, mangoes, guava, prunes, and papayas. Some locales favor homeopathic remedies such as bryonia, calcarea carbonica, lycopodium, or nux vomica.

## CASE SUMMARY

- Forty-eight-year-old female patient presented to her physician complaining of altered stool form and consistency.
- QN's constipation does not appear to be due to organic causes.
- In the recent past, she used psyllium products and a stool softener to self-treat. However, she no longer gets relief from their use.
- QN's presenting medication regimen includes several medications that have been associated with constipation as an adverse effect.

**For more information on the care plan and facilitator's guide please visit http://www.mhpharmacotherapy.com.**

# 22 Alcoholic Cirrhosis

Laurajo Ryan

## CASE LEARNING OBJECTIVES

- Recognize the signs and symptoms of spontaneous bacterial peritonitis (SBP)
- Identify the criteria for diagnosis of SBP
- Develop a treatment plan for ascites and prophylaxis/treatment of SBP
- List common adverse events caused by SBP and develop/identify an appropriate treatment regimen

## PATIENT PRESENTATION

### Chief Complaint

"My stomach is killing me—I think I need to be tapped."

### History of Present Illness

GE is a 48-year-old white female who presents to the emergency department (ED) with complaints of severe abdominal pain and a feeling of fullness. She has a 4-year history of ascites, but is a bit vague about how long her abdomen has been distended; she says that the pain has gotten much worse recently. When questioned more closely about the time frame, she becomes angry and agitated. Although she was diagnosed with alcohol-induced cirrhosis 6 years ago, GE has continued to drink. GE reports subjective fever (she did not take her temperature) this morning and yesterday evening, but says she felt better after she took acetaminophen and ibuprofen. GE says she is mostly compliant with her medications, but has been doubling up on her furosemide for the past few days since she assumed her belly pain was a result of fluid overload.

### Past Medical History

Ethanol-induced cirrhosis × 6 years

Esophageal varices 2 years ago, s/p banding

HTN × 13 years

Gravida 2, para 2

OA of hands × 8 years

### Family History

Father died at age 54 from alcoholic cirrhosis

Mother alive with CAD

Neither brother nor sister have a history of alcohol abuse; sister has type 2 DM

Son with history of alcohol abuse, daughter healthy

### Social History

Lives with husband and adult son

Has worked in her family's restaurant since age 12

### Tobacco/Alcohol/Substance Use

No tobacco, no illicit drugs, began drinking alcohol daily at age 13, currently drinks about seven to eight shots of liquor daily, but denies other forms of alcohol

### Allergies/Intolerances/Adverse Drug Events (ADEs)

Severe hypotension when given IV morphine

### Medications (Current)

Lactulose 15 mL PO twice daily

Propranolol 10 mg PO q 12 h

Furosemide 40 mg PO q AM

Spironolactone 100 mg PO q AM

Acetaminophen 1,000 mg PO PRN

Ibuprofen 600 mg PO PRN

### Review of Systems

(−) Nausea, vomiting, constipation

Frequent diarrhea that she attributes to lactulose use

Occasional bright red blood in her stools (BRBPR), unsure about melena

Subjective fever as above, (−) SOB, cough, hemoptysis

## Physical Examination

### ▶ General

Ill-looking woman who appears much older than stated age
  Rates current pain level at 7 on a scale of 0–10

### ▶ Vital Signs

BP 92/54 mm Hg, HR 104 bpm, RR 16, T 39.3°C

Weight 142 lb (64.5 kg)

Height 67 in. (170 cm)

### ▶ Skin

Dry and jaundiced, with spider angiomata on the upper trunk

### ▶ HEENT

PERRLA, EOMI, (+) scleral icterus

### ▶ Chest

Clear to auscultation bilaterally; breasts tender

### ▶ Cardiovascular

Regular rhythm, tachycardic; no murmurs, rubs, or gallops

### ▶ Abdomen

Very painful and distended with (+) fluid wave, unable to assess for hepatomegaly/splenomegaly due to pain and guarding with palpation, (+) caput medusae, + umbilical hernia

### ▶ Neurology

Grossly intact, some mild confusion and agitation

### ▶ Extremities

No edema

### ▶ Genitourinary

Examination deferred

### ▶ Rectal

Examination deferred

## Laboratory Tests

|        | Conventional Units        | SI Units            |
|--------|---------------------------|---------------------|
| Na     | 125 mEq/L                 | 125 mmol/L          |
| K      | 4.6 mEq/L                 | 4.6 mmol/L          |
| Cl     | 106 mEq/L                 | 106 mmol/L          |
| $CO_2$ | 20 mEq/L                  | 20 mmol/L           |
| BUN    | 17 mg/dL                  | 6.1 mmol/L          |
| Scr    | 1.4 mg/dL                 | 124 μmol/L          |
| Glu    | 96 mg/dL                  | 5.3 mmol/L          |
| Hgb    | 10.4 g/dL                 | 104 g/L; 6.46 mmol/L |

| Hct            | 31%                      | 0.31                         |
|----------------|--------------------------|------------------------------|
| MCV            | 104 μm³                  | 104 fL                       |
| WBC            | $11.2 \times 10^3/mm^3$  | $11.2 \times 10^9/L$         |
| Platelets      | $102 \times 10^3/mm^3$   | $102 \times 10^9/L$          |
| Albumin        | 2.8 g/dL                 | 28 g/L                       |
| Total bilirubin| 6.7 mg/dL                | 114.6 μmol/L                 |
| Alk phos       | 174 IU/L                 | 2.90 μkat/L                  |
| AST            | 317 IU/L                 | 5.28 μkat/L                  |
| ALT            | 142 IU/L                 | 2.37 μkat/L                  |
| GGT            | 167 IU/L                 | 2.78 μkat/L                  |
| LDH            | 206 IU/L                 | 3.43 μkat/L                  |
| PT             | 28 s                     |                              |
| INR            | 1.9                      |                              |

(−) urine toxicology screen

(−) blood alcohol

Paracentesis results

| PMN count | 276 cells/mm³ | $276 \times 10^6$ cells/L |
|-----------|---------------|---------------------------|
| Gram stain negative | | |
| Albumin | 1.3 g/dL | 13 g/L |

## Assessment

Forty-eight-year-old woman with a known history of cirrhosis and ascites (see Fig. 22-1) presents with a painful abdomen and fever, both suggestive of SBP.

**FIGURE 22-1.** Tense ascites in a woman with cirrhosis from her alcoholism. An umbilical hernia is also seen from the increased intraabdominal pressure. (Adapted, with permission, from Usatine RP, Smith MA, Mayeaux Jr EJ, Chumley H, Tysinger J. The Color Atlas of Family Medicine. New York, McGraw-Hill, 2009, Fig 58-5.)

## Student Workup

### Missing Information?

**Evaluate:**    Patient Database

Drug Therapy Problems

Care Plan (by Problem)

## TARGETED QUESTIONS

1. What signs and symptoms of SBP does this patient have?

   *Hint: See p. 413 in PPP*

2. What are the diagnostic criteria for SBP?

   *Hint: See Figure 22-5 in PPP*

3. In what situations would prophylactic treatment for SBP be appropriate?

   *Hint: See p. 417 in PPP*

4. What empiric treatment regimen should be initiated for SBP?

   *Hint: See pp. 417–418 in PPP*

5. What sequelae are associated with SBP? Do any of the patient's laboratory tests indicate that she may be at risk of these complications?

   *Hint: See p. 418 in PPP. Also look closely at her drug regimen and recent self-treatment*

## FOLLOW-UP

6. GE received empiric antibiotic therapy and her abdominal pain is improving. What treatment would be appropriate if the patient progresses to hepatorenal syndrome?

   *Hint: See p. 419 in PPP*

7. Is long-term therapy to prevent SBP warranted? If so, what options are available?

   *Hint: See p. 418 in PPP*

8. What steps can be taken to lower GE's risk of further complications from cirrhosis?

   *Hint: See pp. 419–420 in PPP*

9. What specific counseling would you provide GE to decrease her risk of complications?

   *Hint: See p. 420 in PPP*

## ☽ GLOBAL PERSPECTIVE

In the United States, the majority of cirrhosis cases are caused by overconsumption of alcohol and/or infection with the hepatitis C virus. Worldwide, the primary cause of cirrhosis is hepatitis B; according to the World Health Organization, approximately 2 billion people worldwide are infected. Hepatitis B is preventable by vaccination, and in those countries (such as the United States) that have implemented vaccination programs beginning in infancy, rates of hepatitis B have dropped dramatically. Cirrhosis related to alcohol consumption has increased in industrialized countries, and hepatitis C–related cirrhosis is increasing in many countries since a vaccine is not yet available. In the United States, the prevalence of hepatitis C actually began to decrease in 1992 and has since plateaued despite the lack of a vaccine.

## CASE SUMMARY

- Patient presents with presumptive SBP; ascitic fluid PMN count warrants immediate treatment despite negative Gram stain.

- Antibiotic regimen should cover most common bacteria associated with SBP, both Gram negative and Gram positive.

- Albumin administration can decrease the risk of progression to hepatorenal syndrome.

- Long-term antimicrobial prophylaxis is warranted in those with a history of SBP.

For more information on the care plan and facilitator's guide please visit http://www.mhpharmacotherapy.com.

# 23 Hepatitis B

Juliana Chan

- List modes of transmission and risk factors for hepatitis B
- Identify the signs and symptoms of hepatitis B
- Create treatment goals for treatment of hepatitis B
- Develop a nonpharmacological and pharmacological treatment and monitoring plan for hepatitis B

## PATIENT PRESENTATION

### Chief Complaint

"I have hepatitis B and the medications are not working."

### History of Present Illness

Vivian Lin is a 32-year-old Chinese female referred for further evaluation of her hepatitis B virus (HBV). She is currently being treated for the HBV infection by her primary care physician for the past year and had started lamivudine in March 2006. Her HBV DNA quantitative level was 2,422,348 copies/mL and alanine transaminase (ALT) level was 101 IU/L (1.68 μkat/L). She was born in Hong Kong and immigrated to the United States at the age of 12. She has no complaints of dark urine, pale stools, or yellow eyes or skin.

### Past Medical History

Hepatitis B diagnosed in 2006

### Surgical History

None

### Family History

Mother is deceased and had diabetes and hepatitis B. Father died of heart disease.

### Social History

She is married and has no children. She has been married for 5 years and only has had 1 sexual partner in her lifetime. She currently works in data entry and has no medical insurance.

### Tobacco/Alcohol/Substance Use

She does not drink alcohol, smoke tobacco, or use illicit drugs.

### Allergies/Intolerances/Adverse Drug Events

She denies any allergies.

### Medications (Current)

Multivitamin

Lamivudine 100 mg daily—started March 2006

### Review of Systems

(–) Chest pain, SOB, weight loss, weight gain, dysuria, melena, or hematochezia

### Physical Examination

▸ **General**

The patient is a well-developed, alert and oriented, well-nourished looking woman.

▸ **Vital Signs**

BP 122/80 mm Hg, P 80, RR 20, T 37.1°C

Weight 125 lb (56.8 kg)

Height 69 in. (175 cm)

Pain scale: 0 out of 10

▸ **Skin**

There are no spider angiomata or palmar erythema.

▸ **HEENT**

Eyes anicteric, throat examination normal.

▸ **Neck and Lymph Nodes**

Thyroid not palpable.

▸ **Chest**

Clear to auscultation and percussion.

▶ *Cardiovascular*

RRR, no murmurs or gallops

▶ *Abdomen*

(+) Bowel sounds; (−) ascites; liver and spleen not palpable.

▶ *Neurology*

(−) Asterixis

▶ *Extremities*

(−) Peripheral edema

## Laboratory Tests

*From 5/11/2011*

|  | Conventional Units | SI Units |
|---|---|---|
| Na | 139 mEq/L | 139 mmol/L |
| K | 4.5 mEq/L | 4.5 mmol/L |
| Cl | 103 mEq/L | 103 mmol/L |
| $CO_2$ | 24 mEq/L | 24 mmol/L |
| BUN | 15 mg/dL | 5.4 mmol/L |
| SCr | 0.8 mg/dL | 71 μmol/L |
| Glu | 100 mg/dL | 5.6 mmol/L |
| Ca | 9.3 mg/dL | 2.33 mmol/L |
| Total protein | 8.2 g/dL | 82 g/L |
| Alpha fetoprotein | 3 ng/mL | 3 μg/L |
| Total cholesterol | 148 mg/dL | 3.83 mmol/L |
| LDL cholesterol | 86 mg/dL | 2.22 mmol/L |
| HDL cholesterol | 49 mg/dL | 1.27 mmol/L |
| Triglycerides | 64 mg/dL | 0.72 mmol/L |
| Hgb | 13.4 g/dL | 8.32 mmol/L |
| Hct | 39.7% | 0.397 |
| WBC | $6.1 \times 10^3/mm^3$ | $6.1 \times 10^9/L$ |
| Platelet | $240 \times 10^3/\mu L$ | $240 \times 10^9/L$ |

| Albumin | 4.4 g/dL | 44 g/L |
|---|---|---|
| Total bilirubin | 1 mg/dL | 17.1 μmol/L |
| AST | 22 IU/L | 0.37 μkat/L |
| ALT | 19 IU/L | 0.32 μkat/L |
| Alk phos | 64 IU/L | 1.07 μkat/L |

## Imaging

Abdominal ultrasound 4/2011:

Liver parenchyma shows unremarkable echogenicity. There is no discrete tumor identified. There is no intra- or extrahepatic ductal dilatation. Small polyp is present in the gallbladder, which is otherwise negative. Images of the pancreatic head demonstrate a rounded hypoechoic focus measuring approximately 1.5 cm, which was not clearly present on the comparison study. The right kidney is not hydronephrotic. No ascites is detected.

Impression:

1. Abnormality within the pancreatic head measuring approximately 1.5 cm and for which contrast-enhanced CT is advised

2. No sonographic abnormality of the liver

3. Small gallbladder polyp

## Assessment

Thirty-two-year-old asymptomatic Chinese woman with HBeAg (+) hepatitis B with detectable HBV DNA level suggesting viral resistance.

### Student Workup

**Missing Information?**

| **Evaluate:** | Patient Database |
|---|---|
| | Drug Therapy Problems |
| | Care Plan (by Problem) |

## ADDITIONAL PATIENT LABORATORY DATA

| | HBV DNA Quant. (Normal Range: undetectable <100 copies/mL) | HBsAg | HBcAg | HbeAg | Anti-HBs | Anti-HBe |
|---|---|---|---|---|---|---|
| 5/11/2011 | 27,000 ($27 \times 10^6$/L) | + | | + | | − |
| 5/11/2010 | 400 ($400 \times 10^3$/L) | + | | + | | − |
| 6/21/2009 | <100 (<$100 \times 10^3$/L) | + | + | + | − | − |
| 1/5/2008 | <100 (<$100 \times 10^3$/L) | + | + | − | − | + |
| 9/5/2006 | <100 (<$100 \times 10^3$/L) | + | | + | | − |
| 6/7/2006 | 3,764 ($3.764 \times 10^6$/L) | + | + | + | | − |
| 3/5/2006 | 2,422,348 ($2.422 \times 10^9$/L) | + | + | + | − | − |

## TARGETED QUESTIONS

1. What signs and symptoms of hepatitis B does the patient have?

   *Hint: See p. 436, Table 24-2 in PPP*

2. What are the goals of therapy for the treatment of hepatitis B?

   *Hint: See p. 442 in PPP*

3. What preventative measure can be taken to prevent the spread of hepatitis B and minimize the progression of the liver disease?

   *Hint: See pp. 440–441 in PPP*

4. What are the adverse effects of hepatitis B therapy you would need to discuss with the patient prior to starting treatment?

   *Hint: See pp. 442–444 in PPP*

5. On the basis of these laboratory results, what pharmacological recommendation would you make at this time?

   *Hint: See Tong MJ, Pan CQ, Hann H, et al. The management of chronic hepatitis B in Asian Americans. Dig Dis Sci 2011 56:3143–3162.*

## FOLLOW-UP

Approximately 1 year later, VL continues to be asymptomatic from her hepatitis B infection. An additional anti-HBV agent, entecavir 1 mg daily was added to the current regimen on 5/25/2011. She had been doing well for the past year and returns for follow-up and results of her laboratory tests.

6. Why is this patient no longer responding to the combination hepatitis B treatment? On the basis of these laboratory results, what pharmacological recommendation would you make at this time?

*Hint: See Tong MJ, Pan CQ, Hann H, et al. The management of chronic hepatitis B in Asian Americans. Dig Dis Sci 2011 56:3143–3162.*

## 🌀 GLOBAL PERSPECTIVE

Despite having an effective vaccine to prevent the spread of hepatitis B infection, this disease continues to affect more than 2 billion people in the world. Chronic hepatitis B affects close to 400 million people and 500,000–700,000 may die due to complications associated with the liver disease. Approximately 75% of chronic HBV cases occur in Asia. The hepatitis B–related mortality rate in Asian immigrants to the United States is seven times greater than individuals who are Caucasian. Although the treatment armamentarium for hepatitis B has grown significantly over the past decade, at present the agents available are only effective in suppressing HBV levels and delaying the progression of liver disease to cirrhosis. These agents may not be readily available to patients in developing countries. Since most of these HBV infections are acquired at birth from mothers infected with HBV, providing immunization to include the hepatitis B vaccine with or without immune globulin at birth is the most effective measure to prevent chronic hepatitis B disease.

## CASE SUMMARY

- The patient developed lamivudine resistance while being treated for HBV. Approximately 70% of the patients treated with lamivudine will develop resistance at 5 years of therapy.

### UPDATED PATIENT LABORATORY DATA

| | HBV DNA Quant. (Normal Range: undetectable <100 copies/mL) | HBsAg | HBcAg | HBeAg | Anti-HBs | Anti-HBe | Cr mg/dL (μmol/L) | ALT IU/L (μkat/L) |
|---|---|---|---|---|---|---|---|---|
| 10/5/2012 | 6,316 | + | | + | − | − | 1 (88) | 50 (0.83) |
| 4/30/2012 | 500 | | | + | | | 0.9 (80) | 39 (0.65) |
| 10/27/2011 | <100 | + | | + | − | + | 1 (88) | 17 (0.28) |
| 07/8/2011 | <100 | + | + | + | − | − | 0.8 (71) | 20 (0.33) |
| 5/11/2011 | 27,000 | + | | + | | − | | 19 (0.32) |
| 5/11/2010 | 400 | + | | + | | − | | |
| 6/21/2009 | <100 | + | + | + | − | − | 0.8 (71) | |
| 1/5/2008 | <100 | + | + | − | − | + | | 32 (0.53) |
| 9/5/2006 | <100 | + | + | + | − | − | | 51 (0.85) |
| 6/7/2006 | 3,764 | + | + | + | − | − | 0.9 (80) | |
| 3/5/2006 | 2,422,348 | + | + | + | − | − | 1 (88) | 101 (1.68) |

- The treatment for HBV drug resistance may be to switch or add a HBV antiviral agent from another drug class to the existing regimen (i.e., switch lamivudine to high dose entecavir or add adefovir to lamivudine) or to discontinue the current regimen and switch to a different class of antiviral agent or switch to a more potent antiviral agent within the same class (i.e., switch lamivudine to tenofovir).
- The patient initially developed lamivudine resistance and high dose entecavir was recommended. Several years later, the patient developed entecavir resistance, evident from the elevated HBV DNA level and ALT level.
- Tenofovir has been found to be effective in inhibiting HBV replication in patients who develop lamivudine and entecavir resistance. Therefore, VL's entecavir was discontinued and switched to tenofovir.

For more information on the care plan and facilitator's guide please visit http://www.mhpharmacotherapy.com.

# 24 Hepatitis C

Juliana Chan

## CASE LEARNING OBJECTIVES

- List modes of transmission and risk factors for hepatitis C
- Identify the signs and symptoms of hepatitis C
- Create treatment goals for treatment of hepatitis C
- Develop a nonpharmacological and pharmacological treatment and monitoring plan for hepatitis C

## PATIENT PRESENTATION

### Chief Complaint

"I was referred to you to get started on triple therapy for my hepatitis C."

### History of Present Illness

Victoria Smith is a 42-year-old Caucasian female with no complaints. She is feeling well and is at the clinic because the liver doctor wants her to be worked up for hepatitis C treatment. She has not been treated in the past for the hepatitis C infection. She states that she contracted the hepatitis C infection when she used heroin in the 1980s.

### Past Medical History

Diabetes 2011
Hypertension 2010
Hyperlipidemia 2009
Anxiety
Depression

### Surgical History

None

### Family History

Mother had HTN and type 2 diabetes, died at age 72
Father had a 35 pack-year history of smoking and died of lung cancer at the age of 63
She has one sister and does not know her medical history

### Social History

She was married but now divorced for 12 years. She has two sons who live in the same city as her. She currently works at a law firm.

### Tobacco/Alcohol/Substance Use

She used intravenous drugs including heroin and cocaine starting in her teens and quit in 2001. She was a social drinker and quit in 1993. She does not smoke tobacco.

### Allergies/Intolerances/Adverse Drug Events

Sulfa: hives
Seasonal allergies to pollen

### Medications (Current)

Amlodipine 10 mg daily
Acetaminophen 500 mg, 2 tablets 3 times a day PRN body aches
Lovastatin 20 mg daily
Metformin 1,000 mg, 2 tablets twice daily
Calcium 500 mg with vitamin D 200 international units, take 1 tablet 3 times daily
Glimepiride 2 mg tablet, take 1 tablet once daily
Multivitamin one tablet PO daily

### Review of Systems

Complains of fatigue frequently.

### Physical Examination

▶ *General*

The patient is not in acute distress. She is an obese Caucasian female.

▶ *Vital Signs*

BP 132/92 mm Hg, P 84, RR 20, T 37.1°C
Weight 254 lb (115.5 kg)

Height 69 in. (175 cm)

Pain scale: 0 out of 10

▶ **Skin**

(+) Palmar erythema and some spider angiomas on anterior chest.

▶ **HEENT**

Normocephalic, atraumatic; sclerae anicteric, no gross lesions.

▶ **Neck and Lymph Nodes**

Thyroid not enlarged

▶ **Chest**

Clear to auscultation

▶ **Cardiovascular**

RRR, normal $S_1$, $S_2$

▶ **Abdomen**

(+) Bowel sounds. Obese. Slight hepatomegaly and splenomegaly.

▶ **Neurology**

(−) Asterixis; alert and oriented × 3; DTRs WNL

Extremities: Trace edema bilaterally present

## Laboratory Tests

### Fasting Obtained on 7/15/2012

|  | Conventional Units | SI Units |
| --- | --- | --- |
| Na | 143 mEq/L | 143 mmol/L |
| K | 4.4 mEq/L | 4.4 mmol/L |
| Cl | 108 mEq/L | 108 mmol/L |
| $CO_2$ | 29 mEq/L | 29 mmol/L |
| BUN | 7 mg/dL | 2.5 mmol/L |
| SCr | 0.9 mg/dL | 80 μmol/L |
| Glu | 132 mg/dL | 7.3 mmol/L |
| Ca | 8.6 mg/dL | 2.15 mmol/L |
| TSH | 4.59 μIU/mL | 4.59 mIU/L |
| HCV RNA quant. | 1,401,000 IU/mL | 1,401,000 kIU/L |
| Hepatitis C genotype | 1a | |
| Hgb | 15.2 g/dL | 152 g/L; 9.43 mmol/L |
| Hct | 45.1% | 0.451 |
| WBC | $2.1 \times 10^3/mm^3$ | $2.1 \times 10^9/L$ |
| Platelets | $115 \times 10^3/\mu L$ | $115 \times 10^9/L$ |
| Albumin | 3.4 g/dL | 34 g/L |
| Total bilirubin | 1.2 mg/dL | 20.5 μmol/L |

| AST | 42 IU/L | 0.70 μkat/L |
| --- | --- | --- |
| ALT | 45 IU/L | 0.75 μkat/L |
| Total cholesterol | 134 mg/dL | 3.47 mmol/L |
| LDL cholesterol | 78 mg/dL | 2.02 mmol/L |
| Triglyceride | 116 mg/dL | 1.31 mmol/L |
| HDL cholesterol | 33 mg/dL | 0.85 mmol/L |

## Imaging and Other Studies

Liver biopsy: 03/2012—Mild chronic hepatitis consistent with HCV infection, grade 2 fibrosis, stage 3 disease

Histologic activity index—Portal inflammation: 2, piecemeal necrosis: 2, lobular inflammation: 2, fibrosis: 3

CT of the abdomen with and without contrast: 10/2011— The liver appears to be heterogeneous. In liver segment 2, there is a hypovascular nonenhancing mass in which hepatocellular carcinoma cannot be excluded, but is unlikely. In segment 5, there is a similar mass that is also hypovascular and nonenhancing. The intrahepatic ducts appear slightly enlarged. The spleen is enlarged with a small cyst present within its parenchyma that is too small to characterize. A duodenal diverticulum is present along with esophageal varices and a hiatal hernia. There is no evidence of ascites. A patent portal vein is present.

Treadmill stress echocardiogram: 4/2011—Global LV function at rest is normal. Rest images could not be reviewed real time. Very limited echo imaging without evidence for significant ischemia.

## Assessment

VS is a 42-year-old asymptomatic Caucasian woman with hepatitis C, genotype 1a disease with normal ALT levels and a baseline HCV RNA level of 1,401,000 IU/mL (or kIU/L).

### Student Workup

**Missing Information?**

**Evaluate:**    Patient Database

Drug Therapy Problems

Care Plan (by Problem)

## TARGETED QUESTIONS

1. What signs and symptoms of HCV does the patient have?

   *Hint: See p. 436 in PPP*

2. What are the goals of therapy for the treatment of HCV?

   *Hint: See pp. 438 and 444 in PPP*

3. What preventative measure can be taken to prevent the spread of HCV and minimize the progression of the liver disease?

   *Hint: See p. 444 in PPP*

4. What are the adverse effects of HCV therapy you would need to discuss with the patient prior to starting treatment?

   *Hint: See pp. 444–446 in PPP*

5. Should the patient receive the HCV treatment?

   *Hint: This patient has several comorbidities, which include depression, anxiety, and HTN, and diabetes that must be addressed prior to starting HCV treatment. Additionally, the patient is on several medications that can interact with the hepatitis C medications. These drug interactions must be addressed prior to starting HCV therapy. The HCV medications have many adverse effects that may develop during the course of treatment and could possibly worsen these comorbidities. It would be prudent to treat and stabilize all medical conditions prior to initiating any HCV medications. See p. 444 in PPP.*

## FOLLOW-UP

The patient's depression is stable and is being followed by a psychiatrist. Her diabetes is stable and being followed by an endocrinologist. Her triglyceride levels are elevated. She started HCV treatment and returns today for week 5 of follow-up. She complains of fatigue and headaches. She also states that she is itching more now and never had this type of complaint prior to starting treatment.

## Laboratory Tests

### Fasting Obtained at Wk 4 of Treatment

|  | Conventional Units | SI Units |
|---|---|---|
| Na | 141 mEq/L | 141 mmol/L |
| K | 4 mEq/L | 4 mmol/L |
| Cl | 106 mEq/L | 106 mmol/L |
| $CO_2$ | 30 mEq/L | 30 mmol/L |
| BUN | 9 mg/dL | 3.2 mmol/L |
| SCr | 1 mg/dL | 88 μmol/L |
| Glu | 170 mg/dL | 9.4 mmol/L |
| Ca | 8.3 mg/dL | 2.08 mmol/L |
| HCV RNA quant. | 41 IU/mL | 41 kIU/L |
| Hgb | 11.4 g/dL | 114 g/L; 7.08 mmol/L |
| Hct | 36.7% | 0.367 |
| WBC | $3.1 \times 10^3/mm^3$ | $3.1 \times 10^9/L$ |
| ANC | $0.9 \times 10^3/mm^3$ | $0.9 \times 10^9/L$ |
| Platelets | $61 \times 10^3/\mu L$ | $61 \times 10^9/L$ |

| Albumin | 3.3 g/dL | 33 g/L |
|---|---|---|
| Total bilirubin | 1.3 mg/dL | 22.2 μmol/L |
| AST | 35 IU/L | 0.58 μkat/L |
| ALT | 32 IU/L | 0.53 μkat/L |

6. Why is the patient complaining of these symptoms? Is the patient responding to the HCV regimen? What action should be taken at this time? What other laboratory test(s) should be obtained at this time?

   *Hint: See pp. 444–446 in PPP*

## ☼ GLOBAL PERSPECTIVE

Hepatitis C may affect anyone in the world. There is a higher prevalence of HCV infections in non-Hispanic blacks compared with non-Hispanic whites. Genotype plays an important role in determining the likelihood of the patient's response to hepatitis C treatment. Approximately 75% of those infected with HCV in the United States have genotype 1, and about 14% and 5% have genotypes 2 and 3, respectively. Genotype 4 is predominately found in the Middle East and genotype 6 in Asia. Research efforts continue to focus on determining reason why non-Hispanic whites are less likely to respond to the hepatitis C treatment when compared with Caucasians, especially if the patient has genotype 1 disease. To improve the patient's rate of sustaining virological response, it is prudent to encourage patients to be compliant with their medication regimens, and not miss any doses or discontinue the therapy without notifying their health care provider.

## CASE SUMMARY

- The patient's comorbidities (psychiatric conditions, diabetes hypertension) have been evaluated and cleared by specialists to initiate hepatitis C treatment.

- Treatment would be triple therapy to include ribavirin, pegylated interferon and a direct-acting antiviral (DAA) agent, either boceprevir or telaprevir. The patient would need to be monitored more frequently for DAA and ribavirin-induced anemia.

- Treatment response should be re-evaluated base on the DAA and RGT, typically at weeks 4 and 12 of initiating the hepatitis C medications.

For more information on the care plan and facilitator's guide please visit http://www.mhpharmacotherapy.com.

# 25   Acute Kidney Injury

Lena M. Maynor

## CASE LEARNING OBJECTIVES

- Assess a patient's kidney function based on clinical presentation, laboratory results, and urinary indices
- Identify pharmacotherapeutic outcomes and endpoints of therapy in a patient with acute kidney injury (AKI)
- Apply knowledge of the pathophysiology of AKI to the development of a treatment plan
- Select pharmacotherapy to treat complications associated with AKI

## PATIENT PRESENTATION

### Chief Complaint

"Mom just hasn't been acting like herself for the last few days."

### History of Present Illness

Geraldine Lowry is an 84-year-old Caucasian woman with altered mental status who was brought to the emergency department (ED) by her daughter. She was discharged from the hospital 1 week ago following treatment for an exacerbation of her chronic heart failure. The patient's history of present illness has been relayed by her daughter, as the patient is unable to provide a history at this time. According to the daughter, GL initially felt less fatigued and short of breath following her hospital discharge, which she attributes to the increased dose of her "water pill" that GL has continued to take since her hospital discharge. Her daughter, who is her primary care giver, has noticed that GL has become progressively more confused and lethargic over the last few days. Today, the patient became very dizzy and lightheaded when trying to stand up, and her daughter decided to bring her to the emergency department.

### Past Medical History

Heart failure × 5 years

DM type 2 × 15 years

HTN × 30 years

Osteoarthritis × 35 years

Chronic kidney disease × 7 years

Diabetic gastroparesis, diagnosed 6 months ago

### Family History

Father died of MI at the age of 67 and mother died of breast cancer at the age of 82. Brother has been diagnosed with CAD and has a history of MI and is alive at age 78.

### Social History

Retired, worked as an elementary school teacher for 25 years. Married for 51 years, widowed 7 years ago. Currently lives with daughter.

### Tobacco/Alcohol/Substance Use

(−) Alcohol, tobacco, or illicit drug use

### Allergies/Intolerances/Adverse Drug Events

Macrolide antibiotics (hives)

### Medications (Prior to Admission)

Lisinopril 20 mg PO q 24 h

Metoprolol 50 mg PO q 12 h

Furosemide 40 mg PO twice daily

Metformin 500 mg PO twice daily

Sitagliptin 100 mg PO q 24 h

Ibuprofen 200 mg PO three times daily PRN pain

Multivitamin PO q 24 h

Metoclopramide 10 mg PO with meals and at bedtime

### Review of Systems

Patient is currently unable to contribute to review of systems.

## Physical Examination

▶ *General*

Elderly female in no apparent distress.

▶ *Vital Signs*

BP 134/82 mm Hg, P 72, RR 16, T 36.6°C

Weight 114.4 lb (52.0 kg)

Height 68 in. (173 cm)

▶ *Pain*

Unable to assess

▶ *Skin*

Dry appearing skin; (−) rashes

▶ *HEENT*

Normocephalic, PERRLA

▶ *Chest*

(+) Crackles right lung base

▶ *Cardiovascular*

RRR, (+) S₃

▶ *Abdomen*

(−) Tenderness, distention, organomegaly

▶ *Neurology*

Unable to cooperate for examination

▶ *Genitourinary*

Examination deferred

▶ *Rectal*

Examination deferred

## Laboratory Tests

*Today*

| | Conventional Units | SI Units |
|---|---|---|
| Na | 137 mEq/L | 137 mmol/L |
| K | 5.7 mEq/L | 5.7 mmol/L |
| Cl | 101 mEq/L | 101 mmol/L |
| $CO_2$ | 28 mEq/L | 28 mmol/L |
| BUN | 43 mg/dL | 15.4 mmol/L |
| SCr | 4.12 mg/dL | 364 μmol/L |
| Glu | 119 mg/dL | 6.6 mmol/L |
| Ca | 8.6 mg/dL | 2.15 mmol/L |
| Mg | 2.1 mEq/L | 1.05 mmol/L |
| Phosphate | 4.4 mg/dL | 1.42 mmol/L |
| Hgb | 13.9 g/dL | 139 g/L; 8.63 mmol/L |

| | | |
|---|---|---|
| Hct | 41.3% | 0.413 |
| Platelets | $339 \times 10^3/mm^3$ | $339 \times 10^9/L$ |
| WBC | $9.2 \times 10^3/mm^3$ | $9.2 \times 10^9/L$ |
| Albumin | 2.8 g/dL | 28 g/L |
| Urine osmolality | 614 mOsm/kg | 614 mmol/kg |
| Urine sodium | 15 mEq/L | 15 mmol/L |
| Urine creatinine | 113 mg/dL | 10.0 mmol/L |

Urinalysis

| | | |
|---|---|---|
| Character | Cloudy | |
| Color | Yellow | |
| Specific gravity | 1.011 | |
| Glucose | Negative | |
| Bilirubin | Negative | |
| Ketones | 10 mg/dL | 1.0 mmol/L |
| Blood | Small | |
| pH urine | 5.5 | |
| Protein | 30 mg/dL | 300 mg/L |
| Urobilinogen | Normal | |
| Nitrite | Negative | |
| Leukocytes | Negative | |
| RBC | 12/hpf | |
| WBC | 1/hpf | |
| Bacteria | Occasional | |
| Squamous epithelial cells | Moderate | |

## Assessment

Eighty-four-year-old woman with signs, symptoms, and laboratory tests consistent with acute kidney injury

---

**Student Workup**

**Missing Information?**

| **Evaluate:** | Patient Database |
|---|---|
| | Drug Therapy Problems |
| | Care Plan (by Problem) |

## TARGETED QUESTIONS

1. How would this patient's AKI be classified?

   *Hint: See p. 453 in PPP*

2. Which of the patient's medications could be causing or contributing to the AKI?

   *Hint: See p. 453 in PPP*

3. Which methods of assessing kidney function can be useful in patients with AKI?

   *Hint: See pp. 453–454 in PPP*

4. What signs and symptoms of AKI does the patient have?

   *Hint: See p. 455 in PPP*

5. What potential adverse effects could be caused by the patient's current medications, given the patient's AKI?

   *Hint: Some medications are eliminated renally and, thus, may accumulate during AKI. This accumulation may make patients more susceptible to adverse effects from those particular agents. A review of each medication the patient is receiving should be performed to assess the need for dosing adjustment and potential adverse effects that may occur.*

## FOLLOW-UP

6. One month later, following the resolution of GL's AKI, the patient presents to the emergency department again with complaints of abdominal pain, and her physician orders an abdominal CT scan with IV contrast. What risk factors for contrast-induced nephropathy does this patient have? What measures could be taken to prevent the incidence of contrast-induced nephropathy in this patient?

   *Hint: See p. 461 in PPP*

## ⟳ GLOBAL PERSPECTIVE

It is estimated that the true incidence of AKI is severely underreported in developing countries, due to lack of data reporting and a lack of a global consensus definition of AKI. AKI is thought to differ between developed and developing countries in a number of ways. In developed countries or large urban areas, hospital-acquired AKI predominates. Most of these patients are elderly and have multiple comorbidities that contribute to the development of acute kidney injury. Alternatively, patients that acquire AKI in developing areas are generally younger. AKI in these patients is usually associated with acute, severe volume loss related to a single comorbidity such as gastroenteritis, malaria, leptospirosis, or ingestion of traditional herbal remedies. Reported mortality rates in these patients are generally lower than the reported mortality in developed countries, which is attributed to the younger age and lack of comorbidities in these patients. However, with AKI requiring acute hemodialysis, patients in developing areas are at a definite disadvantage, as access to dialysis is generally limited to only large, urban cities within these countries. In addition, the expense of dialysis generally prohibits the use of dialysis as a treatment option for many patients.

## CASE SUMMARY

- Her current clinical picture is consistent with AKI.
- Treatment of AKI is dependent on the etiology of the injury and whether it is prerenal, intrinsic, or postrenal AKI.
- It is important to evaluate current medications to assess for potential causes of AKI and to determine if any medications may be more likely to cause adverse effects due to decreased elimination.

**For more information on the care plan and facilitator's guide please visit http://www.mhpharmacotherapy.com.**

# 26 Chronic Kidney Disease: Progression Prevention

Melanie Foeppel          Jennifer Jordan

## LEARNING OBJECTIVES

- List the risk factors for development and progression of chronic kidney disease (CKD)
- Explain the mechanisms associated with progression of CKD
- Outline the desired outcomes for treatment of CKD
- Develop a therapeutic approach to slow the progression of CKD, including lifestyle modifications and pharmacologic therapies
- Recommend an appropriate monitoring plan to assess the effectiveness and safety of pharmacotherapy for slowing the progression of CKD

## PATIENT PRESENTATION

### Chief Complaint

"I am worried about going fishing with my grandson. I don't feel like eating supper and have just not felt well lately."

### History of Present Illness

Alfred Statton is a 70-year-old African-American male who presents with complaints of "not feeling well," loss of appetite, and anxiety about his overall wellness. He has had a lack of energy for the past year, but has attributed it to old age. The patient denies nausea or vomiting, but has noticed over the past 6 months that food "just doesn't taste the same," and he has been eating only two small meals a day. He was last seen by a physician approximately 7 years ago, at which time he was started on HCTZ and amlodipine for HTN. The patient reports that he felt worse on the medications, stopped taking them, and decided never to go back. He is very anxious about taking care of his 5-year-old grandson next Saturday and wants to make sure that he is healthy.

### Past Medical History

HTN: diagnosed 20 years ago, untreated

Osteoarthritis: diagnosed 15 years ago

Kidney stones: 1981, 1990, and 1996

### Family History

Father: Deceased from MI in his 80s

Mother: Deceased from cervical cancer in her 60s

### Social History

The patient is retired but volunteers at the local food bank twice a week as a shelf stocker. Currently, he smokes 1½ ppd of cigarettes and denies alcohol or illicit drug use. His physical activity is limited by osteoarthritis.

### Medications

The patient denies taking any prescription, OTC, or herbal medications.

### Allergies

No known drug allergies

### Physical Examination

▶ *General*

Elderly African-American male in no acute distress

► **Vital Signs**

BP 160/98 mm Hg, P 96 bpm, RR 13, T 36.5°C, pain 0

Weight 178 lb (81 kg)

Height 70 in. (178 cm)

► **Skin**

Cool-to-touch, dry-appearing skin and scalp; no rashes/lesions

► **HEENT**

PERRLA; conjunctivae normal; wears bilateral hearing aids

► **Neck and Lymph Nodes**

Thyroid gland smooth, symmetric; (−) thyroid nodules; (−) lymphadenopathy; (−) carotid bruits

► **Chest**

Clear to auscultation

► **Cardiovascular**

RRR, 2/6 systolic murmur heard at apex radiating to axilla

► **Abdomen**

No organomegaly, bruits, or tenderness, (+) bowel sounds

► **Neuro**

Grossly intact; DTRs normal

► **Extremities**

2+ bilateral edema on lower extremities

► **Genitourinary**

Examination deferred

► **Rectal**

(−) Fecal occult blood

## Laboratory Tests (Fasting)

|  | Conventional Units | SI Units |
|---|---|---|
| Sodium | 135 mEq/L | 135 mmol/L |
| Potassium | 4.6 mEq/L | 4.6 mmol/L |
| Chloride | 110 mEq/L | 110 mmol/L |
| Bicarbonate | 18 mEq/L | 18 mmol/L |
| BUN | 45 mg/dL | 16.1 mmol/L |
| Serum creatinine | 2.5 mg/dL | 221 μmol/L |
| Estimated GFR | 31 mL/min/1.73 m² | 0.30 mL/s/m² |
| Glucose | 108 mg/dL | 6.0 mmol/L |
| Total cholesterol | 246 mg/dL | 6.36 mmol/L |
| LDL cholesterol | 175 mg/dL | 4.53 mmol/L |
| HDL cholesterol | 24 mg/dL | 0.62 mmol/L |
| Triglycerides | 235 mg/dL | 2.66 mmol/L |
| Urine albumin | 435 mg/dL | 4.35 g/L |

## Assessment

Seventy-year-old male with untreated HTN due to poor follow-up and adherence, who is now presenting with signs and symptoms of renal insufficiency

### Student Workup

**Missing Information?**

**Evaluate:**    Patient Database

Drug Therapy Problems

Pharmacotherapy Care Plan (by Problem)

## TARGETED QUESTIONS

1. Assuming that the patient's SCr is stable, how would you stage his CKD?

   *Hint: See Table 26-1 in PPP. Staging for CKD is based on the MDRD equation, not Cockcroft-Gault*

2. What signs and symptoms are consistent with CKD?

   *Hint: See p. 472 in PPP*

3. Identify the patient's risk factors for developing CKD and explain how his progression factors may contribute to his eventual kidney failure.

   *Hint: See Table 26-2 in PPP*

4. What nonpharmacologic and pharmacologic treatments are appropriate at this time to slow the patient's progression to ESKD?

   *Hint: See pp. 471–473 in PPP*

5. What is the goal for each pharmacologic intervention listed above?

   *Hint: See pp. 471–473 in PPP*

6. The patient is to be started on lisinopril. Describe an appropriate monitoring plan that includes efficacy and medication safety.

   *Hint: See p. 473 in PPP*

## FOLLOW-UP

7. The patient returns to clinic after taking lisinopril for 10 days. His laboratory tests from this morning reveal a serum creatinine of 2.7 mg/dL (239 μmol/L). On the basis of the pharmacologic effects of an ACE-I in CKD, is this an expected result? What symptoms or findings would prompt you to stop his lisinopril immediately?

   *Hint: See p. 473 in PPP*

## ⟲ GLOBAL PERSPECTIVE

CKD is increasing in prevalence worldwide. It accounts for a major health care expenditure in the developed world, but accounts for considerable morbidity, mortality, and decreased life expectancy in developing countries. Although hypertension and diabetes are the major causes for CKD worldwide, other causes may be significant based on region. In Southeast Asia, there remains a high prevalence of infection-related glomerulonephritis. HIV-related renal disease plays a major role in South Africa and parts of Sub-Saharan Africa. International movements are under way to identify individuals at risk for CKD and prevent progression; however, there are many obstacles including funding, infrastructure, and access to nephrologists.

## CASE SUMMARY

- The patient's presentation and laboratory findings are consistent with CKD.
- Lifestyle and pharmacologic interventions should be initiated to slow the patient's progression to ESKD.
- ACEIs or ARBs are first-line options for decreasing proteinuria. Pharmacists can play a key role in counseling, monitoring, and appropriate titration of these agents.

For more information on the care plan and facilitator's guide please visit http://www.mhpharmacotherapy.com.

# 27 Chronic Kidney Disease: End Stage Renal Disease

Marcella Hoyland        Michael D. Katz
Sophia Vainrub

## CASE LEARNING OBJECTIVES

- Identify specific consequences associated with end-stage renal disease (ESRD)
- Design an appropriate therapeutic approach for specific consequences associated with ESRD
- Recommend an appropriate monitoring plan to assess the effectiveness of pharmacotherapy for ESRD and specific consequences
- Educate patients with CKD about the disease state, the specific consequences, lifestyle modifications, and pharmacologic therapies used for treatment of CKD

## PATIENT PRESENTATION

### Chief Complaint

"I missed my last dialysis session"

### History of Present Illness

Harold Palmer is a 67-year-old Caucasian male who presents to the ED with SOB and nausea. He is relatively compliant with his dialysis appointments but missed his last session because he did not have a ride to the dialysis center. His normal hemodialysis schedule is on Mondays, Wednesdays, and Fridays.

### Past Medical History

HTN: diagnosed 35 years ago

DM type 2: diagnosed 35 years ago

Dyslipidemia: diagnosed 35 years ago

CAD, h/o NSTEMI: 7 years ago

ESRD: began hemodialysis 9 months ago via left AV fistula

### Family History

Father: deceased, MI at age 88 years

Mother: living in a nursing home, HTN, CKD stage 3, and Alzheimer's disease, age 90

### Social History

The patient lives at home with his wife of 45 years. He is a retired plumber. He denies any tobacco use, drinks alcohol only on occasion, and denies any history of illicit drug use.

### Medications

Lisinopril 40 mg PO daily

Candesartan 8 mg PO daily

Carvedilol 25 mg PO twice daily

Insulin glargine 10 units SC at bedtime

Insulin lispro per sliding scale SC before meals

Atorvastatin 20 mg PO at bedtime

Calcium acetate 1334 mg PO three times daily with meals

Multivitamin 1 tablet PO daily

Calcium carbonate/cholecalciferol 500 mg/400 IU 1 tablet PO twice daily

Ferrous sulfate 325 mg PO three times daily

### Allergies

No known drug or food allergies

## Physical Examination

### ▸ General

The patient is a 67-year-old male in no acute distress. He is of normal stature with good hygiene and good affect.

### ▸ Vital Signs

BP 132/78 mm Hg, P 93 bpm, RR 12, T 37°C, pain 0

Weight: 290.4 lb (132 kg)

Height: 73 in. (185 cm)

### ▸ Skin

Dry-appearing skin. No noted scars, bruises, rashes or tattoos.

### ▸ HEENT

Normocephalic and atraumatic. Pupils are equal and reactive to light. Extraocular movements are intact.

### ▸ Neck and Lymph Nodes

No noted neck masses, no tracheal deviation, normal thyroid size.

### ▸ Chest

Slight crackles noted in lung bases bilaterally.

### ▸ Cardiovascular

RRR without murmurs, rubs, or gallops.

### ▸ Abdomen

Positive bowel sounds × 4. Abdomen is soft, non-tender, nondistended.

### ▸ Neurology

Grossly intact bilaterally. Sensation is intact. DTRs normal.

### ▸ Extremities

2+ edema in both lower extremities. No noted muscle weakness. ROM intact.

### ▸ Genitourinary

Deferred.

### ▸ Rectal

Normal sphincter tone noted, no masses noted. Stool occult blood negative.

## Laboratory Tests

### Fasting

|  | Conventional Units | SI Units |
| --- | --- | --- |
| Sodium | 133 mEq/L | 133 mmol/L |
| Potassium | 5.2 mEq/L | 5.2 mmol/L |
| Chloride | 101 mq/L | 101 mmol/L |
| Bicarbonate | 22 mEq/L | 22 mmol/L |
| BUN | 65 mg/dL | 23.2 mmol/L |
| Serum creatinine | 6.3 mg/dL | 5567 μmol/L |
| Estimated CrCl | <10 mL/min | <0.17 mL/s |
| Glucose | 118 mg/dL | 6.5 mmol/L |
| Calcium | 10 mg/dL | 2.50 mmol/L |
| Magnesium | 2 mEq/L | 1.0 mmol/L |
| Phosphorus | 6.5 mg/dL | 2.10 mmol/L |
| Albumin | 3.3 g/dL | 33 g/L |
| WBC | $7.2 \times 10^3/mm^3$ | $7.2 \times 10^9/L$ |
| Hemoglobin | 9.7 g/dL | 97 g/L (6.02 mmol/L) |
| Hematocrit | 29.1% | 0.291 |
| MCV | $85 \ \mu m^3$ | 85 fL |
| Platelets | $298 \times 10^3/mm^3$ | $298 \times 10^9/L$ |
| Total cholesterol | 165 mg/dL | 4.27 mmol/L |
| LDL cholesterol | 98 mg/dL | 2.53 mmol/L |
| HDL cholesterol | 32 mg/dL | 0.83 mmol/L |
| Triglycerides | 113 mg/dL | 1.28 mmol/L |
| Iron | 70 mcg/dL | 12.5 μmicromol/L |
| Transferrin | 215 mg/dL | 2.15 g/L |
| TIBC | 250 mcg/dL | 44.8 μmol/L |
| Ferritin | 378 ng/mL | 378 mcg/L |
| $HbA_{1c}$ | 7.2% | 0.072 (55 mmol/mol Hgb) |
| PTH | 336 pg/mL | 36.0 pmol/L |
| 25-OH, Vit D | 18 ng/mL | 45 nmol/L |

## Assessment

67-year-old male with ESRD on hemodialysis three times per week for the past 9 months, who presents with acute complications after a missed dialysis session and chronic complications from his ESRD.

### Student Workup

**Missing Information?**

**Evaluate:**      Patient Database

Drug Therapy Problems

Care Plan (by Problem)

## TARGETED QUESTIONS

1. Identify the signs and symptoms HP is experiencing as a result of his missed dialysis session?

   *Hint: See p. 472 in PPP*

2. What are the complications that HP has as a result of his ESRD?

   *Hint: See pp. 474–490 in PPP*

3. What nonpharmacologic and pharmacologic options for treatment are appropriate at this time for HP's anemia?

   *Hint: See pp. 477–482 in PPP*

4. What nonpharmacologic and pharmacologic options for treatment are appropriate at this time for HP's bone mineral and metabolism disorder?

   *Hint: See pp. 482–488 in PPP*

5. What are the goals for each pharmacologic intervention listed for questions 3 and 4 above?

   *Hint: See pp. 477–488 in PPP*

6. Describe an appropriate monitoring regimen for a patient with anemia of CKD on ESA therapy.

   *Hint: See p. 482 in PPP*

## FOLLOW-UP

7. The patient follows up with his nephrologist 4 weeks after being discharged from the hospital on epoetin alfa. The day of his appointment, his laboratory tests reveal the following:

|  | *Conventional Units* | *SI Units* |
|---|---|---|
| WBC | $7.2 \times 10^3/mm^3$ | $7.2 \times 10^9/L$ |
| Hemoglobin | 10.1 g/dL | 101 g/L (6.27 mmol/L) |
| Hematocrit | 30% | 0.30 |
| MCV | $80 \ \mu m^3$ | 80 fL |
| Platelets | $310 \times 10^3/mm^3$ | $310 \times 10^9/L$ |
| Iron | 32 mcg/dL | 5.7 μmol/L |
| Transferrin | 110 mg/dL | 1.1 g/L |
| TIBC | 200 mcg/dL | 35.8 μmol/L |
| Ferritin | 179 ng/mL | 179 mcg/L |

   What would be your recommendations on how to proceed with HP's anemia therapy?

   *Hint: See Figure 26-3 in PPP.*

## ⟳ GLOBAL PERSPECTIVE

Dialysis provides an exceptional cost burden worldwide,[1,2] affecting the patient, clinicians, the dialysis facility, the payer, the dialysis manufacturing industry, governments, and society as a whole. In addition, ESRD patients are most likely unemployed shortly prior to dialysis. Peritoneal dialysis (PD) tends to be significantly less costly than hemodialysis (HD) in most regions globally. Since PD requires less technology it would seem to be the preferred method in less developed countries; however, these countries tend to base cost on supplies alone, rather than total care. These cost-benefit analyses are slightly skewed in favor of HD or for less acceptable options such as re-using supplies placing patients at higher risk for infection. Unfortunately, once a patient has progressed to dialysis regardless of modality choice, it becomes an unavoidable cost if the patient's life is to be extended. One of the best ways to reduce the cost of care is early referral to a nephrologist, offering time for the patient and physician to develop a plan that best suits the patient in terms of finance, healthcare access, and convenience.

## REFERENCES

1. Just PM, Th. de Charro F, Tschosik EA, et al. Reimbursement and economic factors influencing dialysis modality choice around the world. Nephrol Dial Transplant 2008 23: 2365–2373.
2. De Vecchi, AF, Dratwa, M, Wiedemann, ME. Healthcare systems and end-stage renal disease (ESRD) therapies – an international review: costs and reimbursement/funding of ESRD therapies. Nephrol Dial Transplant 1999 14(Suppl 6):31-41.

### CASE SUMMARY

- The patient's presentation is consistent with ESRD with a missed dialysis session.
- Pharmacologic interventions should be implemented in addition to dialysis for ESRD patients.
- Pharmacists can help to educate, counsel, and ultimately maximize pharmacotherapy for each complication associated with this complex disease state.

For more information on the care plan and facilitator's guide please visit http://www.mhpharmacotherapy.com.

# 28 Euvolemic Hyponatremia

Mark A. Malesker    Lee E. Morrow

Vijay Gogineni

## CASE LEARNING OBJECTIVES

- Recognize the signs and symptoms of euvolemic hyponatremia
- List common etiologies of euvolemic hyponatremia
- Identify the goals of therapy for euvolemic hyponatremia
- Develop an appropriate treatment and monitoring plan for euvolemic hyponatremia on the basis of individual patient characteristics

## PATIENT PRESENTATION

### Chief Complaint

Fall (per family)

### History of Present Illness

Albert Buterol 89-year-old Caucasian man fell head-first down 5–6 concrete steps. His fall was witnessed by his wife and he had no previous history of falls. He initially lost consciousness for about 5 minutes, after which he was confused. He was taken to a local rural hospital where a CT scan demonstrated an intracranial hemorrhage, chest x-ray showed pneumonia, and he became unresponsive. He was then transferred to a university hospital, where his intracranial hemorrhage was managed with IV nicardipine, mechanical ventilation, antibiotics for suspected pneumonia, and hypertonic saline for hyponatremia. On admission, the patient had no evidence of volume depletion or excess on physical examination. The serum sodium on admission was 119 mEq/L (119 mmol/L) and increased to 129 mEq/L (129 mmol/L) within the first 24 hours.

### Allergies

Antihistamines: Unspecified

Sulfa: Unspecified

Tramadol: Unspecified

Amitriptyline: Unspecified

### Past Medical History

MI, postpercutaneous coronary intervention (PCI)

HTN

Pacemaker for bradycardia

Frequent UTI (enlarged prostate)

### Social History

Quit smoking 10 years ago

Denies alcohol and illicit drug use

### Medications Prior to Admission

HCTZ 50 mg PO daily

Celecoxib 200 mg PO daily

Finasteride 5 mg PO daily

Pantoprazole 40 mg PO daily

Cotrimoxazole PO twice daily

Lorazepam 1 mg PO every 8 h as needed for anxiety

Latanoprost eyedrops, 1 drop in both eyes at bedtime

### Inpatient Medications

Pantoprazole 40 mg IV daily

Piperacillin/tazobactam 3.375 mg IV every 6 h

Levofloxacin 750 mg IV q 24 h

Vancomycin 1 g IV q 24 h

3% saline initiated IV at 15 mL/h

Codeine 15–30 mg per NG tube every 8 h as needed for cough

Metoclopramide 10 mg IV every 6 h as needed for nausea

Nicardipine IV infusion to keep systolic BP <160 mm Hg

Potassium chloride 40 mEq (40 mmol) IV × 1

## Review of Systems

Unattainable as the patient is unresponsive

## Physical Examination

### ▸ General

Frail with some wasting

### ▸ Vital Signs

BP 148/83 mm Hg, P 120, RR 19, T 99.3°F (37.4°C)

Weight 155.5 lb (70.7 kg)

Height 71 in. (180 cm)

Pain—cannot assess because the patient is unresponsive

### ▸ HEENT

PERRLA; large bruise on head but no evidence of depressed skull fracture

### ▸ Neck

Supple; no carotid bruits noted

### ▸ Cardiac

Tachycardic; RRR, no murmur, rub, or gallop

### ▸ Respiratory

Clear to auscultation on right side; decreased breath sounds and crackles in the left lower lung fields. Large ecchymosis overlying the left shoulder and upper chest

### ▸ Abdomen

Soft and nontender; slightly distended; (+) bowel sounds

### ▸ Extremities

Superficial laceration on the left forearm. Bilateral radial pulses and dorsalis pedis and posterior tibial pulses palpable. Cannot assess ROM due to altered mental state

### ▸ Neurologic

Unresponsive

## Laboratory Tests

| | Date | | |
|---|---|---|---|
| | 6/16 at 0600 | 6/16 at 2000 | 6/17 at 0745 |
| Na mEq/L (mmol/L) | 119 | 123 | 129 |
| K mEq/L (mmol/L) | 3.7 | 3.6 | 4.1 |
| Cl mEq/L (mmol/L) | 84 | 84 | 87 |
| $CO_2$/$HCO_3$ mEq/L (mmol/L) | 27 | 27 | 23 |
| BUN mg/dL (mmol/L) | 16 (5.7) | 26 (9.3) | 20 (7.1) |
| Creatinine mg/dL (μmol/L) | 1.0 (88) | 1.0 (88) | 1.3 (115) |
| Glucose mg/dL (mmol/L) | 186 (10.3) | 171 (9.5) | 160 (8.9) |
| Total Ca mg/dL (mmol/L) | 8.3 (2.08) | 8.5 (2.13) | 8.6 (2.15) |
| Hemoglobin g/dL (g/L; mmol/L) | 12.9 (129; 8.01) | | |
| Hematocrit % | 31.2 (0.312) | | |
| WBC × $10^3$/$mm^3$ (×$10^9$/L) | 12.9 | | |
| Platelet × $10^3$/$mm^3$ (×$10^9$/L) | 182 | | |
| Serum osmolality mOsm/kg (mmol/kg) | | 265 | |
| Urine osmolality mOsm/kg (mmol/kg) | 475 | | |
| Urine sodium mEq/L (mmol/L) | <20 | | |

## Assessment

S/P head trauma, intracranial hemorrhage; significant hyponatremia on admission may have been the cause of fall. The patient appeared to be euvolemic on admission. He will be admitted to the ICU with frequent neuro checks. Hypertonic saline is to be initiated at 15 mL/h and replace potassium.

### Student Workup

#### Missing Information?

**Evaluate:**    Patient Database

Drug Therapy Problems

Care Plan (by Problem)

## TARGETED QUESTIONS

1. What are the potential causes of euvolemic hyponatremia in this patient?

   *Hint: See p. 508 in PPP*

2. What is the sodium deficit in this patient?

   *Hint: See p. 508 in PPP*

3. Calculate the change in serum sodium following administration of 1 L of 3% NaCl.

   *Hint: See p. 508 in PPP*

4. What are the safety concerns with sodium replacement?

   *Hint: See p. 509 in PPP*

5. What other therapeutic options are available to correct the euvolemic hyponatremia in this patient?

   *Hint: See p. 508 in PPP*

6. After the patient recovers from his acute problems, what therapeutic options exist if he has chronic euvolemic hyponatremia?

   *Hint: See p. 508 in PPP*

## FOLLOW-UP

Despite ICU management, the patient had progressively worsening neurologic function. Following several days of supportive therapy, the family decided to withdraw care.

### CASE SUMMARY

- 89-year-old male with hypotonic hyponatremia and euvolemic state.
- Possible causes of euvolemic hyponatremia include head trauma, pulmonary disorders, and medications.
- Treatment with 3% NaCl warranted due to unresponsive state.

**For more information on the care plan and facilitator's guide please visit http://www.mhpharmacotherapy.com.**

# 29 Hypovolemic Hyponatremia

Mark A. Malesker      Lee E. Morrow

Vijay Gogineni

## CASE LEARNING OBJECTIVES

- Recognize the signs and symptoms of hypovolemic hyponatremia
- Identify the goals of therapy for hypovolemic hyponatremia
- Develop an appropriate treatment and monitoring plan for fluid replacement based on individual patient characteristics
- Select an appropriate resuscitation fluid
- Recognize what type of patient may be predisposed to fluid overload

## PATIENT PRESENTATION

### Chief Complaint

Diarrhea and altered mental status as per neighbor

### History of Present Illness

Frank Secretion is a 78-year-old Caucasian man who was found by a neighbor wandering outside his residence with his pants saturated with urine and watery stool. The patient appeared intoxicated but he was oriented to person. He was found to have been falling down repeatedly while walking. The patient lives alone and is a widower. His daughter last spoke to him 4 days ago. The patient was unwillingly taken to a university hospital, where he was seen in the emergency department (ED) and admitted to the ICU for further management. In the ED, the following laboratory results were noted: sodium 121 mEq/L (121 mmol/L), potassium 3.0 mEq/L (3.0 mmol/L), chloride 88 mEq/L (88 mmol/L), BUN 47 mg/dL (16.8 mmol/L), creatinine 2.5 mg/dL (221 µmol/L), and ethanol level 150 mg/dL (32.5 mmol/L).

### Past Medical History

HTN for 20 years

Alcoholism (18 beers/d)

Leg wound (new)

### Family History

Father died of MI in his 50s. Mother died at age 92 from Alzheimer's disease. He has one daughter (46 years), who is healthy.

### Social History

Retired carpenter. Completed high school. Married for 50 years. Widower for 1 year. Lives alone.

### Tobacco/Alcohol/Substance Use

Long history of alcoholism; (−) tobacco or illicit drug use

### Allergies/Intolerances/Adverse Drug Events

No known allergies

### Medications (Prior to Admit)

HCTZ 50 mg PO daily

Simvastatin 40 mg PO daily

### Medications (ICU list)

Normal saline

IV potassium chloride 40 mEq (40 mmol) IV × 1

Piperacillin/tazobactam 2.25 g IV q 6 h

Lorazepam 1 mg IV/PO q 1 h PRN (agitation or tremor) per CIWA alcohol-withdrawal protocol

Folic acid 1 mg PO daily

Thiamine 100 mg PO daily

Multivitamin 1 tablet PO daily

Enoxaparin 40 mg SC q 24 h

### Review of Systems

Unobtainable. Patient is extremely drowsy and disoriented.

## Physical Examination (in ED)

▸ *General*

Unshaven unkempt elderly man with clothing saturated with urine and stool. He is oriented to person only.

▸ *Vital Signs*

BP 123/73 mm Hg lying; BP 90/74 sitting, P 122 bpm, RR 18, T 36.7°C

Weight 183 lb (83 kg)

Height 72 in. (183 cm)

Denies pain

▸ *Skin*

Large open area on left lower extremity, (+) cellulitis

▸ *HEENT*

Small pupils, no icterus; mouth appears dry

▸ *Neck and Lymph Nodes*

(−) Neck stiffness, lymphadenopathy, thyromegaly; neck veins flat

▸ *Chest*

Bibasilar wheezes. Otherwise normal

▸ *Cardiovascular*

Tachycardia, normal $S_1/S_2$, heart sounds distant

▸ *Abdomen*

Soft, not distended, (+) bowel sounds, (−) masses, organomegaly

▸ *Neurology*

Sedated, disoriented, incoherent speech; DTRs symmetrical, (−) Babinski

▸ *Genitourinary*

Examination deferred

▸ *Rectal*

Examination deferred

## Laboratory Tests

### Results From ED

|     | Conventional Units | SI Units |
| --- | --- | --- |
| Na | 121 mEq/L | 121 mmol/L |
| K | 3.0 mEq/L | 3.0 mmol/L |
| Cl | 88 mEq/L | 88 mmol/L |
| $CO_2$ | 6 mEq/L | 6 mmol/L |
| BUN | 47 mg/dL | 16.8 mmol/L |
| SCr | 2.5 mg/dL | 221 μmol/L |
| Glu | 128 mg/dL | 7.1 mmol/L |
| Ca | 9.4 mg/dL | 2.35 mmol/L |
| Mg | 4.5 mEq/L | 2.25 mmol/L |
| Phosphate | 9 mg/dL | 2.91 mmol/L |
| Hgb | 12.0 g/dL | 120 g/L; 7.45 mmol/L |
| Hct | 33.6% | 0.336 |
| WBC | $14.4 \times 10^3/mm^3$ | $14.4 \times 10^9/L$ |
| Ethanol | 150 mg/dL | 32.5 mmol/L |
| Albumin | 2.9 g/dL | 29 g/L |
| Total bilirubin | 1.0 mg/dL | 17.1 μmol/L |
| AST | 13 IU/L | 0.22 μkat/L |
| ALT | 10 IU/L | 0.17 μkat/L |

## Assessment

Seventy-eight-year-old man with signs, symptoms, and laboratory tests consistent with hypovolemic hyponatremia

---

### Student Workup

**Missing Information?**

**Evaluate:**  Patient Database

Drug Therapy Problems

Care Plan (by Problem)

---

## TARGETED QUESTIONS

1. What signs and symptoms of hypovolemic hyponatremia does the patient have?

   *Hint: See pp. 503, 507 in PPP*

2. What are potential causes of hypovolemic hyponatremia in this patient?

   *Hint: See p. 508 in PPP*

3. How should the hypovolemic hyponatremia be treated?

   *Hint: See pp. 506, 508 in PPP*

4. What type of monitoring should accompany fluid resuscitation?

   *Hint: See pp. 506, 509 in PPP*

5. What type of patient may be predisposed to fluid overload?

   *Hint: See p. 503 in PPP*

## FOLLOW-UP

This 78-year-old male was admitted in a partially responsive state with altered mental status. Initial evaluation revealed hypovolemic hyponatremia and left lower leg cellulitis. IV fluid and antibiotics were initiated. Alcohol withdrawal prophylaxis was ordered. His leg cultures were negative. Following fluid resuscitation, the patient's mental status improved. Once the patient was fully alert, he was transferred to the general medical floor and antibiotic treatment was continued. It was later decided to discharge the patient on an alternative regimen for hypertension (lisinopril). The patient was discharged with wound care instructions and plans to live with his daughter. He was instructed to take his medications as prescribed and to refrain from alcohol intake.

## ☼ GLOBAL PERSPECTIVE

While intravenous fluid resuscitation is standard of care and readily available for management of severe volume depletion; dehydration; and shock in developed countries, patients in developing countries may not have access to health care facilities, and if they do, those facilities may not have sterile IV access equipment or solutions. Oral rehydration therapy (ORT) is more readily available in these settings and is considered the treatment of choice, particularly for diarrheal illnesses such as rotavirus and cholera. The World Health Organization[1] recommends that oral rehydration solutions be comprised of:

Total osmolality 200–310 mmol/L

Equimolar concentrations of Na and glucose

Glucose concentration not to exceed 20 g/L (111 mmol/L)

Na concentration 60–90 mEq/L (60–90 mmol/L)

K concentration 15–25 mEq/L (15–25 mmol/L)

Citrate concentration 8–12 mmol/L)

Cl concentration 50–80 mEq/L (50–80 mmol/L)

Such products are widely available commercially, but similar formulations can be made with household ingredients (assuming clean water is available). ORT has had a major beneficial impact on childhood mortality in diarrheal illness,[2] and it appears to be as effective as intravenous therapy.

## REFERENCES

1. World Health Organization. Oral Rehydration Salts. Available at: http://www.who.int/maternal_child_adolescent/documents/fch_cah_06_1/en/index.html (Accessed on February 7, 2013).
2. Victora CG, Bryce J, Fontaine O, Monasch R. Reducing deaths from diarrhea through oral rehydration therapy. Bull World Health Organ. 2000;78:1246.

## CASE SUMMARY

- The patient's clinical picture is consistent with hypovolemic hyponatremia, and replacement fluid should be carefully initiated.
- The use of normal saline as the initial fluid replacement is reasonable, with titration based upon follow-up electrolytes and patient response.
- Over-replacement of IV fluids should be avoided, especially considering the patient's advanced age.

**For more information on the care plan and facilitator's guide please visit http://www.mhpharmacotherapy.com.**

# 30 Hyperkalemia

Julie Haase        Lee E. Morrow

Mark A. Malesker

## CASE LEARNING OBJECTIVES

- Recognize the signs and symptoms of hyperkalemia
- List the common etiologies of hyperkalemia
- Identify the goals of therapy for hyperkalemia
- Develop an appropriate treatment and monitoring plan for hyperkalemia on the basis of individual patient characteristics

## PATIENT PRESENTATION

### Chief Complaint

N/V, and associated weakness persisting for 4 days

### History of Present Illness

DS is a 53-year-old Caucasian male who was brought to the emergency department (ED) via ambulance. The patient was unable to provide an in-depth history, but the patient's family noted that he had been experiencing episodes of N/V/D with associated weakness for approximately 4 days. He began feeling worse yesterday morning and had some increased sleepiness. This morning he was nearly unresponsive, so 911 was called. Upon arrival to the ED, the patient was sleepy but arousable, oriented to person and place, with significant bradycardia and hypotension. An ECG done in the ED showed atrial fibrillation.

### Allergies

No known allergies

### Past Medical History

Cardiomyopathy

Heart failure

Atrial fibrillation

Chronic renal insufficiency [baseline SCr 1.8 mg/dL (159 μmol/L)]

### Social History

Smokes ½ ppd of cigarettes

Occasional alcohol use

### Home Medications

Metoprolol tartrate 50 mg PO twice daily

Ciclesonide nasal spray (50 mcg/spray) two sprays in each nostril daily

Digoxin 250 mcg PO daily

Enalapril 5 mg PO daily

Potassium chloride 40 mEq (40 mmol) PO three times daily

APAP 650 mg 1–2 tablets PO every 6 h as needed

Spironolactone 25 mg PO daily

Torsemide 100 mg PO daily

Warfarin 5 mg PO daily

Salt substitute with meals PRN

### Review of Systems

Unattainable due to the patient's decreased mental status

### Physical Examination

▶ *General*

Patient appears to be in moderate distress

▶ *Vital Signs*

ED arrival: BP 68/36 mm Hg, P 34, RR 16, T 96.1°F (35.6°C)

Weight: 229.9 lb (104.5 kg)

Height: 74 in. (188 cm)

Pain: Unknown because the patient does not respond appropriately to questions

▶ *HEENT*

PERRLA, NG tube in place

► *Neck*

Supple; (−) carotid bruits noted; (−) JVD

► *Cardiac*

$S_1$, $S_2$; pulse irregularly irregular; no murmurs noted

► *Respiratory*

Coarse crackles at both bases; chest expansion equal

► *Abdomen*

Soft and nontender; obese; (+) bowel sounds

► *Extremities*

(−) Clubbing, contusions edema; pulses 2+ in all four extremities

► *Neurologic*

The patient is alert and oriented to person and place; cranial nerves II–XII intact; no focal neurologic findings.

## Laboratory Tests

### Obtained Upon Arrival to ED

|  | Conventional Units | SI Units |
|---|---|---|
| Na | 135 mEq/L | 135 mmol/L |
| K | 9.6 mEq/L | 9.6 mmol/L |
| Cl | 112 mEq/L | 112 mmol/L |
| $CO_2$/$HCO_3$ | 6 mEq/L | 6 mmol/L |
| BUN | 95 mg/dL | 33.9 mmol/L |
| SCr | 4.2 mg/dL | 371 μmol/L |
| Glu | 106 mg/dL | 5.9 mmol/L |
| Ca | 9.1 mg/dL | 2.28 mmol/L |
| Mg | 1.6 mEq/L | 0.80 mmol/L |
| $PO_4$ | 7.3 mg/dL | 2.36 mmol/L |
| Hgb | 16 g/dL (160 g/L) | 9.93 mmol/L |
| Hct | 47% | 0.47 |
| WBC | $11.2 \times 10^3$/mm³ | $11.2 \times 10^9$/L |
| INR | 7.9 | |
| Digoxin | 4.4 ng/mL | 5.6 nmol/L |
| ABG | | |
|   pH | 7.08 | |
|   $PO_2$ | 135 mm Hg | 18.0 kPa |
|   $PCO_2$ | 24.6 mm Hg | 3.3 kPa |
|   $HCO_3$ | 7 mEq/L | 7 mmol/L |
| ECG | | |

Atrial fibrillation, ventricular rate 55

## Assessment

Fifty-year-old male with signs/symptoms and laboratory values consistent with acidosis and hyperkalemia

### Student Workup

**Missing Information?**

**Evaluate:**   Patient Database

               Drug Therapy Problems

               Care Plan (by Problem)

## TARGETED QUESTIONS

1. Which s/s of hyperkalemia did this patient present with?

   *Hint: See p. 511 in PPP*

2. What are the most likely causes of this patient's hyperkalemia?

   *Hint: See p. 511 in PPP*

3. What medications likely contributed to the development of hyperkalemia in this patient?

   *Hint: See p. 511 in PPP*

4. What are the treatment options for the management of hyperkalemia?

   *Hint: See p. 511 in PPP*

5. What is the most likely explanation for this patient's increased serum digoxin level?

   *Hint: Consider the pharmacokinetics of digoxin*

## FOLLOW-UP

6. Several days later, the patient is stable and ready to be discharged from the hospital. Important laboratory tests on discharge include INR 2.06, digoxin 0.8 ng/mL (1.0 nmol/L), SCr 1.8 mg/dL (159 μmol/L), and potassium 3.5 mEq/L (3.5 mmol/L). What counseling points should be emphasized on discharge to prevent the patient from presenting in this manner again?

## CASE SUMMARY

- 53-year-old patient with AKI on CKD and severe hyperkalemia
- Hyperkalemia may be related to the AKI, KCl supplements, ACEI, spironolactone, and salt substitutes
- Appropriate treatment is a three-phase process including reversal of the adverse cardiac effects, shifting K into the cells, and ultimately, removing the excess K from the patient

For more information on the care plan and facilitator's guide please visit http://www.mhpharmacotherapy.com.

# 31 Metabolic Acidosis

Lee E. Morrow          Ryan M. Brimeyer

Mark A. Malesker

## PATIENT PRESENTATION

### Chief Complaint

N/V, HA, and decreased appetite

### History of Present Illness

Rachel Willis is a 43-year-old African American female who presented to the emergency department (ED) with the complaints above. On her initial assessment by the ED staff, she was promptly transferred to the ICU for management by the critical care team. The patient reports that she was doing well until 2 days ago, at which time she ran out of her insulin. Since then she has felt dizzy and fatigued. She had two episodes of N/V, and progressive SOB today. The patient is a poor historian who frequently gives conflicting information to different care providers.

### Past Medical History

Type 1 DM for 12 years
History of cesarean section

### Family History

Father deceased from complications of DM and HTN. Mother is alive but has SLE. Her brother and one of her sisters have "emphysema" and another sister takes medications for HTN. The only other family history she knows is that her grandmother took insulin for diabetes and her grandfather died of metastatic colon cancer.

### Social History

She works part time in a local pawn shop and has been intermittently homeless. Because she does not have health care insurance, she does not have a primary care physician and frequently visits the ED for hyperglycemia. The ED records suggest that she does not check her blood sugar at home and that she is not adherent with her insulin therapy.

### Tobacco/Alcohol/Substance Use

She has smoked one ppd of cigarettes for 25 years. She drinks alcohol regularly on the weekends (~12 beers a day) and admits to marijuana use when she is "partying hard."

### Allergies/Intolerances/Adverse Drug Events

Unknown reaction to codeine

### Medications (Outpatient)

Insulin NPH 36 units SC AM and 6 units PM
Insulin regular 15 units SC AM and 6 units PM
Multivitamin PO daily
Loratadine 10 mg PO daily
Omeprazole OTC 10 mg PO as needed

### Review of Systems

Decreased appetite for several days and thinks she has lost about 10 lb (4.5 kg); (–) blurring of vision or disturbances in hearing; (–) chest pain or palpitations; (+) shortness of breath; (−) cough, sputum expectoration, or hemoptysis; chronic nausea and bloating after eating; no bowel movement for 2 days; markedly increased urinary frequency for the past week but has had minimal urination in past 24 hours; (−) dysuria, urgency, or incontinence; (+) diffuse weakness and fatigue; (+) numbness and tingling in her feet for several months; (+) diffuse myalgias

## Physical Examination

### ▶ General

African American woman appearing her stated age, uncomfortable appearing, mildly dyspneic, but in no acute respiratory distress

### ▶ Vital Signs

BP 108/73 mm Hg, P 124, RR 19, T 99.3°F (37.4°C), $O_2$ sat 99% (0.99) on room air

Weight 115.7 lb (52.6 kg)

Height 66 in. (168 cm)

Headache pain 2/10

### ▶ Skin

Warm and dry; (−) rash, lesions; (+) decreased turgor with skin tenting, multiple tattoos

### ▶ HEENT

PERRLA; EOMI; (−) scleral icterus; (−) sinus tenderness; oral mucous membranes dry; TMs normal

### ▶ Neck and Lymph Nodes

Supple with full ROM; (−) adenopathy, goiter, JVD

### ▶ Chest

Clear to auscultation bilaterally

### ▶ Breasts

Examination deferred

### ▶ Cardiovascular

Tachycardic but regular rhythm; normal $S_1$, $S_2$; (−) $S_3$ or $S_4$

### ▶ Abdomen

Soft, mild diffuse tenderness; (−) distention, organomegaly; normally active bowel sounds

### ▶ Neurology

Awake, alert, and oriented; neurologic examination is grossly intact with normal DTRs.

### ▶ Genitourinary and Rectal

Examination deferred; however, the nurse notes that the patient has made no urine in the 6 hours she has been in the ED and that catheterization was required to obtain the urine drug screen.

## Laboratory Tests

| Blood | Day 1—04:35 | Day 1—10:20 | Day 1—20:00 |
|---|---|---|---|
| Na mEq/L (mmol/L) | 130 | 140 | 139 |
| K mEq/L (mmol/L) | 6.0 | 5.1 | 3.8 |
| Cl mEq/L (mmol/L) | 91 | 103 | 117 |
| $CO_2$ mEq/L (mmol/L) | 5 | 5 | 16 |
| BUN mg/dL (mmol/L) | 19 (6.8) | 18 (6.4) | 7 (2.5) |
| SCr mg/dL (μmol/L) | 1.7 (150) | 1.4 (124) | 0.7 (62) |
| Calcium mg/dL (mmol/L) | 9.9 (2.48) | 8.0 (2.00) | 7.3 (1.83) |
| Phosphorous mg/dL (mmol/L) | | | 1.5 (0.48) |
| Glucose mg/dL (mmol/L) | 649 (36.0) | 352 (19.5) | 108 (6.0) |
| WBC × $10^3$/ mm³ (× $10^9$/L) | 16.4 | | 7.6 |
| Hemoglobin g/dL (g/L; mmol/L) | 14.4 (144; 8.94) | | 10.7 (107; 6.64) |
| Hematocrit (%) | 43.6 (0.436) | | 31.0 (0.310) |
| Platelets × $10^3$/mm³ (× $10^9$/L) | 352 | | 221 |
| ABG | | | |
| pH | 7.05 | | |
| $PCO_2$ mm Hg (kPa) | 17 (2.3) | | |
| $PO_2$ mm Hg (kPa) | 157 (20.9) | | |

| | | | |
|---|---|---|---|
| HCO₃ mEq/L (mmol/L) | 2 | | |
| Hgb A₁c % | 16.6% (0.166; 158 mmol/ mol Hgb) | | |
| INR | 1.18 | | |
| Alk phos IU/L (μkat/L) | 175 (2.92) | | |
| AST IU/L (μkat/L) | 16 (0.27) | | |
| ALT IU/L (μkat/L) | 16 (0.27) | | |
| Total bilirubin mg/dL (μmol/L) | 0.2 (3.4) | | |
| Albumin g/dL (g/L) | 4.6 (46) | | |
| Amylase IU/L (μkat/L) | | 59 (0.98) | |
| Lipase IU/L (μkat/L) | | 13 (0.22) | |
| CK IU/L (μkat/L) | 135 | 91 (1.52) | |
| CK-MB ng/mL (μg/L) | 3.3 | 2.8 | |
| Troponin I ng/mL (μg/L) | 0.1 | 0.00 | 0.00 |
| Urine ketones | Positive (1:16) | | |
| Urine drug screen | (+) cocaine | | |

## Assessment

43-year-old woman with DKA, likely caused by nonadherence with her insulin.

### Student Workup

**Missing Information?**

**Evaluate:**     Patient Database

Drug Therapy Problems

Care Plan (by Problem)

## TARGETED QUESTIONS

1. What acid–base disturbance does this patient demonstrate on presentation?

   *Hint: See pp. 519–522 in PPP*

2. Calculate the anion gap in this patient using the initial (04:35) laboratory tests. Is this value abnormal?

   *Hint: See p. 521 in PPP*

3. What is the likely cause of this patient's acid–base disorder?

   *Hint: See Table 28-4 in PPP*

4. What is the best laboratory value to indicate this patient's fluid status? What do you think her fluid status is and why?

   *Hint: See pp. 502–503 in PPP*

5. Calculate this patient's creatinine clearance (CrCl) at 04:35 and 20:00 using the Cockcroft–Gault equation. Why are the values different? What disorder caused this difference?

   *Hint: See Table 25-2 in PPP*

6. Why did the potassium value change in this patient between 04:35 and 20:00? Explain your answer in reference to facts regarding potassium and to total body stores of potassium.

   *Hint: See p. 511 in PPP*

## FOLLOW-UP

7. Upon arrival to the ICU, the patient had a central line placed for fluid resuscitation and hemodynamic monitoring (CVP transduction). She was given 4 L of normal saline as a bolus and is now receiving a continuous infusion at 250 mL/h. She was started on an IV insulin infusion protocol, including hourly glucose measurements, and the infusion rate is being titrated. How quickly should we correct her hyperglycemia? What should be our plan regarding the IV fluids and her electrolytes?

   *Hint: See pp. 780–781 in PPP*

8. Because she has remained nauseated, metoclopramide 10 mg IV every 6 hours was prescribed. DVT prophylaxis with heparin 5,000 units SC every 8 hours has been initiated. Her home doses of omeprazole and loratadine have been continued. Acetaminophen 325 mg PO every 4 hours as needed was also ordered for her ongoing myalgias and headache. What therapy should be prescribed for her anion gap metabolic acidosis? What additional laboratory tests should be sent? What recommendations can be made regarding her discharge plan?

   *Hint: See pp. 780–781 in PPP*

## CASE SUMMARY

- The patient's clinical presentation and laboratory studies are consistent with DKA, leading to significant volume depletion.

- The presence of severe acidosis affects various electrolytes, particularly potassium, and may have pharmacokinetic and/or pharmacodynamic implications.

- Appropriate treatment of the patient's DKA should resolve her acid–base disorder. Specific therapy for the observed acidosis is typically not required.

**For more information on the care plan and facilitator's guide please visit http://www.mhpharmacotherapy.com.**

# 32 Metabolic Alkalosis

Lee E. Morrow        Ryan M. Brimeyer

Mark A. Malesker

## CASE LEARNING OBJECTIVES

- Correctly interpret ABG values
- Identify risk factors for acid–base and electrolyte disorders
- Develop an appropriate treatment and monitoring plan for a patient with metabolic alkalosis and critical hypokalemia
- Understand the clinical implications of hypophosphatemia
- Integrate magnesium repletion into the care plan of a patient with hypokalemia that is refractory to conventional correction

## PATIENT PRESENTATION

### Chief Complaint

Altered mental status

### History of Present Illness

Helen Baker is a 78-year-old woman transferred from a local nursing home for weakness and confusion. For several days she has had "the flu" according to the nursing home staff. The patient is delirious and unable to provide any history: nursing notes show at least 3 days of N/V/D, and poor oral intake. Several other residents at the nursing home have been ill with similar symptoms. A review of the patient's records shows that she was recently discharged from another hospital after being treated for pneumonia for 7 days. Although she was previously living independently, she had agreed to a temporary stay in the nursing home's acute care area to complete an additional 7 days of intravenous ciprofloxacin and gentamicin for a resistant *Pseudomonas* strain. Her current symptoms began within the first 24 hours of hospital discharge. The hospital discharge note indicates that the only other change to her medications during that hospitalization was the addition of 40 mEq (40 mmol) of oral potassium supplementation taken twice daily for persistent hypokalemia.

### Past Medical History

Hyperlipidemia with CAD

MI (1999, 2005); three-vessel CABG (2001)

Angioplasty with stent placement (2009)

Ischemic cardiomyopathy with a left ventricular ejection fraction of 20% (0.20)

HTN

PVD

CKD: baseline serum creatinine 1.5 mg/dL (133 µmol/L)

GERD

Idiopathic bronchiectasis

Recurrent TIAs

Arthritis

### Family History

Unknown, as the patient was adopted

### Social History

The patient is a lifelong resident of a rural Iowa farming community. She is a widow and lives with her son. She was employed as a bank teller for 19 years before retiring 5 years ago for health reasons. She has no recent travel history.

### Tobacco/Alcohol/Substance Use

The patient is a lifelong nonsmoker. Although she denied alcohol consumption to medical staff during her recent hospitalization and at the time of nursing home admission, her son reports ingestion of a pint of vodka daily for the past 25 years. Her recent hospital records document moderate alcohol withdrawal, requiring short-term benzodiazepine therapy.

## Allergies/Intolerances/Adverse Drug Events

NKDA

## Medications

Aspirin 81 mg PO daily

Ciprofloxacin 400 mg IV q 8 h

Clopidogrel 75 mg PO daily

Furosemide 40 mg PO bid

Gentamicin 130 mg IV every 24 h

Isosorbide mononitrate 60 mg PO at bedtime

Nitroglycerin 0.4 mg SL as needed for chest pain

Pantoprazole sodium 40 mg PO bid

KCl 40 mEq PO bid

Prednisone 5 mg PO daily, alternating with 7.5 mg PO daily

Simvastatin 40 mg PO at bedtime

## Review of Systems

Unable to obtain an ROS at present given her altered mental status. Although the nursing home staff who accompany her are not particularly familiar with her, they do not remember any symptoms other than those outlined above. Her vaccinations are current.

## Physical Examination

### ▶ General

Elderly Caucasian woman with fluctuating consciousness. She is weak and appears acutely ill.

### ▶ Vital Signs

BP 103/45 mm Hg; P 121; RR 9; T 97.7°F (36.5°C); SpO$_2$ 100% (0.100) on 2 L via nasal cannulae

Weight 105 lb (47.7 kg)

Height 65 in. (165 cm)

Pain—does not respond to question about her level of pain

### ▶ Skin

Warm, dry skin without apparent rashes or breakdown; poor turgor with tenting when pinched

### ▶ HEENT

PERRL; no scleral icterus; TMs appear normal; nares with small amount of old, crusted blood; oropharynx pink and moist without lesions

### ▶ Neck

Supple with full passive ROM; neck veins flat; no lymphadenopathy or goiter; a soft carotid bruit heard on the right

### ▶ Chest

Symmetric thoracic movement and resonance to percussion; clear to auscultation throughout

### ▶ Cardiovascular

Tachycardic with normal S$_1$ and S$_2$; no S$_3$ or S$_4$; PMI not displaced; peripheral pulses diminished

### ▶ Abdomen

Soft; not tender or distended; no guarding or rebound; no organomegaly; bowel sounds hyperactive

### ▶ Neurology

Moves all four extremities with intent when stimulated; DTRs normal throughout

### ▶ Genitourinary

Unremarkable; urinary catheter draining minimal dark-yellow urine

### ▶ Rectal

No palpable abnormalities; watery stool in rectal vault

## Laboratory Tests

Fecal occult blood negative

Stool ova and parasites negative

*Clostridium difficile* toxin negative

|  | Conventional Units | SI Units |
|---|---|---|
| Na | 141 mEq/L | 141 mmol/L |
| K | 1.9 mEq/L | 1.9 mmol/L |
| Cl | 87 mEq/L | 87 mmol/L |
| CO$_2$ | 44 mEq/L | 44 mmol/L |
| BUN | 55 mg/dL | 19.6 mmol/L |
| SCr | 2.1 mg/dL | 186 μmol/L |
| Glu | 101 mg/dL | 5.6 mmol/L |
| Ca | 8.6 mg/dL | 2.15 mmol/L |
| Mg | 1.5 mg/dL | 0.75 mmol/L |
| PO$_4$ | 1.8 mg/dL | 0.58 mmol/L |
| Troponin I | 0.06 ng/mL | 0.06 mcg/L |
| Hgb | 15.2 g/dL | 152 g/L; 9.43 mmol/L |
| Hct | 46.6% | 0.466 |
| WBC | 12.7 × 10$^3$/mm$^3$ | 12.7 × 10$^9$/L |
| Platelets | 519 × 10$^3$/mm$^3$ | 519 × 10$^9$/L |
| pH | 7.57 | |
| PCO$_2$ | 50 mm Hg | 6.7 kPa |
| PO$_2$ | 106 mm Hg | 14.1 kPa |

## Assessment

Seventy-eight-year-old woman receiving antibiotic therapy for pneumonia presents with N/V/D, possibly due to gastroenteritis, antibiotic-associated diarrhea, or *C. difficile*–associated diarrhea. Her poor oral intake coupled with her excessive GI losses and ongoing diuretic therapy has resulted in volume depletion and metabolic alkalosis. She also has critical hypokalemia (despite supplementation) and hypophosphatemia. Given her comorbidities, this combination of metabolic disorders has resulted in delirium.

## Student Workup

### Missing Information?

**Evaluate:**   Patient Database

Drug Therapy Problems

Care Plan (by Problem)

## TARGETED QUESTIONS

1. What medications need to be adjusted on the basis of her calculated creatinine clearance?

   *Hint: See standard drug information reference for renal drug dosing adjustments*

2. What acid–base disorder(s) do you recognize?

   *Hint: See pp. 524–525 in PPP*

3. What electrolyte disorder(s) do you recognize?

   *Hint: See Chapter 27 in PPP*

4. What factors may have contributed to these disorders?

   *Hint: See p. 525 in PPP*

5. Why would the admitting team members be concerned about the phosphate deficiency?

   *Hint: See pp. 512–513 in PPP*

6. Describe your treatment plan to correct the patient's electrolyte abnormalities.

   *Hint: See Chapter 27 in PPP*

7. What medications can contribute to a potential magnesium deficiency?

   *Hint: See p. 514 in PPP*

8. Would you give magnesium to this patient?

   *Hint: See p. 514 in PPP*

9. What other recommendations do you have to maximize her current medications?

## CASE SUMMARY

- The patient has metabolic alkalosis as a consequence of poor oral intake, excessive GI losses, and inappropriate diuretic therapy.

- She also has two electrolyte disorders (hypokalemia and hypophosphatemia), which are frequently encountered in this setting. These must be carefully corrected while monitoring serum levels.

- This patient has risk factors for magnesium deficiency and her suboptimal clinical response to potassium supplementation suggests that magnesium should be given despite the normal serum value.

**For more information on the care plan and facilitator's guide please visit http://www.mhpharmacotherapy.com.**

# 33 Epilepsy: Chronic Management

Timothy E. Welty

## CASE LEARNING OBJECTIVES

- Differentiate and classify seizure types when provided a description of the clinical presentation of the seizure and EEG
- Identify key therapeutic decision points in the treatment of epilepsy
- Establish therapeutic goals for pharmacotherapy in a patient with epilepsy
- Recommend an appropriate pharmacotherapeutic regimen for the treatment of epilepsy
- Select appropriate monitoring parameters for a pharmacotherapeutic regimen of epilepsy
- Devise a plan for switching a patient from one antiepileptic regimen to a different regimen
- Recognize complications of pharmacotherapy for epilepsy
- Analyze potential drug interactions with antiepileptic drugs (AEDs)
- Determine when and how to discontinue AED therapy
- Educate a patient or caregiver on epilepsy and pharmacotherapy for this disorder

## PATIENT PRESENTATION

### Chief Complaint

"I keep having spells where I don't remember things. My friends tell me I act weird at times, but I do not remember this."

### History of Present Illness

James Young is a 24-year-old man who presents to his primary care physician complaining of episodes of "lost memory" for the past 3–4 months. His last routine visit was 18 months ago, and he had a normal physical examination and laboratory values at that time. He explains that these spells occur randomly and last no longer than a few minutes. From his friends, he has been told that he talks funny, smacks his lips, and his right arm jerks. When asked if he remembers these spells, he insists that he hears people talking but is unable to respond. However, he does not recall anything about what he does during these spells. Immediately after a spell he feels sleepy and somewhat confused. In addition to this description, he volunteers that he awoke a month ago feeling sore and had wet the bed.

### Past Medical History

Multiple episodes of otitis media as a child
Fractured arm at age 18

### Family History

His father is 58 and has HTN and dyslipidemia. Mother is 54 and has hypothyroidism. He has two siblings in good health.

### Social History

He was married a year ago. His wife is 5 months pregnant. He graduated from college and works at a local bank as an assistant branch manager.

### Tobacco/Alcohol/Substance Use

Social drinker, but every few months will binge drink on a weekend; (–) tobacco or illicit drug use

### Allergies

Sulfa (rash)

### Medications (Current)

Multivitamin PO daily
Loratadine 10 mg PO as needed for seasonal allergies
Ibuprofen 200 mg PO PRN headache

## Physical Examination

▶ *General*

WDWN, white male in no acute distress

▶ *Vital Signs*

BP 118/72 mm Hg, P 70, RR 12, T 37°C

Weight 194 lb (88.2 kg)

Height 73 in. (185 cm)

Denies pain

▶ *Skin*

Normal color and turgor; (−) rashes or lesions

▶ *HEENT*

PERRLA, EOMI

▶ *Neck and Lymph Nodes*

Normal thyroid; (−) lymphadenopathy; (−) carotid bruits

▶ *Chest*

Clear to auscultation

▶ *Cardiovascular*

RRR; (−) murmurs or gallops

▶ *Abdomen*

Not tender or distended; (−) organomegaly

▶ *Neurology*

Alert and oriented × 3; CN II–XII intact; DTR 3+ and brisk; (−) Romberg; (−) plantar reflex; strength 5/5 in all extremities; normal gait; able to tandem walk; finger to nose intact; normal sensation to touch, pin prick, and vibration.

▶ *Genitourinary*

Examination deferred

▶ *Rectal*

Examination deferred

## Laboratory Tests

### Fasting Obtained Same Day

|  | Conventional Units | SI Units |
|---|---|---|
| Na | 140 mEq/L | 140 mmol/L |
| K | 4.0 mEq/L | 4.0 mmol/L |
| Cl | 105 mEq/L | 105 mmol/L |
| $CO_2$ | 24 mEq/L | 24 mmol/L |
| BUN | 9 mg/dL | 3.2 mmol/L |
| SCr | 0.8 mg/dL | 71 μmol/L |
| Glu | 80 mg/dL | 4.4 mmol/L |
| Ca | 9.8 mg/dL | 2.45 mmol/L |
| Mg | 1.7 mEq/L | 0.85 mmol/L |
| Phos | 3.9 mg/dL | 1.26 mmol/L |
| Albumin | 4.0 g/dL | 40 g/L |
| AST | 35 IU/L | 0.58 μkat/L |
| ALT | 32 IU/L | 0.53 μkat/L |
| GGT | 25 IU/L | 0.42 μkat/L |
| Hgb | 14.2 g/dL | 8.81 mmol/L; 142 g/L |
| Hct | 40.2% | 0.402 |
| WBC | $6.5 \times 10^3/mm^3$ | $6.5 \times 10^9/L$ |
| Platelets | $325 \times 10^3/\mu L$ | $325 \times 10^9/L$ |

## Assessment

Twenty-four-year-old man with possible seizures

---

**Student Workup**

**Missing Information?**

**Evaluate:**  Patient Database

Drug Therapy Problems

Care Plan (by Problem)

---

## TARGETED QUESTIONS

1. What s/s of seizures does this patient have?

   *Hint: See pp. 560–561 in PPP*

2. What information is needed prior to making a decision to starting an AED and selecting the drug to start?

   *Hint: See p. 562 in PPP*

3. What medications can be used in treating this patient's apparent seizure disorder?

   *Hint: See Table 31-2 in PPP*

4. For the AEDs most likely to be used in this patient, what are the common starting dose regimens?

   *Hint: See Table 31-3 in PPP*

5. For the AEDs most likely to be used in this patient, what are the most common adverse effects that need to be discussed with the patient?

   *Hint: See pp. 566–573 in PPP*

6. What additional items should be discussed with this patient during this clinic visit?

   *Hint: See pp. 573–574 in PPP*

## FOLLOW-UP

7. Two weeks later, the patient returns to clinic having completed a MRI scan of his head and an EEG. The MRI scan is read as left mesial temporal sclerosis and the EEG is read as left temporal spike waves consistent with a seizure disorder. Should long-term AED therapy be given to this patient? What actions, if any, would you take at this point?

   *Hint: See pp. 561–562 in PPP*

8. Six years later, the patient returns to clinic for a visit 9 months after a left temporal lobectomy for seizures. He has been seizure free since surgery. Prior to surgery, he continued to have two to three seizures per month despite multiple AEDs and drug combinations. At the time of surgery and currently, he is receiving carbamazepine extended-release capsules 200 mg in the AM and 300 mg in the PM, and levetiracetam 1,000 mg twice daily. Should AEDs be discontinued in this patient? What actions, if any, would you take at this point?

   *Hint: See pp. 573–574 in PPP*

## ⟳ GLOBAL PERSPECTIVE

The World Health Organization[1] estimates that there are approximately 50 million people with epilepsy throughout the world. The annual incidence in third-world nations is twice that of the United States (2/100 compared to 1/100). In many countries it remains a stigmatizing condition surrounded with mystical beliefs and social taboos.

On a global basis, an astonishing three-fourths of people with epilepsy receive no treatment for their seizures. Such lack of treatment is related to the above-mentioned social stigma as well as lack of access to medical care and medications. Patients may be treated with local traditional remedies in lieu of standard AED therapy. Also, the array of antiepileptic medications available in developing countries is more limited, so patients with seizures who do not respond to older first-line agents may have few options.

## REFERENCE

1. World Health Organization http://www.who.int/media-centre/factsheets/fs999/en/index.html, accessed February 8, 2013

### CASE SUMMARY

- His clinical presentation, MRI scan, and EEG are consistent with complex partial seizures.
- An AED useful in first-line therapy of partial seizures and with an adverse-effect profile that minimizes the influence of adverse effects on the patient's lifestyle should be selected.
- Ongoing monitoring of efficacy and toxicity is essential to further treatment decisions.

**For more information on the care plan and facilitator's guide please visit http://www.mhpharmacotherapy.com.**

# 34 Epilepsy: Status Epilepticus

Eljim P. Tesoro    Gretchen M. Brophy

## CASE LEARNING OBJECTIVES

- Explain the urgency of diagnosis and treatment of status epilepticus
- Recognize the signs and symptoms of status epilepticus
- Identify the treatment options available for termination of status epilepticus
- Formulate an initial treatment strategy for a patient in generalized convulsive status epilepticus
- Recommend monitoring parameters for a patient in status epilepticus

## PATIENT PRESENTATION

### History of Present Illness

James Lee is a 48-year-old African American male who was admitted to the hospital 2 days ago for treatment of a subdural hematoma that he incurred after falling down the steps in front of his home and hitting his head. He had surgical evacuation of the hematoma on the day of admission and is recovering in the surgical step-down unit. He had been loaded with phenytoin postoperatively to prevent seizures. The nurse went into his room to take his vital signs and found him unarousable with all his extremities shaking. He was seen talking on the phone 10 minutes before.

### Past Medical History

HTN
Type 2 DM
Dyslipidemia
Asthma

### Past Surgical History

Cholecystectomy 15 years ago
Appendectomy 21 years ago
Left-knee repair 5 years ago

### Family History

HTN in father
DM in mother

### Social History

He lives at home with his wife and two children, and works as a city bus driver.

He smokes ½ ppd of cigarettes; he drinks wine socially and denies any illicit drug use.

### Allergies/Intolerances

Sulfa (hives)

### Current Medications

Lisinopril 20 mg PO daily
Glyburide 5 mg PO daily
HCTZ 25 mg PO daily
Simvastatin 20 mg PO at bedtime
Phenytoin ER 300 mg PO at bedtime
Docusate 100 mg PO twice daily
Acetaminophen 500 mg/hydrocodone 5 mg tablet PO every 4 h as needed for pain or HA

### Review of Systems

Deferred; patient is now unresponsive

### Physical Examination

▶ *General*

Slightly overweight, middle-aged male with continuous convulsions of the extremities

141

▶ *Vital Signs*

BP 173/98 mm Hg, P 112, RR 20, T 38.0°C

Weight 220 lb (100 kg)

Height 62 in. (157 cm)

Unable to evaluate pain

▶ *Skin*

Sweaty skin and scalp; (−) rashes or lesions

▶ *HEENT*

Persistent upward gaze

▶ *Cardiovascular*

Tachycardic, RRR, normal $S_1$, $S_2$; (−) $S_3$ or $S_4$

▶ *Abdomen*

Not tender/not distended; (−) organomegaly

▶ *Neurology*

Unresponsive; unarousable; actively convulsing

▶ *Genitourinary*

Incontinent of stool and urine

## Laboratory Tests

|  | Conventional Units | SI Units |
|---|---|---|
| Na | 142 mEq/L | 142 mmol/L |
| K | 4.1 mEq/L | 4.1 mmol/L |
| Cl | 100 mEq/L | 100 mmol/L |
| $CO_2$ | 24 mEq/L | 24 mmol/L |
| BUN | 7 mg/dL | 2.5 mmol/L |
| SCr | 0.9 mg/dL | 80 μmol/L |
| Glu | 104 mg/dL | 5.8 mmol/L |
| Ca | 9.6 mg/dL | 2.40 mmol/L |
| Mg | 1.2 mEq/L | 0.60 mmol/L |
| Phosphate | 4.1 mg/dL | 1.32 mmol/L |
| Hgb | 12.5 g/dL | 125 g/L; 7.76 mmol/L |
| Hct | 37.7% | 0.377 |
| WBC | $9.6 \times 10^3/mm^3$ | $9.6 \times 10^9/L$ |
| MCV | 88 μm$^3$ | 88 fL |
| Albumin | 3.4 g/dL | 34 g/L |
| Phenytoin level | 7.8 mcg/mL | 31 μmol/L |

## Assessment

Forty-eight-year-old black male s/p head trauma and evacuation of subdural hematoma with signs of acute status epilepticus

## TARGETED QUESTIONS

1. What signs of status epilepticus does this patient have?

   *Hint: See p. 581 in PPP*

2. What are some possible causes of status epilepticus in this patient?

   *Hint: See p. 580 in PPP*

3. What medication(s) would you recommend to stop this patient's status epilepticus?

   *Hint: See Tables 32-1 and 32-2 in PPP*

4. What medication(s) would you recommend for preventing future seizures in this patient?

   *Hint: See Tables 31-2, 31-3 in PPP*

## FOLLOW-UP

Thirty minutes later, the patient continues to have generalized seizures. An endotracheal tube is inserted by anesthesiology, and the patient is transported to the neurology ICU.

5. What therapy for the patient's continued seizures would you recommend now?

   *Hint: See Tables 32-1 and 32-2 in PPP*

6. What if the patient stops convulsing but does not wake up?

   *Hint: Consider the possibility of non-convulsive status epilepticus*

7. What if the patient was a 26-year-old female who was 32 weeks pregnant?

   *Hint: See p. 587 in PPP*

## 🌀 GLOBAL PERSPECTIVE

According to the World Health Organization[1], the incidence of seizures is greater in developing countries compared to the United States, and a large proportion of patients receive no treatment due to social taboos and lack of access to care. Given the higher incidence of seizure disorders and lack of access to therapy in many patients, it is likely that there is a higher incidence of status epilepticus in developing countries. Although the overall therapeutic approach would be the same, patients in developing countries may have poor access to emergency medical care. While first-line medications such as benzodiazepines, phenytoin, and phenobarbital may be available, newer intravenous medications may not be available for refractory status epilepticus.

## REFERENCE

1. World Health Organization http://www.who.int/mediacentre/factsheets/fs999/en/index.html, Accessed February 8, 2013

## CASE SUMMARY

- Status epilepticus is a medical emergency and should be assessed and treated immediately.

- Intravenous benzodiazepines (lorazepam or diazepam) are the first drugs of choice to stop seizure activity.
- Anticonvulsants are used after benzodiazepines to prevent future seizures.
- Prolonged status epilepticus can lead to nonconvulsive status epilepticus if not treated.

**For more information on the care plan and facilitator's guide please visit http://www.mhpharmacotherapy.com.**

# 35 Parkinson's Disease

Jack J. Chen

## CASE LEARNING OBJECTIVES

- Identify motor and nonmotor symptoms of Parkinson's disease (PD) as well as symptoms that indicate disease progression
- Explain the desired therapeutic goals for patients with PD
- Recommend lifestyle modifications and pharmacotherapy interventions for treating motor symptoms of patients with PD
- Recommend drug and nondrug interventions for treating the nonmotor symptoms of patients with PD
- Develop a monitoring plan to assess the effectiveness and adverse effects of nonpharmacologic therapy and pharmacotherapy for PD
- Educate patients about the disease state, appropriate lifestyle modifications, and drug therapy required for effective treatment

## PATIENT PRESENTATION

### Chief Complaint

"My primary care physician says I might have Parkinson's disease."

### History of Present Illness

Oliver Covey is a 62-year-old, right-handed man who is referred to a neurologist by his primary care physician. He was visiting his primary care physician for a routine checkup appointment. At that time, his primary care physician noted that the patient had a mild, right-hand tremor and walked with reduced arm swing. His primary care physician felt that these signs and symptoms were compatible with possible Parkinson's disease (PD) and referred him to a neurologist for further assessment. At the neurologist visit, the patient is accompanied by his wife. He states that he is in good spirits. He admits noticing the tremor in his right hand about 1 year ago, but did not think much of it. His wife has also noticed the tremor. The patient states no other problems. However, his wife reports he walks a bit slower and that his "tennis game has gotten worse." She states that he used to be very agile on the tennis court but during the past year has "slowed considerably and often misses shots." The patient admits this is true. When asked about his employment and work capabilities, he states the movement problems do not interfere. The neurologist asks, "If there is one thing we can make better about your movement, what would it be?" The patient replies, "I want to be able to swing the tennis racket like I used to a year ago." He is willing to start drug therapy to help improve his movement.

### Past Medical History

BPH × 1 y
GERD × 1 y
Hyperlipidemia × 5 y
Nephrolithiasis in the past
Tonsillectomy

### Family History

He is an only child. His father died of MI. Mother died of some other type of cardiac problem. No family history of neurologic conditions.

### Social History

He was born in Arizona and lives in Los Angeles. He has a college education. He is married and lives with his wife of 32 years, and has two children aged 30 and 25. He works as an agricultural irrigation consultant.

### Tobacco/Alcohol/Substance Use

(−) Alcohol, tobacco, or illicit drug use

## Allergies/Intolerances/Adverse Drug Events

Sulfonamides (severe rash as a teenager)

## Medications (Current)

Omeprazole 20 mg PO q 24 h

Silodosin 8 mg PO q 24 h

Simvastatin 20 mg PO q 24 h

Multivitamin one tablet PO q 24 h

## Review of Systems

(–) Cancer, cardiac disease, falls, loss of consciousness, psychiatric conditions, respiratory disease, seizures, stroke, syncope, or vertigo

## Physical Examination

### ▸ General

WDWN Caucasian man in no acute distress. Oriented to person, place, and time. Mood and affect appropriate

### ▸ Vital Signs

BP 128/76 mm Hg, P 76, RR 16, T 36.4°C

Weight 180 lb (81.8 kg)

Height 71 in. (180 cm)

Denies pain

### ▸ HEENT

PERRLA, EOMI, (–) nystagmus, (–) gaze palsy, (–) olfactory deficit

### ▸ Neck and Lymph Nodes

Neck supple; (–) adenopathy

### ▸ Chest

Clear to auscultation

### ▸ Cardiovascular

Deferred

### ▸ Abdomen

Deferred

### ▸ Extremities

Pedal pulses are 2+ and equal

### ▸ Skin

Warm and dry; (–) rashes or lesions

### ▸ Neurology

**Cranial nerves**

II: Normal visual acuity, visual fields, fundi

III, IV, VI: PERRL, EOMI

V: Facial sensation intact

VII: Normal facial asymmetry and strength

VIII: Whisper test normal

IX: Uvula midline with "Ah"

XI: Shoulder shrug strength normal

XII: Tongue midline with protrusion

No masked facies. Mild hypophonia. Slightly stooped posture. DTRs normal. No tremor on finger to nose test

Positive micrographia (Fig. 35-1)

Resting tremor right arm = 2; no tremor in left arm or legs

Rigidity right arm = 2, left arm = 1; no rigidity of lower extremities

Finger taps right = 2, left = 1

Hand movements right = 1, left = 1

Leg agility right = 0, left = 0

Ability to arise from seated position in chair with arms folded across the chest: Normal

Gait normal and steady. Slightly reduced arm swing on right. No postural instability observed upon pull test

### ▸ Genitourinary

Deferred

### ▸ Rectal

Deferred

**FIGURE 35-1.** Micrographia. (Reprinted with permission from Jack J. Chen, PharmD, Loma Linda University Movement Disorders Center, Loma Linda, CA.)

## Laboratory Tests

### Fasting Obtained 1 Month Ago

|  | Conventional Units | SI Units |
|---|---|---|
| Na | 140 mEq/L | 140 mmol/L |
| K | 4 mEq/L | 4 mmol/L |
| Cl | 99 mEq/L | 99 mmol/L |
| $CO_2$ | 29 mEq/L | 29 mmol/L |
| BUN | 14 mg/dL | 5.0 mmol/L |
| SCr | 1 mg/dL | 88 μmol/L |
| Glu | 90 mg/dL | 5.0 mmol/L |
| Ca | 9.5 mg/dL | 2.38 mmol/L |
| Mg | 2.2 mEq/L | 1.10 mmol/L |
| Phosphate | 3.5 mg/dL | 1.13 mmol/L |
| Albumin | 3.7 g/dL | 37 g/L |
| WBC | $8.5 \times 10^3/mm^3$ | $8.5 \times 10^9/L$ |
| RBC | $5.63 \times 10^6/\mu L$ | $5.63 \times 10^{12}/L$ |
| Hgb | 16.4 g/dL | 164 g/L; 10.18 mmol/L |
| Hct | 48.7% | 0.487 |
| MCV | $86.4 \mu m^3$ | 86.4 fL |
| Platelet | $300 \times 10^3/\mu L$ | $300 \times 10^9/L$ |
| Total cholesterol | 180 mg/dL | 4.65 mmol/L |
| LDL cholesterol | 100 mg/dL | 2.59 mmol/L |
| HDL cholesterol | 38 mg/dL | 0.98 mmol/L |

## Assessment

Sixty-two-year-old man with signs and symptoms consistent with early stage idiopathic PD

### Student Workup

**Missing Information?**

**Evaluate:** Patient Database

Drug Therapy Problems

Care Plan (by Problem)

## TARGETED QUESTIONS

1. What motor and nonmotor signs and symptoms of PD does the patient have?

   *Hint: See pp. 593–594 in PPP*

2. What is the severity of s/s rated by the neurologist?

   *Hint: See Unified Parkinson's Disease Rating Scale (UPDRS) Section III Motor Examination (http://www.mdvu.org/ library/ratingscales/pd/updrs.pdf)*

3. What are common medications that can cause PD and should be queried during the patient interview?

   *Hint: See p. 593 in PPP*

4. If pharmacotherapy is desired, what are the classes of medications that can be initiated?

   *Hint: See pp. 596–600 in PPP*

5. For each class of anti-Parkinson medication, what are the benefits versus risks/adverse effects that you should consider for this specific patient?

   *Hint: See pp. 596–600 in PPP*

6. Which specific pharmacotherapy regimen would you recommend for this patient and why?

   *Hint: See pp. 596–600 in PPP*

7. What nonpharmacologic recommendations should this patient receive?

   *Hint: See p. 595 in PPP*

## FOLLOW-UP

8. Eight weeks later, the patient returns for follow-up. He is in good spirits and feels his tremor has improved while on the medication. On examination, his tremor, rigidity, and bradykinesia are still present, but they are improved. His handwriting is still the same. He also reports that his tennis game seems somewhat improved and is happy about that. He has not experienced any unpleasant side effects. Are any pharmacologic interventions required at this time?

   *Hint: See pp. 596–600 in PPP*

## REFERENCES

1. Drugs for Parkinson's disease. Treat Guidel Med Lett 2011 9:1–6.
2. Fox SH, Katzenschlager R, Lim SY, Ravina B, Seppi K, Coelho M, et al. The Movement Disorder Society evidence-based medicine review update: treatments for the motor symptoms of Parkinson's disease. Mov Disord 2011 26(Suppl 3):S2–41.
3. Seppi K, Weintraub D, Coelho M, Perez-Lloret S, Fox SH, Katzenschlager R, et al. The Movement Disorder Society evidence-based medicine review update: treatments for the non-motor symptoms of Parkinson's disease. Mov Disord 2011 26(Suppl 3):S42–80.

## ⟳ GLOBAL PERSPECTIVE

PD affects individuals worldwide. Regional figures showing differences in both incidence and prevalence[1] probably reflect the existence of factors that may be demographic (variations in life expectancy across countries), health care–related (lack of proper and widespread recognition of the disorder, variations in access to health care), genetic, and environmental, together with methodologic differences. In addition, early studies had shown variations in prevalence at the international level attributed to ethnic differences across regions. Higher rates were reported for Caucasians in Europe and North America, intermediate rates for Asians in China and Japan, and the lowest rates for blacks in Africa. However, more recent studies from Asia do not show significant differences in prevalence compared with studies in Caucasians

## REFERENCE

1. World Health Organization. Neurological Disorders: Public Health Challenges; www.who.int/mental_health/neurology/neurodiso/en/index.html, accessed August 2, 2012.

## CASE SUMMARY

- His current clinical picture is consistent with idiopathic PD. The patient desires treatment, so it is justified to initiate pharmacotherapy.

- This patient should be informed that there is no cure of PD and that if left untreated, his movements will likely worsen over time. Several medications are available to make the movements better.

- Several pharmacotherapy options exist for this relatively young patient with early PD, including carbidopa/levodopa, dopamine agonists, and rasagiline. Amantadine and anticholinergics should be avoided due to the patient's history of BPH.

- The advantages, disadvantages, and side effects of amantadine, carbidopa/levodopa, dopamine agonists, and MAO-B inhibitors should be considered when discussing therapeutic options with the patient. An initial trial of rasagiline or a dopamine agonist would be appropriate. However, amantadine and carbidopa/levodopa are also justifiable choices.

- Nonpharmacologic suggestions include encouraging this patient to continue his physical exercise, such as tennis. If the patient and his wife desires, educational material on PD and support groups can be recommended.

- At this stage of his PD, it is unnecessary to provide information about advanced-stage PD or surgical options.

**For more information on the care plan and facilitator's guide please visit http://www.mhpharmacotherapy.com.**

# 36 Acute Pain Management

Asad E. Patanwala

## CASE LEARNING OBJECTIVES

- Recognize components of a comprehensive pain assessment
- Recommend an appropriate choice of analgesic, dose, and monitoring plan for a patient on the basis of type and severity of pain and other patient-specific parameters
- Identify the goals of therapy for the management of acute pain
- Properly educate patients when opioid analgesia is initiated

## PATIENT PRESENTATION

### Chief Complaint

"This is the worst pain I have ever had. It is like a 10 out of 10."

### History of Present Illness

Jose Garcia is a 44-year-old man who is admitted to the hospital after a motorcycle collision. He lost control of his motorcycle and hit a parked vehicle when traveling at approximately 40 mph (64 km/h). He was wearing a helmet at the time of the collision. This occurred at 2 AM today after he left a local bar to go home. According to the paramedics, he did not have any loss of consciousness, was unable to move his right leg, and had a definite odor of alcohol. In the emergency department, he was given 100 mcg of IV fentanyl for pain and 2 L of IV NS. He was subsequently taken to the operating room for an open reduction internal fixation (ORIF) of his right lower extremity fracture. Soon after surgery he was transferred to a general surgical ward for postoperative care.

### Past Medical History

PUD × 2 years (had a GI bleed 6 months ago)

Seizure disorder × 10 years

Chronic shoulder pain × 5 years (from previous motorcycle collision)

### Family History

His father died at age 60 from alcoholic cirrhosis and mother died at age 50 from a motor vehicle collision. He has no siblings.

### Social History

He is single, has no children, and works at a construction company.

### Tobacco/Alcohol/Substance Use

Drinks six beers daily; smokes one ppd; (−) illicit drug use

### Allergies/Intolerances/Adverse Drug Events

Morphine (itching); oxycodone (constipation)

### Medications (Current)

Famotidine 40 mg PO q h (home medication)

Promethazine 25 mg IV q 4–6 h PRN

Tramadol 100 mg PO q 4–6 h PRN

Meperidine 50 mg PO q 2–4 h PRN

Phenytoin 100 mg PO q 8 h (home medication)

Ibuprofen 400 mg PO q 6 h PRN (home medication)

Aspirin 325 mg PO q 24 h (home medication)

Docusate 100 mg PO q 12 h

Heparin 5,000 units SC q 24 h

### Review of Systems

He has severe leg pain that is not relieved by current therapy; his shoulder is also hurting again from his previous injury; his back is sore from road rash; (+) abdominal distension, constipation, and nausea; vomited twice this morning; feels drowsy.

## Physical Examination

▸ *General*

Well-developed, middle-aged, Hispanic male grimacing in pain

▸ *Vital Signs*

BP 160/110 mm Hg, P 102, RR 16, T 37.2°C

Weight 187 lb (85 kg)

Height 70 in. (178 cm)

Pain score 10/10

▸ *Skin*

(+) Road rash on back and right thigh; no penetrating injuries

▸ *HEENT*

PERRLA, EOMI; TMs appear normal, normocephalic, atraumatic

▸ *Neck and Lymph Nodes*

Supple; (−) bruits; (−) thyromegaly; (−) lymphadenopathy; trachea midline

▸ *Chest*

Clear breath sounds bilaterally; (−) crackles

▸ *Cardiovascular*

Tachycardic, RRR, normal $S_1$, $S_2$; (−) $S_3$ or $S_4$

▸ *Abdomen*

Soft, nontender, distended; (+) bowel sounds; (−) masses; (−) hepatomegaly

▸ *Neurology*

Oriented × 3; neurologic examination grossly intact, DTRs normal

▸ *Extremities*

Right tibia fracture

▸ *Genitourinary*

No abnormalities

▸ *Rectal*

(+) Rectal tone; (−) gross blood

## Laboratory Tests
### Obtained this Morning

|  | Conventional Units | SI Units |
| --- | --- | --- |
| Na | 141 mEq/L | 141 mmol/L |
| K | 3.9 mEq/L | 3.9 mmol/L |
| Cl | 101 mEq/L | 101 mmol/L |
| $CO_2$ | 23 mEq/L | 23 mmol/L |
| BUN | 11 mg/dL | 3.9 mmol/L |
| SCr | 1.1 mg/dL | 97 μmol/L |
| Glu | 95 mg/dL | 5.3 mmol/L |
| Ca | 8.7 mg/dL | 2.18 mmol/L |
| Mg | 0.9 mEq/L | 0.45 mmol/L |
| Phosphate | 3.5 mg/dL | 1.13 mmol/L |
| Hgb | 14.1 g/dL | 8.75 mmol/L; 141 g/L |
| Hct | 42.5% | 0.425 |
| WBC | $8.2 \times 10^3/mm^3$ | $8.2 \times 10^9/L$ |
| Platelets | $240 \times 10^3/mm^3$ | $240 \times 10^9/L$ |
| Albumin | 3.7 g/dL | 37 g/L |
| Total bilirubin | 1.1 mg/dL | 18.8 μmol/L |
| Direct bilirubin | 0.3 mg/dL | 5.1 μmol/L |
| AST | 82 IU/L | 1.37 μkat/L |
| ALT | 53 IU/L | 0.88 μkat/L |
| Alk phos | 96 IU/L | 1.60 μkat/L |

## Assessment

Forty-four-year-old man s/p trauma with right tibia fracture and ORIF now with s/s of severe acute postoperative pain

### Student Workup

**Missing Information?**

**Evaluate:**   Patient Database

Drug Therapy Problems

Care Plan (by Problem)

## TARGETED QUESTIONS

1. What s/s of this patient are consistent with poor pain control?

   *Hint: See pp. 608–609 in PPP*

2. Why is IV opioid analgesia the treatment of choice for most patients with severe acute pain in the hospital setting?

   *Hint: See pp. 613–614 in PPP*

3. How does the potency of commonly used opioids differ?

   *Hint: See p. 613 in PPP*

4. What risks and adverse effects of opioid therapy would you discuss with this patient?

   *Hint: See pp. 614–615 in PPP*

5. Is this patient a candidate for PCA? Explain.

   *Hint: See p. 614 in PPP*

## FOLLOW-UP

6. Three days after surgery the patient is being discharged from the hospital. While in the hospital he was treated only with IV opioids. He now needs to be switched to an oral medication for pain control. What are some of the pertinent pieces of information that you would need to create a regimen that this patient can take at home? What counseling and adjunctive therapy may be required if this patient is sent home with prescriptions for oral opioid analgesia?

   *Hint: See pp. 614–615 in PPP*

## ☼ GLOBAL PERSPECTIVE

Morphine is metabolized in the liver via hepatic conjugation with glucuronic acid. There are significant ethnic differences with regard to morphine metabolism. Morphine clearance is higher in Chinese men compared with Caucasian men. This is likely due to an increase in partial metabolic clearance by glucuronidation in the Chinese population. There is no physiologic or laboratory parameter for accurate pain assessment. Hence, providers must rely on the patient's self-reported pain to make treatment decisions. There are cultural, behavioral, and age-related differences with regard to how patients report their pain. This ranges from expressing their pain in a stoic manner to being very expressive. Also, there is evidence that patients from ethnic minorities or cultures that are different from the health care provider are more likely to receive inadequate analgesia. All of this must be incorporated in the decision-making process with regard to pain assessment and treatment.

## CASE SUMMARY

- His clinical picture is consistent with severe acute postoperative pain.
- He is currently on pain medications that are suboptimal and contraindicated due to his seizure disorder and peptic ulcer disease.
- He is experiencing opioid-induced adverse effects, such as sedation, constipation, N/V.

For more information on the care plan and facilitator's guide please visit http://www.mhpharmacotherapy.com.

# 37 Chronic Pain Management

Michael D. Katz    Claire A. Simister

## CASE LEARNING OBJECTIVES

- Recognize the signs and symptoms of various etiologies of pain
- Identify the goals of therapy for chronic pain management
- Identify actual and potential side effects of drugs utilized in pain management
- Develop an appropriate treatment regimen and monitoring plan for chronic pain based on individual patient characteristics
- Select an appropriate drug regimen for chronic pain, including scheduled, as-needed, and adjunctive therapy
- Select appropriate therapy for prevention and treatment of opioid side effects
- Properly educate a patient on pain management therapies

## PATIENT PRESENTATION

### Chief Complaint

"This back pain is unbearable. What other pain pills are available that won't cause constipation?"

### History of Present Illness

Jean Walter is a 58-year-old woman with stage IV ductal breast carcinoma who presents anxiously to the cancer clinic after having run out of her previous prescription for oxycodone/acetaminophen 1 week prior. Three weeks ago, she was prescribed oxycodone SR 10 mg twice daily and oxycodone 5 mg/acetaminophen 325 mg as needed (#120 tablets); however, she decided to only fill her oxycodone/acetaminophen prescription since she didn't think she needed two different pills to control her pain. After taking all of the oxycodone/acetaminophen over the course of 2 weeks, she began to supplement her pain regimen with OTC acetaminophen (averaging 12 tablets per day) for her worsening lower back pain. She describes the back pain as throbbing and constant and rates the severity as a 9 on a scale of 1 to 10, but also notes a "pins and needles" sensation that radiates from her lower back down her left leg to her knee and some weakness in her left leg. JW was initially diagnosed with breast cancer in 2006 after which she underwent a lumpectomy, radiation therapy, and adjuvant chemotherapy. During the past year, a CT scan showed recurrence of a breast tumor and spinal metastases in the L4–S2 region, which is consistent with her complaints of increasing back pain and immobility.

### Past Medical History

Stage IV ductal breast carcinoma (diagnosed 2006) s/p chemotherapy and radiation

DM type 2 × 12 y

HTN × 17 y

### Past Surgical History

Left breast lumpectomy (2008)

Hysterectomy (2002)

Cholecystectomy (1989)

### Family History

Father had DM type 2 and CAD and died of MI at the age of 70. Mother had breast cancer and died at the age of 62 secondary to metastatic disease. She has two brothers who are alive with hypertension and DM type 2.

### Social History

Married and lives with her husband of 34 years; has three adult children. She previously worked as a social worker, but had to retire secondary to her disease progression.

## Tobacco/Alcohol/Substance Use

(−) Alcohol, tobacco, or illicit drug use

## Allergies/Intolerances/Adverse Drug Events

Sulfa (rash), codeine (nausea)

## Medications (Current)

Metformin 500 mg PO twice daily

Atorvastatin  40 mg PO daily

Lisinopril 20 mg PO daily

Metoprolol 50 mg PO daily

Calcium carbonate/vitamin D 1,000 mg/400 IU PO
  twice daily

Oxycodone/acetaminophen 5 mg/325 mg, two tablets PO
  every 4–6 h PRN pain

Acetaminophen 650 mg PO PRN headache

Citalopram 20 mg PO daily

Tamoxifen 20 mg PO daily

## Review of Systems

(+) Chronic back pain from metastases, occasionally relieved
with oxycodone/acetaminophen, not relieved with acetaminophen; decreased appetite with some nausea; (+) "pins and
needles" sensation in left leg that radiates to the knee; slight
weakness upon standing; (+) constipation not relieved with
OTC stool softeners.

## Physical Examination

### ▶ General

WDWN anxious-appearing middle-aged woman in no apparent acute distress

### ▶ Vital Signs

BP 132/84 mm Hg, P 82, RR 16, T 37.1°C

Weight 142 lb (64.5 kg)

Height 65 in. (165 cm)

Lower back pain and tingling, which radiates down the back
  of her left leg to the knee

### ▶ Skin

Warm and dry; no evidence of rash

### ▶ HEENT

PERRLA, EOMI; TMs clear bilaterally

### ▶ Neck and Lymph Nodes

No lymphadenopathy; no tenderness to palpation of the
cervical spine

### ▶ Chest

Clear to auscultation; no wheezes, crackles, or rhonchi

### ▶ Breasts

Well-healed scar on lateral aspect of left breast, and palpable
mass on medial side of left breast; no masses or nipple discharge noted on right breast

### ▶ Cardiovascular

RRR; no murmurs, rubs, or gallops

### ▶ Abdomen

Soft, slight tenderness with mild distension; bowel sounds
positive; no organomegaly

### ▶ Neurology

Cranial nerves II–XII grossly intact; slight weakness in the
left leg upon standing; DTRs are normal; decreased pinprick
sensation on posterior aspect of the left thigh

### ▶ Genitourinary

Examination deferred

### ▶ Rectal

Examination deferred

## Laboratory Tests

| | Conventional Units | SI Units |
|---|---|---|
| Na | 139 mEq/L | 139 mmol/L |
| K | 3.9 mEq/L | 3.9 mmol/L |
| Cl | 104 mEq/L | 104 mmol/L |
| $CO_2$ | 23 mEq/L | 23 mmol/L |
| BUN | 14 mg/dL | 5.0 mmol/L |
| SCr | 1.1 mg/dL | 97 μmol/L |
| Glu | 160 mg/dL | 8.9 mmol/L |
| Ca | 8.4 mg/dL | 2.10 mmol/L |
| Mg | 2.0 mEq/L | 1.00 mmol/L |
| Phosphate | 3.6 mg/dL | 1.16 mmol/L |
| Hgb | 13.5 g/dL | 135 g/L; 8.38 mmol/L |
| Hct | 39.7% | 0.397 |
| WBC | $6.5 \times 10^3/mm^3$ | $6.5 \times 10^9/L$ |
| MCV | 87 μm$^3$ | 87 fL |
| Platelets | $178 \times 10^3/mm^3$ | $178 \times 10^9/L$ |
| Albumin | 3.5 g/dL | 35 g/L |
| Alk phos | 95 U/L | 1.58 μkat/L |
| AST | 37 U/L | 0.62 μkat/L |
| ALT | 68 U/L | 1.13 μkat/L |
| Total bilirubin | 0.7 mg/dL | 12 μmol/L |

## Assessment

Fifty-eight-year-old woman with ductal breast carcinoma with metastatic lesions on the spine and associated chronic pain and neuropathic pain syndromes

### Student Workup

**Missing Information?**

**Evaluate:**    Patient Database

Drug Therapy Problems

Care Plan (by Problem)

## TARGETED QUESTIONS

1. What other information would be useful in characterizing, assessing, and treating this patient's pain?

   *Hint: See pp. 608–609 in PPP*

2. What signs and symptoms of neuropathic pain does the patient have, and how does treatment of neuropathic pain differ from other types of chronic pain?

   *Hint: See p. 608 in PPP*

3. What is the rationale behind the use of both scheduled and PRN medications in chronic pain?

   *Hint: See p. 613 in PPP*

4. What common adverse effects of opioid medications are dose-dependent, and what are appropriate methods to prevent and treat such adverse effects?

   *Hint: See pp. 614–615 in PPP*

5. What nonpharmacologic therapies may be useful for this patient?

   *Hint: See p. 611 in PPP*

Also see Swarm R, Abernathy AP, Anghelescu DL, et al. NCCN clinical practice guidelines in oncology: Adult cancer pain. National Comprehensive Cancer Network, version 1.2012. http://www.nccn.org/professionals/physician_gls/f_guidelines.asp#supportive, accessed June 7, 2012.

## FOLLOW-UP

6. Six months later, the patient returns for a follow-up pain visit. She is s/p palliative chemotherapy treatment. Three months ago she developed sepsis from an infected central venous catheter and acute kidney injury, and her renal function never fully recovered. Her most recent laboratory work shows a BUN of 41 mg/dL (14.6 mmol/L) and SCr of 2.3 mg/dL (203 μmol/L). At her visit 1 month prior, her pain medication regimen was as follows: MS Contin 100 mg q 8 h, fentanyl patch 50 mcg/hour to be changed every 72 hours, and morphine immediate release (IR) 5–10 mg PO every 4–6 hours as

needed. She presents in a wheelchair with her husband who states that she has been more lethargic, and he is concerned that it may be related to her medications. What changes would you make to her current pain regimen?

*Hint: See pp. 614–616 in PPP*

## ⟲ GLOBAL PERSPECTIVE

For more than 20 years, the World Health Organization (WHO) has promoted adequate control of cancer-related pain through the application of key therapeutic principles shown to improve pain relief. Opioids are the mainstay of treating moderate to severe pain associated with cancer and other life-threatening conditions associated with chronic pain (e.g., HIV/AIDS). There are a variety of barriers that may interfere with successful pain control in such patients, and one such barrier is availability of and patient access to opioid medications. International research[1] has shown that a country's per capita consumption of opioids is a marker of adequate pain management. There are very large disparities in per capita opioid consumption among regions and individual countries. Some, but not all, of the disparities are related to per capita income. Fifteen percent of the world's population accounts for 87% of the morphine consumption. The United States, which comprises 4.7% of the world's population, accounts for 49% of global morphine consumption (77 mg/capita). Other developed countries consume significantly less morphine: Australia 46 mg/capita, France 34 mg/capita, Germany 23 mg/capita, United Kingdom 57 mg/capita, and Japan 3 mg/capita. Consumption in developing countries is strikingly lower (Brazil 2.3 mg/capita, Thailand 0.8 mg/capita, Ghana 0.075 mg/capita, Mexico 0.36 mg/capita, and Niger 0.0004 mg/capita). There are several reasons for such disparities in opioid consumption beyond simple economics. Because of concerns about opioid addiction and diversion of prescription drugs, many countries have implemented regulations that severely restrict patient access to such drugs. In some countries, potent opioids can be used only in severe cancer-related pain when other agents have failed. Also, there may be cultural or religious differences in how pain and suffering are interpreted and therefore how pain is managed. The WHO and the United Nations are working with countries around the world to develop balanced national policies that deal not only with drug abuse and diversion but also improve the care of patients who are needlessly suffering[2]. However, changes in governmental policies will not by itself improve pain control. Education of health professionals in effective palliative care and changing the attitudes of professionals and patients also will be needed.

## REFERENCES

1. Joranson DE, Ryan KM. Ensuring opioid availability: Methods and resources. J Pain Sympt Manage 2007 33:527–532.

2. World Health Organization. Pain and Policy Studies Group, University of Wisconsin Carbone Cancer Center and WHO. www.painpolicy.wisc.edu/. Accessed February 18, 2013.

## CASE SUMMARY

- Her clinical picture is consistent with chronic malignant pain secondary to metastatic disease.

- Her current regimen is not providing adequate pain relief, and she is experiencing adverse effects, including constipation.

- The patient would benefit from an individualized regimen, which includes pharmacologic agents to treat both somatic and neuropathic pain. An appropriate regimen should include scheduled and as-needed medications as part of her opioid pain regimen and bowel regimen to prevent opioid-induced adverse effects.

For more information on the care plan and facilitator's guide please visit http://www.mhpharmacotherapy.com.

# 38 Headache

Brendan S. Ross          Leigh Ann Ross

## CASE LEARNING OBJECTIVES

- Differentiate among types of headaches (HAs) based on symptoms and signs
- List underlying causes and precipitating factors of different types of HA disorders
- Recommend appropriate nonpharmacologic measures for HA treatment and prevention
- On the basis of patient-specific data, determine when pharmacologic therapy is indicated for HA
- Propose individualized pharmacologic treatment regimens for the acute and chronic management of HA syndromes
- Construct therapeutic and adverse effect monitoring plans for patients with HA
- Discuss pertinent patient education points for patients with HA disorders

## PATIENT PRESENTATION

### Chief Complaint

"My headaches just won't go away no matter how many pills I take."

### History of Present Illness

XA is a 54-year-old man who is evaluated by the outpatient neurology service of an academic medical center due to chronic daily HA, which has recently grown more severe. He reports that his HAs are bitemporal and that the pain radiates into his neck and upper back, but that they are not associated with stiffness or weakness: "It feels like a heavy weight on my head and shoulders." The pain is nonpulsatile, grows steadily over hours until it is 8/10 in intensity; and it lasts most of the day, if left untreated. "Almost anything" can bring on a HA, but they are more frequent and more intense when he is under significant "stress." He reports that worry over recent marital problems makes it difficult for him to fall asleep. Bright lights can make the pain worse, but he has not experienced nausea or any neurologic deficits prior to or during an attack. The pain makes it difficult to concentrate, though he rarely misses business or family obligations. He has experienced HA since his teenage years, but they had previously been easy to treat with the use of OTC analgesics. Over the past several years, his HAs have become more difficult to control. His primary care physician (PCP) provided him prescription-strength NSAIDs for PRN use without much relief: "I take them every day; they don't seem to do much good." His other health issues remain stable, although he is scheduled for a prostate biopsy to further evaluate an elevated screening PSA test.

### Past Medical History

Dyslipidemia

Gastritis, s/p treatment for *Helicobacter pylori*

Generalized anxiety disorder (GAD), diagnosed at age 44 years, stable on medication therapy for 2 years

HTN

Seasonal allergic rhinitis

### Family History

Mother aged 79 years has diabetes and suffers from migraine HA. His father had an open prostatectomy for cancer at age 64 years, and died of a stroke at 84 years. His daughter, age 23 years, is treated for recurrent depression.

### Social History

He was divorced from his wife of 25 years 6 months prior to presentation. He is a retired naval aviator, currently an attorney. His only child is attending law school. He has few leisure or sports interests, though he used to be an avid golfer.

### Tobacco/Alcohol/Substance Use

He smokes 1/2–1 ppd of low-tar, filtered cigarettes. He has an occasional beer on weekends. He drinks 5–6 caffeinated beverages per day. No current or history of illicit drug use.

### Medication Allergies

Sulfa (rash)

## Medications

Acetaminophen 500 mg 1–2 PO PRN headache, to q 6 h ("I pop them around-the-clock.")

Benazepril 10 mg/HCTZ 12.5 mg PO q day

Cetirizine 10 mg PO PRN allergy symptoms q day

Escitalopram 10 mg PO q day

Meloxicam 7.5 mg PO PRN headache to q 12 h ("But 'when needed' means I'm using them everyday.")

Pantoprazole 20 mg PO q day

Simvastatin 40 mg PO q day

## Review of Systems

(+) Unintended weight loss of 5 lb (2.3 kg) over recent months. A recent optometric examination led to an adjustment in his lens prescription, but no evidence of glaucoma was noted. (–) Dizziness or vertigo with HAs reported. (+) Rhinorrhea in spring and autumn. (–) Chest pain or palpitations. (+) Morning "smoker's" cough, but (–) sputum production; (+) dyspnea with strenuous exertion. (–) Reflux complaints on daily antacid medication. (+) Nocturia once each night; (–) hesitancy or dribbling. (+) Left knee arthralgia associated with previous sports injury. (–) Lower extremity edema.

## Physical Examination

### ▸ General

Well-developed, anxious, middle-aged white male, in no acute distress

### ▸ Vital Signs

BP 132/84 mm Hg, HR 78, RR 20, T 37°C

Weight 189 lb (86 kg)

Height 70 in. (178 cm)

Pain 4/10, "mild" neck tenderness

### ▸ Skin

No rash or other lesions

### ▸ HEENT

PERRLA, EOMI, funduscopic examination benign, conjunctivae injected, nares with gray, boggy mucosa, (–) mucopurulent nasal discharge, external auditory canals and TMs clear, oropharynx without erythema, (–) temporal artery tenderness, occipital prominences tender bilaterally, without referred pain

### ▸ Neck and Lymph Nodes

Tender over trapezius without discrete trigger points, (–) stiffness with passive motion, thyroid without enlargement or nodularity, (–) carotid bruit, (–) JVP elevation, (–) adenopathy

### ▸ Chest

Minimal late expiratory wheezes bilaterally, resonant to percussion throughout

### ▸ Cardiovascular

RRR, (–) murmur or gallop

### ▸ Abdomen

Nontender, (–) organomegaly; normal bowel sounds

### ▸ Genitourinary/ Rectal

Examination deferred

### ▸ Neurology

Appears nervous, but not agitated. Alert and fully oriented. Cranial nerves intact. Motor and sensory examinations without focality. No cerebellar abnormalities. Speech and thought appropriate to situation.

## Laboratory Tests

### Nonfasting Obtained at PCP Office 2 Weeks Previously

|        | Conventional Units | SI Units            |
| ------ | ------------------ | ------------------- |
| Na     | 139 mEq/L          | 139 mmol/L          |
| K      | 4.2 mEq/L          | 4.2 mmol/L          |
| CL     | 102 mEq/L          | 102 mmol/L          |
| $CO_2$ | 24 mEq/L           | 24 mmol/L           |
| BUN    | 12 mg/dL           | 4.3 mmol/L          |
| SCr    | 0.9 mg/dL          | 80 mmol/L           |
| Glu    | 96 mg/dL           | 5.3 mmol/L          |
| Hgb    | 14.4 g/dL          | 144 g/L; 8.94 mmol/L |
| Hct    | 46.2%              | 0.462               |
| TSH    | 2.8 μIU/mL         | 2.8 mIU/L           |
| Urine toxicology | (+) cotinine |                 |

## Assessment

Chronic tension-type headache (TTH) with pericranial muscle tenderness complicated by analgesic medication overuse headache (MOH)

### Student Workup

**What clinical or diagnostic information is missing?**

**Evaluate:**  Patient Database Form

Drug Therapy Problem Worksheet

Pharmacotherapy Care Plan

## TARGETED QUESTIONS

1. What signs and symptoms allow the practitioner to differentiate this TTH syndrome from others, such as migraine HA or cluster headache?

   *Hint: See pp. 623–624 in PPP*

2. What lifestyle issues may be contributing to the development or perpetuation of HA symptoms in this patient, and what nonpharmacologic measures might be recommended to provide pain relief and HA prevention?

   *Hint: See p. 625 in PPP*

3. What medical comorbidities or medication therapies may be contributing to this patient's distress?

   *Hint: Uncontrolled HTN and poorly managed emotional distress can precipitate or potentiate HA. Sinusitis and rhinitis may present as HA, so these conditions should be fully addressed in people with HA. Many drugs list HA as an adverse treatment effect, so any newly added medication therapy should be suspected of contributing to HA pain.*

4. Will this patient require prophylactic pharmacologic treatment, as well as acute drug therapy?

   *Hint: See pp. 627–628 in PPP*

5. How will the practitioner assess the outcome of the interventions, assess the need for alterations or additions in the chosen treatment regimen?

   *Hint: See p. 630 in PPP*

## FOLLOW-UP

6. MRI of the patient's brain did not reveal any pathologic lesions, an ESR was within normal limits, and the prostate biopsy only demonstrated benign hyperplasia. Allergy testing revealed reactivity to household dust, and anti-allergy treatment was added with good symptomatic results. Concurrently, the patient was advised to wean caffeine intake and to seek talk therapy for stress reduction. He declined tobacco cessation assistance. An HA diary was completed by the patient, which identified the frequency and severity of his HAs, presumed precipitates and associated symptoms, and his symptomatic response to analgesics. It was believed that acetaminophen and NSAID overuse had "transformed" his episodic TTH into a chronic daily HA syndrome. His use of around-the-clock analgesics was discontinued and, to limit the development of withdrawal HAs, prednisone 50 mg PO per day was added with a rapid taper. He was provided an opiate compound for use, but was instructed that it should be reserved for debilitating pain only. To limit HA recurrence and to improve sleep, amitriptyline 10 mg PO per night was added, with an expected upward dosage titration based on tolerability and treatment benefit.

   If the patient had diabetes, how might this impact the choice of therapies? How can a practitioner tell if an anxiety disorder is adequately treated? What risks are assumed with the concurrent use of an SSRI and a TCA? How would one counsel a patient to monitor and to appropriately react to the development of this potential drug–drug interaction? What is an alternative prevention strategy in a patient who reports headache with muscle pain or stiffness? Are any HTN medications associated with the development or even prevention of headache?

## ☞ GLOBAL PERSPECTIVE

Headache is the most common condition seen by neurologists, and TTH is the most prevalent HA syndrome. More than 80% of individuals report having experienced a TTH. The episodic subtype predominates, though most of those affected experience infrequent HAs of mild to moderate intensity; the societal impact of TTH is much less than migraine. Heredity may play an important role in the development of the chronic TTH variant, which places a greater burden on the patient and the health care system. As with migraine, women predominate in chronic TTH cohorts. The peak incidence for TTH is in middle age, with some data suggesting that attacks diminish with age. The distribution of TTH among countries and populations of varying ethnic and socioeconomic groups has not identified clear distinctions, but there is some evidence to suggest that Caucasians in developed countries and those with advanced educational achievement are more prone to suffer from TTH. Complementary and alternative medicine approaches to HA treatment and prevention are more commonly employed in non-Western societies, with acupuncture demonstrating benefit in limiting headache frequency in clinical trials. Multiple herbal remedies, including feverfew, valerian, and chamomile are purported to have analgesic, antispasmodic, and anxiolytic properties that might be beneficial for TTH sufferers. Herbal therapies must be used cautiously when prescription drugs are employed, so as to avoid adverse pharmacokinetic or pharmacodynamic interactions, such as the cytochrome (CYP) and serotonin interactions with the concurrent use of St. John's wort and SSRIs.

## CASE SUMMARY

- The clinical presentation is most consistent with TTH, which, due to the frequency of attacks, more than two per week, meets the International Headache Society (IHS) criteria for chronicity; due to the presence of occipital and neck tenderness on manual palpation this pain syndrome can be more fully described as chronic TTH with pericranial tenderness.

- Given the patient's age, family history of prostate cancer, and his elevated PSA level, increase in pain severity, and analgesic refractoriness, neuroimaging is indicated: either a contrasted CT scan or an MRI.

- The daily use of analgesic agents may be complicating definitive diagnostic classification, as unrestrained pain medication use can transform episodic TTH into a chronic daily HA syndrome, the so-called MOH; analgesic withdrawal may be difficult and protracted in either chronic TTH or MOH cases.

- The patient's comorbidities and current medication use may complicate the choice of therapeutic options to limit HA frequency and severity, his HTN and use of an anxiolytic for instance. But they may also serve to direct drug and nonpharmacologic choices, so that the targeted HA therapies chosen benefit the other conditions as well, such as the use of a CCB for his HTN or stress-reducing massage therapy for his GAD.

**For more information on the care plan and facilitator's guide please visit http://www.mhpharmacotherapy.com.**

# 39 Alzheimer's Disease

Megan J. Ehret

## PATIENT PRESENTATION

### Chief Complaint

"I want to die. I hate forgetting all the important things."

### History of Present Illness

Barbara O'Neil is a 65-year-old woman who presents with her husband to the primary care clinic. She does not state any other information when asked what has brought her to the clinic for this visit. Her husband describes how over the past several months since their last visit, his wife has had increased memory loss. He notices that she frequently forgets to complete her normal daily activities, such as brushing her teeth, combing her hair, and getting dressed for the day. Several nights ago, he found her wandering down the street looking for their dog that passed away last month. When he tried to bring her home, she became tearful and withdrawn. Additionally, she has always taken her own medications without any help, but the pharmacy has been calling stating that she is late on her refills. He has found multiple bottles of unused medications in their bedroom. Over the past few months, their daughter has also mentioned that her mother appears depressed. She has noticed her decreased appetite, decreased concentration, and a lack of interest in her mother's favorite activities. The husband and daughter are wondering if the patient is suffering from depression.

### Past Medical History

Mild cognitive decline diagnosed 6 months ago

HTN

Type 2 DM

Hyperlipidemia

### Family History

Mother had dementia and died of pneumonia at age 85. Father died of a MI at age 73. She has one brother, age 62, with HTN and diabetes.

### Social History

Married and lives with her husband of 40 years; has one daughter aged 35; retired grade-school teacher

### Tobacco/Alcohol/Substance Use

Thirty-three pack-year history; denies alcohol and illicit drug use

### Allergies/Intolerance/Adverse Drug Events

Enalapril (cough)

Galantamine (N/V); she self-discontinued the medication at 8 mg twice daily

## Medications (Current)

Amlodipine 10 mg PO daily

Metformin 750 mg PO twice daily

Atorvastatin 20 mg PO daily

Multivitamin PO daily

Calcium carbonate 600 mg PO twice daily

## Review of Systems

Appears tearful and unable to answer many questions during the mental status examination; (–) history of seizures, head injuries, or loss of consciousness; (+) loss of appetite

## Physical Examination

### ▶ General

Mildly disheveled African American woman who is slightly tearful

### ▶ Vital Signs

BP 140/90 mm Hg, P 70, RR 14, T 36.4°C

Weight 145 lb (65.9 kg)

Height 68 in. (173 cm)

Denies any physical pain

### ▶ Skin

Moist skin; (–) rashes or lesions

### ▶ HEENT

PERRLA, EOMI; (–) sinus tenderness, TMs appear normal

### ▶ Neck and Lymph Nodes

Normal

### ▶ Chest

Clear to auscultation

### ▶ Breasts

Examination deferred

### ▶ Cardiovascular

RRR, normal $S_1$, $S_2$, (–) $S_3$ or $S_4$

### ▶ Abdomen

Not tender/not distended; (–) organomegaly

### ▶ Neurology

Folstein Mini-Mental Status Examination Score (MMSE) 20/30; unable to count backward from 100 by 7, recalled one out of three items; unable to read paper and follow command; unable to make up a sentence and write it; unable to copy a picture; poor registration with impaired attention and short-term memory

### ▶ Psychiatry

Tearful expression, mood congruent; (–) auditory and visual hallucinations; (–) delusion; (+) suicidal ideations

### ▶ Genitourinary

Examination deferred

### ▶ Rectal

Examination deferred

## Laboratory Tests

CT scan: Mild-to-moderate generalized cerebral atrophy

|  | Conventional Units | SI Units |
|---|---|---|
| Na | 140 mEq/L | 140 mmol/L |
| K | 4.2 mEq/L | 4.2 mmol/L |
| Cl | 100 mEq/L | 100 mmol/L |
| $CO_2$ | 24 mEq/L | 24 mmol/L |
| BUN | 8 mg/dL | 2.9 mmol/L |
| SCr | 0.9 mg/dL | 80 μmol/L |
| Glu | 150 mg/dL | 8.3 mmol/L |
| Vitamin $B_{12}$ | 600 pg/mL | 443 pmol/L |
| Total cholesterol | 240 mg/dL | 6.21 mmol/L |
| LDL cholesterol | 200 mg/dL | 5.17 mmol/L |
| HDL cholesterol | 30 mg/dL | 0.78 mmol/L |
| Triglycerides | 210 mg/dL | 2.37 mmol/L |
| ALT | 20 IU/L | 0.33 μkat/L |
| AST | 18 IU/L | 0.30 μkat/L |
| TSH | 3.1 μIU/mL | 3.1 mIU/L |
| Free $T_4$ | 1.1 ng/dL | 14.2 pmol/L |

## Assessment

Sixty-five-year-old woman with s/s, and laboratory tests consistent with Alzheimer's disease and depression

## Student Workup

### Missing Information?

**Evaluate:**  Patient Database

Drug Therapy Problems

Care Plan (by Problem)

## TARGETED QUESTIONS

1. What signs and symptoms of Alzheimer's disease does the patient have?

   *Hint: See pp. 530–531 in PPP*

2. What s/s of depression does the patient have?

   *Hint: Differentiating between depression and dementia can be difficult, so symptoms of depression should be documented for several months prior to the initiation of therapy for the treatment of de pression with Alzheimer's disease. Signs of depression that the patient displays, which make her a candidate for therapy for depression, include suicidal thoughts, anhedonia, withdrawal from activities, and a poor appetite. See p. 679 in PPP*

3. Why is a cholinesterase inhibitor in conjunction with nonpharmacologic strategies the treatment of choice for most patients with Alzheimer's disease?

   *Hint: See pp. 532–533 in PPP*

4. What are indications for the use of antidepressants in the treatment of depression with dementia?

   *Hint: See pp. 536–537 in PPP*

5. What risks and adverse effects of therapy would you discuss with the patient?

   *Hint: See pp. 533–535 in PPP*

## FOLLOW-UP

6. Four weeks later, the patient returns for a follow-up. She feels somewhat better, with more energy, but still some symptoms of sadness. Her MMSE score is 22/30. Why did her MMSE score not improve more? What actions would you take regarding the residual depressive symptoms and the MMSE score?

   *Hint: See pp. 534–536 in PPP*

## GLOBAL PERSPECTIVE

Overall prevalence rates for dementia have been reported to be substantially higher for African Americans than for Caucasians. Studies have demonstrated prevalence rates from 14% to 500% higher for African Americans than for Caucasians. Preliminary evidence has shown that the relative contributions of several genetic risk factors for the Alzheimer's-type dementia at a molecular level appear to differ between African Americans and Caucasians, particularly with regard to APOE-ε4, which is a potent risk factor in Caucasians, but not in African Americans. However, potential flaws in the research design of the studies may have led to the increased prevalence rates. Cultural factors have led to a relative over-reporting of cognitive disability in studies with African Americans, which have utilized self-report or caregiver report of cognitive functioning. Additionally, some investigators have proposed that the lower mean educational level of African American study subjects may account for the difference in cognitive test scores achieved by the older African-American sample versus the Caucasian sample. Research into the actual difference in prevalence rates may affect the clinical practice and future policy planning in the treatment of dementia worldwide.

## CASE SUMMARY

- Her current clinical picture is consistent with mild-to-early stage Alzheimer's disease. Cholinesterase inhibitor therapy should be reinitiated.

- She also has a clinical picture consistent with a major depressive episode, which meets criteria for treatment with an antidepressant.

**For more information on the care plan and facilitator's guide please visit http://www.mhpharmacotherapy.com.**

# Alcohol Withdrawal

Krina H. Patel

## CASE LEARNING OBJECTIVES

- Identify signs and symptoms associated with alcohol withdrawal
- Recommend appropriate agents for the treatment of alcohol withdrawal on the basis of specific individualized needs
- Design a comprehensive treatment plan and monitoring program to treat alcohol withdrawal, prevent relapse, and maintain abstinence

## PATIENT PRESENTATION

### Chief Complaint

"My son needs help, he is really sick. He is really shaky and nervous, and he has also been vomiting since last night!"

### History of Present Illness

Michael Jones is a 23-year-old male who has a history of alcoholism. His father died 6 months ago and since then he has been drinking on a daily basis. The patient's family states that he is not the same. Recently he has been extremely pessimistic about life, is generally sad, and only gets out of his bed to drink. His mother is getting really frustrated because it has now been 6 months and the patient has still not accepted his father's death and continues to drink. Yesterday afternoon the patient's mother and sister got into an argument with him regarding his drinking. He is tired of all the nagging and wanted to show them that he does not need alcohol and therefore he stopped drinking.

### Past Medical History

Perennial allergies × 4 years

Chronic pain × 6 months

Alcohol dependence × 3 years

Bipolar disorder I × 4 years

### Family History

Father died at the age of 49 due to a motor vehicle accident. Mother is 51 and has a diagnosis of HTN, generalized anxiety disorder, and migraine. He has an older brother and younger sister; both are healthy.

### Social History

The patient has a history of alcohol dependence for 3 years. He had been sober for the past 2 years until recent death of his father. The patient and father were in a motor vehicle accident. The patient survived, but father did not. Currently, he lives with mother and 2 siblings. He is an elementary school teacher; however, he has not worked since the accident.

### Tobacco/Alcohol/Substance Use

Denies tobacco use; drinks one bottle (750 mL) of vodka daily; occasional illicit drug use (marijuana); denies abuse of prescription medications

### Allergies/Intolerances/Adverse Drug Events

None

### Medications (Prior to Admission)

Cetirizine 10 mg PO daily

Acetaminophen 500 mg PO every 4–6 hours PRN pain

Lithium carbonate 300 mg PO in morning and 600 mg at bedtime

### Review of Systems

(−) Chest pain, (−) palpitations, (+) nausea and vomiting since last drink, (+) decreased appetite for past 3 months; (+) tremors, appeared about 6 hours after last drink, (−) seizures; (+) anxiety since last drink, (−) hallucinations, (+) headache

### Physical Examination

▶ *General*

Twenty-three-year-old Caucasian male who appears malnourished and thin. Presents with signs of acute distress.

The patient is alert and oriented, and is cooperative with clear speech.

▶ **Vital Signs**

BP 147/98 mm Hg, P 114, RR 20, T 37°C

Weight 120 lb (54.5 kg)

Height 67 in. (170 cm)

Pain level 0/10

▶ **Skin**

Moist, (−) rash, (−) pruritus

▶ **HEENT**

PERRLA, EOMI

▶ **Neck and Lymph Nodes**

(−) Lymphadenopathy

▶ **Chest**

Lung auscultation clear, (−) crackles, rhonchi, or wheezing

▶ **Cardiovascular**

Tachycardic, RRR, (−) murmurs

▶ **Abdomen**

Normal bowel sounds, (+) enlarged liver, (−) abdominal pain

▶ **Neurology**

Alert and oriented × 3; tremulous; DTRs normal; CN II to XII intact

▶ **Extremities**

(+) Tremors in fingers and hands

▶ **Genitourinary**

Examination deferred

▶ **Rectal**

Examination deferred

## Laboratory Tests

|  | Conventional Units | SI Units |
|---|---|---|
| Na | 137 mEq/L | 137 mmol/L |
| K | 3.5 mEq/L | 3.5 mmol/L |
| Cl | 101 mEq/L | 101 mmol/L |
| $CO_2$ | 23 mEq/L | 23 mmol/L |
| BUN | 9 mg/dL | 3.2 mmol/L |
| SCr | 0.8 mg/dL | 71 μmol/L |
| CrCl | 110 mL/min | 1.84 mL/s |
| Glu | 99 mg/dL | 5.5 mmol/L |
| Ca | 9.0 mg/dL | 2.25 mmol/L |
| Mg | 1.6 mEq/L | 0.80 mmol/L |
| Phosphate | 2.5 mg/dL | 0.81 mmol/L |
| Albumin | 3.5 g/dL | 35 g/L |
| PT | 12.0 s | |
| Platelet | $200 \times 10^3/mm^3$ | $200 \times 109/mm^3$ |
| GGT | 122 IU/L | 2.03 μkat/L |
| LDH | 200 IU/L | 3.33 μkat/L |
| AST | 250 IU/L | 4.17 μkat/L |
| ALT | 123 IU/L | 2.05 μkat/L |
| Alk phos | 41 IU/L | 0.68 μkat/L |
| Total bilirubin | 0.7 mg/dL | 12.0 μmol/L |
| Direct bilirubin | 0.2 mg/L | 3.4 μmol/L |
| Ammonia | 35 mcg/dL | 21 μmol/L |
| Lithium | 0.3 mEq/L | 0.3 mmol/L |

## Assessment

Twenty-three-year-old male with history and current signs, symptoms, and laboratory tests consistent with alcohol withdrawal

### Student Workup

**Missing Information?**

**Evaluate:**    Patient Database

Drug Therapy Problems

Care Plan (by Problem)

## TARGETED QUESTIONS

1. What signs and symptoms of alcohol withdrawal is this patient presenting with?

   *Hint: See Table 36-4 in PPP*

2. How should alcohol withdrawal be managed for this patient?

   *Hint: See pp. 642–644 in PPP*

3. What are some risks of not appropriately managing alcohol withdrawal?

   *Hint: See pp. 643–644 in PPP*

4. What psychiatric symptoms does this patient present with? How does this psychiatric illness relate to alcohol dependence?

   *Hint: The patient is presenting with symptoms of depression. The patient appears to have cycled into an acute depressive episode. The prevalence of psychiatric illnesses among the substance-abuse population is quite high. Many patients who have bipolar disorder also have coexisting alcohol dependence. Additionally, alcohol may be a secondary cause for inducing depression. See Chapter 39 Bipolar Disorder in PPP.*

## FOLLOW-UP

5. A few days later, the patient is doing much better and free of all withdrawal symptoms. However, the patient does mention that he is still experiencing the urge to go out and drink once he is released from the hospital. He states his intention is not to drink; however, he is not sure if can abstain from alcohol. What nonpharmacologic and pharmacologic treatment option would you recommend for this patient?

*Hint: See pp. 646–649 in PPP*

## 🌐 GLOBAL PERSPECTIVE

Substance-related disorders, such as alcohol dependence, are quite prevalent not only in the United States but also in countries around the world. There are some cultures that do tend to have a lower prevalence rate of alcoholism, such as in certain Asian countries. It is believed that genetically determined aldehyde dehydrogenase deficiency might be the reason for the lower prevalence rate among Asian populations. Patients with this type of deficiency may refrain from alcohol intake due to the unwanted effects, such as facial flushing and palpitations, which may occur with alcohol intake. Western countries, in general, tend to have a higher prevalence rate of alcohol dependence. One of the populations in the United States that tends to have a higher prevalence rate of alcohol dependence is the male Latino population. Overall, genetic, environmental, and cultural factors play a significant role in the difference of prevalence rates among different countries and cultures.

## CASE SUMMARY

- The patient should be treated for alcohol withdrawal since he is exhibiting signs and symptoms of withdrawal.
- Benzodiazepine treatment should be initiated for alcohol withdrawal. In addition, this patient should also receive thiamine supplementation.

**For more information on the care plan and facilitator's guide please visit http://www.mhpharmacotherapy.com.**

# 41 Schizophrenia

Heidi J. Wehring        Deanna L. Kelly

## CASE LEARNING OBJECTIVES

- Recognize the signs and symptoms of schizophrenia and be able to distinguish among positive, negative, and cognitive symptoms of the illness
- Identify the treatment goals for a patient with schizophrenia
- Recommend appropriate antipsychotic medications using patient-specific data
- Develop an appropriate treatment and monitoring plan for the treatment of symptoms of schizophrenia
- Educate a patient about antipsychotic medications and the importance of adherence to the treatment

## PATIENT PRESENTATION

### Chief Complaint

"I'm being poisoned because I'm going to be a TV star."

### History of Present Illness

Carla Lee is a 24-year-old woman who presents to the clinic after being brought in by a family member. Her family has noted that she has become more withdrawn within the past 8 months, and she rarely comes out of her room at the family home. CL has been seen muttering to herself for the past 6 weeks and when questioned, has been telling family members that her "TV agent" has been talking to her all day and all night. By her own report, she is not sleeping as much as usual so that she can get through these important conferences with her agent. CL's family has become worried since she has been refusing to eat food in the family home. She has been suspicious of all the food that her mother cooks, and complains that her mother and others in the house may be trying to poison her food due to their jealousy over her upcoming celebrity status. She now refuses to eat any food that is not prepackaged or shrink-wrapped, and has started complaining that even that is not a guarantee that her food has not been altered. CL recently lost her job as a clerk at a convenience store because she missed too many shifts. Other employees saw her as disruptive since she would carry on conversations, apparently with herself, while ringing up customers. CL stated that she used to like to work at the store, but lately she has noticed people staring at her and talking about her. She attributes this to their jealousy about her role in the TV show *The Carla Show* which is all about her life. CL presents as unkempt and malodorous, wearing several different layers of clothes and a large hat, which she refuses to take off since it is keeping her fans from recognizing her. She has not showered for several days and has not brought along the correct medical paperwork, although she has brought along her journal, which she uses to track her thoughts for script ideas. Although she complains of being thirsty, she refuses a drink of water as the paper cup may have been tampered with.

### Past Medical History

CL has a history of acne in adolescence, which was treated with oral antibiotics from age 17 to 19. She has been treated for GERD in the past year, first with ranitidine and most currently with esomeprazole, with reportedly good symptom control. She is also prescribed an oral contraceptive and occasionally, she takes desloratadine 5 mg daily as needed for allergic rhinitis.

### Family History

CL's mother and one of her maternal aunts have type 2 DM, and her paternal grandfather reportedly suffered from an unspecified mental illness.

### Social History

CL is a single, never-married female who lives in her mother's house. She reportedly had some friends and a boyfriend in high school, but over the past several years, she has been seeing fewer people socially, which does not seem to bother her. CL was a good student in high school and completed several years at a local college before seeming to lose interest in her studies. She left college and worked a series of jobs before the most recent position as a clerk in a convenience store.

## Tobacco/Alcohol/Substance Use

Social drinker, generally 1–2 beers once weekly, although she denies any intake in past month; smokes 1 ppd of cigarettes since age 16; history of illicit drug use (marijuana)

## Allergies/Intolerances/Adverse Drug Events

Intolerance to tetracycline due to GI upset and diarrhea

## Medications (Current)

Esomeprazole 20 mg PO daily

Norethindrone and ethinyl estradiol 1 mg/20 mcg PO daily

Desloratadine 5 mg PO daily as needed

Admits to missing doses of her medications "here and there"

## Review of Systems

(–) History of head injury or loss of consciousness; (–) tinnitus, vertigo, or infections; (–) history of seizures or syncope

## Physical Examination

### ▶ General

Disheveled and unkempt, young adult woman in no acute distress

### ▶ Vital Signs

BP 110/84 mm Hg, P 74, RR 14, T 36.8°C

Weight 131 lb (59.5 kg)

Height 64 in. (163 cm)

Denies pain

### ▶ Skin

Dry-appearing skin and scalp; (–) rashes or lesions

### ▶ HEENT

PERRLA, EOMI

### ▶ Neck and Lymph Nodes

(–) Thyroid nodules; (–) lymphadenopathy; (–) carotid bruits

### ▶ Chest

Clear to auscultation

### ▶ Breasts

Examination deferred

### ▶ Cardiovascular

RRR, normal $S_1$, $S_2$

### ▶ Abdomen

Not tender, not distended; (–) organomegaly

### ▶ Neurology

Grossly intact; DTRs normal

### ▶ Genitourinary

Examination deferred

### ▶ Rectal

Examination deferred

## Laboratory Tests

### Fasting Obtained 2 days ago

|  | Conventional Units | SI Units |
|---|---|---|
| Na | 146 mEq/L | 146 mmol/L |
| K | 4.8 mEq/L | 4.8 mmol/L |
| Cl | 102 mEq/L | 102 mmol/L |
| $CO_2$ | 24 mEq/L | 24 mmol/L |
| BUN | 9 mg/dL | 3.2 mmol/L |
| SCr | 0.9 mg/dL | 80 μmol/L |
| Glu | 98 mg/dL | 5.4 mmol/L |
| Ca | 9.6 mg/dL | 2.40 mmol/L |
| Mg | 1.6 mEq/L | 0.80 mmol/L |
| Phosphate | 4.1 mg/dL | 1.32 mmol/L |
| Hgb | 12.7 g/dL (127 g/L) | 7.88 mmol/L |
| Hct | 40.3% | 0.403 |
| WBC | $5.6 \times 10^3$/mm³ | $5.6 \times 10^9$/L |
| MCV | 80 μm³ | 80 fL |
| Albumin | 4.3 g/dL | 43 g/L |
| TSH | 2.4 μIU/mL | 2.4 mIU/L |
| Total cholesterol | 195 mg/dL | 5.04 mmol/L |

## Mental Status Examination

CL is a 24-year-old female of average build, appearing stated age, disheveled, unkempt, malodorous, and wearing inappropriately layered clothes. She is somewhat guarded in conversation, but will answer questions when asked. Eye contact is sporadic and she seems to be distracted by and responding to internal stimuli periodically throughout the interview. CL describes her mood as "just fine." Her range of affect is somewhat blunted, though appropriate. She is alert and oriented to person, place, and time. Intellectual functioning appears average, although, at times, it is difficult to assess due to her tendency to become distracted during the interview. Thought processes are coherent and goal directed; however, her conclusions that people are trying to poison her and her belief in her impending fame are illogical. Prominent delusions are apparent, including her belief that people want to poison her and that she is starring in her own television series. CL endorses auditory hallucinations of hearing the voice of her

"TV agent." She denies suicidal or homicidal ideation. Her insight and judgment are poor.

## Assessment

Twenty-four-year-old woman with signs and symptoms consistent with a psychotic disorder such as schizophrenia

### Student Workup

**Missing Information?**

**Evaluate:**     Patient Database

Drug Therapy Problems

Care Plan (by Problem)

## TARGETED QUESTIONS

1. What signs and symptoms of schizophrenia does the patient have?

   *Hint: See pp. 656–658 in PPP*

2. What will be the goals of treatment for CL?

   *Hint: See pp. 658–659 in PPP*

3. What types of nonpharmacologic interventions should be implemented in the treatment plan for a person with schizophrenia?

   *Hint: See pp. 659–660 in PPP*

4. What first-line pharmacologic options are available for the treatment of CL's symptoms of psychosis?

   *Hint: See pp. 660–664 in PPP*

5. Which of the options from above would you recommend for CL, including titration schedule and monitoring plan?

   *Hint: See Tables 37-2 in PPP*

6. What risks and adverse effects of therapy would you discuss with the patient?

   *Hint: See pp. 660–664 and Table 37-3 in PPP*

## FOLLOW-UP

Three months later after CL's initial visit and her formal diagnosis of schizophrenia, she returns for follow-up. You learn that in the 2 weeks following her initial visit, CL's symptoms exacerbated to the point that she was hospitalized. During this time, the regimen you selected was discontinued and a regimen of quetiapine 100 mg 3 times daily was implemented. CL has now been prescribed this regimen for approximately 2 months. She is complaining that she still hears her agent talking to her and still feels somewhat paranoid about her family. She is upset about the fact that she has gained 12 lb (5.5 kg), and admits to missing several doses of the medication every week because it is hard for her to remember taking the medication several times a day. She states that if she keeps gaining weight, she will stop taking the medication completely.

7. What reason(s) may be contributing to CL's continuing symptoms?

   *Hint: See pp. 662, 666 in PPP*

8. What action would you take?

   *Hint: See Table 37-3 in PPP*

## GLOBAL PERSPECTIVE

Schizophrenia is a disorder that is present worldwide. However, when assessing for the signs and symptoms of schizophrenia (delusions, hallucinations, etc.), it is important to take cultural and religious beliefs into consideration as what is considered within the norm for a certain ethnic group may not be considered within normal limits for another group also. Differences in response to antipsychotic treatment may exist due to differences in genetic makeup of persons with schizophrenia, from both an efficacy and adverse effect standpoint, although information is limited. Antipsychotic medications are the treatment of choice for schizophrenia; however, the particular agents available in various countries may differ. In addition, the treatment algorithms may differ widely depending on the location of treatment.

## CASE SUMMARY

- CL's current clinical picture is consistent with the symptoms of schizophrenia and warrants treatment with antipsychotic medication.

- An initial second-generation antipsychotic such as aripiprazole, risperidone, quetiapine, or ziprasidone at appropriate doses would be appropriate for the treatment of CL's symptoms.

- Upon her representation to the clinic 3 months later, either an increase in dose of quetiapine (≤800 mg) or switching to an antipsychotic that may offer once-daily dosing and a lower weight gain burden (such as aripiprazole or risperidone) would be appropriate.

**For more information on the care plan and facilitator's guide please visit http://www.mhpharmacotherapy.com.**

# 42 Depression

Cherry W. Jackson

## CASE LEARNING OBJECTIVES

- Identify the symptoms and clinical features of major depressive disorder
- Outline the goals of therapy for depression
- Develop an appropriate treatment plan for a patient with depression on the basis of individual patient characteristics
- Educate patients and caregivers on the proper use of antidepressants

## PATIENT PRESENTATION

### Chief Complaint

"I can't keep living like this."

### History of Present Illness

Melvin Collie is a 36-year-old male who presents to the primary care clinic for the management of his depression. He was diagnosed with major depressive disorder (MDD) by his primary care physician and is presenting for initiation of medication treatment. During the past month, he experienced a depressed mood, anhedonia, poor sleep and appetite, isolative behavior, and crying spells. In addition, he reports having a passive death wish. There have been no precipitating events and he states "I felt like this two years ago." He states that he initially took an over-the-counter medication for depression, but it did not work. He states that at that point he went to see his physician; he diagnosed him with depression and he has been taking sertraline 50 mg faithfully since then. He states that initially he felt better, but then the medication seemed to stop working and his original symptoms returned. He also states that his friend said that she gained weight on her antidepressant and that he does not want to take any medications that will make him gain weight.

### Past Medical History

Depression diagnosed 2 years ago

Tonsillectomy age 14 years

Right-knee arthroscopy in 2002

### Family History

Mother suffers from depression, and alcohol and cocaine dependence. Father died from suicide at age 57 years.

### Social History

Thirty-six-year-old male who is divorced. Has one son in high school. Works in sales at a local business.

### Tobacco/Alcohol/Substance Abuse

Smokes 1½ packs of cigarettes per week; recently increased alcohol intake (6–8 beers daily); no current illicit drug use, smoked marijuana in high school

### Allergies/Intolerances/Adverse Drug Events

Penicillin (pruritus, last exposure at age 4)

### Medications (Current)

Tramadol ER 100 mg daily for low back pain

Centrum multivitamin one tablet PO daily

Sertraline 50 mg PO daily

Ibuprofen 200 mg two tablets PO as needed for pain

### Prior Medication Use

St. John's wort 300 mg PO tid for 3 months, with no effect

### Review of Systems

Chronic low back pain, currently using ibuprofen 200 mg two tablets as needed for pain, and tramadol ER 100 mg daily for low back pain. Depressed mood, anhedonia, poor sleep and appetite, isolative behavior, crying spells, and suicidal ideation.

### Physical Examination

▶ *Vital Signs*

BP 130/87 mm Hg, P 70, RR 12, T 36.0°C

Weight 217 lb (98.6 kg)

Height 68 in. (173 cm)

Chronic low back pain

Physical examination 2 days ago by primary care physician was entirely normal and is not repeated today.

## Mental Status Examination

▶ *Appearance*

The patient is a 36-year-old white male, who appears older than stated age; clothing is wrinkled and dirty. Hair appears disheveled.

▶ *Movement/Behavior*

The patient has poor eye contact and is intermittently tearful. (+) Psychomotor retardation.

▶ *Speech*

The patient has slow rate and prosody, and he speaks very softly. He was asked to repeat answers several times because of the volume. He clearly understands the questions, and his answers are appropriate.

▶ *Affect*

Restricted, tearful.

▶ *Mood*

"Sad." The patient appears withdrawn and isolative. He reports poor sleep and appetite as well as anhedonia.

▶ *Thought content*

The patient denies paranoia, delusions, hallucinations, obsessions, compulsions, or strange impulses. He reports thinking about his father's suicide. He states that it used to make him angry, but now he understands why he did it. He reports having a passive death wish. He does not have a plan to commit suicide at this time.

▶ *Thought process*

The patient is logical and coherent, but has some thought blocking.

▶ *Cognition*

A + O × 3. The patient has poor concentration, and is tearful and distracted throughout the interview, but he could perform serial 7s. His memory is intact. He has average intellect, evidenced by his response to the interviewer, but not thoroughly assessed. Abstract reasoning is intact, evidenced by, How are an apple and orange similar? "Both are fruit." Different? "One is red and one is orange, they taste different, and they grow in different parts of the country."

▶ *Judgment/Insight*

The patient has some understanding of his illness. He has poor insight and judgment, feeling that "suicide may be the only way out."

## Laboratory Tests

| | Conventional Units | SI Units |
|---|---|---|
| Na | 140 mEq/L | 140 mmol/L |
| K | 3.9 mEq/L | 3.9 mmol/L |
| Cl | 103 mEq/L | 103 mmol/L |
| $CO_2$ | 24 mEq/L | 24 mmol/L |
| BUN | 11 mg/dL | 3.9 mmol/L |
| SCr | 0.93 mg/dL | 82 µmol/L |
| Glu | 72 mg/dL | 4.0 mmol/L |
| Ca | 9.7 mg/dL | 2.43 mmol/L |
| Mg | 2.4 mEq/L | 1.20 mmol/L |
| Phosphate | 4.3 mg/dL | 1.39 mmol/L |
| Hgb | 14.3 g/dL | 8.88 mmol/L (143 g/L) |
| Hct | 42.6% | 0.426 |
| WBC | $4.0 \times 10^3/mm^3$ | $4.0 \times 10^9/L$ |
| MCV | $90.6 \ \mu m^3$ | 90.6 fL |
| Albumin | 4.6 g/dL | 46 g/L |
| Total cholesterol | 191 mg/dL | 4.94 mmol/L |
| LDL cholesterol | 83 mg/dL | 2.15 mmol/L |
| HDL cholesterol | 97 mg/dL | 2.51 mmol/L |

## Assessment

36-year-old man with symptoms indicative of major depressive disorder (MDD)

### Student Workup

**Missing Information?**

**Evaluate:**      Patient Database

Drug Therapy Problems

Care Plan (by Problem)

## TARGETED QUESTIONS

1. What symptoms and clinical features of MDD does the patient have?

   *Hint: See p. 679 in PPP*

2. What is the time course of response for antidepressant therapy and what is the response rate with antidepressants?

   *Hint: See p. 687 in PPP*

3. What medication therapy might the patient use to treat chronic low back pains and depression?

   *Hint: See p. 615 in PPP*

4. How do you treat partial response to an antidepressant?

   *Hint: See pp. 687, 689 in PPP*

5. What risks and adverse effects of antidepressants would you discuss with the patient?

   *Hint: See pp. 687–689 in PPP*

## What If's?

6. What if the patient complained of sexual dysfunction with his antidepressant?

   *Hint: See Table 38-3 in PPP*

7. What if the patient was a female and was receiving Ortho Tri-Cyclen Lo in addition to St. John's wort?

   *Hint: See p. 682 in PPP*

8. What if the patient was taking an SSRI and needed to be transitioned to an MAOI?

   *Hint: See pp. 685–686 in PPP*

9. What if the patient was initiated on Robitussin DM for cough?

   *Hint: See Table 38-6 in PPP*

10. What if the patient was concerned about all of the media attention about antidepressants making you "want to kill yourself"?

    *Hint: See pp. 682–683 in PPP*

## ☉ GLOBAL PERSPECTIVE

Depression is a common mental disorder that presents with depressed mood, loss of interest or pleasure, feelings of guilt or low self-worth, disturbed sleep or appetite, low energy, and poor concentration. These problems can become chronic or recurrent, and may lead to substantial impairment in an individual's ability to take care of his or her everyday responsibilities. At its worst, depression can lead to suicide, with the loss of about 850,000 lives every year.

Depression in the year 2000 was the leading cause of disability worldwide as measured by years lived with disability (YLD) and the fourth leading contributor to the global burden of disease on the basis of disability-adjusted life-years (DALYs).[1] By the year 2020, depression is projected to reach second place of the ranking of DALYs calculated for all ages, both sexes. Today, depression is already the second cause of DALYs worldwide in the age category 15–44 years for both sexes combined. According to the World Health Organization, fewer than 25% of depressed patients have access to care and in some countries, fewer than 10%. Barriers to effective care include the lack of resources, lack of trained providers, and the social stigma associated with mental disorders, including depression.

## REFERENCE

1. World Health Organization. www.who.int/mental_health/management/depression/definition/en/index1.html. Accessed February 20, 2013.

## CASE SUMMARY

- The patient's clinical picture is consistent with MDD, and an antidepressant medication should be used.
- Sertraline 50 mg is a reasonable initial dose, but the dose needed is to be maximized to a therapeutic dose, especially in the case of partial response.
- Tricyclic antidepressants are one of the treatments of choice for chronic migraine and should be considered in patients who need treatment for both chronic migraine and depression.

**For more information on the care plan and facilitator's guide please visit http://www.mhpharmacotherapy.com.**

# 43 Bipolar Disorder

Brian L. Crabtree

- Recognize the signs and symptoms of an acute manic episode and bipolar disorder
- Identify the goals of therapy for an acute manic episode and bipolar disorder
- Develop an appropriate treatment and monitoring plan for the pharmacotherapy of bipolar disorder using a specific patient presentation
- Educate a patient on taking medications for bipolar disorder

## PATIENT PRESENTATION

### Chief Complaint

"My mind's going too fast."

### History of Present Illness

Lisa Walking is a 34-year-old woman who has been admitted to a psychiatric hospital. She was brought to the hospital by her husband after she stopped sleeping, would stay up all night praying, could not be redirected, and would say simply, "I am communicating with God." The husband reports LW had become more agitated during the past week with rapid speech, irritability, and now bizarre ideas about special powers and abilities. He indicates that "she explodes, anything sets her off, she was talking to people who are not there and has been hitting herself." She has poor insight into why she was brought to the hospital, but states, "I have problems with nerves and I don't sleep." She is seen on team rounds by a psychiatrist, nurse, pharmacist, psychologist, and social worker.

### Past Medical History

LW had all of the usual childhood illnesses.

She has a history of psychiatric illness with four hospitalizations dating to 1990, but this is the first admission to this hospital and none of the previous records are immediately available. She is followed on an outpatient basis at a community mental health center.

She has a history of HTN. The husband reports that the patient had "low blood" on her previous medication and this was one reason she stopped taking it.

### Family History

Father healthy, except HTN, well controlled on medication. Mother has depression, takes paroxetine. She has three siblings, two brothers and one sister. One brother is alcoholic. She has no children.

### Social History

Married, lives with husband. Unemployed; worked previously as a checkout clerk at a supermarket, but has not worked in over a year. High school graduate, but has difficulty with reading and writing. Receives supplemental security income payments and supported by husband. Receives Medicaid coverage. No pending legal problems. No special diet. No regular exercise program.

### Tobacco/Alcohol/Substance Use

Occasional binge-drinking episodes. Smokes 1 ppd with approximately 20 pack-year history. Denies illicit substances. Drinks several cups of caffeinated coffee daily.

### Allergies/Intolerances/Adverse Drug Events

Diazepam (nausea and vomiting after injection) during a previous hospitalization.

### Medications

Paroxetine 20 mg PO daily × 3 months, started during previous hospitalization

Clonazepam 0.5 mg PO three times daily × 3 months, started during previous hospitalization

HCTZ 25 mg PO daily × 4 years

Acetaminophen 500 mg PO as needed, about twice weekly

Previously treated with olanzapine 20 mg PO at bedtime, divalproex 750 mg PO twice daily, stopped approximately 3 months prior to current admission. Denies other prescription and nonprescription medication

Denies herbal or other complementary and alternative therapies

## Review of Systems

The patient states she feels "energized" and is impatient with people who do not listen to her ideas. (–) Headaches or dizziness, but states dizziness was a problem when she was taking divalproex. No history of asthma or other lung disease. Says she had a TB skin test recently, but does not know results. (–) Chest pain, palpitations, or heart disease other than HTN. Appetite has been less lately. "I don't need to eat. God will provide." Denies weight loss. (–) Genitourinary complaints. Says some of the medications interfere with her sex drive. Has regular menses. (–) History of sexually transmitted diseases. (–) Neuromuscular complaints. Says, "Strength is getting better every day."

## Physical Examination

### ▶ General

Well-developed, well-nourished Caucasian female in no acute distress; appears stated age, disheveled, and mildly obese

### ▶ Vital Signs

BP 154/105 mm Hg sitting, P 102, RR 22, T 97.9°F (36.6°C)

Weight 197 lb (89.5 kg)

Height 66 in. (168 cm)

Denies pain

### ▶ Skin

Unremarkable

### ▶ HEENT

PERRLA, EOMI, periorbital bruising apparent; discs sharp, AV nicking noted; TMs normal, normal hearing to conversational volume; several missing teeth, poor oral hygiene

### ▶ Neck and Lymph Nodes

Supple; (–) thyromegaly, JVD, or lymphadenopathy

### ▶ Chest

Clear to auscultation

### ▶ Breasts

No tenderness, no lumps or masses, no discharge

### ▶ Cardiovascular

Tachycardia, RRR, no murmurs, rubs, or gallops

### ▶ Abdomen

Nontender, nondistended, (+) bowel sounds, (–) hepatosplenomegaly

### ▶ Neurology

Mental status—behavior is childlike, mood is elevated and irritable, affect is animated; speech is loud and pressured; thoughts indicate flight of ideas, looseness of associations, ideas of reference, delusions; reports she feels others plot against her because of jealousy over her superior intellectual and physical powers and her ability to receive special messages from God; denies auditory and visual hallucinations; denies suicidal and homicidal ideas; alert and oriented to person, year, not place; shows deficits in long- and short-term memory; concentration poor; judgment poor; insight poor.

Cranial nerves II to XII grossly intact; normal gait; (–) nystagmus, facial weakness, tremor; DTRs normal.

### ▶ Genitourinary

Deferred

### ▶ Rectal

Deferred

## Laboratory Tests

Urine for toxicology collected the day of hospital admission; ECG and blood obtained fasting at 6:30 AM day after admission.

|  | Conventional Units | SI Units |
|---|---|---|
| Na | 137 mEq/L | 137 mmol/L |
| K | 3.5 mEq/L | 3.5 mmol/L |
| Cl | 100 mEq/L | 100 mmol/L |
| $CO_2$ | 24 mEq/L | 24 mmol/L |
| BUN | 12 mg/dL | 4.3 mmol/L |
| SCr | 0.9 mg/dL | 80 μmol/L |
| Glu | 108 mg/dL | 6.0 mmol/L |
| Mg | 1.6 mEq/L | 0.80 mmol/L |
| Ca | 10.2 mg/dL | 2.55 mmol/L |
| Phos | 3.8 mg/dL | 1.23 mmol/L |
| Total protein | 7.7 g/dL | 77 g/L |
| Albumin | 4.2 g/dL | 42 g/L |
| ALT | 54 IU/L | 0.90 μkat/L |
| AST | 48 IU/L | 0.80 μkat/L |
| TSH | 0.97 μIU/mL | 0.97 mIU/L |
| Total cholesterol | 168 mg/dL | 4.34 mmol/L |
| Triglycerides | 72 mg/dL | 0.81 mmol/L |
| HDL cholesterol | 35 mg/dL | 0.91 mmol/L |
| LDL cholesterol | 119 mg/dL | 3.08 mmol/L |
| Serum pregnancy test | (–) | |
| RBC | $5.3 \times 10^6/mm^3$ | $5.3 \times 10^{12}/L$ |
| WBC | $9.7 \times 10^3/mm^3$ | $9.7 \times 10^9/L$ |
| Hgb | 15.9 g/dL | 9.87 mmol/L (159 g/L) |
| Hct | 46.7% | 0.467 |
| MCV | 88 μm$^3$ | 88 fL |

| MCH | 29 pg | |
|---|---|---|
| Platelets | $283 \times 10^3/mm^3$ | $283 \times 10^9/L$ |

Urinalysis

| Glucose | (−) |
|---|---|
| Ketone | Trace + |
| pH | 5.5 |
| Specific gravity | 1.013 |
| Protein | 1+ |
| Blood | (−) |

Toxicology screen

| Cannabinoids | (−) |
|---|---|
| Opiates | (−) |
| Phencyclidine | (−) |
| Amphetamines | (−) |
| Cocaine | (−) |
| Benzodiazepines | (+) |
| Other substances | (+) cotinine |

ECG

Sinus tachycardia, otherwise normal

## Assessment

Bipolar I disorder, most recent episode was manic, with psychotic features; hx of HTN

### Student Workup

**Missing Information?**

**Evaluate:**     Patient Database

Drug Therapy Problems

Care Plan (by Problem)

## TARGETED QUESTIONS

1. What signs and symptoms of bipolar disorder does this patient have?

   *Hint: See pp. 698–699 in PPP*

2. What prescribed or nonprescribed drugs could be exacerbating this patient's illness?

   *Hint: See Table 39-3 in PPP*

3. What is the purpose of the laboratory examination?

   *Hint: See Table 39-1 in PPP*

4. Should drug therapy be initiated with mood-stabilizing monotherapy, antipsychotic drug monotherapy, or mood-stabilizing and antipsychotic drug combination therapy?

   *Hint: See Table 39-2 in PPP*

5. What risks of drug therapy would you discuss with this patient when she is appropriate for patient education?

   *Hint: See pp. 705–711 in PPP*

## FOLLOW-UP

6. Drug therapy is initiated with the combination of lithium, titrated to a dosage of 900 mg PO at bedtime and a serum concentration of 1.02 mEq/L (1.02 mmol/L), aripiprazole 20 mg PO at bedtime, and clonazepam 2 mg PO twice daily. The clonazepam is tapered and discontinued prior to hospital discharge. She is continued on HCTZ 25 mg PO daily, and amlodipine 5 mg PO daily is added. She responded well to this regimen, but experienced polyuria, including bothersome nocturia, and a mild tremor. The polyuria improved with consolidating lithium to single-daily dosing instead of divided dosing. The tremor was treated with the addition of propranolol 10 mg PO twice daily. Her hospital discharge drug therapy regimen was lithium 900 mg PO at bedtime, aripiprazole 20 mg PO at bedtime, HCTZ 25 mg PO in the morning, and amlodipine 5 mg PO in the morning. She was counseled to moderate her caffeine intake. Her length of stay in the hospital was 17 days. After 6 months, still feeling well with a generally euthymic mood state, she and her husband are interested in starting a family. During a routine outpatient follow-up visit, she asks about the risks of medications for bipolar disorder and pregnancy. How should she be advised about this issue?

   *Hint: See pp. 712–713 in PPP*

### ☼ GLOBAL PERSPECTIVE

The assessment and treatment of bipolar disorder has been largely standardized through the use of common diagnostic criteria and widely available mood-stabilizing and antipsychotic medication. In all countries, financial considerations influence the choice of treatment. Hospital care may not be readily available and length of stay restricted. In rural or poorly developed regions where access to frequent outpatient follow-up may be limited, use of medications with a narrow therapeutic index, such as lithium or drugs that require regular laboratory monitoring, may be less practical. Additionally, although this case presents as a patient experiencing a manic episode, her history indicates a likely prior history of depressive episodes. Epidemiologic data indicate that depressive episodes are more common than manic episodes in both bipolar disorders I and II. Although research data sometimes conflict, activation of manic episodes by antidepressant drugs may be a risk, as may have happened in this patient's case, and appears as a risk in prescribing information for antidepressant drugs. Teratogenic risks of drug therapy during pregnancy are significant, especially with antiepileptic mood-stabilizing drugs and, to a lesser extent, with lithium. Careful education of the patient about risks and benefits and whether pregnancy is planned or unplanned is an important consideration. The judgment about continuing or stopping drug therapy will be influenced by these factors, the history of the individual patient, and the risk to the fetus in the medicated versus unmedicated condition.

## CASE SUMMARY

- This patient's clinical presentation and history are consistent with bipolar disorder I in a manic episode.
- Treatment with mood-stabilizing and antipsychotic medication is appropriate for the acute manic episode.

Maintenance therapy may attempt consolidating to mood-stabilizing monotherapy, but research supports reduced relapse with continued combination therapy.

- Antidepressant therapy should be avoided if possible in this patient as she appears to have a history of a pharmacologically induced mood switch.
- Treatment of bipolar disorder during pregnancy must balance the risks of exposure of prescribed drugs to the developing fetus with the risks of relapse of bipolar disorder if not adequately treated. Antiepileptic mood-stabilizing drugs such as divalproex and carbamazepine carry the greatest teratogenic risks.

For more information on the care plan and facilitator's guide please visit http://www.mhpharmacotherapy.com.

# 44 Anxiety

Sheila R. Botts

## CASE LEARNING OBJECTIVES

- List common presenting symptoms of panic disorder
- Identify the desired therapeutic outcomes for patients with panic disorder
- Discuss appropriate lifestyle modifications and over-the-counter medication use
- Develop a monitoring plan for anxiety patients placed on specific medications
- Educate patients about their disease state and appropriate lifestyle modifications, psychotherapy, and pharmacotherapy for effective treatment

## PATIENT PRESENTATION

### Chief Complaint

"I think I'm going crazy. I get this tightness in my chest, my heart races and I feel like I am going to die."

### History of Present Illness

Angela Brown is a 32-year-old woman who presents to her primary care physician complaining of sudden episodes of fearfulness accompanied by a tightening in her chest and intense anxiety. During these episodes she has heart palpitations, nausea, sweating, and a fear "that I'm going to die." They "just come out of nowhere" and last 10–15 minutes. She reports experiencing 2–3 episodes a week for the past few months. She recalls having her first episode like this approximately 3 years ago after the death of her father. Over the past 6–8 months they have increased in frequency and intensity. She has gone to the ED twice in the past 6 months as she felt something was wrong with her heart, but was told her heart was fine and it was probably stress. Her "ECG and blood tests were normal." She was given a prescription for diazepam 5 mg PO as needed and told she should schedule an appointment with her regular doctor.

She reports worrying a lot about her job, finances, children, and her health. She reports feeling sad, irritable and tense, and has difficulty sleeping. She is very fearful of having another episode and has started to avoid places like Wal-mart, and the mall, where these have occurred. She has difficulty attending after school events where "everyone is in the gymnasium and I'm afraid I can't get out." She called in sick the day of the holiday performance but fears she will be in trouble at work if this continues.

### Past Medical History

Migraine headaches diagnosed 5 years ago

Depression 3 years ago following father's death; resolved with psychotherapy

### Family History

Father died at age 54 in a motor vehicle accident. Mother diagnosed Stage 1 breast cancer 14 months ago, s/p lumpectomy with good prognosis. She has one sister who has "anxiety" and is on citalopram.

### Social History

She grew up in southern Colorado with both parents and one younger sibling. College graduate with a degree in secondary education. Currently employed as an art teacher at the local high school. Happily married with a 2-year-old daughter. Few social activities outside of work.

### Tobacco/Alcohol/Substance Use

Drinks 2–3 glasses wine each evening to relax and help with sleep. Denies tobacco or illicit substance use. Avoids caffeine.

### Allergies/Intolerances/Adverse Drug Events

Fluoxetine (was started on 20 mg daily for depressive episode 3 years ago); stopped after 3 doses due to extreme agitation and anxiety)

### Medications (Current)

Zolmitriptan 2.5 mg PO PRN for migraine headache

Diazepam 5 mg PO PRN anxiety

Ibuprofen 400 mg PO PRN headache, menstrual pain

Multivitamin w/Iron PO daily

## Review of Systems

Frequent non-migraine type headaches relieved by ibuprofen; migraine headaches 2–3 per month; soreness in the jaw which she attributes to grinding her teeth; muscle ache in shoulders

## Physical Examination

### ▶ General

Mildly anxious 32-year-old woman in no acute distress

### ▶ Vital Signs

BP 118/76 mm Hg, P 88, RR 18, T 37.1°C

Weight 145 lb (65.9 kg)

Height 65 in. (165 cm)

Denies pain

### ▶ Skin

(−) rashes or lesions

### ▶ HEENT

PERRLA, EOMI; normal fundi; TMs appear normal

### ▶ Neck and Lymph Nodes

Supple, thyroid normal size without nodules; (–) adenopathy

### ▶ Chest

Clear to auscultation

### ▶ Breasts

Exam deferred

### ▶ Cardiovascular

Tachycardia, normal $S_1$, $S_2$

### ▶ Abdomen

Not tender / Not distended; (−) organomegaly

### ▶ Neurology

Grossly intact; mild tremor in hands; deep tendon reflexes normal

## Medical Status Examination

A 32-year-old cooperative, casually dressed, well-groomed female. Appears anxious and has moderate psychomotor agitation. Speech is normal in rate and volume. Mood is "worried" and "sometimes sad," affect congruent to mood. No apparent delusions or hallucinations. Denies suicidal or homicidal ideation. She appears to have good attention and concentration.

### ▶ Genitourinary

Examination deferred

### ▶ Rectal

Examination deferred

## Laboratory Tests

|  | Conventional Units | SI Units |
|---|---|---|
| Na | 142 mEq/L | 142 mmol/L |
| K | 4.1 mEq/L | 4.1 mmol/L |
| Cl | 100 mEq/L | 100 mmol/L |
| $CO_2$ | 24 mEq/L | 24 mmol/L |
| BUN | 10 mg/dL | 3.6 mmol/L |
| SCr | 0.7 mg/dL | 62 μmol/L |
| Glu | 98 mg/dL | 5.4 mmol/L |
| AST | 22 U/L | 0.37 μkat/L |
| ALT | 28 U/L | 0.47 μkat/L |
| Alk phos | 40 IU/L | 0.67 μkat/L |
| Hgb | 14.5 g/dL (145 g/L) | 9.00 mmol/L |
| Hct | 42% | 0.42 |
| WBC | $6.8 \times 10^3/mm^3$ | $6.8 \times 10^9/L$ |
| Albumin | 3.8 g/dL | 38 g/L |
| TSH | 1.2 μIU/mL | 1.2 mIU/L |
| Total cholesterol | 178 mg/dL | 4.60 mmol/L |
| LDL cholesterol | 89 mg/dL | 2.30 mmol/L |
| HDL cholesterol | 36 mg/dL | 0.93 mmol/L |

Urine pregnancy test (−); urine drug screen (+) benzodiazepine

### ▶ ECG

Sinus tachycardia

## Assessment

Panic disorder with agoraphobia

### Student Workup

**Missing Information?**

**Evaluate:**    Patient Database

Drug Therapy Problems

Care Plan (by Problem)

## TARGETED QUESTIONS

1. What signs and symptoms of panic disorder (PD) does the patient have?

   *Hint: See p. 725 in PPP*

2. What nonpharmacologic interventions might be useful for this patient?

   *Hint: See p. 726 in PPP*

3. Why is an antidepressant the drug therapy of choice in PD?

   *Hint: See pp. 726–728 in PPP*

4. What adverse effects of therapy would you discuss with this patient?

   *Hint: See pp. 726–728 in PPP*

5. What if the patient fails the first choice of antidepressant treatment?

   *Hint: See p. 728 in PPP*

## FOLLOW-UP

The patient returns 8 weeks later and reports a significant reduction in panic attacks but she still worries she'll have another one. She continues to avoid shopping malls and Wal-mart.

6. What is the expected time frame for improvement in anticipatory anxiety and phobic avoidance? How long should the patient be maintained on drug therapy for her PD?

## ☉ GLOBAL PERSPECTIVE

Treatment guidelines for panic disorder are similar worldwide to that used in the United States. Culture is expected to play a role in clinical presentation of panic symptoms and should be considered when individualizing cognitive behavioral treatments. Panic symptoms are reported in other cultures but not always referred to as "panic." For example, Cambodian and Vietnamese cultures often refer to panic as "sore neck" and "wind overload", respectively. In the United States, African Americans seem to have a higher prevalence of agoraphobia and are more likely to seek treatment in primary care settings.

## CASE SUMMARY

- Her clinical presentation includes panic attacks, anticipatory anxiety, and agoraphobic avoidance resulting in functional impairment, and treatment should be initiated.
- SSRI antidepressants reduce panic attack frequency and severity, anticipatory anxiety, and agoraphobia. Initial doses should be much lower than that used in depression but titrated to a similar target daily dose.
- Antidepressant therapy should be continued for least one year after achieving response to minimize the risk of relapse.

**For more information on the care plan and facilitator's guide please visit http://www.mhpharmacotherapy.com.**

# 45 Sleep Disorder

Amy M. Lugo          Amy L. Stump

## CASE LEARNING OBJECTIVES

- Recommend and optimize appropriate sleep hygiene and nonpharmacologic therapies for the management and prevention of sleep disorders
- Recommend and optimize appropriate pharmacotherapy for sleep disorders
- Describe the components of a monitoring plan to assess safety and efficacy of pharmacotherapy for common sleep disorders
- Educate patients about preventive behavior, appropriate lifestyle modifications, and drug therapy required for effective treatment and control of sleep disorders

## PATIENT PRESENTATION

### Chief Complaint

"I'm so tired, can't talk right, feel shaky and my arms and legs don't want to work."

### History of Present Illness

Miriam Weber is a 61-year-old woman who presents to the pharmacotherapy clinic complaining of feeling tired, uncoordinated, shaky, anxious, and mentally "foggy" for the past 4 days. In addition, she states that her speech has become slurred, which prompted her to go to the emergency department (ED) earlier today. At the ED, she was told to make an appointment with her regular physician as there were no urgent problems identified, but she has no medical insurance and typically receives all of her care and medications from the local free clinic, which is not open until tomorrow. On hearing of the situation, the physician in charge of the free clinic directed her to you for a medication evaluation. She presents with her husband and a basket full of medications. She asks you if you can recommend something for her to take for sleep. She has been taking a new medication, amitriptyline, for the past week and it does not seem to be working as she still cannot fall asleep at night.

### Past Medical History

Hypothyroidism
GERD
Depression
HTN
Gastritis/duodenitis

Migraine headache
Insomnia

### Past Surgical History

Total hysterectomy 20 years ago

### Family History

Father had a history of DM and stroke. Mother has unknown cancer. Brother has "kidney problems" and alcoholism.

### Social History

The patient is married and lives with and cares for her disabled husband and son as well as her elderly mother. She is currently unemployed. Family income consists of social security benefits from husband, son, and mother. She has no medical or prescription drug insurance.

### Tobacco/Alcohol/Substance Use

(−) Tobacco and alcohol; (+) methamphetamine, patient has not used in 10 years after going through rehabilitation program.

### Allergies/Intolerances/Adverse Drug Events

Cephalexin—hives; latex—rash

### Medications (Current)

Citalopram 20 mg PO daily
Amitriptyline 25 mg PO q hs
Estradiol 1 mg PO daily

Quinapril 20 mg PO daily

HCTZ 25 mg PO daily

Levothyroxine 100 mcg PO daily

Rizatriptan 10 mg PO PRN headache

Dicyclomine 20 mg PO daily

## Review of Systems

Complains of fatigue and sleep disorder; (−) fever and sweats; (−) chest pain, racing heart, or light-headedness; (−) cough and SOB; (+) falling down, poor balance, disturbances in coordination, tremors, and slurred speech; (−) fainting, seizures, and numbness; (+) anxiety; (−) depressed mood; (−) nocturia, urinary urgency, and urinary frequency.

## Physical Examination

### ▶ General

Well-developed patient in mild distress, unkempt, noticeable slurred speech, looks older than stated age

### ▶ Vital Signs

BP 117/73 mm Hg, P 86, RR 20, T 36.9°C

Weight 185 lb (84 kg)

Height 62 in. (157 cm)

Denies pain

### ▶ Skin

No clubbing, cyanosis, edema, or lesions noted

### ▶ HEENT

PERRLA, pupils slightly enlarged; EOMI; dry oral mucosa

### ▶ Neck and Lymph Nodes

No thyromegaly

### ▶ Chest

Lungs clear to auscultation bilaterally

### ▶ Breasts

Examination deferred

### ▶ Cardiovascular

RRR, no murmurs, rubs, or gallops

### ▶ Abdomen

Examination deferred

### ▶ Neurology

(+) Ataxia; no hyperreflexia noted

### ▶ Genitourinary

Examination deferred

### ▶ Rectal

Examination deferred

## Laboratory Tests

### From Her ED Visit This Morning

|  | Conventional Units | SI Units |
|---|---|---|
| Na | 137 mEq/L | 137 mmol/L |
| K | 4.2 mEq/L | 4.2 mmol/L |
| Cl | 105 mEq/L | 105 mmol/L |
| $CO_2$ | 22 mEq/L | 22 mmol/L |
| BUN | 18 mg/dL | 6.4 mmol/L |
| SCr | 0.82 mg/dL | 72 mmol/L |
| Glu | 104 mg/dL | 5.8 mmol/L |
| WBC | $6.6 \times 10^3/mm^3$ | $6.6 \times 10^9/L$ |
| Hgb | 14.2 g/dL | 8.81 mmol/L (142 g/L) |
| Hct | 42.6% | 0.426 |
| Plt | $428 \times 10^3/mm^3$ | $428 \times 10^9/L$ |
| MCV | $84 \ \mu m^3$ | 84 fL |
| TSH | 0.05 μIU/mL | 0.05 mIU/L |
| Acetaminophen | <1 mcg/mL | <7 μmol/L |
| Salicylate | <4 mcg/mL | <0.03 mmol/L |
| Ethanol | <10 mg/dL | <2.2 mmol/L |
| Urine drug screen | (−) | |

## Assessment

Sixty-one-year-old female with signs and symptoms, consistent with possible anticholinergic delirium due to initiation of amitriptyline for insomnia

## Student Workup

### Missing Information?

**Evaluate:**   Patient Database

Drug Therapy Problems

Care Plan (by Problem)

## TARGETED QUESTIONS

1.  What signs and symptoms of anticholinergic delirium does this patient have?

    *Hint: Older patients are much more susceptible to the anticholinergic effects of medications.[1] Pharmacists can play a key role in recognizing these drug-induced problems and preventing the addition of a new drug to the patient's regimen to treat the adverse effect. See p. 597 in PPP*

2. Why is amitriptyline the most likely cause of anticholinergic delirium in this patient?

   *Hint: See pp. 682–683 in PPP*

3. What medication would be the best choice to recommend for this patient to treat her insomnia?

   *Hint: See Table 41-2 in PPP*

4. How might you counsel this patient on nonpharmacologic management of her insomnia?

   *Hint: See Table 41-1 in PPP*

## FOLLOW-UP

5. Two weeks later, the patient returns for follow-up. She feels "back to normal," with no tremor, slurred speech, or coordination problems. However, she is still having trouble falling asleep. She has not taken anything for sleep since her last physician visit because she is scared that she will have another adverse effect to the medication. The patient wishes to use an OTC or herbal product to help her sleep, stating that she feels they are safer because they are not as strong as prescription medications. How will you respond to the patient? What OTC or herbal product(s), if any, would you tell her not to use? What product(s), if any, would you recommend?

   *Hint: See p. 740 in PPP*

## REFERENCES

1. The American Geriatrics Society 2012 Beers Criteria Update Expert Panel. AGS updated Beers Criteria for potentially inappropriate medication use in older adults. J Am Geriatr Soc 2012 60:616–631.

## GLOBAL PERSPECTIVE

Melatonin is a naturally occurring endogenous hormone produced by the pineal gland. Exogenous melatonin has been shown to help regulate circadian rhythm sleep disorders. Many travelers experience a circadian rhythm disorder, commonly known as jet lag. When traveling across time zones, the traveler's sleep–wake cycle becomes out of sync with the time of day. Jet lag severity is determined by direction of travel (traveling east is often worse than traveling west), age of the traveler, and number of time zones crossed. Manipulating factors such as exposure to bright light, social contact, and activity are nonpharmacologic options to improve jet lag. Supplementing with 3–5 mg of exogenous melatonin hormone 30 minutes prior to the local bedtime can expedite sleep–cycle normalization.

## CASE SUMMARY

- The patient is experiencing anticholinergic adverse effects likely due to the addition of amitriptyline to her medication regimen for the treatment of insomnia. All anticholinergic medications should be discontinued (amitriptyline and dicyclomine).

- A thorough sleep history should be taken from the patient and she should be counseled about nonpharmacologic treatments for insomnia.

- Product selection for sleep aids, both prescription and OTC, should be made with care. Patient-specific factors such as age, comorbid conditions, concomitant medications, and pharmacoeconomic issues should be considered.[1]

**For more information on the care plan and facilitator's guide please visit http://www.mhpharmacotherapy.com.**

# 46 Attention-Deficit Hyperactivity Disorder

John Erramouspe     Kevin W. Cleveland

## CASE LEARNING OBJECTIVES

- Recognize the signs and symptoms of attention deficit/hyperactivity disorder (ADHD) that respond to therapy
- Select appropriate stimulant preparations for a patient with ADHD displaying an adverse effect to another stimulant preparation
- Propose ways of improving the effectiveness and/or minimizing the cost of medications used for ADHD and other common comorbid childhood problems (i.e., encopresis/constipation, sleep latency problems, allergic rhinitis, asthma)
- Recommend an appropriate monitoring plan for stimulant therapy on the basis of individual patient characteristics and past adverse side-effect profile
- Properly educate a patient taking stimulants for ADHD therapy

## PATIENT PRESENTATION

### Chief Complaint

"I still have this rash where I stick my Daytrana patch. Using my hay fever spray before I stick on the patch helps a lot but my mom says it is getting kind of expensive."

### History of Present Illness

Rev Williams is a 12½-year-old male who presents with his mother to the pediatrician's clinic office for a refill request of Nasonex. His mother works as a receptionist at an adult medicine clinic in a neighboring town. One month ago, after reading a magazine advertisement for Daytrana and talking with various medical staff at her clinic, she requested that her pediatrician switch RW from Vyvanse to the patch. Her reasons for switching were that RW was a little more fidgety on Vyvanse (although this was tolerable), to take advantage of the flexibility in dosing of Daytrana according to her son's schedule, and that Daytrana costs about the same as Vyvanse. She incurs the same monthly $50 co-pay for both ADHD medications since they both are available only as brand name and nonpreferred tier 3 agents on her current prescription insurance plan. RW was switched to Daytrana and soon afterward began manifesting a bumpy red rash with slight swelling

at the application site. RW's mother began applying Nasonex (also nonpreferred tier 3 agent on RW's prescription plan with a $50 co-pay) to her son's application site for the patch as a temporary measure until she could talk to her pediatrician. RW just finished the sixth grade and did very well in his charter school. His teacher says he has a high IQ, is on task, finishes his work quickly, and might benefit from the gifted program. Since beginning stimulant therapy over the last 4½ years (Ritalin LA → Concerta → Vyvanse → Daytrana + methylphenidate PRN), there has been a marked decrease in his level of forgetfulness (e.g., homework, lunch box), aggressiveness, temper tantrums, anger, frustration, and in hitting and kicking fellow classmates. Prior to stimulant therapy, RW hated to read but now has acquired a desire to read after years of treatment for ADHD and continues to read avidly at almost a ninth-grade level. His favorite class is physical education, especially when they play soccer. This occurs the first hour of the day, immediately after arriving at school. He will be changing to a public junior high school next year due to his parents' desire to increase his range of friends. RW feels like he presently has a sufficient number of friends but seems okay with this change. Some teachers have noted a slight oddity to his behavior and social interactions. He feels like his mood is fine and things are going well within his family. RW states that Daytrana helps him focus and remember better and that the only side effect he has is the bumpy red rash with slight swelling, but that Nasonex has helped lessen this problem. He states that he takes an ADHD pill every weekday at about 5 PM, so he can complete his homework after dinner. RW's pediatrician contacts you, the pharmacist, and asks you if it is okay to continue both the Nasonex and the Daytrana as they are presently being used.

## Past Medical History

ADHD for 4½ years

Encopresis/constipation for 8 years

Sleep problems (difficulty falling asleep)

Allergic rhinitis and mild asthma for 7 years

Migraine headache with aura in last month

Chest pain occurred at 9 years (likely musculoskeletal in origin and not cardiac per pediatric cardiologist)—resolved

Sporadic high blood pressure on three occasions at 6–8 years—resolved

Nummular eczema on shoulder at 4 years—resolved following use of Eucerin and triamcinolone 0.025% cream for 1 month

Secondarily infected molluscum contagiosum at 4 years—resolved

Meatal stenosis at 4 years—surgically resolved with meatotomy and cystoscopy

## Family History

Biological parents are alive and healthy. Mother has migraines and father displays inattentiveness concurrent with ADHD but has never been medically evaluated for ADHD. RW has a biological 8-year-old sister who is co-managed by RW's pediatrician and a pediatric psychologist for ADHD (on Concerta).

## Social History

Lives with biological parents (married) and younger sister. Presently attends a charter school, but will be changing to a public junior high school next year in an effort to increase his range of friends.

## Tobacco/Alcohol/Substance Use

None

## Allergies/Intolerances/Adverse Drug Events

Daytrana—rash (local contact rash vs. sensitivity?)

## Medications (Current)

Daytrana 30 mg patch applied daily in the morning with breakfast at 7 AM (remove by 4 PM)

Methylphenidate 5 mg tablet PO in the late afternoon PRN

Lactulose 30 mL PO twice daily (RW does not like the sweet/syrupy taste and admits to frequently taking the product on a PRN basis due to taste and forgetfulness.)

Melatonin 3 mg tablet PO in the evening PRN

Cetirizine 5 mg tablet PO daily

Nasonex two sprays in each nostril once daily

Naproxen sodium 220 mg tablets, 1–2 tablet(s) PO initially and then 1 tablet q 8 h until migraine resolves (do not exceed 3 tablets per day)

## Review of Systems

(−) Migraine or other headache symptoms since 1 month ago; (−) vision changes; (−) appetite problems, normal at breakfast, lunch, and dinner (feels hungrier around bedtime), weight is stable; (+) chronic constipation symptoms with infrequent, slightly hard, mildly painful bowel movements every other day; minimal to no complaints of pruritus with rash; (+) difficulty falling asleep often until midnight (plays Pokémon and watches television in his bedroom following completion of homework until he feels sleepy enough to fall asleep); denies any inability to concentrate on school assignment while at school.

## Physical Examination

▶ *General*

Well-appearing 12½-year-old male who is not very interested in talking with the pediatrician today

▶ *Vital Signs*

BP 110/70 mm Hg, P 85, RR 16, T 37°C

Weight 94 lb (42.7 kg)

Height 61.4 in. (156 cm)

▶ *Skin*

Faint circumferential erythematous raised rash on left hip where Daytrana patch was located from yesterday; same rash with slight swelling evident beneath patch located on right hip today

▶ *HEENT*

Normocephalic, atraumatic, tympanic membranes and oropharynx WNL, conjunctivae clear

▶ *Neck and Lymph Nodes*

Supple without lymphadenopathy

▶ *Chest*

Clear to auscultation bilaterally

▶ *Cardiovascular*

*Heart:* RRR without murmurs

*Extremities:* Normal pulses

▶ *Abdomen*

Soft, nontender without hepatosplenomegaly

> *Neurology*

WNL

> *Genitourinary*

Normal Tanner stage III male, both testes descended

> *Rectal*

Examination deferred

## Laboratory Tests

Last assessed at 9 years of age when evaluated by pediatric cardiologist

|  | Conventional Units | SI Units |
|---|---|---|
| Na | 140 mEq/L | 140 mmol/L |
| K | 4.2 mEq/L | 4.2 mmol/L |
| Cl | 100 mEq/L | 100 mmol/L |
| Total $CO_2$ | 28 mEq/L | 28 mmol/L |
| BUN | 14 mg/dL | 5.0 mmol/L |
| SCr | 0.7 mg/dL | 62 μmol/L |
| Glu | 101 mg/dL | 5.6 mmol/L |
| Ca | 9.6 mg/dL | 2.40 mmol/L |
| Mg | 1.9 mEq/L | 0.95 mmol/L |
| Phosphate | 4.1 mg/dL | 1.32 mmol/L |
| Hgb | 13.1 g/dL | 8.13 mmol/L (131 g/L) |
| Hct | 39.0% | 0.390 |
| WBC | $9.1 \times 10^3/mm^3$ | $9.1 \times 10^9/L$ |
| MCV | 83 μm³ | 83 fL |
| Albumin | 4.5 g/dL | 45 g/L |
| TSH | 1.9 μIU/mL | 1.9 mIU/L |
| Free $T_4$ | 1.07 ng/dL | 13.8 pmol/L |
| Total cholesterol | 161 mg/dL | 4.16 mmol/L |
| LDL cholesterol | 94 mg/dL | 2.43 mmol/L |
| HDL cholesterol | 55 mg/dL | 1.42 mmol/L |

## Assessment

A 12½-year-old preadolescent male with probable local Daytrana-induced contact dermatitis

## Student Workup

### Missing Information?

**Evaluate:** Patient Database

Drug Therapy Problems

Care Plan (by Problem)

## TARGETED QUESTIONS

1. What signs and symptoms of ADHD has this patient manifested in the past and which ones does he presently display that may respond to stimulant therapy?

   *Hint: See pp. 748–749 in PPP*

2. Why are stimulants the treatment of choice for most patients with ADHD?

   *Hint: See pp. 749–753 in PPP, References 1 and 2*

3. What adverse effects of stimulant therapy would you discuss with this patient and his parent(s) and what remedies would you offer to decrease them?

   *Hint: See Table 42-3 in PPP*

4. If this patient was to be switched from Daytrana to a different stimulant formulation, what should it be?

   *Hint: The patient probably does not require a stimulant preparation with both a rapid onset and an extended duration because his ADHD symptoms have been responding well to Daytrana (an extended-acting stimulant with slow onset) and his first class of the school day, physical education, may not require as much attentiveness as classes later in the school day. Therefore, a less expensive intermediate-acting stimulant might be the best replacement for Daytrana (see Table 42-4 in PPP). In the future, the patient's schedule could change so that more attention would be required earlier in the school day. A stimulant formulation with both rapid- and extended action might be necessary at this point.*

5. Are any laxatives that are used chronically for children with encopresis more palatable and less frequently administered than lactulose?

   *Hint: Many laxatives are considered to have an unpleasant taste by children and/or require dosing multiple times per day (e.g., lactulose, mineral oil, magnesium hydroxide, sorbitol 70%). Polyethylene glycol (PEG) 3350 (MiraLax) was approved as a prescription laxative in the United States in 1999 and subsequently changed to OTC in 2006. PEG 3350 is currently available both OTC and by prescription. Over the last decade it has been investigated in a variety of childhood constipation disorders and found to consistently have good outcomes. In some childhood studies, it has demonstrated greater efficacy than lactulose or improved tolerability compared to magnesium hydroxide.[3] Many providers consider PEG 3350 a preferred laxative for chronic use in children owing to the fact that it has no taste, can be mixed with a child's preferred beverage, and typically requires dosing only once daily.*

6. Is there a preferred medication for treating ADHD children who have difficulty falling asleep despite proper adjustment of their stimulant therapy and an adequate trial of behavioral therapy?

   *Hint: Benzodiazepines are frequently avoided in children with chronic sleep disorders due to concerns of excessive sedation and addiction. In randomized controlled trials of children with various sleep disorders, diphenhydramine and zolpidem were shown to have no difference from placebo.[4] Other newer nonbenzodiazepine hypnotics (i.e., zaleplon, eszopiclone, ramelteon) have not been rigorously investigated in children.[4] Clonidine or guanfacine are sometimes added to existing stimulant therapy in an effort to facilitate proper nighttime sleep and improve control of ADHD symptoms (see Table 42-3 in PPP). Melatonin has been shown to be effective in children with sleep problems and various comorbid problems including ADHD (e.g., learning difficulties, visual impairment, neurodevelopmental disabilities).[4,5]*

## FOLLOW-UP

7. RW was switched to methylphenidate ER in the morning plus methylphenidate RR in the afternoon prior to 3 PM as needed for his ADHD. At 1-month follow-up, the local reaction he experienced with Daytrana has resolved and he continues to do well in school and in completing his homework. His transition to public school initially was somewhat traumatic due to some bullying behavior he encountered from one classmate. However, now he has established a group of three good friends who play soccer together and the bullying no longer occurs. His bowel function is much improved, and he has been faithfully adhering to laxative therapy on a daily basis and his stool pattern has become more normal with a daily soft bowel movement every morning just following breakfast. He does not like the new nasal spray quite as well as the Nasonex (says it causes his nose to bleed approximately once in a while). However, his hay fever symptoms remain adequately controlled. RW's mother is ecstatic about the savings in medications since she now incurs only a $5 co-pay for each methylphenidate prescription. What action, if any, would you take?

## ☼ GLOBAL PERSPECTIVE

ADHD is a behavioral disorder that affects up to 1 in 20 children in the United States. The predominance of American research into this disorder over the past 40 years has led to the impression that ADHD is largely an American disorder and much less prevalent elsewhere. This impression was reinforced by the perception that ADHD may stem from social and cultural factors that are most common in American society. However, another school of thought suggested that ADHD is a behavioral disorder common to children of many different races and societies worldwide, but that is not recognized by the medical community, perhaps due to confusion regarding its diagnosis and/or misconceptions regarding its adverse impact on children, their families, and society as a whole. Studies performed in United States and non-United States populations suggest that the prevalence of ADHD is at least as high in many non-United States children as in United States children, with the highest prevalence rates being seen when using *DSM-IV* diagnostic criteria. Recognition that ADHD is not purely an American disorder and that the prevalence of this behavioral disorder in many countries is in the same range as that in the United States will have important implications for the psychiatric care of children. Although the treatment strategies and medication availability may differ among countries, most published ADHD treatment guidelines from Europe and other parts of the world show similar approaches to managing this disorder.[6]

## REFERENCES

1. Subcommittee on Attention-Deficit/Hyperactivity Disorder; Steering Committee on Quality Improvement and Management, Wolraich M, Brown L, Brown RT, et al. ADHD: clinical practice guideline for the diagnosis, evaluation, and treatment of attention-deficit/hyperactivity disorder in children and adolescents. Pediatrics 2011 128:1007–1022.
2. American Academy of Pediatrics. Supplemental information implementing the key action statements: an algorithm and explanation for process of care for the evaluation, diagnosis, treatment, and monitoring of ADHD in children and adolescents. http://pediatrics.aappublications.org/content/suppl/2011/10/11/peds.2011-2654.DC1/zpe611117822p.pdf. Accessed February 20, 2013.
3. Candy D, Belsey J. Macrogol (polyethylene glycol) laxatives in children with functional constipation and faecal impaction: A systematic review. Arch Dis Child 2009 94:156–160.
4. Sweis D. The uses of melatonin. Arch Dis Child Educ Pract Ed 2005 90:ep74–ep77.
5. Gringras P. When to use drugs to help sleep. Arch Dis Child 2008 93:976–981.
6. Faraone SV, Sergeant J, Gillberg C, Biederman J. The worldwide prevalence of ADHD: Is it an American condition? World Psychiatr 2003 2:104–113.

## CASE SUMMARY

- RW's current clinical picture is consistent with a probable local drug-induced contact dermatitis to Daytrana that is being mismanaged by continuance of the patch and misuse of the Nasonex.

- It is reasonable to replace Daytrana with a single 7 AM dose of generic methylphenidate extended release.

- The as-needed afternoon dose of methylphenidate regular-release 5 mg tablet should be continued but given no later than 3 PM in an effort to avoid possible drug-induced difficulties in falling asleep from the afternoon stimulant dose.

- RW's chronic laxative needs to be changed to a more palatable, less frequently administered preparation.

- RW's treatment of migraine with naproxen sodium is appropriate and should be continued. He does not yet require a maintenance medication.

**For more information on the care plan and facilitator's guide please visit http://www.mhpharmacotherapy.com.**

# 47 Drug-Seeking Behavior

Lisa W. Goldstone

## CASE LEARNING OBJECTIVES

- Identify the typical signs and symptoms of withdrawal associated with the use of opioids
- Determine the appropriate treatment measures to produce a desired outcome following an episode of opiate withdrawal
- Determine when a patient meets criteria for substance dependence
- Choose specific pharmacotherapeutic options based on patient-specific factors

## PATIENT PRESENTATION

### Chief Complaint

"I hurt my knee playing with the kids yesterday. I'm in a lot of pain."

### History of Present Illness

RG is a 44-year-old man who presents to the emergency department (ED) on a Sunday afternoon complaining of knee pain. The patient states that he was playing with his girlfriend's children yesterday and accidentally stepped into a hole in the yard and "twisted" his right knee. Per the patient, he tried acetaminophen but it did not work for him. He rates his pain as a 9 on a 10 point scale. The patient states that he has had problems with this knee before and is concerned that he may have triggered an old injury. He offers that he has had prior success with both oxycodone and hydromorphone for a similar injury.

### Past Medical History

Knee surgery 3 years ago

Depression × 8 years

Generalized anxiety disorder (GAD) × 6 years

### Family History

Patient was adopted and does not have any health-related information regarding his birth family

### Social History

The patient is divorced and lives with his girlfriend and her two children. He is currently employed as an insurance agent.

### Tobacco/Alcohol/Substance Use

Social drinker; denies tobacco or illicit substance use.

### Allergies/Intolerances/Adverse Drug Events

Patient states that he has anaphylaxis to all NSAIDs

### Medications (Current)

Bupropion 75 mg PO daily

Sertraline 50 mg PO daily

Lorazepam 2 mg PO q 6 h prn

Zolpidem 15 mg PO q hs prn

### Review of Systems

Overall physical health good; (+) mild abdominal cramping; (−) chest pain, shortness of breath; (+) depression, anxiety

### Physical Examination

▶ *General*

Patient is a well-developed, 44-year-old male who appears to be in mild distress and is moderately agitated.

▶ *Vital Signs*

BP 152/93 mm Hg, P 93, RR 18, T 37.5°C, pain score = 9

Weight 164.6 lb (74.8 kg)

Height 72 in. (183 cm)

▶ *HEENT*

(+) Rhinorrhea, lacrimation, dilated pupils

▸ *Chest*

Clear to auscultation

▸ *Cardiovascular*

Tachycardic, RRR, (–) murmurs

▸ *Abdomen*

(+) bowel sounds

▸ *Neurology*

Alert and oriented × 3; (+) muscle twitching

▸ *Skin*

(+) wet sweaty palms, diaphoresis; (–) swelling or redness in right knee

## Laboratory Tests

|  | Conventional Units | SI Units |
|---|---|---|
| Na | 143 mEq/L | 143 mmol/L |
| K | 3.3 mEq/L | 3.3 mmol/L |
| Cl | 106 mEq/L | 106 mmol/L |
| CO$_2$ | 24 mEq/L | 24 mEq/L |
| BUN | 30 mg/dL | 10.7 mmol/L |
| SCr | 1.2 mg/dL | 106 μmol/L |
| Glu | 86 mg/dL | 4.8 mmol/L |
| Hgb | 14.2 g/dL | 142 g/L (8.81 mmol/L) |
| Hct | 42.6% | 0.426 |
| WBC | 11.4 × 10$^3$/mm$^3$ | 11.4 × 10$^9$/L |
| Platelets | 336 × 10$^3$/mm$^3$ | 336 × 10$^9$/L |
| Albumin | 3.6 g/dL | 36 g/L |
| Total bilirubin | 0.5 mg/dL | 8.6 μmol/L |
| AST | 23 IU/L | 0.38 μkat/L |
| ALT | 28 IU/L | 0.47 μkat/L |
| Alk phos | 74 IU/L | 1.23 μkat/L |

▸ *Urine Toxicology*

Patient refused

▸ *X-Ray of Right Knee*

No significant findings

▸ *State Prescription Drug Monitoring Database*

Patient has received opioid prescriptions from four different emergency care or urgent care prescribers and filled the prescriptions at four different pharmacies over the past month.

## Assessment

Patient is a 44-year-old male who has signs and symptoms of opioid withdrawal. Although he complains of knee pain, no redness or swelling is present. An X-ray did not reveal any significant findings. Based upon the information contained with the state-controlled substance database, the patient has utilized multiple physicians and pharmacies to obtain pain medication within the past month. It appears that the patient may be engaging in drug seeking behaviors.

## TARGETED QUESTIONS

1. What signs and symptoms is the patient experiencing that may indicate that he is going through opiate withdrawal?

    *Hint: See Table 36-4 in PPP*

2. What type of treatment(s) should be initiated to address symptoms of opiate withdrawal?

    *Hint: See pp. 644–645 in PPP*

3. Does the patient have sufficient criteria to warrant a diagnosis of opiate dependence?

    *Hint: See Table 36-1 in PPP*

## FOLLOW-UP

The patient is discharged with prescriptions to aid in his detoxification from opiates and is referred for an evaluation at a community mental health center that offers substance abuse treatment programming. At this appointment, he is diagnosed with opiate dependence. What type of treatment modalities (pharmacological and nonpharmacological) should be used to treat this opiate dependence?

## ⊙ GLOBAL PERSPECTIVE

Amphetamine-like substances continue to be the major psychotropic substance trafficked and used throughout the world. However, there have been reports of opioid prescription drug abuse in countries such as Bolivia, Brazil, Chile, Australia, New Zealand, India, Nepal, Bangladesh, and South Africa[1]. The most commonly abused prescription opioids worldwide (excluding the United States) include codeine products, buprenorphine, and morphine. Despite evidence of misuse in other countries, the United States appears to have the most significant prescription opioid drug abuse problem at this time.

## REFERENCE

1. International Narcotics Control Board. Report of the International Narcotics Control for 2011. http://incb.org/incb/en/publications/annual-reports/annual-report.html. Accessed February 21, 2013.

## CASE SUMMARY

- The patient is displaying drug-seeking behavior that may be indicative of an opioid abuse or dependence. He requires an evaluation by a trained professional to determine his diagnosis for treatment planning purposes.

- He is also experiencing opioid withdrawal and should receive treatment to lessen the distress of these symptoms. Opioid withdrawal, in general, is not life threatening and therefore does not require hospitalization unless the patient has other medical comorbidities.

- Psychiatric comorbidities need to be properly treated to aid in the patient's recovery.

For more information on the care plan and facilitator's guide please visit http://www.mhpharmacotherapy.com.

# 48 Type 1 Diabetes Mellitus: Diabetic Ketoacidosis

Hanna Phan        Christopher J. Edwards

## CASE LEARNING OBJECTIVES

- Recognize the signs and symptoms of diabetic ketoacidosis (DKA)
- Identify the goals of therapy for the treatment of DKA and type 1 diabetes mellitus (T1DM)
- Develop an appropriate treatment and monitoring plan for DKA using individual patient characteristics
- Properly educate a patient newly diagnosed with T1DM to prevent possible future incidents of DKA

## PATIENT PRESENTATION

### Chief Complaint

"I've been vomiting for 2 days."

### History of Present Illness

Jimmy Wilkinson is a 20-year-old Caucasian male university student with known T1DM who comes into the emergency department with a 2-day history of N/V. Two weeks ago, he noticed that he was drinking water and urinating more frequently than usual. He also mentions that recently he has been having some difficulty waking up in the morning and staying awake and alert throughout the day. These symptoms began 2 weeks ago and have gotten progressively worse. He mentions that he has been feeling "a bit down" since his last round of final examinations approximately 3 weeks ago. When asked about his insulin therapy, he states that he "has not felt like using it for a while." He came to the emergency department after he missed 2 days of school and work due to N/V. He states that he has not been able to eat or drink without vomiting for about 36 hours. He reports that he has not seen his home physician in 8 months, and he does not currently have a primary care provider on campus. He is currently insured through the university's campus insurance plan. He denies any recent history of weight loss, diarrhea, changes in vision, or dysuria.

### Past Medical History

Type 1 DM
Major depressive disorder

Seasonal allergic rhinitis
Tonsillectomy at age 4 years

### Family History

Father is alive at age 43 and has a history of T1DM, hypertension, and hyperlipidemia. Uncle on father's side is alive at age 50 and has a history of T1DM and stroke. Grandfather on father's side died at age 63 of MI. He had a history of T1DM. Mother is alive at age 38 with a major depressive disorder and systemic lupus erythematous.

### Social History

Currently a junior in college and has a part-time job at a book store.

### Tobacco/Alcohol/Substance Use

Admits to occasional alcohol and marijuana use at social gatherings; denies use of tobacco and other illicit drugs.

### Allergies/Intolerances/Adverse Drug Events

NKDA

### Medications Prior to Admission

Loratadine 10 mg PO daily
Diphenhydramine 50 mg PO every 6 to 8 hours PRN allergies
Fluticasone one spray each nostril daily

Escitalopram 10 mg PO daily

Insulin glargine 20 units SC at bedtime

Insulin lispro 5 units SC with meals (e.g., three times a day)

## Review of Systems

### ▶ General

(–) Fevers, chills, rigors, or weight loss

### ▶ HEENT

(–) Visual changes, diplopia, tinnitus, vertigo

### ▶ Respiratory

(+) Tachypnea; (–) SOB and cough

### ▶ Cardiovascular

(–) Rapid heartbeat or palpitations, chest pain

### ▶ Gastrointestinal

(+) Polydipsia, nausea, and vomiting; (–) abdominal pain

### ▶ Genitourinary

(+) Urinary frequency, urgency, polyuria; (–) dysuria

### ▶ Musculoskeletal

(–) Joint or muscle pain

### ▶ Neurology

(+) Fatigue; (–) HA, numbness, weakness, or tingling

## Physical Examination

### ▶ General

Thin, healthy looking young male in no acute distress. Acetone breath noted during examination

### ▶ Vital Signs

BP 87/62, P 124, RR 27, T 37.2°C

Weight 139 lb (63.2 kg)

Height 68 in. (173 cm)

Denies pain

### ▶ Skin

Warm and dry, mild acne on face and back. No rashes, petechiae, ecchymosis, or jaundice

### ▶ HEENT

Normocephalic; PERRLA, EOMI intact; TMs benign bilaterally; oropharynx benign; mucous membranes dry

### ▶ Neck and Lymph Nodes

Supple; no thyroid nodules, lymphadenopathy, or carotid bruits; neck veins flat

### ▶ Chest

Breathing unlabored; mild tachypnea; breath sounds equal bilaterally; no wheezes, crackles, or rhonchi

### ▶ Cardiovascular

RRR, normal $S_1$, $S_2$; no $S_3$ or $S_4$ detected

### ▶ Abdomen

Nontender, nondistended; no organomegaly; bowel sounds present

### ▶ Neurology

No deficits appreciated

### ▶ Genitourinary

Examination deferred

### ▶ Rectal

Examination deferred

## Laboratory Tests

### Fasting Obtained on Admission

|  | Conventional Units | SI Units |
|---|---|---|
| Na | 130 mEq/L | 130 mmol/L |
| K | 3.0 mEq/L | 3.0 mmol/L |
| Cl | 104 mEq/L | 104 mmol/L |
| $HCO_3$ | 11 mEq/L | 11 mmol/L |
| BUN | 40 mg/dL | 14.3 mmol/L |
| SCr | 1.5 mg/dL | 133 μmol/L |
| Glu | 550 mg/dL | 30.5 mmol/L |
| Ca | 9.3 mg/dL | 2.33 mmol/L |
| Mg | 2.1 mEq/L | 1.05 mmol/L |
| Phosphate | 2.0 mg/dL | 0.65 mmol/L |
| Hgb | 15.5 g/dL | 9.62 mmol/L (155 g/L) |
| Hct | 44.7% | 0.447 |
| WBC | $8.2 \times 10^3/mm^3$ | $8.2 \times 10^9/L$ |
| AST | 29 IU/L | 0.48 μkat/L |
| ALT | 20 IU/L | 0.33 μkat/L |
| Alk phos | 516 IU/L | 8.60 μkat/L |
| T bili | 2 mg/dL | 34.2 mmol/L |
| D bili | 0.2 mg/dL | 3.4 mmol/L |
| $HbA_{1c}$ | 10.3% | 0.103 (89 mmol/mol Hgb) |

Venous blood gas

| | | |
|---|---|---|
| pH | 7.17 | |
| pCO$_2$ | 25 mm Hg | 3.3 kPa |
| pO$_2$ | 58 mm Hg | 7.7 kPa |
| Calculated HCO$_3$ | 9.1 mEq/L | 9.1 mmol/L |
| Urinalysis | Urine, dark yellow | |
| pH | 5 | |
| Specific gravity | 1.017 | |
| White blood cells | (−) | |
| Nitrite | (−) | |
| Glucose | 890 mg/dL | 49.4 mmol/L |
| Ketone | 150 mg/dL | 14.7 mmol/L |
| Red blood cells | (−) | |
| Protein | (−) | |

## Assessment

The patient is a 20-year-old male with signs, symptoms, and laboratory tests consistent with DKA secondary to T1DM. He is currently awaiting treatment in a room in the emergency department. The nurse is currently placing a peripheral IV line.

### Student Workup

**Missing Information?**

Evaluate:    Patient Database

Drug Therapy Problems

Care Plan (by Problem)

## TARGETED QUESTIONS

1. What signs and symptoms of DKA does the patient have?

    *Hint: See pp. 780–781 in PPP*

2. What happens at the cellular level when insulin is given to a patient with DKA?

    *Hint: Consider how insulin treats hyperglycemia and how this may affect ketone production. See p. 781 in PPP*

3. What electrolyte changes are likely to occur as the patient's blood glucose levels normalize following insulin therapy?

    *Hint: Consider side effects of insulin and glucose metabolism end product. Also see Table 43-12 in PPP*

4. What potential adverse effects of insulin therapy during treatment of DKA and as part of T1DM maintenance therapy would you discuss with the patient?

    *Hint: See p. 774 and Table 43-12 in PPP*

5. What long-term complications may be avoided with better glycemic control?

    *Hint: See pp. 763–764 in PPP*

## FOLLOW-UP

6. Three months after the patient is discharged from the hospital, he returns to the emergency department. He states that has been feeling much better lately, until he became light-headed, tachycardic, and began to sweat profusely while working out in the gym earlier that day. He was found to have a blood glucose level of 54 mg/dL (3.0 mmol/L) on admission to the emergency department. What should be discussed with the patient to help him recognize, prevent, and treat hypoglycemia?

    *Hint: See p. 780 in PPP*

## ⟳ GLOBAL PERSPECTIVE

Worldwide, approximately 70,000 children develop type 1 diabetes mellitus (T1DM) each year, equating to nearly 20 children per day. According to global statistics released by the International Diabetes Federation, 3.8 million deaths are related to type 1 diabetes mellitus.[1] This is a fairly conservative estimate as data were not available from several countries. This study reports some interesting information regarding the global incidence of T1DM. The incidence rate of T1DM seems to vary greatly among different populations. In parts of Asia, Central America, and South America, the incidence is as low as 4 cases per 100,000 in people younger than 14 years. In Scandinavia and some parts of Europe, the incidence is closer to 20 cases per 100,000 in people younger than 14 years.[2] As of 2010, over 200,000 people younger than 20 years in the United States of America have been diagnosed with T1DM.[3] The exact cause of T1DM is not fully understood. Current theories involve genetic predisposition for the disease coupled with viral-induced autoimmune response to insulin-producing β-cells.[4] These genetic and environmental factors may help to explain variations in the global incidence and prevalence of this disease.

## REFERENCES

1. Type 1 Diabetes Facts and Statistics. Juvenile Diabetes Research Foundation. http://www.jdrf.ca/news-and-media/fact-sheets/. Accessed February 22, 2013.

2. Daneman D. State of the world's children with diabetes. Pediatr Diabetes. 2009 10(2):120–126.

3. US Department of Health and Human Services. National Diabetes Statistics, 2011. National Diabetes Information Clearinghouse Web site http://diabetes.niddk.nih.gov/statistics/index.aspx. Accessed February 22, 2013.

4. Achenbach P, Bonifacio E, Koczwara K, Ziegler AG. Natural history of type 1 diabetes. Diabetes 2005 54:S25–S31.

## CASE SUMMARY

- The patient's current clinical picture is consistent with DKA and he should be started on an insulin drip, with dextrose, fluid, and electrolyte replacement as needed.

- Care should be taken to avoid rapid fluctuations in serum electrolyte levels when correcting the patient's serum glucose level.

- The patient will require extensive education on diabetes, the proper use of insulin, and the importance of adherence with insulin therapy.

For more information on the care plan and facilitator's guide please visit http://www.mhpharmacotherapy.com.

# 49 Type 2 Diabetes Mellitus

Susan Cornell

## CASE LEARNING OBJECTIVES

- Assess the signs and symptoms of hyperglycemia
- Differentiate diabetes-related complications
- Evaluate the goals of therapy for type 2 diabetes (T2DM) mellitus
- Develop an appropriate diabetes self-management education, treatment, and monitoring plan for a patient with T2DM and its related conditions

## PATIENT PRESENTATION

### Chief Complaint

"My physician told me I need to control my sugar better. I'm feeling okay, but I think I have another urinary infection. I am going to the bathroom more frequently and sometimes it burns. Will cranberry juice help?"

### History of Present Illness

AL is a 36-year-old woman who presents to the community pharmacy/clinic complaining of frequent and burning urination. She reports having recurrent UTIs and vaginal yeast infections for the past 8 years, ever since the birth of her second child. She is adherent to her physician appointments every 3 months since she was diagnosed with T2DM 3 years ago. She is aware that her glucose and $A_{1c}$ are not at goal and she needs to control her diabetes. She states that she takes her medications daily as prescribed and only misses an occasional dose. She checks her fasting blood glucose almost every day. She tries to monitor the amount and type of food she eats; but often "cheats," especially during tax season when she and her husband are very busy with their business. She walks 3–4 days per week for 20–30 minutes, depending on the weather. She denies any feelings of dizziness, lightheadedness, or fatigue.

### Past Medical History

Dyslipidemia × 5 years

T2DM × 3 years

Obesity × 20 years

Recurrent UTI and yeast infections × 8 years

Gestational DM in two pregnancies (10 and 8 years ago)

### Family History

Father had T2DM, dyslipidemia, and hypertension, and died from a myocardial infarction at the age of 56. Mother is alive at age 60 and has T2DM, dyslipidemia, sleep apnea, and GERD. Brother is alive at age 40 and has T2DM and HTN. Sister is alive at age 33 and is healthy.

### Social History

She came to the United States from Puerto Rico at the age of 6, speaks Spanish and English. She is married for 13 years and lives with husband and two children aged 9 and 7. Works as an administrative assistant for her husband's accounting business. He is self-employed.

### Tobacco/Alcohol/Substance Use

Social drinker (one to two glasses of wine two to three times per week); (–) tobacco or illicit drug use.

### Allergies/Intolerances/Adverse Drug Events

No known drug or food allergies

### Medications (Current)

Metformin 1,000 mg PO q 24 h (with dinner)

Atorvastatin 20 mg PO q 24 h (at bedtime)

ASA 81 mg PO q 24 h (with dinner)

Ortho Tri-Cyclen-28 PO q day (at bedtime)

Tylenol 500 mg PRN

## Review of Systems

Occasional body aches relieved with acetaminophen. (+) Increased frequency and burning upon urination. (−) Vaginal discharge or dyspareunia; (−) tinnitus, vertigo, dizziness, lightheadedness, or fatigue. (+) Dry skin, minor bruises on (r) upper arm.

## Physical Examination

### ▶ General

Well-appearing, young Hispanic woman in no acute distress

### ▶ Vital Signs

BP 136/78 mm Hg, P 68, RR 14, T 36.8°C

Weight 225.5 lb (102.5 kg)

Height 63 in. (160 cm)

BMI 40 kg/m²

Waist circumference 37 in. (94 cm)

Denies pain other than burning on urination

### ▶ Skin

Dry appearing skin, two visible bruises on right upper arm which patient states have been there for several weeks after "bumping into a door"

### ▶ HEENT

PERRLA, (−) sinus tenderness, TMs normal

### ▶ Chest

Clear to auscultation

### ▶ Breast

Examination deferred

### ▶ Cardiovascular

RRR, normal $S_1$, $S_2$, (−) $S_3$ or $S_4$

### ▶ Abdomen

Not tender/not distended; (−) organomegaly

### ▶ Extremities

No edema, (+) pedal pulses, (−) lesions or callus, (+) hair on first toe at the interphalangeal joint on both feet; normal monofilament examination bilaterally

### ▶ Genitourinary

Examination deferred

### ▶ Rectal

Examination deferred

## Laboratory Tests

### Fasting

|  | Conventional Units | SI Units |
|---|---|---|
| Na | 137 mEq/L | 137 mmol/L |
| K | 4.7 mEq/L | 4.7 mmol/L |
| Cl | 101 mEq/L | 101 mmol/L |
| $CO_2$ | 22 mEq/L | 22 mmol/L |
| BUN | 9 mg/dL | 3.2 mmol/L |
| SCr | 0.8 mg/dL | 71 mmol/L |
| Glu | 168 mg/dL | 9.3 mmol/L |
| $HbA_{1c}$ | 8.2% | 0.082 (66 mmol/mol Hgb) |
| AST | 22 U/L | 0.37 μkat/L |
| ALT | 44 U/L | 0.73 μkat/L |
| Total cholesterol | 184 mg/dL | 4.76 mmol/L |
| LDL cholesterol | 112 mg/dL | 2.90 mmol/L |
| HDL cholesterol | 29 mg/dL | 0.75 mmol/L |
| Triglycerides | 217 mg/dL | 2.45 mmol/l |
| Hgb | 13.5 g/dL | 135 g/L; 8.38 mmol/L |
| Hct | 37.7% | 0.377 |
| RBC | $4.47 \times 10^6/mm^3$ | $4.47 \times 10^{12}/L$ |
| WBC | $11.2 \times 10^3/mm^3$ | $4.47 \times 10^9/L$ |
| Platelets | $172 \times 10^3/mm^3$ | $172 \times 10^9/L$ |

Urinalysis: Trace (+) protein, (−) heme, (+) nitrite, WBC 10–20/HPF

## Assessment

Thirty-six-year old woman with obesity, T2DM and inadequate glycemic control, dyslipidemia, and dietary nonadherence. She has signs and symptoms suggestive of UTI, and she has a history of recurrent UTIs and vaginal infections.

## Student Workup

### Missing Information?

**Evaluate:**   Patient Database

Drug Therapy Problems

Care Plan (by Problem)

## TARGETED QUESTIONS

1. What signs and symptoms is the patient experiencing that may indicate her diabetes is not controlled?

    *HINT: See pp. 761–763 and Table 43-7 in PPP*

2. What diabetes-related complications does the patient have?

    *HINT: See p. 758 in PPP*

3. What are the therapeutic goals for this patient?

    *HINT: See pp. 763–765 in PPP*

4. What modifications should be made to her drug therapy and diabetes self-management plans?

    *HINT: See Tables 43-8, 9, 10 in PPP*

5. How should the patient's therapeutic plan be monitored?

    *HINT: See Figure 43-2 and Tables 43-7, 8, 10 in PPP*

## ⊙ GLOBAL PERSPECTIVE

T2DM is growing at an epidemic rate.[1] Worldwide more than 285 million people have diabetes, and more than 3.2 million people die each year from diabetes-related problems. Almost 80% of deaths due to diabetes occur in low- to middle-income countries. Almost half of the deaths (mostly from heart disease and stroke) occur in people younger than 70 years, and it is projected that diabetes deaths will double between 2005 and 2030. As many developing countries adopt a Western diet and lifestyle, increased rates of obesity are associated with increased diabetes morbidity and mortality. The approach to T2DM is similar in all countries, including eating a healthy diet and exercise. However, low-income patients may have poor access to health care and may not be able to afford or have access to healthier foods and medications.[1,2]

## REFERENCES

1. CDC National Diabetes Fact Sheet, 2011. Available at: http://www.cdc.gov/diabetes/pubs/pdf/ndfs_2011.pdf. Accessed February 22, 2013.
2. International Diabetes Federation Atlas 2012. Available at: http://www.idf.org/diabetesatlas/5e/Update2012. Accessed February 22, 2013.

### CASE SUMMARY

- The patient needs diabetes self-management education. She is unaware of the relationship between her recurrent UTIs, delayed wound healing, and cardiovascular complications and her type 2 diabetes.
- If the patient's BP stays above the desired target, starting the patient on hypertension pharmacotherapy is warranted. Adding a second blood glucose-lowering agent may be warranted. Considerations regarding adverse effects and drug/disease interactions must be addressed.
- Lifestyle modifications must be aggressively addressed to achieve improved control of diabetes, hypertension, cholesterol, and weight.

**For more information on the care plan and facilitator's guide please visit http://www.mhpharmacotherapy.com.**

# 50 Diabetes and Pain

Amy K. Kennedy

## CASE LEARNING OBJECTIVES

- Assess the signs and symptoms of diabetic neuropathy
- List the goals of treatment for patients with diabetic neuropathy
- Select appropriate nonpharmacologic and pharmacologic treatment regimens for patients presenting with diabetic neuropathy
- Develop a monitoring plan that assesses the safety and efficacy of the patient's diabetic neuropathy management

## PATIENT PRESENTATION

### Chief Complaint

"My feet are on fire and I cannot sleep."

### History of Present Illness

Andrew Carter is a 60-year-old African-American male with type 2 diabetes who presents to your ambulatory care clinic with burning pain in both feet. He reports that "nothing has helped, even the medication I took for surgery last year." The pain has worsened over the past several months and is preventing him from falling asleep. Patient also says that in the past he could eat anything put in front of him, but lately he has been nauseated and felt full with a small amount of food. When asked, patient says that he takes all of his medicine at the same time on an empty stomach.

### Past Medical History

Type 2 diabetes diagnosed at age 39

Benign essential HTN diagnosed at age 44

Dyslipidemia diagnosed at age 39

ACL surgery 1 year ago

### Family History

Father had HTN and died from a stroke at age 67

Mother is alive at age 82 and has HTN and asthma

Sister is alive at age 57 with a history of asthma

### Social History

Widowed 2 years ago, lives alone and is working at a grocery store. Son and daughter-in-law live out of state.

### Tobacco/Alcohol/Substance Use

(–) alcohol, but he does smoke 2 ppd of cigarettes.

### Allergies/Intolerances/Adverse Drug Events

Lisinopril: Cough

### Medications (Current)

Aspirin 81 mg daily

Insulin glargine 10 units daily

Losartan 100 mg daily

Metformin 500 mg twice daily

Pravastatin 40 mg daily

Diphenhydramine 50 mg daily at bedtime as needed (has used over the past several days without relief)

### Medications (Prior)

Was on glipizide and metformin when he was first diagnosed, but insulin was started 3 months ago.

### Review of Systems

Feet: (+) paresthesia (burning, tingling) and allodynia that is worse at night, (–) for ulcer, cuts, sores, or deformities, (+) dry skin. (+) nausea and bloating, (+) for insomnia, (–) chest pain, SOB or dizziness.

### Physical Examination

▶ *General*

The patient is a healthy looking individual who is alert and oriented ×3 in moderate distress due to his insomnia.

▶ **Vital Signs**

BP 118/76 mm Hg, P 98 bpm, RR 20, T 36.8°C

Height 5'8" (173 cm), weight 151 lb (68.6 kg)

Pain 8/10

▶ **Skin**

Dry, warm, intact

▶ **HEENT**

PERRLA

▶ **Chest**

(−) for pain, lungs are clear to auscultation without rhonchi, rales, or wheezing

▶ **Cardiovascular**

RRR without $S_3$, $S_4$

▶ **Abdomen**

Positive bowel sounds, soft, nontender

▶ **Neurology**

CNs II–XII intact

▶ **Extremities**

Dry, intact skin. (+) pedal pulses, (+) allodynia, paresthesia, (−) cuts, sores or lesions. Semmes–Weinstein 10 g monofilament exam normal except for decreased sensation on second metatarsal bilaterally. Toronto Neuropathy Scoring System = 6, patient reported pain 8/10.

▶ **Genitourinary**

Deferred

▶ **Rectal**

(−) hemorrhoids

## Laboratory and Other Diagnostic Tests

| | Conventional Units | SI units |
|---|---|---|
| Na | 137 mEq/L | 137 mmol/L |
| K | 4.4 mEq/L | 4.4 mmol/L |
| Cl | 102 mEq/L | 102 mmol/L |
| $CO_2$ | 25 mEq/L | 25 mmol/L |
| BUN | 18 mg/dL | 6.4 mmol/L |
| SCr | 1.1 mg/dL | 97 μmol/L |
| Glu | 257 mg/dL | 14.3 mmol/L |
| Hgb | 15.6 g/dL | 135 g/L; 9.68 mmol/L |
| Hct | 48.2% | 0.48 |
| WBC | $8.3 \times 10^3/mm^3$ | $8.3 \times 10^9/L$ |
| Platelets | $186 \times 10^3/mm^3$ | $186 \times 10^9/L$ |
| Albumin | 3.9 g/dL | 39 g/L |
| AST | 24 U/L | 0.4 μkat/L |
| ALT | 36 U/L | 0.6 μkat/L |
| Alk Phos | 124 U/L | 2.07 μkat/L |
| $HbA_{1c}$ | 13.2% | 0.132; 121 mmol/mol Hgb |
| Total cholesterol | 190 mg/dL | 4.91 mmol/L |
| Triglycerides | 270 mg/dL | 3.05 mmol/L |
| HDL cholesterol | 40 mg/dL | 1.03 mmol/L |
| LDL cholesterol | 96 mg/dL | 2.48 mmol/L |
| TSH | 0.89 uIU/ml | 0.89 mIU/ml |
| Vitamin $B_{12}$ | 547 pg/mL | 404 μmol/L |

## Assessment

60-year-old male with hypertension, dyslipidemia and poorly controlled type 2 diabetes. He presents today with new onset painful diabetic peripheral neuropathy and possible diabetic gastroparesis.

## Student Workup

**Missing Information?**

**Evaluate:**    Patient Database

Drug Therapy Problems

Care Plan (by Problem)

## TARGETED QUESTIONS

1. What signs, symptoms, and laboratory data support the diagnosis of peripheral neuropathy?

   *Hint: See p. 782 in PPP*

2. What other diabetes-related neuropathies should be ruled out at this time?

   *Hint: See p. 782 in PPP*

3. What are the treatment goals for this patient?

   *Hint: See p. 610 in PPP*

4. What would be the most appropriate course of treatment for this patient? Please address pharmacological and nonpharmacological aspects. For the pharmacological agent, please include dose, route, frequency and duration. Please explain your rationale.

   *Hint: See pp. 616, 782 in PPP*

## FOLLOW-UP

AC returns 3 months later for follow-up labs. $HbA_{1c}$ is 8.3% (0.083; 67 mmol/mol Hgb). He reports that he is doing much better, but he notices that his feet are cold a lot of the time and that there is less hair on them.

5. What might AC have developed?

> *Hint: It is also a major risk factor for diabetic foot infections and see p. 782 in PPP*

## ⟳ GLOBAL PERSPECTIVE

Peripheral neuropathy is one of the most common diabetic complications[1,2] with a prevalence of 30–50%. This prevalence increases in developing countries. Even in developed countries, peripheral neuropathies account for more hospitalizations than all other neuropathies combined and is a major risk factor for complications. Additionally, common prescribing patterns lag behind treatment guidelines.[3] In one study, almost 40% of patients reported that they were never treated and 33% were treated with medications with no known efficacy for neuropathy.

## REFERENCES

1. Daousi C, MacFarlane IA, Woodward A, et al. Chronic painful peripheral neuropathy in an urban community: a controlled comparison of people with and without diabetes. Diabet Med 2004 21:976–982.

2. Vinik AI, Mehrabyan A. Diabetic neuropathies. Med Clin North Am 2004 88:947–999.

3. Bril V, England J, Franklin GM, et al. Evidence-based guideline: treatment of painful diabetic neuropathy: report of the American Academy of Neurology, the American Association of Neuromuscular and Electrodiagnostic Medicine, and the American Academy of Physical Medicine. Neurology 2011 76:1758–1769.

### CASE SUMMARY

- The patient's clinical presentation was consistent with peripheral diabetic neuropathy characterized by paresthesias and allodynia.
- Treatment for peripheral neuropathy is symptomatic in nature with control of hyperglycemia the best mechanism for prevention of complications.
- When a patient presents with peripheral neuropathy, it is prudent to assess whether other neuropathies are present.

**For more information on the care plan and facilitator's guide please visit http://www.mhpharmacotherapy.com**

# 51 Hyperthyroidism: Graves' Disease

Andrea N. Traina    Michael P. Kane

## CASE LEARNING OBJECTIVES

- Recognize the signs and symptoms of subclinical and overt hyperthyroidism
- Identify the goals of treatment for hyperthyroidism
- Develop an appropriate pharmacotherapy care plan for the management of hyperthyroidism based on individual patient characteristics and appropriate clinical judgment
- Properly educate a patient being treated for hyperthyroidism

## PATIENT PRESENTATION

### Chief Complaint

"My neck is swollen and I am having a hard time swallowing!"

### History of Present Illness

Michael Vera is a 60-year-old female who presents to the clinic complaining of swelling and tenderness in her neck with difficulties swallowing solids and liquids, as well as 5 days of watery diarrhea. She appears anxious and is having a hard time sitting still during the interview. She explains that she has not felt like herself in well over a year, but things have gotten significantly worse over the last 4 months. She has had an unintentional weight loss of approximately 70 lb (32 kg) over the past year despite an increase in appetite. She attributes this weight loss to be the reason she is so exhausted and why her muscles have felt so weak of late. She also complains that she is heat intolerant and perspires with very little activity. Finally, she inquires about allergy eye drops as her eyes have been bothering her for the last several months since they are so itchy and watery, "feeling as if they are ready to pop out of my head."

### Past Medical History

Seasonal allergies

Systolic hypertension × 1 year

Atrial fibrillation × 6 months

s/p total abdominal hysterectomy/bilateral salpingo-oophorectomy (TAH/BSO) at age 45

### Family History

Maternal grandmother with goiter and subsequent thyroidectomy. Mother with hyperthyroidism (treated with medication) and osteoporosis. Father with coronary artery disease and type 2 diabetes mellitus.

### Social History

Married and lives with her husband of 37 years; has two dogs, and no children. She works as a kindergarten teacher at the local elementary school.

### Tobacco/Alcohol/Substance Use

(+) Tobacco 45-pack year history (currently 1.5 ppd); (−) alcohol or illicit drug use.

### Allergies/Intolerances/Adverse Drug Events

NKDA

### Medications (Current)

Loratadine 10 mg PO daily PRN

Verapamil 240 mg PO daily

Digoxin 0.125 mg PO daily

Warfarin 2.5 mg PO daily

Calcium citrate with D (315 mg calcium with 200 IU Vitamin $D_3$) two tablets PO three times daily

## Review of Systems

Denies chest pain, shortness or breath, abdominal pain, hematochezia, dysuria, hematuria, changes in urinary frequency or urgency.

## Physical Examination

### ▶ General

Pleasant, middle-aged, Caucasian woman in no acute distress

### ▶ Vital Signs

BP 140/80 mm Hg, P 110, RR 18

Weight 118 lb (53.6 kg)

Height 63 in. (160 cm)

Denies pain

### ▶ Skin

Warm, moist to touch; (−) rashes or lesions

### ▶ HEENT

PERRLA, EOMI; (+) lid lag; mild proptosis without diplopia on upper outward gaze

### ▶ Neck and Lymph Nodes

Thyroid gland approximately 3 × normal size; minimally tender; (+) bruit versus radiated murmur over thyroid; symmetric and non-nodular

### ▶ Chest

Clear

### ▶ Cardiovascular

Tachycardia, irregular rate regular rhythm, 1/6 systolic murmur, (−) gallop or rub

### ▶ Abdomen

Soft, nontender; (−) organomegaly

### ▶ Neurology

Nonfocal; (+) bilateral resting tremor; increased DTRs

### ▶ Extremities

(−) Cyanosis, clubbing or edema

## Laboratory Tests

### Fasting Obtained Yesterday

|  | Conventional Units | SI Units |
| --- | --- | --- |
| Na | 138 mEq/L | 138 mmol/L |
| K | 4.3 mEq/L | 4.3 mmol/L |
| Cl | 98 mEq/L | 98 mmol/L |
| $CO_2$ | 25 mEq/L | 25 mmol/L |
| BUN | 9 mg/dL | 3.2 mmol/L |
| SCr | 0.9 mg/dL | 80 μmol/L |
| Glu | 84 mg/dL | 4.7 mmol/L |
| Ca | 9.2 mg/dL | 2.30 mmol/L |
| Mg | 2.0 mEq/L | 1.00 mmol/L |
| Phosphate | 3.0 mg/dL | 0.97 mmol/L |
| ALP | 123 IU/L | 2.05 μkat/L |
| AST | 24 IU/L | 0.40 μkat/L |
| ALT | 64 IU/L | 1.07 μkat/L |
| 25-OH vitamin D | 4.8 ng/mL | 12 nmol/L |
| INR | 2.7 | |
| Hgb | 12.2 g/dL | 122 g/L; 7.57 mmol/L |
| Hct | 39.4% | 0.394 |
| WBC | $10.4 \times 10^3/mm^3$ | $10.4 \times 10^9/L$ |
| Neutrophils | 57% | 0.57 |
| MCV | 83 μm³ | 83 fL |
| PLT | $305 \times 10^3/mm^3$ | $305 \times 10^9/L$ |
| Albumin | 3.6 g/dL | 36 g/L |
| Anti-thyroid peroxidase (TPO) antibody | (+) | |
| Thyrotropin receptor (TSHR)-S antibody | (+) | |
| TSH | <0.01 μU/mL | <0.01 mU/L |
| $T_3$ | 876 ng/dL | 13.5 nmol/L |
| Free $T_4$ | 6.71 ng/dL | 86.4 pmol/L |
| Total cholesterol | 110 mg/dL | 2.84 mmol/L |
| LDL cholesterol | 42 mg/dL | 1.09 mmol/L |
| HDL cholesterol | 38 mg/dL | 0.98 mmol/L |

## Assessment

Sixty-year-old woman with signs, symptoms, and laboratory tests consistent with severe Graves' disease

### Student Workup

#### Missing Information?

**Evaluate:**    Patient Database

Drug Therapy Problems

Care Plan (by Problem)

## TARGETED QUESTIONS

1.  What signs and symptoms of hyperthyroidism does the patient have?

    *Hint: See p. 798 in PPP*

2.  What are the advantages and disadvantages of thioamide therapy, radioactive iodine (RAI), and surgery for Graves' disease treatment?

    *Hint: See pp. 799–801 in PPP*

3.  What medications can cause hyperthyroidism?

    *Hint: See p. 803 in PPP*

4.  What risks and adverse effects of thioamide therapy would you discuss with the patient?

    *Hint: See pp. 799–800 in PPP*

5.  What complications of hyperthyroidism is this patient experiencing or at risk for?

    *Hint: See pp. 797–798 in PPP*

## FOLLOW-UP

6.  Three weeks later, the patient returns for follow-up. She feels much better, she has regained a bit of weight (4 lb [1.8 kg]), notes improved energy, less weakness, and tremulousness, and denies palpitations. She is no longer having difficulty swallowing and denies neck pain. Her TSH, drawn today, is still undetectable at <0.01 μIU/mL (<0.01 mIU/L); however, her $T_3$ and free $T_4$ have markedly improved at 213 ng/dL (3.3 nmol/L) and 1.48 ng/dL (19.0 pmol/L), respectively. At what point would you recheck thyroid function tests? When would you expect her to reach a euthyroid state? Once a euthyroid state is achieved what, if any, dosage changes would you recommend in her thioamide therapy? At what point would you consider RAI? What medication changes need to be considered prior to RAI therapy?[1]

    *Hint: See pp. 799–801 in PPP*

## REFERENCES

1.  Bahn RS, Burch HB, Cooper DS, et al. Hyperthyroidism and other causes of thyrotoxicosis: Management guidelines of the American Thyroid Association and American Association of Clinical Endocrinologists. Thyroid 2011 21:593–646.

2.  U.S. Food and Drug Administration FDA drug safety communication: New boxed warning on severe liver injury with propylthiouracil; http://www.fda.gov/Drugs/DrugSafety/Postmarket Drug SafetyInformationforPatientsandProviders/ucm209023. htm. Accessed May 7, 2012.

### ⟳ GLOBAL PERSPECTIVE

Iodine deficiency is a common cause of hypothyroid disease in developing countries. Percentages of hyperthyroid patients treated with RAI, surgery, or drug therapy vary among countries. Several drugs are associated with thyroid disease.

### CASE SUMMARY

*   Patient's current clinical picture is consistent with severe Graves' disease and treatment needs to be initiated.

*   Given the severity of disease methimazole 20 mg PO every 8 hours should be initiated. The patient should return in 1–2 weeks and thyroid function tests should be drawn with the methimazole dose titrated accordingly. Once euthyroid state has been reached (approximately 6–8 weeks) a maintenance dose of 5 to 15 mg/d should be given to avoid hypothyroidism.

*   Symptomatic relief should also be provided by initiating propranolol 20 mg PO four times daily. Discontinuation of verapamil and digoxin can be considered (with monitoring) after adequate treatment of her hyperthyroidism (the systolic hypertension and atrial fibrillation will likely resolve). In anticipation of reaching a euthyroid state, a discussion of the pros and cons of definitive treatment should take place (*see Table 44-1*).

*   Patient needs to follow-up with ophthalmology for evaluation, and be urged to quit smoking prior to considering RAI therapy as to avoid or minimize the risk of exacerbating her Graves' eye disease.

**For more information on the care plan and facilitator's guide please visit http://www.mhpharmacotherapy.com.**

# 52 Hypothyroidism

Michael D. Katz

## PATIENT PRESENTATION

### Chief Complaint

"I'm so tired lately. I have no energy. Maybe I need some vitamins or something."

### History of Present Illness

Yi-Ling Wang is a 49-year-old woman who presents to her new physician complaining of feeling tired, lethargic, and "not thinking straight" for the last 6 months. She has seen her previous primary care physician several times and has been told that her symptoms are probably due to anemia from menorrhagia, stress, depression, and/or impending menopause. She was not entirely satisfied with those explanations, and despite treatment with iron (and resultant improvement of her anemia), a hormonal contraceptive to help regulate her menstrual cycle, and an antidepressant, her symptoms have slowly worsened. Two years ago at a pharmacy student-run health fair, she was told her TSH was 6.2 μIU/mL (6.2 mIU/L) and her total cholesterol was 246 mg/dL (6.36 mmol/L). Y-L's primary care physician felt the TSH value was compatible with subclinical hypothyroidism and therefore could not explain her symptoms at that time. She has been wondering if she really is depressed and why the depression medication is not helping. Over the past few months, she has also noticed that her skin seems a little more dry and itchy and that she has difficulty keeping warm even in warm weather. Finally, she asks you what is good for constipation since the Chinese herbs her mother gave her are not helping.

### Past Medical History

Iron-deficiency anemia diagnosed 6 months ago

Depression × 6 months

Menorrhagia diagnosed 6 months ago

Osteopenia × 1 year

### Family History

Father had CAD and died of gastric cancer at age 74. Mother is alive at age 70 with osteoporosis and hypothyroidism. She has one older brother who is healthy.

### Social History

Came to the United States from China at age 15. Speaks Mandarin and English. Married and lives with her husband of 24 years; has two children, aged 22 and 19. Works as a language instructor at a local community college.

### Tobacco/Alcohol/Substance Use

Social drinker; (–) tobacco or illicit drug use

### Allergies/Intolerances/Adverse Drug Events

Penicillin (rash as child)

### Medications (Current)

MOM 30 mL PO q 24 h PRN constipation

Rhubarb (Chinese herbal product) PO PRN constipation

Sertraline 50 mg PO q 24 h

Ortho Tri-Cyclen 28 PO q day

$FeSO_4$ 300 mg PO q day

Calcium carbonate 1,000 mg PO bid

Alendronate 35 mg PO weekly

Acetaminophen 650 mg PO PRN headache, body aches

## Review of Systems

Occasional HA relieved with nonaspirin pain reliever; (–) tinnitus, vertigo, or infections; frequent body aches, which she attributes to lack of exercise; (–) change in urinary frequency, but she has noticed an increase in the number of episodes of constipation in the past year; reports cold extremities; (–) history of seizures, syncope, or loss of consciousness; (+) dry skin.

## Physical Examination

▶ **General**

Well-appearing, Asian woman in no acute distress

▶ **Vital Signs**

BP 112/76 mm Hg, P 64, RR 12, T 36.2°C

Weight 127.6 lb (58 kg)

Height 62 in. (157 cm)

Denies pain

▶ **Skin**

Dry-appearing skin and scalp; (–) rashes or lesions

▶ **HEENT**

PERRLA, EOMI; trace periorbital edema; (–) sinus tenderness; TMs appear normal

▶ **Neck and Lymph Nodes**

Thyroid gland smooth, slightly enlarged symmetrically; (–) thyroid nodules; (–) lymphadenopathy; (–) carotid bruits

▶ **Chest**

Clear to auscultation

▶ **Breasts**

Examination deferred (previous breast exam 3 months ago)

▶ **Cardiovascular**

RRR, normal $S_1$, $S_2$; (–) $S_3$ or $S_4$

▶ **Abdomen**

Not tender/not distended; (–) organomegaly

▶ **Neurology**

Grossly intact; DTRs normal

▶ **Genitourinary**

Examination deferred

▶ **Rectal**

Examination deferred

## Laboratory Tests

### Fasting Obtained 2 Days Ago

|  | Conventional Units | SI Units |
|---|---|---|
| Na | 142 mEq/L | 142 mmol/L |
| K | 4.1 mEq/L | 4.1 mmol/L |
| Cl | 100 mEq/L | 100 mmol/L |
| $CO_2$ | 24 mEq/L | 24 mmol/L |
| BUN | 7 mg/dL | 2.5 mmol/L |
| SCr | 0.7 mg/dL | 62 μmol/L |
| Glu | 104 mg/dL | 5.8 mmol/L |
| Ca | 9.4 mg/dL | 2.35 mmol/L |
| Mg | 1.8 mEq/L | 0.90 mmol/L |
| Phosphate | 3.8 mg/dL | 1.23 mmol/L |
| Hgb | 13.5 g/dL | 135 g/L; 8.38 mmol/L |
| Hct | 39.7% | 0.397 |
| WBC | $7.6 \times 10^3$/mm³ | $7.6 \times 10^9$/L |
| MCV | 83 μm³ | 83 fL |
| Albumin | 3.8 g/dL | 38 g/L |
| Anti-TPO antibody | (+) | |
| TSH | 12.8 μIU/mL | 12.8 mIU/L |
| Free $T_4$ | 0.71 ng/dL | 9.1 pmol/L |
| Total cholesterol | 268 mg/dL | 6.93 mmol/L |
| LDL cholesterol | 142 mg/dL | 3.67 mmol/L |
| HDL cholesterol | 36 mg/dL | 0.93 mmol/L |

## Assessment

Forty-nine-year-old woman with signs, symptoms, and laboratory tests consistent with hypothyroidism

---

### Student Workup

**Missing Information?**

**Evaluate:**   Patient Database

Drug Therapy Problems

Care Plan (by Problem)

---

## TARGETED QUESTIONS

1. What s/s of hypothyroidism does the patient have?
   *Hint: See pp. 791–792 in PPP*

2. Why is levothyroxine ($LT_4$) the treatment of choice for most patients with hypothyroidism?
   *Hint: See p. 793 in PPP*

3. What medications can cause hypothyroidism?
   *Hint: See p. 803 and Table 44-2 in PPP*

4. What risks and adverse effects of therapy would you discuss with the patient?

   *Hint: See p. 796 in PPP*

5. Should the patient receive specific lipid-lowering pharmacotherapy?

   *Hint: Hypothyroidism is commonly associated with elevated LDL cholesterol, and adequate LT$_4$ replacement may significantly lower LDL. Since the patient has no other cardiovascular risk factors, it would be reasonable to withhold specific lipid-lowering pharmacotherapy until she has been euthyroid for several months.*

## FOLLOW-UP

6. Eight weeks later, the patient returns for follow-up. She feels much better, with more energy and less depressed feelings. Her TSH, drawn yesterday, is 0.2 µIU/mL (0.2 mIU/L). What are some reasons why her TSH might now be low and what are the risks associated with a suppressed TSH? What actions, if any, would you take?

   *Hint: See pp. 795–797 in PPP*

## 🌐 GLOBAL PERSPECTIVE

Goiter, an enlargement of the thyroid gland, is caused by a variety of conditions, and can be associated with normal, excessive, or deficient thyroid function (Figure 52-1). In developed countries, enlargement of the thyroid gland is most often associated with nodular goiter, autoimmune thyroiditis, and Grave's disease. However, in developing countries, iodine-deficient diet is commonly associated with goiter. Iodine deficiency and endemic goiter are especially common in women of childbearing age since pregnancy increases iodine requirements. Substances in the diet can also serve as goitrogens. Diets high in foods or herbal products containing cyanoglucosides (cassava, lima beans, maize, bamboo shoots, and sweet potatoes) release cyanide, which is then metabolized to thiocyanate, an agent

**FIGURE 52-1.** Goiter. (Adapted, with permission, from Gardner DG, Shoback D. Greenspan's Clffinical & Basic Endocrinology, 8th ed. New York, McGraw-Hill, 2007, Fig. 8-27A.)

that inhibits iodine transport. Foods or herbal products high in thioglucosides (cruciferous vegetables) can have a thionamide-like effect on the thyroid gland. Endemic goiter is easily treated with iodine supplementation (often in the form of iodized salt) and avoidance of dietary goitrogens.

## CASE SUMMARY

- The patient's current clinical picture is consistent with overt hypothyroidism, and thyroid replacement therapy should be initiated.
- An initial levothyroxine dose of 50 mcg daily is reasonable, with dose titration to target TSH (0.5–2.5 µIU/mL [0.5–2.5 mIU/L]) using TSH values obtained at least 6 weeks after any change in the dose.
- Overreplacement of thyroid hormone should be avoided, especially with her history of osteopenia.

**For more information on the care plan and facilitator's guide please visit http://www.mhpharmacotherapy.com.**

# 53 Cushing's Syndrome

Devra K. Dang          Jiehyun Lee

## CASE LEARNING OBJECTIVES

- Recognize the clinical presentation of Cushing's syndrome and the physiologic consequences of cortisol excess
- Describe the pharmacologic and nonpharmacologic management of patients with Cushing's syndrome
- Recommend strategies to prevent the development of Cushing's syndrome associated with exogenous glucocorticoid administration
- Recommend therapy-monitoring parameters for patients with Cushing's syndrome

## PATIENT PRESENTATION

### Chief Complaint

"Doctor, something is wrong with me. I'm gaining so much weight and I'm always so tired and weak."

### History of Present Illness

JT is a 48-year-old female who presents to her primary care physician's (PCP) office with complaints of increasing fatigue and muscle weakness over the last 3 months. She states that she feels so tired and weak some mornings that she is not able to get herself out of bed. She also reports having gained about 10 lb (~4.5 kg) over the last 3 months and has been experiencing menstrual irregularity since then. She is not pregnant and not currently attempting to become pregnant. JT was diagnosed with RA 2 years ago, at which point she was placed on hydroxychloroquine 400 mg daily and celecoxib 200 mg daily to relieve joint pain and stiffness. Within the last year, she had been experiencing more flare-ups of her RA. Hydroxychloroquine and celecoxib were discontinued and she was placed on prednisone approximately 4 months ago. Since being diagnosed with RA, the patient also reports having episodes of depressed mood. Her depression had been well controlled on sertraline 50 mg PO daily, but she reports increasing number of depressive episodes recently.

### Past Medical History

RA × 2 years

Depression × 1½ years

HTN × 1 year

Dyslipidemia × 1 year

### Family History

Mother is alive at age 72 with type 2 DM; father is alive at age 75 with type 2 DM and HTN. She has one sister, who is healthy.

### Social History

Married and lives with husband. Has a healthy 19-year-old son in college. Works as an assistant manager at a local grocery store

### Tobacco/Alcohol/Substance Use

(−) Alcohol, tobacco, or illicit drug use

### Allergies/Intolerances/Adverse Drug Events

No known drug/food allergies/intolerances/ADEs

### Medications (Current)

Prednisone 10 mg PO q AM

Sertraline 50 mg PO q AM

Lisinopril/HCTZ 20 mg/12.5 mg PO q AM

Atorvastatin 20 mg PO q AM

### Review of Systems

(+) Fatigue and frequent body aches with muscle weakness in major muscle groups; (+) pain in joints of hands, ankles, and knees; reports weight gain in her abdomen, face, and around her neck and shoulders; (+) excess hair growth on face; (+) generalized depressed mood and insomnia; (+) thin, dry skin with occasional bruising; notes irregular light periods; (+) increased urination; (+) increased thirst

## Physical Examination

### ▶ General

Cushingoid-appearing, obese, middle-aged Caucasian woman in slight distress

### ▶ Vital Signs

BP 144/86 mm Hg, P 80, RR 16, T 37°C

Weight 188.1 lb (85.5 kg)

Height 63 in. (160 cm)

Pain 3/10 in joints of hands, ankles, and knees

### ▶ Skin

Thin, dry-appearing skin with several small bruises; (−) rashes; pink and purple striae visible on abdomen and bilateral breasts

### ▶ HEENT

Round face; excess facial hair; PERRLA, EOMI; (−) sinus tenderness; TMs appear normal

### ▶ Neck and Lymph Nodes

(−) Lymphadenopathy; (−) carotid bruits, JVD, or thyromegaly

### ▶ Chest

Clear to auscultation bilaterally

### ▶ Breasts

Normal with some pink and purple striae bilaterally; (−) lumps

### ▶ Cardiovascular

RRR, normal $S_1$, $S_2$; (−) $S_3$ or $S_4$

### ▶ Abdomen

Soft; not tender; obese with pink and purple striae; (−) organomegaly

### ▶ Neurology

Grossly intact; DTRs normal

### ▶ Genitourinary

Examination deferred

### ▶ Rectal

Examination deferred

### ▶ Musculoskeletal/Extremities

Decreased muscle strength in upper and lower extremities bilaterally; bilateral symmetrical tenderness at metacarpophalangeal (MCP) and proximal interphalangeal (PIP) joints of the hands and joints of ankles

## Laboratory Tests

### Collected as Fasting at 9 am

|  | Conventional Units | SI Units |
|---|---|---|
| Na | 139 mEq/L | 139 mmol/L |
| K | 3.6 mEq/L | 3.6 mmol/L |
| Cl | 102 mEq/L | 102 mmol/L |
| $CO_2$ | 24 mEq/L | 24 mmol/L |
| BUN | 13 mg/dL | 4.6 mmol/L |
| SCr | 0.8 mg/dL | 71 μmol/L |
| Glu | 133 mg/dL | 7.4 mmol/L |
| Ca | 9.6 mg/dL | 2.40 mmol/L |
| Mg | 1.9 mEq/L | 0.95 mmol/L |
| Phosphate | 3.7 mg/dL | 1.20 mmol/L |
| Total cholesterol | 228 mg/dL | 5.90 mmol/L |
| LDL cholesterol | 142 mg/dL | 3.67 mmol/L |
| HDL cholesterol | 48 mg/dL | 1.24 mmol/L |
| Triglycerides | 190 mg/dL | 2.15 mmol/L |
| Hgb | 13.5 g/dL | 135 g/L; 8.38 mmol/L |
| Hct | 38.7% | 0.387 |
| MCV | 86 μm³ | 86 fL |
| WBC | $6.6 \times 10^3$/mm³ | $6.6 \times 10^9$/L |
| Platelets | $280 \times 10^3$/mm³ | $280 \times 10^9$/L |
| Albumin | 3.8 g/dL | 38 g/L |
| Total bilirubin | 0.5 mg/dL | 8.6 μmol/L |
| Direct bilirubin | 0.1 mg/dL | 1.7 μmol/L |
| AST | 32 IU/L | 0.53 μkat/L |
| ALT | 26 IU/L | 0.42 μkat/L |
| Alkaline phosphatase | 112 IU/L | 1.87 μkat/L |
| Rheumatoid factor | (+) | |

## Assessment

Forty-eight-year-old woman with clinical presentation consistent with Cushing's syndrome

## Student Workup

### Missing Information?

**Evaluate:**   Patient Database

Drug Therapy Problems

Care Plan (by Problem)

## TARGETED QUESTIONS

1. What signs and symptoms of Cushing's syndrome does the patient exhibit?

   *Hint: See p. 818 in PPP*

2. What is the likely etiology of Cushing's syndrome in this patient?

   *Hint: See pp. 816–817 and Table 45-5 in PPP*

3. How would you treat Cushing's syndrome in this patient?

   *Hint: See pp. 817, 819, and 821 and Table 45-7 in PPP*

4. What are the potential risks of therapy that need to be discussed with the patient?

   *Hint: See pp. 819 and 821 and Table 45-7 in PPP*

5. Should the patient receive drug treatment for her hyperglycemia?

   *Hint: Does she have a diagnosis of diabetes mellitus? See pp. 762–763 in PPP*

## FOLLOW-UP

6. JT was tapered off the prednisone and started on methotrexate 10 mg once a week, along with folic acid 1 mg once daily to prophylax against the side effects of methotrexate. She will follow-up with her rheumatologist in 2 weeks for further assessment of her therapy for RA. Four weeks after her initial PCP visit, JT returns for a follow-up with the PCP. She has more energy, can sleep better, and has less depressed feelings. Laboratory evaluation of her HPA axis function reveals a serum cortisol concentration of 16 mcg/dL (441 nmol/L). What could be the reason why her cortisol concentration is slightly low? What are the risks associated with a suppressed cortisol concentration? What actions, if any, would you take?

   *Hint: See pp. 821 and 822 and Table 45-8 in PPP*

## 🌐 GLOBAL PERSPECTIVE

Cushing's syndrome is most commonly caused by chronic administration of exogenous glucocorticoids. Endogenous Cushing's syndrome is an uncommon disorder. According to European population-based studies, the incidence of endogenous Cushing's syndrome is two to three cases per 1 million inhabitants per year.[1] A study conducted in Spain reports that Cushing's disease due to a pituitary adenoma is the most frequent cause of endogenous Cushing's syndrome, which is 5–6 times more frequent than adrenal Cushing's syndrome, with an incidence of 1.2–2.4 cases per 1 million inhabitants per year.[2] Treatment options for various types of endogenous Cushing's syndrome include surgery and pharmacotherapeutic options, which are discussed in Chapter 45 of PPP.

## REFERENCES

1. Nieman LK, Biller BM, Findling JW, et al. The diagnosis of Cushing's syndrome: An Endocrine Society Clinical Practice Guideline. J Clin Endocrinol Metab 2008 93:1526–1540.
2. Lindholm J, Juul S, Jorgensen AO, et al. Incidence and late prognosis of Cushing's Syndrome: A population-based study. J Clin Endocrinol Metab 2001 86:117–123.

## CASE SUMMARY

- The patient's current clinical presentation and history point toward a diagnosis of corticosteroid-induced Cushing's syndrome. Gradual tapering and discontinuation of prednisone therapy should be initiated. Her Cushing's symptoms should resolve on discontinuation of prednisone therapy.

- After prednisone has been tapered down to 5 mg daily for 2 weeks, perform testing to assess for recovery of HPA axis function to determine the need for continued slow taper or if prednisone can be discontinued at that time.

- The patient should be educated about the possibility of adrenal insufficiency and symptoms of an acute adrenal crisis during the period when her adrenal function is thought to be suppressed.

- Alternative treatment for RA should be initiated while prednisone is being tapered.

- The patient's depression and menstrual irregularity need further evaluation and work-up if not resolved upon discontinuation of prednisone.

**For more information on the care plan and facilitator's guide please visit http://www.mhpharmacotherapy.com.**

# 54 Pregnancy

Ema Ferreira          Caroline Morin
Évelyne Rey

## CASE LEARNING OBJECTIVES

- Develop an appropriate treatment plan during pregnancy
- Properly educate a patient taking drugs during pregnancy
- Identify the risks of epilepsy during pregnancy
- Identify the risks of anticonvulsants during pregnancy and lactation

## PATIENT PRESENTATION

### Chief Complaint

"I think I am pregnant."

### History of Present Illness

Loretta Baldwin is a 26-year-old woman who presents to her primary care physician after completing a pharmacy pregnancy test that was positive 2 days ago. Her period is 3 weeks late. Her menstrual cycle is usually 28–32 days. She stopped her medications yesterday because she has been told that they may cause fetal malformations. She has never been pregnant before.

### Past Medical History

Epilepsy (generalized tonic–clonic seizures) for 13 years following viral encephalitis. No seizures since one episode last year. Last visit to her neurologist 6 months ago.

Overweight since childhood

Chronic HAs

Occasional constipation

### Family History

Mother is alive at age 51 with DM, obesity, and HTN. Father is alive at age 53 with hypothyroidism. She has one brother who is healthy and two sisters who had normal pregnancies. There have been no multiple pregnancies in the family.

### Social History

Born in the United States. Married and lives with her husband. Works full time as a clerk. Dislikes fruit and vegetables, eats two meals a day, often in fast-food restaurants. (–) Exercise. No pets.

### Tobacco/Alcohol/Substance Use

Social drinker; (–) tobacco or illicit drug use

### Allergies/Intolerances/Adverse Drug Events

Phenytoin (unknown reaction at age 13)

### Medications (Current)

Lamotrigine 200 mg PO twice daily, stopped yesterday

Carbamazepine CR 400 mg PO twice daily, stopped yesterday

MOM 30 mL PO once daily as needed for constipation

Feverfew herbal tea two to five times a week

Ibuprofen 400 mg PO as needed for HA, twice weekly in the last month

### Review of Systems

No seizure; occasional HA relieved with ibuprofen; increased urinary frequency and constipation in the past 2 weeks; occasionally SOB; tiredness and mild nausea.

## Physical Examination

► **General**

Overweight young Caucasian woman in no acute distress

► **Vital Signs**

BP 112/76 mm Hg, P 89, RR 12, T 36.2°C

Weight 207.2 lb (94.2 kg)

Height 67 in. (170 cm)

Denies pain

► **Skin**

Normal

► **HEENT**

PERRLA, EOMI; TMs normal

► **Neck and Lymph Nodes**

Thyroid gland not palpable

► **Chest**

Clear to auscultation

► **Breasts**

Slight tenderness; no nodule, discharge, or skin deformation

► **Cardiovascular**

RRR, normal $S_1$, $S_2$; (−) $S_3$ or $S_4$; systolic ejection murmur (2/6) at the left second intercostal space without radiation

► **Abdomen**

Not tender/not distended; (−) organomegaly

► **Neurology**

Grossly intact; DTRs normal

► **Genitourinary**

(−) discharge or lesions; cervix closed; bimanual examination normal; no urinary symptoms

► **Rectal**

Examination deferred

## Laboratory Tests

Nonfasting, obtained the same day

Urinalysis: bacteria (+ +), nitrite (+); culture pending

|  | Conventional Units | SI Units |
|---|---|---|
| Urine pregnancy test | (+) | |
| Hgb | 12.3 g/dL | 123 g/L; 7.63 mmol/L |
| Hct | 37.8% | 0.378 |

| | | |
|---|---|---|
| WBC | $5.4 \times 10^3/mm^3$ | $5.4 \times 10^9/L$ |
| MCV | $82 \, \mu m^3$ | 82 fL |
| Platelets | $203 \times 10^3/mm^3$ | $203 \times 10^9/L$ |
| SCr | 0.63 mg/dL | 56 μmol/L |
| Glu | 101 mg/dL | 5.6 mmol/L |
| Lamotrigine | Not done | |
| Urinalysis | Bacteria (2+) | |
| | Nitrite (+) | |
| Urine culture | Pending | |
| Blood group/rhesus type | O⁺ | |
| Rubella antibody | (+) | |
| Hepatitis B surface antigen | (−) | |
| HIV antibody | (−) | |
| Vaginal culture | (−) | |
| Carbamazepine | 4.2 mcg/mL | 18 μmol/L |

## Assessment

Twenty-six-year-old woman, 7 weeks pregnant, wanting to stop her antiepileptic therapy

### Student Workup

**Missing Information?**

**Evaluate:**     Patient Database

Drug Therapy Problems

Care Plan (by Problem)

## TARGETED QUESTIONS

1. What risks and adverse effects of epilepsy therapy would you discuss with the patient?

   *Hint: See Tables 47-3 and 47-4 and pp. 848 and 850 in PPP*

2. How should headaches be treated?

   *Hint: See Table 47-4 in PPP*

3. Should other medication be added?

   *Hint: See Table 47-7 and p. 852 in PPP*

4. How could nausea affect the actual therapy? What is the approach of nausea?

   *Hint: See Table 47-7 and p. 856 in PPP*

5. How are you going to address the urinalysis results?

   *Hint: See Table 47-7 and p. 861 in PPP*

## FOLLOW-UP

Two weeks later, the patient returns for follow-up. She is taking her usual anticonvulsants and folic acid as recommended by a fetomaternal obstetrician who asked for fetal ultrasounds at 12 and 20 weeks and carbamazepine and lamotrigine blood concentrations. every month. Despite a diet rich in fiber and psyllium supplement, she complains of constipation. A follow-up urinalysis is normal.

6. Why are carbamazepine and lamotrigine concentrations assessed and how should the results be interpreted?

    *Hint: See Table 47-5 in PPP*

7. What do you suggest for persistent constipation?

    *Hint: See Table 47-7 and p. 856 in PPP*

## ⚘ GLOBAL PERSPECTIVE

Anticonvulsants should not be stopped during pregnancy because it puts the woman at risk of seizures. Triggers of seizures, such as tiredness and vomiting, should be avoided. Anticonvulsants increase the risk of fetal malformations, a topic that should be discussed with the woman. In general, pregnant women overestimate the teratogenic risk of drugs. Lifestyle modifications should be discussed, and folic acid 4 mg should be prescribed at the first prenatal visit (if not already taken). Planning a pregnancy is especially important in women with epilepsy because folic acid is more efficient in preventing fetal malformations when started 3 months before pregnancy (general population). Multivitamins, containing vitamin D, calcium, and iron, should be considered in women with a poor diet or lack of sun exposure. Other drugs, for which proven safe alternatives are available or that have no proven efficacy, should be stopped. Urinary tract infections, including asymptomatic bacteriuria, are associated with complications during pregnancy and need to be treated appropriately.

## CASE SUMMARY

- The current clinical picture is consistent with pregnancy.
- The risks and benefits of anticonvulsants were not well understood before pregnancy.
- The anticonvulsants should not be stopped.
- Pregnancy causes a decrease in total anticonvulsant blood concentrations.
- Even though at 7 weeks pregnancy, the neural tube is already closed. Folic acid 4 mg should be added to current medications to decrease the risk of congenital malformations.
- Ibuprofen and NSAIDs should not be used regularly during pregnancy, and should be stopped at 26 weeks of pregnancy. Acetaminophen is the first-line drug for aches.
- Herbal medications should not be used in pregnancy unless their safety has been proved.
- N/V can affect drug absorption and efficacy.
- Asymptomatic bacteriuria has to be treated during pregnancy. Check urinary cultures regularly.
- Constipation and nausea of pregnancy could be relieved by diet modifications. Psyllium preparations are the first-line drugs for constipation.

**For more information on the care plan and facilitator's guide please visit http://www.mhpharmacotherapy.com.**

# 55 Contraception

Shareen Y. El-Ibiary

## CASE LEARNING OBJECTIVES

- Assess patient needs for hormonal contraceptives
- Manage and minimize side effects associated with hormonal contraceptives on the basis of patient needs
- Identify drug interactions and contraindications associated with hormonal contraceptives
- Recommend an appropriate contraceptive method on the basis of patient characteristics and needs
- Properly educate a patient using a recommended contraceptive method

## PATIENT PRESENTATION

### Chief Complaint

"I'm getting married soon, and I need to start birth control."

### History of Present Illness

Carrie Anderson is a 36-year-old woman who presents to her primary care physician (PCP) for a routine follow-up appointment and excitedly states that she is getting married in 4 months and "needs to start birth control." She has been seeing her PCP regularly for the management of HTN and depression. She and her fiancé are currently using condoms for pregnancy prevention, but states that she wants "something easier." She would like to have children "in a year or so." She was treated for depression 1 year ago with sertraline 50 mg PO daily for 6 months and her BP is controlled with HCTZ 25 mg PO daily and recent addition of ramipril 5 mg PO 6 weeks ago. Overall, she is feeling well and very happy. She admits to a nagging cough that started about 2 weeks ago, but otherwise, she is seeking to start on a hormonal contraceptive.

### Past Medical History

HTN diagnosed 2 years ago

Depression treated successfully 1 year ago (6-month treatment course)

### Family History

Father is alive at age 67 with HTN. Mother is alive at age 65 with osteoporosis and HTN. She has one brother and one sister who are healthy.

### Social History

Single, planning to get married for the first time in 4 months, no children, but plans to have children in 1 year. Caucasian, English speaking, United States born

### Tobacco/Alcohol/Substance Use

Social drinker; admits to smoking ½ ppd, but would like to quit

### Allergies/Intolerances/Adverse Drug Events

NKDA

### Medications (Current)

HCTZ 25 mg PO daily

Ramipril 5 mg PO daily

Ibuprofen 200 mg PO PRN menstrual cramps

Dextromethorphan/guaifenesin 5 mL PO q 6 h PRN cough

### Review of Systems

Noticed dry cough, attributes it to possibly new allergies; (−) fever, chills, sore throat; otherwise feeling well

### Physical Examination

▶ *General*

Obese, well-appearing, Caucasian woman in no acute distress

▸ **Vital Signs**

BP 137/82 mm Hg, P 84, RR 12, T 36.2°C

Weight 202.4 lb (92 kg)

Height 67 in. (170 cm)

▸ **Skin**

Supple, normal appearance

▸ **HEENT**

PERRLA, EOMI; (–) sinus tenderness; TMs appear normal

▸ **Neck and Lymph Nodes**

Thyroid gland smooth, slightly enlarged symmetrically; (–) thyroid nodules; (–) lymphadenopathy; (–) carotid bruits

▸ **Chest**

Clear to auscultation

▸ **Breasts**

Slight tenderness; no nodule, discharge, or skin deformation

▸ **Cardiovascular**

RRR, normal $S_1$, $S_2$; (–) $S_3$ or $S_4$

▸ **Abdomen**

Not tender/not distended; (–) organomegaly

▸ **Neurology**

Grossly intact; DTRs normal

▸ **Genitourinary**

(–) Discharge or lesions; bimanual examination normal; no urinary symptoms

▸ **Rectal**

Examination deferred

## Laboratory Tests

### Fasting Obtained this Morning

|  | Conventional Units | SI Units |
|---|---|---|
| Na | 139 mEq/L | 139 mmol/L |
| K | 4.3 mEq/L | 4.3 mmol/L |
| Cl | 101 mEq/L | 101 mmol/L |
| $HCO_3$ | 25 mEq/L | 25 mmol/L |
| BUN | 10 mg/dL | 3.6 mmol/L |
| SCr | 0.62 mg/dL | 55 μmol/L |
| Glu | 104 mg/dL | 5.8 mmol/L |
| Ca | 9.1 mg/dL | 2.28 mmol/L |
| Hgb | 13.5 g/dL | 135 g/L; 8.38 mmol/L |
| Hct | 39.7% | 0.397 |
| WBC | $5.1 \times 10^3/mm^3$ | $5.1 \times 10^9/L$ |
| Albumin | 4.1 g/dL | 41 g/L |
| AST | 29 U/L | 0.48 μkat/L |
| ALT | 30 U/L | 0.50 μkat/L |
| Alk phos | 63 U/L | 1.05 μkat/L |

## Assessment

Thirty-six-year-old woman with history of depression, HTN, obesity, smoking, and mild cough requesting a hormonal contraceptive

### Student Workup

**Missing Information?**

**Evaluate:** Patient Database

Drug Therapy Problems

Care Plan (by Problem)

## TARGETED QUESTIONS

1. What hormonal contraceptives should be avoided in this patient and why?

    *Hint: See Table 48-3 in PPP*

2. Why is smoking in women older than 35 years and uncontrolled HTN contraindicated with combined hormonal contraceptives?

    *Hint: See p. 874 in PPP*

3. What medications interact with hormonal contraceptives based on this patient's medication regimen?

    *Hint: See p. 878 and Table 48-4 in PPP*

4. What risks and adverse effects of hormonal contraceptives would you discuss with this patient?

    *Hint: See pp. 874–877 in PPP*

5. How do this patient's needs influence the choice of hormonal contraceptive agents?

    *Hint: Important to consider this patient's desire to have children in the near future and her age of 36 years. Consider the return to fertility of different contraceptive agents in this patient. The patient is also obese and contraceptive agents that heavily contribute to weight gain should also be avoided. See pp. 876–877 in PPP*

## FOLLOW-UP

6. Eight weeks later, the patient returns for follow-up. Her cough has resolved after discontinuing ramipril and starting losartan 50 mg PO daily. She has been taking her

progestin-only pills every morning right after brushing her teeth, but missed a dose when she went out of town for a night. What are some reasons her cough went away after discontinuing ramipril? What counseling would you provide the patient with regard to missing a progestin-only pill?

*Hint: See p. 877 in PPP*

## ☼ GLOBAL PERSPECTIVE

Hormonal contraception is mainly used for pregnancy prevention, but has other uses as well, such as treating acne, hirsutism, dysmenorrhea, menorrhagia, polycystic ovary syndrome, iron-deficiency anemia, premenstrual dysphoric disorder, and premenstrual syndrome. In the developing world, however, hormonal contraceptives are mainly desired for pregnancy prevention. Information provided by the Guttmacher institute (http://www.guttmacher.org/pubs/Abortion-Worldwide.pdf Accessed May 15, 2013) states that in Africa 22% of childbearing age women have an unmet need for contraception. The report also states that 30–50% of women ages 15–24 years in Latin America and the Caribbean do not use contraceptives. The number is even higher in Sub-Saharan Africa with 24–60% of women ages 15–24 not using birth control. The information also cites that approximately half of all reproductive age women (818 million women) in developing countries would like to prevent pregnancies. Of those women, approximately 17% are not using any birth control method, with 9% using a suboptimal method. Reasons for not using birth control included fear of side effects, inaccessible methods, and partner disapproval.

Contraception in developing countries may be particularly important in preventing abortions of unplanned babies, decreasing the spread of diseases such as HIV from partner to partner and mother to infant, preventing pregnancies in areas where risks of nonconsensual intercourse is high, and preventing pregnancies in women who have multiple children and cannot afford to have another. Increasing education and improving access related to contraception whether barrier, hormonal, or surgical in developing countries and in the United States may help to decrease unplanned pregnancies and prevent the associated consequences.

## CASE SUMMARY

- The patient's contraceptive needs include an easier birth control method than condoms. Ideally, this method could be a hormonal contraceptive that includes the following characteristics: effective with her current weight, does not increase her weight significantly, does not increase her risk of stroke and CV risk because of her HTN and smoker status, does not increase her potassium level, and has a quick return to fertility.

- A progestin-only pill or IUD would be appropriate in this patient with monitoring of mood symptoms in case the progestin induces depression symptoms.

**For more information on the care plan and facilitator's guide please visit http://www.mhpharmacotherapy.com.**

# 56 Menstrual Disorder

Jacqueline M. Klootwyk    Elena M. Umland

## PATIENT PRESENTATION

### Chief Complaint

"My cramps are unbearable!"

### History of Present Illness

Anita Jacob is a 21-year-old Caucasian woman who presents to the clinic complaining of painful menses for the past few months. Her menses last between 6 and 8 days on average and have become increasingly painful. The pain begins 1 day prior to the onset of menses and lasts 2–3 days. The pain is "crampy" in nature. She has heavy menses for 2 days that require her to change feminine hygiene products every 2–3 hours. She has a history of iron-deficiency anemia secondary to menorrhagia that has been successfully treated with iron supplementation. She has tried OTC products that contain ibuprofen without success. Today, she is also complaining of abdominal pain, but denies vaginal discharge.

### Past Medical History

Iron-deficiency anemia × 6 months

Menorrhagia × 6 months

Seasonal allergic rhinitis × 2 years

### Family History

Father is alive at age 56 with CHD, H/O MI at age 55, dyslipidemia, HTN, and osteoarthritis. Mother is alive at age 54 with osteopenia, HTN, and H/O ovarian cancer. She has one older brother (age 30) and one older sister (age 27) who are both alive and well.

### Social History

The patient is a single, heterosexual, sexually active female. She has been sexually active since age 15. She does not desire pregnancy at this time. She has had vaginal intercourse with multiple partners (approximately 10–12 men). Her partners use condoms only occasionally. She has been in a monogamous relationship for the past 8 months. She is a student at the local university.

### Tobacco/Alcohol/Substance Use

Social drinker (3–5 drinks per weekend); (+) tobacco use (1 ppd); (−) illicit drug use. The patient is not ready to quit smoking at this time.

### Allergies/Intolerances/Adverse Drug Events

Penicillin (rash)

### Medications (Current)

Fexofenadine 180 mg PO once daily

Ferrous sulfate 325 mg PO twice daily

Ibuprofen 200 mg two tablets PO PRN headache and menstrual cramps

Midol Menstrual Complete two tablets PO PRN menstrual cramps

### Medications (Past)

Kava kava root capsules 500 mg PO two to three times daily PRN menstrual cramps

## Review of Systems

Occasional HA relieved with NSAID medication; seasonal allergies relieved with antihistamine; (−) GI upset, heartburn, or constipation, but (+) abdominal pain; (−) change in urinary frequency; (−) dysuria; (−) vaginal discharge; (+) menorrhagia, (+) dysmenorrhea; LMP 27 days ago; age at menarche 14 years.

## Physical Examination

### ▶ General

Overweight-appearing, young, Caucasian woman in no apparent distress

### ▶ Vital Signs

BP 114/72 mm Hg, P 76, RR 12, T 37.0°C

Weight 170 lb (77.3 kg)

Height 65 in. (165 cm)

Pain score 2/10

### ▶ Skin

Normal-appearing skin and nails; (−) rashes or lesions

### ▶ HEENT

PERRLA, EOMI; TMs appear normal

### ▶ Neck and Lymph Nodes

No nodules

### ▶ Chest

Clear to auscultation bilaterally; (−) chest pain

### ▶ Breasts

Nontender; (−) masses

### ▶ Cardiovascular

RRR, normal $S_1$, $S_2$; (−) $S_3$ or $S_4$

### ▶ Abdomen

Soft, tender, nondistended; (−) hepatosplenomegaly

### ▶ Neurology

Grossly intact; DTRs normal

### ▶ Genitourinary

Normal external appearance of labia; (−) lesions on cervix; (−) cervical motion tenderness; (−) vaginal discharge

### ▶ Rectal

Examination deferred

## Laboratory and Other Diagnostic Tests

### Today

- Urine pregnancy test: Negative
- Urine gonorrhea/chlamydia screening: Pending

### Fasting Obtained 3 Months Ago

|  | Conventional Units | SI Units |
|---|---|---|
| Na | 138 mEq/L | 138 mmol/L |
| K | 4.8 mEq/L | 4.8 mmol/L |
| Cl | 104 mEq/L | 104 mmol/L |
| $CO_2$ | 25 mEq/L | 25 mmol/L |
| BUN | 12 mg/dL | 4.3 mmol/L |
| SCr | 0.9 mg/dL | 80 µmol/L |
| Glu | 85 mg/dL | 4.7 mmol/L |
| Hgb | 12.8 g/dL | 128 g/L; 7.94 mmol/L |
| Hct | 37.2% | 0.372 |
| MCV | 84 µm³ | 84 fL |
| WBC | $6.9 \times 10^3/mm^3$ | $6.9 \times 10^9/L$ |
| Platelet | $255 \times 10^3/mm^3$ | $255 \times 10^9/L$ |
| Iron | 54 mcg/dL | 9.7 µmol/L |
| Ferritin | 45 ng/mL | 45 mcg/L |
| TIBC | 382 mcg/dL | 68.4 µmol/L |
| Transferrin saturation | 26% | 0.26 |

### Fasting Obtained 6 Months Ago

|  | Conventional Units | SI Units |
|---|---|---|
| Na | 140 mEq/L | 140 mmol/L |
| K | 4.5 mEq/L | 4.5 mmol/L |
| Cl | 102 mEq/L | 102 mmol/L |
| $CO_2$ | 24 mEq/L | 24 mmol/L |
| BUN | 11 mg/dL | 3.9 mmol/L |
| SCr | 0.8 mg/dL | 71 µmol/L |
| Glu | 78 mg/dL | 4.3 mmol/L |
| AST | 23 IU/L | 0.38 µkat/L |
| ALT | 17 IU/L | 0.28 µkat/L |
| Hgb | 9.8 g/dL | 98 g/L; 6.08 mmol/L |
| Hct | 30.9% | 0.309 |
| MCV | 72 µm³ | 72 fL |
| WBC | $5.5 \times 10^3/mm^3$ | $5.5 \times 10^9/L$ |
| Platelet | $220 \times 10^3/mm^3$ | $220 \times 10^9/L$ |
| Iron | 20 mcg/dL | 3.6 µmol/L |

| Ferritin | 6 ng/mL | 6 mcg/L |
| TIBC | 465 mcg/dL | 83.2 μmol/L |
| Transferrin saturation | 12% | 0.12 |

Diagnostic tests, 6 months ago

Pap smear: (−) cervical changes

Pelvic ultrasound: (−) masses or lesions, (−) ovarian cysts or endometriomas

## Assessment

Twenty-one-year-old woman with signs and symptoms consistent with dysmenorrhea secondary to menorrhagia

### Student Workup

**Missing Information?**

**Evaluate:** Patient Database

Drug Therapy Problems

Care Plan (by Problem)

## TARGETED QUESTIONS

1. What signs and symptoms of dysmenorrhea does the patient have?

   *Hint: See p. 886 in PPP*

2. Why are NSAIDs the treatment of choice for most patients with dysmenorrhea?

   *Hint: See pp. 886 and 888 in PPP*

3. What nonpharmacologic therapies have been shown to be beneficial in the treatment of dysmenorrhea?

   *Hint: See p. 886 in PPP*

4. What risks and adverse effects of therapy would you discuss with the patient?

   *Hint: See Table 49-1 in PPP*

## FOLLOW-UP

5. Three months later, the patient returns for follow-up. Her symptoms have improved dramatically with a reduction in menstrual flow and pain. Her iron studies, drawn last week, are iron 85 mcg/dL (15.2 μmol/L), ferritin 70 ng/mL (70 mcg/L), TIBC 325 mcg/dL (58.2 μmol/L), and transferrin saturation 32% (0.32). Would you recommend discontinuing the iron supplementation?

   *Hint: See pp. 1163–1165 in PPP*

## GLOBAL PERSPECTIVE

Reports of primary dysmenorrhea have been shown to vary among different cultures. It has been reported by 15.8% of Japanese women,[1] 65% of African American adolescents,[2] 48% of Mexican adolescents,[3] 85% of Hispanic adolescents,[4] and more than 80% of Caucasian women.[5] It has been proposed that some of these variations can be explained by the cultural perceptions of menstruation. Those cultures that have a more negative view of menstruation appear to report higher levels of dysmenorrhea.[5] Further, these negative expectations also seem to impact and be associated with higher levels of absenteeism.[2] Knowledge of such cultural differences may be of benefit in the assessment and treatment of women presenting with complaints consistent with dysmenorrhea.

## REFERENCES

1. Ohde S, Tokuda Y, Takahashi O, Yanai H, Hinohara S, Fukui T. Dysmenorrhea among Japanese women. Int J Gynecol Obstet 2008 100:13–17.
2. Houston AM, Abraham A, Huang Z, D'Angelo LJ. Knowledge, attitudes, and consequences of menstrual health in urban adolescents. J Pediatr Adolesc Gynecol 2006 19:271–275.
3. Ortiz MI, Rangel-Flores E, Carrillo-Alarcon LC, Veras-Godoy HA. Prevalence and impact of primary dysmenorrhea among Mexican high school students. Int J Gynecol Obstet 2009 107(3):240–243.
4. Banikarim C, Chacko MR, Kelder SH. Prevalence and impact of dysmenorrhea on Hispanic female adolescents. Arch Pediatr Adolesc Med 2000 154:1226–1229.
5. Bettendorf B, Shay S, Tu F. Dysmenorrhea: Contemporary perspectives. Obstet Gynecol Surv 2008 63:597–603.

## CASE SUMMARY

- The patient's current clinical picture is consistent with dysmenorrhea and menorrhagia, and an oral contraceptive should be initiated.
- Given the patient's family history of ovarian cancer and her occasional use of a barrier contraceptive, a combination oral contraceptive would be a good alternative to NSAIDs.
- Resolution of symptoms (both dysmenorrhea and menorrhagia) should occur within one to three menstrual cycles.

For more information on the care plan and facilitator's guide please visit http://www.mhpharmacotherapy.com.

# 57 Menopause

Leigh V. Maine

## CASE LEARNING OBJECTIVES

- Identify the signs and symptoms associated with menopause
- Explain how to evaluate a patient for the appropriate use of HT
- Recommend nonpharmacologic therapy for menopausal symptoms
- Differentiate between topical and systemic forms of HT
- Educate a patient regarding the proper use and potential adverse effects of HT

## PATIENT PRESENTATION

### Chief Complaint

"It has been very painful to have intercourse recently; nothing I've tried from the drugstore seems to help."

### History of Present Illness

Shirley Davis is a 52-year-old Caucasian woman who presents to her primary care physician complaining of dyspareunia for the last 2 months. Due to her embarrassment over the issue, she has tried several OTC lubricants in order to relieve her problem rather than seek medical attention. Within the last year, she has informed her physician that her menstrual cycle has stopped. She denied having hot flashes or mood changes approximately a year ago. Currently, she admits to interruptions in her day several times per week due to profuse sweating and mood swings. She states it usually happens after having hot tea or soup for lunch.

### Past Medical History

Amenorrhea × 1 year

HTN × 3 years

Hyperlipidemia × 4 years

### Past Surgical History

Hysterectomy 1 year ago

Oophorectomy (left ovary) 32 years ago

Tonsillectomy 44 years ago

### Family History

Father is 78 and has CHD and DM. Mother is 76 and is in overall good health, is a survivor of breast cancer, and had a double mastectomy 20 years ago. SD has no siblings.

### Social History

SD is a married mother of 3 children, ages 27, 25, and 23. She has been married for 27 years. She works as a librarian.

### Tobacco/Alcohol/Substance Use

Three to five alcoholic drinks/wk; states she drinks wine to help her cholesterol; (−) tobacco or illicit drug use

### Allergies/Intolerances/Adverse Drug Events

HCTZ (hypokalemia)

### Medications (Current)

Amlodipine/benazepril 5 mg/10 mg PO q 24 h

Fenofibrate 145 mg PO q 24 h

Calcium with vitamin D 600 mg/400 IU PO bid

Multivitamin one tablet PO q 24 h

Ibuprofen 200 mg PO PRN joint pain after gardening

### Review of Systems

Several incidences of painful intercourse; (+) dyspareunia; also episodes of increased body temperature and irritability; (+) vasomotor symptoms; (−) night sweats; (−) chest pain; (−) palpitations; (−) tachycardia

## Physical Examination

▶ *General*

Fifty-two-year-old Caucasian woman in no acute distress

▶ *Vital Signs*

BP 104/70 mm Hg, P 70, RR 18, pulse O$_2$ 97% (0.97),
    T 96.7°F (35.9°C)

Weight 141.2 lb (64.2 kg)

Height 62.8 in. (159.5 cm)

Pain score 0/10

▶ *Skin*

Denies history of skin cancer. No rashes or new or unusual skin lesions

▶ *HEENT*

PERRLA, EOMI; intact without nystagmus, conjunctivas clear, sclera anicteric, canals clear, oropharynx clear without exudate

▶ *Neck and Lymph Nodes*

No masses or crepitance, symmetric, thyroid without nodularity, midline trachea

▶ *Breasts*

No discrete nodules

▶ *Cardiovascular*

Regular rate and rhythm, no murmurs, no jugular venous distention

▶ *Lungs*

Clear to auscultation

▶ *Abdomen*

No tenderness, organomegaly, or masses

▶ *Neurology*

No history of seizures, migraines, falls, or vertigo

▶ *Genitourinary*

No urinary problems, negative for renal stones

▶ *External Genitalia*

No unusual findings

▶ *Vagina*

Atrophic, erythematous mucosa

▶ *Psychiatric*

Mood swings, irritability

## Laboratory Tests

### Fasting Obtained this Morning

|  | Conventional Units | SI Units |
|---|---|---|
| Na | 137 mEq/L | 137 mmol/L |
| K | 5 mEq/L | 5 mmol/L |
| Cl | 106 mEq/L | 106 mmol/L |
| CO$_2$ | 22 mEq/L | 22 mmol/L |
| BUN | 7 mg/dL | 2.5 mmol/L |
| SCr | 0.7 mg/dL | 62 μmol/L |
| Glu | 78 mg/dL | 4.3 mmol/L |
| Ca | 8 mg/dL | 2 mmol/L |
| Mg | 1.6 mEq/L | 0.80 mmol/L |
| Phosphate | 3.7 mg/dL | 1.20 mmol/L |
| Hgb | 12.8 g/dL | 128 g/L; 7.93 mmol/L |
| Hct | 37.5% | 0.375 |
| WBC | 5 × 10$^3$/mm$^3$ | 5 × 10$^9$/L |
| MCV | 87 μm$^3$ | 87 fL |
| Albumin | 3.8 g/dL | 38 g/L |
| TSH | 3.5 μIU/mL | 3.5 mIU/L |
| Free T$_4$ | 0.84 ng/dL | 10.8 pmol/L |
| Total cholesterol | 213 mg/dL | 5.51 mmol/L |
| LDL cholesterol | 114 mg/dL | 2.95 mmol/L |
| HDL cholesterol | 80 mg/dL | 2.07 mmol/L |
| TG | 94 mg/dL | 1.06 mmol/L |

## Assessment

Fifty-two-year-old woman with s/s consistent with menopause

### Student Workup

**Missing Information?**

**Evaluate:**     Patient Database

Drug Therapy Problems

Care Plan (by Problem)

## TARGETED QUESTIONS

1. What s/s of menopause does SD have?

   *Hint: See p. 903 in PPP*

2. What factors in SD's medical history must we consider when deciding medication therapy?

   *Hint: See pp. 903–905 in PPP*

3. What pharmacologic/nonpharmacologic therapy would be recommended in SD's case?

   *Hint: See pp. 903–904 and 906 in PPP*

4. What risks and adverse effects of therapy would you discuss with SD?

   *Hint: See Table 50-2 and pp. 908–910 in PPP*

## FOLLOW-UP

5. Six weeks later, SD is back for a follow-up appointment. She denies dyspareunia and reports her vasomotor symptoms have improved. If started on hormone replacement therapy, when should discontinuation be considered?

   *Hint: See p. 910 in PPP*

## 🌐 GLOBAL PERSPECTIVE

Menopause happens to every woman in the world when considering menopause as a physiologic change. However, when comparing how menopause manifests itself through signs and symptoms across cultures, the results differ greatly. Signs and symptoms of menopause can differ in quality and duration depending on the culture. Use of medication or alternative therapies can vary considerably as well.

## CASE SUMMARY

- SD's clinical condition is consistent with menopause and therapy should be initiated.
- Use of topical estrogen and an SSRI are acceptable given her PMH of hysterectomy and risk factors for CHD and breast cancer.
- Close follow-up (4–6 weeks) may be desired initially to ensure success of medication therapy, and then 6-month follow-up would be acceptable.

For more information on the care plan and facilitator's guide please visit http://www.mhpharmacotherapy.com.

# 58 Erectile Dysfunction

Nicole J. Brandt      Allison A. Chilipko

## CASE LEARNING OBJECTIVES

- Differentiate between organic and psychogenic erectile dysfunction (ED) with regard to etiology and pathophysiology
- Identify the drug classes most likely to contribute to ED
- Define the essential components of history, physical examination, and laboratory data needed to evaluate the patient presenting with ED
- Describe current nonpharmacologic and pharmacologic options for ED treatment to determine an appropriate first-line therapy for a specific patient
- Compare and contrast the benefits and risks for current phosphodiesterase inhibitors
- Recommend an appropriate treatment approach for patients with ED and significant cardiovascular risk factors

## PATIENT PRESENTATION

### Chief Complaint

"I am having trouble in the bedroom."

### History of Present Illness

JM is a 67-year-old African American male who comes to your medication management clinic complaining about "not getting it up." He has a new girlfriend, and he is frustrated that they cannot be intimate. He has not been sexually active for at least 10 years, yet really wants to get back "on the horse," but needs help. He wants to know if he can get one of those pills he saw on television. In terms of his other medications, he admits to not taking his depression medication regularly as well as his cholesterol medication.

### Past Medical History

HTN × 25 years

Angina × 10 years

Hyperlipidemia × 20 years

Depression × 5 years

### Family History

Father died at age 75 from lung cancer. Mother died at age 70 from complications of diabetes. He has one brother who is healthy (age 61) and one sister who has diabetes and HTN (age 56). He has two sons (ages 42 and 27) who both have HTN and diabetes.

### Social/Work History

The patient retired from the real estate business to take care of his wife about 10 years ago. For the last 3 years, he has been living in an apartment within a retirement community. Prior to this transition, he was living in his own home; however, he was lonely due to his wife's death 7 years ago from cancer. He has completed a few years of college but was unable to graduate. Now, he has a new girlfriend in his building.

### Tobacco/Alcohol/Substance Use

He has a history of smoking about ½ to 1 ppd for the last 50 years. He admits he is trying to cut back. Currently, he regularly drinks about two cans of beer per night and occasionally more during "Happy Hours" at the facility on Friday.

### Allergy/Intolerance/Adverse Event History

No known drug allergies

### Medications (Current)

HCTZ 25 mg PO q 24 h (for the past 6 years)

Paroxetine 40 mg PO daily (for the past 3 years)

Isosorbide mononitrate 60 mg PO daily (for the past 10 years)

Atorvastatin 40 mg once daily (for the past 10 years)

Clonidine 0.2 mg PO twice daily (for the past 10 years)

Multivitamin one tablet PO daily

Enteric-coated aspirin 81 mg PO daily

## Current Insurance Plan

Rx payment: Medicare Part D plan

## Review of Systems

The patient has occasional dry mouth and stuffy nose with occasional cough. He denies any chest pain or tightness, but admits to occasional DOE when walking up a hill and with exercise. The patient denies any urinary hesitancy, but some issues with urgency due to the water pill. He notes it is hard for him to get and maintain an erection. He describes suffering from depressive episodes since his wife died. Now, though, the patient is happy to have made a new friend, but he is anxious about intimacy. He notes history of pain and tingling in both feet.

## Physical Examination

### ▸ General

Pleasant, well-groomed and dressed male in no apparent distress, accompanied by his "friend."

### ▸ Vital Signs

BP 126/76 mm Hg (left arm, sitting), P 62 (regular), RR 20 (unlabored), T 98.0°F (36.7 °C) (oral)

Weight 225 lb (102 kg)

Height 73 in. (185 cm)

Pain 0/10

### ▸ HEENT

PERRLA, EOMI

### ▸ Chest

Clear to auscultation bilaterally

### ▸ Cardiovascular

RRR, nl $S_1$, $S_2$; no murmurs, rubs, or gallops

### ▸ Abdomen

Nontender, nondistended, normal bowel sounds

### ▸ Neurology

Cranial nerves intact, normal reflexes, good strength throughout

### ▸ Genitourinary

Slightly enlarged prostate gland, smooth, no nodules, tenderness, or warmth

### ▸ Extremities

Good muscle strength and tone throughout, with no decrease in range of motion noted

## Laboratory Tests

### Measured Today After 12-h Fasting

|  | Conventional Units | SI Units |
|---|---|---|
| Na | 135 mEq/L | 135 mmol/L |
| K | 4 mEq/L | 4 mmol/L |
| Cl | 100 mEq/L | 100 mmol/L |
| $CO_2$ | 22 mEq/L | 22 mmol/L |
| BUN | 38 mg/dL | 13.6 mmol/L |
| SCr | 1.1 mg/dL | 97 μmol/L |
| Glu | 92 mg/dL | 5.1 mmol/L |
| Urinalysis | (−) | |
| TSH | 2.8 μIU/mL | 2.8 mIU/L |
| Hgb | 13.5 g/dL | 135 g/L; 8.38 mmol/L |
| Hct | 39.7% | 0.397 |
| WBC | $7.6 \times 10^3/mm^3$ | $7.6 \times 10^9/L$ |
| Albumin | 3.8 g/dL | 38 g/L |
| PSA | 3.6 ng/mL | 3.6 mcg/L |
| Free testosterone | 10 ng/dL | 0.35 nmol/L |
| Total cholesterol | 185 mg/dL | 4.78 mmol/L |
| LDL cholesterol | 98 mg/dL | 2.53 mmol/L |
| HDL cholesterol | 45 mg/dL | 1.16 mmol/L |
| Triglycerides | 128 mg/dL | 1.45 mmol/L |

## Assessment

This is a 67-year-old African American man with ED who is not currently receiving treatment.

## Student Workup

### Missing Information?

**Evaluate:**  Patient Database

Drug Therapy Problems

Care Plan (by Problem)

## TARGETED QUESTIONS

1.  What potential etiologies may be responsible for this patient's ED?

    *Hint: See pp. 917 and 918 and Table 51-1 in PPP*

2.  What medications may be causing or contributing to this patient's ED?

    *Hint: See Table 51-2 in PPP*

3.  Why are phosphodiesterase inhibitors not a treatment consideration for this patient?

    *Hint: See pp. 920 and 921 and Table 51-4 in PPP*

4.  Why should a vacuum erection device, representative of nonpharmacologic means, be considered with drug therapy in this patient?

    *Hint: See p. 920 in PPP*

5.  What risks and adverse effects of therapy would you discuss with this patient?

    *Hint: See pp. 920 and 921 in PPP*

## FOLLOW-UP

6.  One year later, JM comes back to your clinic to follow-up with you. Over the last year, he underwent a three-vessel CABG for his heart disease and since his angina has resolved. He underwent extensive cardiac rehab, and his cardiologist notes that he is stable off of his isosorbide mononitrate. He wants to know if he can now take "Viagra" because he was not satisfied with the results from the previous recommendation. On the basis of the changes in his comorbid conditions and medications, how would you change your treatment recommendations?

    *Hint: See Table 51-4 in PPP*

## GLOBAL PERSPECTIVE

ED may not be incorporated into conventional screening measures for older men despite its prevalence of occurrence. This omission may be due to the health care providers' level of comfort with the topic or lack of time to properly evaluate the patient given the potential for multiple etiologies. The increasing prevalence of ED could be due to physiologic changes that occur with aging, the onset of chronic disease states associated with ED (e.g., HTN, DM), increased medication use (e.g., antihypertensives, antidepressants), lifestyle factors (e.g., smoking, drinking, obesity), or a combination of the above influences. Although there appears to be a difference in reporting among certain cultures (e.g., Hispanic men), overall, it seems that the prevalence may be more attributable to the interplay of above-mentioned risk factors.

## CASE SUMMARY

- ED is very common in older adults but is often not discussed or treated appropriately.
- All potential etiologies (e.g., vasculogenic, psychogenic medications) need to be considered and investigated before starting treatments with unrealistic expectations for symptomatic improvement.
- Monitoring patients over time is essential to assess the efficacy, toxicity, and need for alternative treatment options.

For more information on the care plan and facilitator's guide please visit http://www.mhpharmacotherapy.com.

# 59 Benign Prostatic Hypertrophy

Mary Lee                     Roohollah Sharifi

## CASE LEARNING OBJECTIVES

- Recognize the symptoms and signs of benign prostatic hyperplasia (BPH) in individual patients
- List the desired treatment outcomes for a patient with BPH
- Identify the factors that guide selection of a particular α-adrenergic antagonist for an individual patient
- Compare and contrast the α-adrenergic antagonists versus 5-α-reductase inhibitors in terms of mechanism of action, treatment outcomes, adverse effects, and interactions when used for management of BPH
- Describe the indications, advantages and disadvantages of single versus combination drug treatment of BPH
- Describe the indications for surgical treatment of BPH
- Formulate a monitoring plan for a patient on a given drug treatment regimen based on patient-specific information and formulate appropriate counseling information for patients receiving drug treatment for BPH

## PATIENT PRESENTATION

### Chief Complaint

"I'm taking 2 drugs for my big prostate, but my urine flow is still too slow. I have urinary frequency day and night. I feel like I can't empty my bladder. Sometimes I can't get to the bathroom on time and I leak on myself."

### History of Present Illness

George Gold is a 73-year-old male with long-standing lower urinary tract symptoms (LUTS) who is referred to the urology service after failing maximal medication therapy for BPH. He has been taking terazosin 20 mg orally daily and finasteride 5 mg orally daily for 9 months. His current complaints include urgency with urge incontinence, nocturia 2–3 times a night, a weak urinary stream, and small-volume voids. He denies hematuria, dysuria, suprapubic or flank pain. He has no fever, chills, nausea, or vomiting. His American Urological Association (AUA) symptom score is 30.

### Past Medical History

Essential HTN × 10 years

Hyperlipidemia × 10 years

Obesity, BMI 35 kg/m$^2$

OA with chronic lower back pain × 5 years

History of a bleeding ulcer secondary to aspirin overuse

S/p transurethral incision of the prostate (TUIP) in 2005

### Family History

Father died of a stroke. Mother died of breast cancer. Sister, alive, has breast cancer.

### Social History

Married for 45 years; has 2 children: a son and a daughter, both alive and healthy.

### Tobacco/Alcohol/Substance Use

Negative for all

### Allergies/Intolerances/Adverse Drug Events

Sulfonamides; develops hives and shortness of breath when exposed. Cannot use Bactrim or Septra (trimethoprim/sulfamethoxazole)

## Medications (Current)

Docusate 100 mg PO daily

Finasteride 5 mg PO daily

Furosemide 40 mg PO daily

Lisinopril 40 mg PO daily

Metoprolol 50 mg PO twice a day

Nifedipine 60 mg extended release 2 tablets PO daily

Terazosin 20 mg PO at bedtime

Simvastatin 80 mg PO at bedtime

Hydrocodone 5 mg/acetaminophen 500 mg 2 tablets PO twice a day

## Review of Systems

The patient has chronic moderately severe low back pain that is only slightly relieved with analgesic. He takes narcotic analgesic only as needed; he is worried about addiction. To prevent constipation, he takes docusate and eats a high-fiber diet. Medications for HTN make him dizzy, particularly when he kneels down or suddenly changes body positions. He is most bothered by urinary incontinence. He has had to curb some social activities because of it.

## Physical Examination

### ▶ General

Well-developed, well-nourished male in no apparent distress

### ▶ Vital Signs

BP 132/64 mm Hg, P 62, RR 14, T 37°C

Weight 222 lb (101 kg)

Height 66.5 in. (168.9 cm)

### ▶ Skin

(–) Rashes or lesions

### ▶ HEENT

PERRLA, EOMI

### ▶ Neck and Lymph Nodes

Thyroid gland is smooth and symmetrical; (–) thyroid nodules; (–) lymphadenopathy; (–) carotid bruits

### ▶ Chest

Clear to auscultation and percussion

### ▶ Cardiovascular

RRR; no murmurs

### ▶ Abdomen

Soft, not tender, or distended; no masses or organomegaly

### ▶ Neurology

Grossly intact; deep tendon reflexes normal

### ▶ Extremities

Trace bilateral lower extremity edema; good range of motion; normal pedal pulses

### ▶ Genitourinary

Digital rectal examination shows a large (50 g), soft, symmetric nontender prostate, no nodules, and no areas of induration. Normal external genitalia. No costovertebral angle tenderness. No rectal pathology.

### ▶ Rectum

No hemorrhoids

### Laboratory Tests

| | Conventional Units | SI Units |
|---|---|---|
| Na | 143 mEq/L | 143 mmol/L |
| K | 4.6 mEq/L | 4.6 mmol/L |
| Cl | 107 mEq/L | 107 mmol/L |
| $CO_2$ | 27.1 mEq/L | 27.1 mmol/L |
| BUN | 30 mg/dL | 10.7 mmol/L |
| SCr | 1.6 mg/dL | 141 µmol/L |
| Glu fasting | 95 mg/dL | 5.3 mmol/L |
| Ca | 8.7 mg/dL | 2.18 mg/dL |
| Urinalysis—yellow, clear | | |
| pH | 5 | |
| Specific gravity | 1.027 | |
| WBC | 2/lpf | |
| RBC | 0/lpf | |
| Protein | Trace | |
| Glucose | (–) | |
| Ketones | (–) | |
| Blood | (–) | |
| Hyaline casts | 6–10/lpf | |
| Hgb | 13.8 g/dL | 138 g/L; 8.57 mmol/L |
| Hct | 40.7% | 0.407 |
| WBC | $6.7 \times 10^3/mm^3$ | $6.7 \times 10^9/L$ |
| Platelets | $167 \times 10^3/mm^3$ | $167 \times 10^9/L$ |
| Albumin | 3.8 g/dL | 38 g/L |
| Total cholesterol | 123 mg/dL | 3.18 mmol/L |
| LDL cholesterol | 63 mg/dL | 1.63 mmol/L |
| HDL cholesterol | 32 mg/dL | 0.83 mmol/L |

| | | |
|---|---|---|
| PSA | 1.6 ng/mL | 1.6 mcg/L |
| PSA (1 yr ago) | 3.0 ng/mL | 3.0 mcg/L |

## Assessment

The patient has severe LUTS, s/p TUIP, and is not responding to maximum doses of terazosin and finasteride after 9 months. He has urinary incontinence and impaired renal function, and is at risk of additional complications of BPH on the basis of size of the prostate and PSA. Patient to undergo preoperative testing for a prostatectomy, which will include uroflowmetry, postvoid residual volume, and transrectal ultrasound (TRUS) of the prostate.

### Student Workup

**Missing Information?**

Evaluate:     Patient Database

Drug Therapy Problems

Care Plan (by Problem)

## TARGETED QUESTIONS

1. What symptoms and signs of BPH does this patient have?

    *Hint: See pp. 929 and 930 in PPP*

2. Explain the mechanism of terazosin and finasteride in the management of BPH. Contrast their onset of action, clinical benefits, and adverse effects.

    *Hint: See pp. 934–938 and Table 52-5 in PPP*

3. Was this patient given an adequate medication treatment trial? Explain your answer.

    *Hint: See pp. 934–938 in PPP*

4. Interpret the change in this patient's PSA over the past year.

    *Hint: See pp. 939–940 in PPP*

5. In view of this patient's renal impairment, are the doses of terazosin and finasteride appropriate?

    *Hint: See Tables 52-6 and 52-7 in PPP*

## FOLLOW-UP

Preoperative testing is done. Test results reveal the following: maximum urinary flow rate 8 mL/s (normal, at least 10–14 mL/s) with a voided volume of 150 mL, postvoid residual urine volume 150 mL (normal, 0 mL), and TRUS shows a prostate size of 50 cm³. One week after this clinic visit, the patient is scheduled for an outpatient transurethral resection of the prostate (TURP). Surgery is uneventful. Three months after the TURP, the patient returns to the clinic. AUA symptom score is 9, maximum urinary flow rate is 18 mL/s, and postvoid residual urine volume is 0 mL. The patient reports that he is able to sleep through the night without having to wake up to urinate. He has noticed no blood clots or red coloring of his urine. He has urinary frequency and urgency.

6. Interpret the preoperative and postoperative assessments performed on this patient. Are the postoperative tests consistent with improvement in the symptoms and signs of BPH?

    *Hint: See Table 52-2 in PPP*

7. Postoperatively, the patient has moderately severe urinary urgency and frequency. What drug treatment would be useful for improving these symptoms?

    *Hint: See Table 52-5 in PPP*

## 🌐 GLOBAL PERSPECTIVE

Treatment of BPH may differ in countries outside the United States because of the use of herbals to control obstructive or irritative voiding symptoms. The American Urological Association and the Food and Drug Administration have concluded that clinical evidence is not sufficient to document the efficacy of any herbal product for this disorder, which should dissuade physicians from prescribing such agents. However, in other countries, widespread use of herbals including saw palmetto, pygeum (African plum), *Secale cereale* (rye pollen), and *Hypoxis rooperi* (South African star grass) is common. Such agents may be taken on their own, in combination with other herbals, or in common with prescription medications.

## CASE SUMMARY

- First-line drug treatment for moderate-to-severe BPH is an α-adrenergic antagonist. A uroselective α-adrenergic antagonist or an extended-release α-adrenergic antagonist is preferred in patients who cannot tolerate the cardiovascular side effects of immediate-release terazosin or doxazosin. All α-adrenergic antagonists quickly relieve voiding symptoms and have comparable efficacy in relieving voiding symptoms.

- For a patient with a moderately enlarged prostate, 40 g or more, a 5-α-reductase inhibitor may be considered. However, these agents require a minimum clinical trial of 6 months. Onset is delayed as the prostate gland must shrink in size and this takes time.

- Combination drug therapy with an α-adrenergic antagonist and a 5-α-reductase inhibitor is considered in those patients with moderate-to-severe disease who also have an enlarged prostate gland of at least 30–40 g and a PSA greater than 1.5 ng/mL (1.5 mcg/L). In such patients, combination therapy may relieve LUTS, slow disease progression, and reduce the need for prostatectomy.

- For patients who fail drug therapy or for those with complications of BPH, surgery is the treatment of choice.

- Anticholinergic agents (e.g., tolterodine or oxybutynin) may be used to relieve irritative voiding symptoms including urinary urgency and frequency. By causing relaxation of the detrusor muscle, anticholinergic agents decrease detrusor muscle contraction in response to small volumes of urine in the bladder. This can be problematic in patients with detrusor muscle hypertrophy resulting from long standing bladder outlet obstruction.

For more information on the care plan and facilitator's guide please visit http://www.mhpharmacotherapy.com.

# 60 Incontinence

Andrea S. Franks

## CASE LEARNING OBJECTIVES

- Contrast the pathophysiology of overactive bladder with other major types of urinary incontinence (i.e., stress, overflow, functional)
- Recognize the signs and symptoms of overactive bladder
- List the treatment goals for a patient with urinary incontinence, including overactive bladder
- Compare and contrast anticholinergics/antispasmodics, vaginal estrogens, tricyclic antidepressants, and α-adrenoceptor antagonists in terms of mechanism of action, treatment outcomes, adverse effects, and drug–drug interaction potential when used to manage overactive bladder
- Identify the factors that guide drug selection for an individual patient
- Formulate a monitoring plan for a patient on a given treatment regimen using patient-specific information
- Describe the indicators for combination drug therapy of urinary incontinence
- Describe the nonpharmacologic treatment approaches (including surgery) for overactive bladder
- Formulate appropriate patient-counseling information for patients undergoing drug therapy for overactive bladder

## Chief Complaint

"I tried bladder medicine but it didn't help my overactive bladder very much. Do you have any better pads than these to protect me when I need it?"

## History of Present Illness

Phoebe J. Engling, a 72-year-old woman, comes to the pharmacy for a refill of her pain medicine. She was recently hospitalized for dehydration and possible head injury after falling. Despite behavioral therapy and regular use of absorbent pads and undergarments, she is embarrassed and bothered by uncontrollable wetting of her clothing for at least a couple of years. She was initially told by her physician not to worry about urine leakage, that this can be expected with aging. With trepidation, she revealed she may have become dehydrated while trying to relieve her wetting accidents by limiting her fluid consumption and doubling the dose of her prescribed diuretic. This led to being hospitalized last month for severe dehydration with a fall without hitting head or bone fracture. At hospital discharge, she was given a prescription for oxybutynin. In a hurry to get home before she had another "accident" she declined medication counseling from the pharmacist. She stopped taking oxybutynin after a few days' use due to the lack of substantial improvement in her urinary symptoms.

## Past Medical History

Overactive bladder (diagnosed 2 years ago)

Type 2 DM (diagnosed 4 years ago)

HTN (for over 10 years)

OA (diagnosed last year)

Dehydration (one month ago) (resolved)

Fall (last month, and twice more the past year)

Depression (diagnosed 6 months ago)

Insomnia (diagnosed 6 months ago)

Cerebrovascular disease (stroke 5 years ago) with gait disturbance

Glaucoma, open angle (diagnosed 1987)

Chronic constipation

## Family History

No details

## Social History

Widowed, 3 children, worked as a hospital laboratory phlebotomist for 40 years

## Tobacco/Ethanol/Substance Use

Denies tobacco; drinks one glass of wine at bedtime to help sleep; 3–5 cups of caffeinated coffee daily

## Allergies/Intolerances/Adverse Drug Events

Amoxicillin (rash), tetracycline (GI discomfort)

## Medications (Current)

Immediate-release oxybutynin 5 mg PO bid

Acetaminophen 650 mg PO q 6 h

Senna 8.6 mg PO q hs

HCTZ 25 mg PO q 24 h

Metformin 500 mg PO bid

Enteric-coated aspirin 81 mg PO q 24 h

Lisinopril 10 mg PO q 24 h

Citalopram 20 mg PO q 24 h

Simvastatin 40 mg PO every evening

Acetaminophen 500 mg/diphenhydramine 25 mg PO hs
   PRN insomnia

Bimatoprost ophthalmic solution 0.03% one drop both eyes
   every night

Timolol maleate ophthalmic solution 0.5% one drop in the
   right eye every morning

## Review of Systems

Overall, the patient's appetite is adequate. Her cataracts are stable, but she is hard of hearing. She has had insomnia for a couple of years; she has recently started taking a glass of wine nightly to help her relax, and believes that can prevent urinary urgency that awakens her during the night. The patient uses an absorbent pad. She has chronic urinary incontinence (incontinent several times per week). She needs to void within a couple of minutes or large urine loss. She urinates as frequently as every 1–2 hours during the day. She wakes up as many as 5 times nightly with a strong urge to void. The patient also has pain in knees and hips; balance is fine with walker (uses all the time), but unsteady gait. She has right-hand weakness.

## Physical Examination

### ▸ General

Obese white female in no acute distress. Decreased normal fluid intake

### ▸ Vital Signs

BP 129/78 mm Hg, P 72, RR 18, T 36.3°C

Weight 182 lb (82.7 kg)

Height 62 in. (157 cm)

### ▸ Skin

Dry-appearing skin

### ▸ HEENT

PERRLA, EOMI; dry oral mucosal membranes

### ▸ Neck and Lymph Nodes

No masses

### ▸ Chest

Clear lung fields

### ▸ Breasts

No masses

### ▸ Cardiovascular

RRR; no murmurs heard

### ▸ Abdomen

Obese; bowel sounds

### ▸ Neurology

Motor strength 5/5 symmetrical

### ▸ Genitourinary

Incontinence

### ▸ Rectal

Examination deferred

## Laboratory Tests

Postvoid residual urine volume 89 mL (2 days ago)

|  | Conventional Units | SI Units |
|---|---|---|
| Na | 137 mEq/L | 137 mmol/L |
| K | 4.5 mEq/L | 4.5 mmol/L |
| Cl | 100 mEq/L | 100 mmol/L |
| $CO_2$ | 24 mEq/L | 24 mmol/L |
| BUN | 17 mg/dL | 6.1 mmol/L |
| SCr | 0.52 mg/dL | 46 mmol/L |
| Glucose (fasting) | 162 mg/dL | 9 mmol/L |
| Ca | 8.8 mg/dL | 2.20 mmol/L |
| Hgb | 13.9 g/dL | 139 g/L; 8.63 mmol/L |
| HCT | 39.7% | 0.397 |
| MCV | 93 um$^3$ | 93 fL |
| WBC | $7.2 \times 10^3/mm^3$ | $7.2 \times 10^9/L$ |
| Platelets | $156 \times 10^3/mm^3$ | $156 \times 10^9/L$ |
| Albumin | 3.8 g/dL | 38 g/L |
| $A_{1c}$ | 8.8% | 0.088 (73 mmol/mol Hgb) |
| TSH | 2.25 mIU/mL | 2.25 mIU/L |

## Assessment

Seventy-two-year-old woman with signs and symptoms consistent with overactive bladder along with numerous other comorbid conditions

## Student Workup

### Missing Information?

**Evaluate:**     Patient Database

Drug Therapy Problems

Care Plan (by Problem)

## TARGETED QUESTIONS

1. What signs and symptoms of overactive bladder does the patient have?

   *Hint: See pp. 944 and 945 in PPP*

2. Why is antimuscarinic medication the pharmacologic treatment of choice for patients with overactive bladder?

   *Hint: See p. 950 in PPP*

3. What medications can aggravate overactive bladder?

   *Hint: See Table 53-1 in PPP*

4. What risks and adverse effects of pharmacotherapy would you discuss with the patient?

   *Hint: See p. 955 and Table 53-4 in PPP*

5. Should the patient receive specific (other) pharmacotherapy that could indirectly improve overactive bladder symptoms?

   *Hint: See p. 954 and Table 53-2 in PPP*

## FOLLOW-UP

6. One month later, the patient returns for a refill of oxybutynin. She reports moderate improvement in her overactive bladder symptoms, with this documented in a bladder diary. However, she complains of dry mouth and worsened constipation. What actions, if any, would you take?

   *Hint: See p. 955 in PPP*

## 🌐 GLOBAL PERSPECTIVE

It is estimated by the World Health Organization that more than 200 million people worldwide have some type of bladder-control issue. Considering pathophysiology, it is not surprising that there is no evidence of significant international differences in the prevalence of overactive bladder or other types of urinary incontinence and their symptoms and drug response. The female sex and older age are associated with a higher risk of development of bladder-control issues, likely due to the stress and hormonal changes of childbirth and menopause. Differences in continence services for managing urinary incontinence outside of North America are attributed to government policies.

## CASE SUMMARY

- Her current clinical presentation is consistent with overactive bladder with urge urinary incontinence.

- The patient's glaucoma is a contraindication for use of an antimuscarinic agent, therefore, requires clarification regarding its type and whether her intraocular pressures are controlled by her current ophthalmic medicine. Because the use of an antimuscarinic agent with uncontrolled narrow-angle glaucoma could potentially cause serious damage to the optic nerve, this therapy should be confirmed with her ophthalmologist before starting therapy.

- If the antimuscarinic medication cannot be used, transient factors and elements of functional incontinence should be managed.

- Antimuscarinic therapy should be started at the lowest recommended dose during or after amelioration of transient factors and potential functional incontinence in the patient, especially with her advanced age. If bothersome adverse effects occur, if possible, the dose should be reduced or the current antimuscarinic agent replaced with the lowest dose of a different antimuscarinic agent, preferably an extended-release or transdermal formulation.

- An excessive dose of the antimuscarinic agent should be avoided, especially with her advanced age, history of falls, history of constipation, diuretic use that predisposes to dry mouth, constipation, and falls, and glaucoma that predisposes to vision disturbances.

For more information on the care plan and facilitator's guide please visit http://www.mhpharmacotherapy.com.

# 61  Drug Allergy

Lauren S. Schlesselman

- Recognize the signs and symptoms of anaphylaxis
- Identify the goals of therapy for anaphylaxis
- Develop an appropriate treatment and monitoring plan for anaphylaxis based on individual patient characteristics
- Select an appropriate product for treating the underlying condition on the basis of patient's allergic history
- Properly educate a patient with a history of drug allergies

## PATIENT PRESENTATION

### Chief Complaint

"I was walking back from the mailbox when I heard a rustling sound in the woods. A raccoon came charging out of the woods at me. I tried to run but he caught up to me and bit my leg."

### History of Present Illness

Faith Stevens is a 19-year-old woman who presents to the emergency department with a raccoon bite to her left leg. While walking in her yard during daylight hours, a raccoon (whose whereabouts are currently unknown) raced across the lawn to bite her. The patient describes attempting to shake the raccoon from her leg. Damage to the leg confirms raccoon-inflicted significant damage to the skin and muscles on the left calf.

On arrival at the hospital, cleaning of the wound began with soap and water, followed by povidine–iodine. During this time, a single dose of amoxicillin/clavulanate 875/125 mg was orally administered. Within 30 minutes of the dose, the patient began complaining of SOB, abdominal pain, itchiness, nausea, and rapid heart rate. Nurse noted audible wheezing and pruritis on trunk and arms.

### Past Medical History

History of Stevens–Johnson syndrome with sulfa

### Family History

Father is alive with no significant medical history at age 44. Mother is alive with no significant medical history at age 42. She has two young sisters who are healthy.

### Social History

College student pursuing a degree in psychology. Single, lives with her parents and sisters; has no children. Works part-time at a local library

### Tobacco/Alcohol/Substance Use

Social drinker; (–) tobacco or illicit drug use

### Allergies/Intolerances/Adverse Drug Events

Sulfa-induced Stevens–Johnson syndrome

Codeine-induced nausea

Ibuprofen (GI upset and abdominal pain)

Meperidine (hallucinations)

### Medications (Current)

No outpatient medications

### Physical Examination

▶ *General*

Teenaged, Caucasian woman in acute distress

▶ *Vital Signs*

BP 90/45 mm Hg, P 98, RR 16, T 37.2°C

Weight 134.2 lb (61 kg)

Height 68 in. (173 cm)

Pain 7 (scale 0–10)

**FIGURE 61-1.** Rash after administration of a beta-lactam agent. (Adapted, with permission, from Usatine RP, Smith MA, Mayeaux Jr EJ, Chumley H, Tysinger J. The Color Atlas of Family Medicine. New York, McGraw-Hill, 2009, Fig 196-1.)

▶ **Skin**

Clammy skin

Laceration of left calf 4 inch (10 cm) in diameter with underlying tissue and muscle damage; significant bleeding at site; (+) urticaria on trunk and arms (Figure 61-1)

▶ **HEENT**

PERRLA, EOMI; (−) trace periorbital edema; (−) sinus tenderness

▶ **Neck and Lymph Nodes**

(−) Lymphadenopathy; (−) carotid bruits

▶ **Chest**

Audible wheezing

▶ **Breasts**

Examination deferred

▶ **Cardiovascular**

Normal rhythm; tachycardia; normal $S_1$, $S_2$; (−) $S_3$ or $S_4$

▶ **Abdomen**

Not tender/not distended; (−) organomegaly

▶ **Neurology**

Grossly intact; deep tendon reflexes normal

▶ **Genitourinary**

Examination deferred

▶ **Rectal**

Examination deferred

## Laboratory Tests

*Nonfasting*

|  | Conventional Units | SI Units |
|---|---|---|
| Na | 140 mEq/L | 140 mmol/L |
| K | 4 mEq/L | 4 mmol/L |
| Cl | 100 mEq/L | 100 mmol/L |
| $CO_2$ | 24 mEq/L | 24 mmol/L |
| BUN | 8 mg/dL | 2.9 mmol/L |
| SCr | 0.7 mg/dL | 62 μmol/L |
| Glu | 105 mg/dL | 5.8 mmol/L |
| Ca | 9.4 mg/dL | 2.35 mmol/L |
| Mg | 1.8 mEq/L | 0.90 mmol/L |
| Phosphate | 3.8 mg/dL | 1.23 mmol/L |
| Hgb | 13.5 g/dL | 135 g/L; 8.38 mmol/L |
| Hct | 39.7% | 0.397 |
| WBC | $9.2 \times 10^3/mm^3$ | $9.2 \times 10^9/L$ |
| MCV | 83 μm³ | 83 fL |
| Albumin | 4.3 g/dL | 43 g/L |

## Assessment

Nineteen-year-old woman with signs and symptoms consistent with anaphylaxis following antibiotic administration; also with signs consistent for animal bite

**Student Workup**

**Missing Information?**

**Evaluate:** Patient Database
Drug Therapy Problems
Care Plan (by Problem)

## TARGETED QUESTIONS

1. What signs and symptoms of anaphylaxis does the patient have?

   *Hint: See Clinical Presentation and Diagnosis of Allergic and Pseudoallergic Drug Reactions in PPP*

2. What are the treatments of choice for patients with anaphylaxis?

   *Hint: See Table 54-3 in PPP*

3. What classes of medications are frequently associated with anaphylaxis?

   *Hint: See Table 54-2 in PPP*

4. What are the odds of cross-reactivity with β-lactams?

   *Hint: See pp. 968–969 in PPP*

5. In a patient like this with multiple medication allergies, how can the health care professional determine which medications are safe to use?

   *Hint: See p. 968 and Table 54-5 in PPP*

## FOLLOW-UP

6. After administration of her five doses of rabies vaccine, the patient is seen by her primary care provider for follow-up. She feels much better with significant wound healing and limited discomfort. Is the patient a candidate for desensitization to penicillin or sulfa? If so, how would this be done?

   *Hint: See pp. 972–973 and Table 54-6 in PPP*

## ⟲ GLOBAL PERSPECTIVE

Drug allergy is an adverse immune response to a stimulus. Such responses, categorized utilizing the Gell and Coombs categories, can be type I, II, III, IV, or a combination of these. Classes of medications frequently associated with anaphylaxis include penicillins, sulfa, vaccines, NSAIDs, and radiocontrast media. Available medications commonly associated with allergies and skin tests vary by country. For example, penicillin minor-determinant skin tests are not available in the United States, but are used in Europe. Additionally, many medication-related allergic reactions have been associated with impurities in medication solutions, which depend on manufacturing procedures and regulations in different countries.

## CASE SUMMARY

- Her current clinical picture is consistent with anaphylaxis and epinephrine and fluid replacement should be initiated.

- An initial epinephrine dose of 0.2–0.5 mg IM or SC, repeated every 5 minutes as needed, is appropriate. This should be accompanied by 1–2 L of normal saline at 5–10 mL/kg in the first 5 minutes followed by a slower infusion.

- Anaphylaxis can reoccur 6–8 hours after presentation, so patients should be monitored for at least 12 hours.

- Documentation of allergies in the patient's medical records in the hospital, physician's office, and pharmacy is a critical component in preventing exposure to these medications in the future. Differentiation between true allergies and adverse reactions is also essential.

**For more information on the care plan and facilitator's guide please visit http://www.mhpharmacotherapy.com.**

# 62 Solid Organ Transplantation

Basma Sadaka          Rita R. Alloway

## CASE LEARNING OBJECTIVES

- Identify signs and symptoms of cytomegalovirus (CMV) infection for renal transplant recipients post rejection
- Develop a comprehensive treatment plan for renal transplant recipients with CMV infection
- Determine the appropriate duration of treatment and appropriate dose for CMV infection
- Formulate a medication counseling plan for a renal transplant recipient

## PATIENT PRESENTATION

### Chief Complaint

"I'm just here for a my regular checkup"

### History of Present Illness

Karen Smith is a 35-year-old African American female with a history of end stage renal disease (ESRD) secondary to hypertension (HTN) and type 2 diabetes mellitus. She underwent a 4 antigen mismatched deceased donor kidney transplant 11 months ago. This was her second transplant. Prior to her second transplant, she was on peritoneal dialysis 5 times a week for 1 year. She received blood transfusions due to anemia on two occasions while she was on dialysis as well as had two prior pregnancies. Pre-transplant testing revealed a peak cytotoxic PRA of 44% and current cytotoxic PRA of 20%. She received induction with rabbit anti-thymocyte globulin (rATG) and a rapid steroid taper. Pre-transplant viral serologies showed that Ms. Smith was cytomegalovirus (CMV) IgG negative and the donor was CMV IgG positive. Maintenance immunosuppression includes tacrolimus and mycophenolate mofetil. She was on sulfamethoxazole/trimethoprim for 6 months and nystatin for 2 months for infectious prophylaxis. She was prescribed valganciclovir for 6 months post-transplant; however, she reported missing "a couple of weeks" of this medication due to issues with insurance co-pays. Post-transplant, her serum creatinine nadir was 1.1 mg/dL (97 μmol/L) and has remained relatively constant. However, 7 months post-transplant, she had an elevation in her serum creatinine (2.5mg/dL [221 μmol/L]) and a biopsy was obtained. Her biopsy revealed a grade 1B acute cellular rejection. She was treated with a course of 4 doses of rATG and a steroid pulse (500 mg × 3 doses) followed by a rapid taper for 7 days.

She was last seen in the renal transplant clinic 3 weeks prior. She states that she has been feeling tired and has had constant diarrhea and abdominal pain for the past 2 weeks. She was not sure if it was from something that she had eaten or if she caught a virus. She has also noticed a slight decrease in her urine output, which she attributes to not drinking enough water and dehydration from the weather humidity.

### Past Medical History

ESRD s/p deceased donor kidney transplant in 2011 (rATG induction × 4 doses)

Acute cellular rejection in 2012 (treated with rATG and steroid pulse)

Hypertension × 10 years

Diabetes mellitus type 2 × 8 years

Hyperlipidemia × 6 years

Diabetic gastroparesis

### Past Surgical History

S/p living donor kidney transplant in 2009 that was lost due to non-compliance (rATG induction × 4 doses at time of transplant)

11 months s/p deceased donor kidney transplant

Tonsillectomy at age 9

### Family History

Mother is alive at 67 years with HTN and diabetes mellitus type 2; Father had HTN and hyperlipidemia and he died last year due to myocardial infarction at the age of 68.

## Social/Work History

She is married with 2 children (aged 7 and 4), both of whom are alive and well. She worked as a retail store manager, but is currently on disability and is not working.

## Tobacco/Alcohol/Substance Use

Previously social drinker (last approximately 4 years ago); denies tobacco use and illicit drug use.

## Allergies

NKDA

## Medications (current)

Tacrolimus 9 mg PO twice daily

Mycophenolate mofetil 1,500 mg PO twice daily

Sulfamethoxazole/trimethoprim 400 mg/80mg PO daily

Metoprolol 100 mg PO twice daily

Nifedipine ER 60 mg PO daily

Lisinopril 10 mg PO daily

Aspirin EC 81 mg PO daily

Metoclopramide 5 mg PO three times daily before meals

Omeprazole 20 mg PO daily

Simvastatin 20 mg PO at bedtime

Insulin glargine 12 units subcutaneous at bedtime

## Review of Systems

Denies dysuria; denies nausea/vomiting, chest pain, or shortness of breath; endorses subjective decrease in urinary output. Reported 7–8 episodes of diarrhea per day for the past 2 weeks.

## Physical Exam

### ▶ General

Well-nourished, middle-aged, African-American female complaining of abdominal pain

### ▶ Vital Signs

BP 138/86 mmHg; P 74; RR 16; T 37.2°C; Pain 4/10
Height 63 in. (160 cm); Weight 165 lbs (75 kg)

### ▶ HEENT

PERRLA; EOMI

### ▶ Chest

Clear to auscultation bilaterally

### ▶ Cardiovascular

RRR; (+) S1, S2; (−) murmurs

### ▶ Abdomen

Tender; distended; (+) bowel sounds

### ▶ Neurology

Alert and oriented × 3; CN II-XII intact; no focal deficits

### ▶ Genitourinary/Rectal

Colonoscopy performed

## Laboratory Assessment

### Fasting

| | Conventional Units | SI Units |
|---|---|---|
| Na | 143 mEq/L | 143 mmol/L |
| K | 5.3 mEq/L | 5.3 mmol/L |
| Cl | 107 mEq/L | 107 mmol/L |
| $CO_2$ | 20 mEq/L | 20 mmol/L |
| BUN | 38 mg/dL | 14 mmol/L |
| SCr | 1.9 mg/dL | 168 μmol/L |
| Glu | 112 mg/dL | 6.2 mmol/L |
| Ca | 8.6 mg/dL | 2.15 mmol/L |
| Mg | 1.7 mEq/L | 0.85 mmol/L |
| Hgb | 11.3 g/dL | 113 g/L; 7.01 mmol/L |
| Hct | 32.7% | 0.327 |
| WBC | $2.5 \times 10^3/mm^3$ | $2.5 \times 10^9/L$ |
| Neutrophil | 42.1% | 0.42 |
| MCV | $87.0 \ \mu m^3$ | 87.0 fL |
| Albumin | 3.6 g/dL | 36 g/L |
| Phos | 3.8 mg/dL | 1.23 mmol/L |
| eGFR | 36 mL/min | $1.73 \ m^2$ (MDRD) |
| Total cholesterol | 172 mg/dL | 4.45 mmol/L |
| Tacrolimus | 24 ng/mL or mcg/L | 30 nmol/L |
| LDL cholesterol | 93 mg/dL | 2.40 mmol/L |
| HDL cholesterol | 51 mg/dL | 1.32 mmol/L |
| C. difficile toxin A/B | Negative | |
| CMV quant (PCR) | 280,895 cells/mL | $281 \times 10^6$ copies /L |
| BK quant (PCR) | 0 cells/mL | 0 copies/L |
| EBV quant (PCR) | 0 cells/mL | 0 copies/L |

## Renal Biopsy Pathology

No acute cellular rejection

## Colonoscopy

Invasive CMV infection in the colon

## Assessment

Ms. Smith is a 35-year-old female who is 11 months s/p deceased donor kidney transplant and presents with symptoms of diarrhea, abdominal pain, and abnormal laboratory tests that are consistent with CMV viremia.

### Student Workup

**Missing Information?**

**Evaluate:**     Patient Database

Drug Therapy Problems

Care Plan (by Problem)

## TARGETED QUESTIONS

1. Was Ms. Smith prescribed the appropriate dose and duration of valganciclovir for infectious prophylaxis post-transplant?

    *Hint: See pp. 995–996 in PPP*

2. What risk factors for CMV does Ms. Smith have?

    *Hint: See p. 995 in PPP*

3. What therapies could be used for the treatment of CMV?

    *Hint: See pp. 995–996 in PPP*

4. What clinical parameters should be monitored for efficacy of CMV treatment and resolution of CMV?

    *Hint: See pp. 995–996 in PPP*

## FOLLOW-UP

Ms. Smith was started on ganciclovir sodium 190 mg IV daily 2 weeks ago. She presents to the renal transplant clinic today for a follow-up visit. Serum CMV PCR was checked and was reduced to 25,000 cell copies/mL ($25 \times 10^6$ copies/L). Renal function from today's clinic visit had improved to 1.1 mg/dL (97 µmol/L) (her baseline serum creatinine) and patient reports that she no longer has diarrhea or abdominal pain. RBC was 8 g/dL (80 g/L; 4.97 mmol/L) and WBC is stable at $2.5 \times 10^3$/mm³ ($2.5 \times 10^9$/L). She reports that she has been adherent to her medication regimen and has not missed any doses.

5. What would be the next step for the patient in terms of the therapeutic option chosen above to treat CMV? Should it be continued at the current dose or should it be changed, and why?

    *Hint: See Table 55-6 in PPP*

## ⟳ GLOBAL PERSPECTIVE

Immunosuppression, as well as infectious prophylaxis practices, varies widely from region to region and country to country. In general, as more potent immunosuppressive agents are utilized, infectious complications increase. The increased incidence of infectious complications as a result of increased immunosuppression is typically viral infections, (e.g., CMV, EBV, BKV). CMV is a common viral infection post-transplant. CMV infections are concerning due to the severity spectrum of the disease and because they are immunomodulatory, thus causing rejection.

Techniques of testing the donor and recipient CMV serologies have allowed clinicians to identify patients at the greatest risk of CMV infection. The greatest risk of CMV is associated with the transmission of CMV infection from a CMV positive donor by the transplanted kidney to a naïve CMV recipient.

The use of potent immunosuppressive drugs post-transplant and for treating rejection further increases the risk of developing CMV disease. T-cell depleting antibody therapies are principally associated with an increased risk of viral infections.

The preferred treatment regimen for CMV disease is antiviral therapy and immunosuppressive dose reduction management. Medications used to treat CMV infection depend upon disease severity and likelihood of resistance. Medications may include valganciclovir, ganciclovir sodium, valacyclovir, CMV hyperimmune globulin, cidofovir, or foscarnet sodium.

## CASE SUMMARY

- There is a risk of opportunistic infection in immunosuppressed patients. Therefore, appropriate prophylaxis and surveillance should be employed to improve patient outcomes.

- Initial clinical presentation is consistent with CMV infection in a kidney transplant recipient. Clinical laboratory monitoring as well as the appropriate use of medication is crucial to treat the infection.

**For more information on the care plan and facilitator's guide please visit http://www.mhpharmacotherapy.com.**

# 63 Osteoporosis

Beth Bryles Phillips      Shelley King McIntire

Alexis E. Horace

## CASE LEARNING OBJECTIVES

- Identify risk factors that predispose patients to osteoporosis
- Recommend appropriate lifestyle modifications to prevent bone loss
- Compare and contrast the effect of available treatment options on reduction of fracture risk
- Recommend an appropriate treatment regimen for a patient with osteoporosis and develop a monitoring plan for the selected regimen
- Educate patients on osteoporosis and drug treatment, including appropriate use, administration, and adverse effects

## PATIENT PRESENTATION

### Chief Complaint

"I am here to see my new doctor."

### History of Present Illness

DS is a 72-year-old Caucasian woman who presents to the internal medicine clinic to establish care at the urging of her daughter. She had been followed for a number of years by her previous physician who recently retired. She reports she has been taking calcitonin nasal spray for the past 5 years when her doctor ordered a bone density test. She remembers asking her physician if she should take aldendronate instead because she knew several women in her book club who took the medication. She reports they discussed it but he felt calcitonin may be a better choice due to her loss of height and presence of heartburn. She tries to walk on a regular basis for exercise but finds that her speed and distance are not what they used to be since her hip was replaced 6 months ago. She reports consuming milk on a daily basis with her cereal. She only rarely takes in other dairy products. She drinks 5–6 cups of coffee daily and has been a heavy coffee drinker all of her life. She has had problems with heartburn "on and off" over the years. She currently takes omeprazole for her heartburn and feels that her symptoms are well controlled.

### Past Medical History

Osteoporosis status post (s/p) vertebral fractures and left hip fracture with hip replacement 6 months ago

Gastroesophageal reflux disease (GERD) × 20 years

Hypertension × 5 years

Peripheral artery disease (PAD) (Duration: 3 years)

Hypothyroidism × 21 years

Nicotine dependence × 55 years

Osteoarthritis s/p total knee replacement 10 years ago

S/p deep venous thrombosis (DVT) after knee surgery 10 years ago

### Family History

Father deceased at age 94 due to cancer (type unknown). Mother deceased at age 92, history of hip fracture. She has one brother and one sister who are both healthy.

### Social History

Married and lives with her husband of 44 years; has 5 children. She is a retired social worker.

### Tobacco/Alcohol/Substance Use

Social drinker; (+) tobacco 1 ppd × 54 years, (−) illicit drug use

### Allergies/Intolerances/Adverse Drug Events

No known drug allergies (NKDA)

### Medications (Current)

Calcitonin nasal spray 200 IU alternating nostrils daily

Omeprazole 20 mg PO daily

Hydrochlorothiazide 25 mg PO daily

Aspirin 325 mg PO daily

Levothyroxine 125 mcg PO daily

Naproxen 500 mg BID

Calcium carbonate 500 mg daily AM prn

## Review of Systems

(+) For heartburn treated with omeprazole, denies difficulty swallowing or burning in her throat; Denies back or hip pain but reports 2.5-in. decrease in height since young adulthood, (+) kyphosis; Denies heat intolerance, weight loss, or changes in texture of hair or skin

## Physical Exam

▶ *General*

Thin, elderly woman who looks older than her stated age, mild kyphosis present

▶ *Vital Signs*

BP 132/76 mm Hg, P 78, RR 16, T 36.2°C

Weight 117 lb (53.2 kg)

Height 69 inches (175 cm)

Denies pain

▶ *Skin*

Normal turgor and color; warm

▶ *HEENT*

PERRLA, EOMI; disks flat; fundi with no hemorrhages or exudates

▶ *Neck and Lymph Nodes*

No lymphadenopathy, thyromegaly, or carotid bruits

▶ *Chest*

Clear to auscultation bilaterally

▶ *Breasts*

Exam deferred

▶ *Cardiovascular*

RRR; normal $S_1$ and $S_2$; no $S_3$ or $S_4$; no m/r/g

▶ *Abdomen*

Not tender/not distended; (–) organomegaly

▶ *Neurology*

A & O × 3; CN II–XII intact; DTR 2+

▶ *Extremities*

Cool, normal color, dorsalis pedis pulse weak

▶ *Genitourinary*

Exam deferred

▶ *Rectal*

Exam deferred

## Laboratory Tests

### Fasting Obtained 2 Days Ago

|  | Conventional Units | SI Units |
|---|---|---|
| Na | 139 mEq/L | 139 mmol/L |
| K | 4.7 mEq/L | 4.7 mmol/L |
| Cl | 101 mEq/L | 101 mmol/L |
| $CO_2$ | 30 mEq/L | 30 mmol/L |
| BUN | 14 mg/dL | 5.0 mmol/L |
| SCr | 0.8 mg/dL | 70.1 µmol/L |
| Glu | 99 mg/dL | 5.5 mmol/L |
| Ca | 9.3 mg/dL | 2.33 mmol/L |
| TSH | 0.2 µIU/mL | 0.2 mIU/L |
| 25(OH)D | 31 ng/mL | 77 nmol/L |
| Hgb | 15.5 g/dL | 9.62 mmol/L |
| Hct | 48% | 0.48 |
| WBC | $7.6 \times 10^3/mm^3$ | $7.6 \times 10^9/L$ |
| MCV | 79 µm³ | 79 fL |
| Albumin | 3.8 g/dL | 38 g/L |
| Total cholesterol | 184 mg/dL | 4.76 mmol/L |
| LDL cholesterol | 96 mg/dL | 2.48 mmol/L |
| HDL cholesterol | 48 mg/dL | 1.24 mmol/L |
| Triglyceride | 184 mg/dL | 2.08 mmol/L |

### Other:

Bone mineral density

| | | |
|---|---|---|
| *5 years ago* | | |
| Total hip | T score –1.8 | |
| Lumbar spine | T score –2.1 | |
| *3 months ago* | | |
| Total hip | T score –2.3 | |
| Lumbar spine | T score –2.95 | |

## Assessment

72-year-old female with signs and bone densitometry consistent with osteoporosis; recurrent osteoporotic fracture on current therapy

## Student Workup

### Missing Information?

| Evaluate: | Patient Database |
|---|---|
| | Drug Therapy Problems |
| | Care Plan (by Problem) |

## TARGETED QUESTIONS

1. What signs and symptoms of osteoporosis does the patient have?

   *Hint: See pp. 1010 and 1011 in PPP*

2. What risk factors does this patient have for osteoporosis?

   *Hint: See p. 1012 in PPP*

3. What non-pharmacologic recommendations are important for her treatment plan?

   *Hint: See pp. 1013–1015 in PPP*

4. What are her calcium and vitamin D requirements? Is she a candidate for calcium and/or vitamin D supplementation? If so, which one would you recommend and why?

   *Hint: See pp. 1015 and 1016 in PPP*

5. Is her current osteoporosis treatment effective? What alternative medications would you recommend for this patient?

   *Hint: See p. 1021 in PPP*

## FOLLOW-UP

1. What if a follow-up bone mineral density scan in two years shows no improvement in T scores and the patient has not had any recurrent fractures? Should her therapy be changed at that time?

2. What if the patient develops adverse gastrointestinal effects on therapy in 6 months? What alternative therapies are appropriate?

3. What if the patient had a history of breast cancer? Would that influence your choice of agent to treat osteoporosis?

## ⟳ GLOBAL PERSPECTIVE

Osteoporosis is the most common skeletal disorder caused by an imbalance of bone remodeling which results in overall bone loss. The development of bone loss can lead to painful and debilitating bone fractures. Though osteoporosis affects over 10 million Americans, the World Health Organization reports that osteoporosis affects approximately 75 million people in America, Europe, and Japan combined. The lifetime risk for developing wrist, vertebral, and hip fractures are 30–40% for these combined populations. Osteoporosis primarily affects the Caucasian ethnicity; however, significant risk has been reported for all ethnic backgrounds. Asian and non-Hispanic Caucasian women aged 50 years or greater diagnosed with osteoporosis approximate 20% of Americans. Approximately 5% of American non-Hispanic black women within the same age group have osteoporosis. An estimated 35% of women in all three of these ethnic groups are estimated to have low bone mass. The risk of osteoporosis is increasing more in American Hispanic women when compared to other ethnic/racial groups. Ten percent of American Hispanic women aged 50 years and older are diagnosed with osteoporosis with 23% of those women estimated to have low bone mass. To add to the significance of these statistics for American Hispanic women, experts predict an increase in cost related to osteoporotic fractures from $754 million in 2005 to $2 billion in 2025. To help decrease the mortality associated with osteoporosis, it is important to educate all patient populations irrelevant of race/ethnicity of the importance of proper nutrition, pharmacotherapy, and yearly bone mineral density screenings.

## CASE SUMMARY

- ·Current pharmacotherapy for the treatment of osteoporosis has been ineffective in preventing fractures. Alternative therapy should be considered.

- Adequate calcium and vitamin D supplementation is needed to optimize osteoporosis treatment. A calcium supplement whose absorption is not dependent on an acidic gastric environment is needed.

- Over suppression of thyroid can promote bone loss and increase risk for osteoporotic fracture and should be avoided.

**For more information on the care plan and facilitator's guide please visit http://www.mhpharmacotherapy.com.**

# 64 Rheumatoid Arthritis

Susan P. Bruce          Elaine M. Greifenstein

## CASE LEARNING OBJECTIVES

- Discuss the comorbidities associated with rheumatoid arthritis (RA)
- Recognize the typical clinical presentation of RA
- Create treatment goals for a patient with RA arthritis on the basis of global disease activity
- Compare and contrast the available pharmacotherapeutic options, selecting the most appropriate regimen for a given patient
- Propose a patient education plan that includes nonpharmacologic and pharmacologic treatment measures
- Formulate an initial prescreening and a long-term monitoring plan to evaluate the safety and efficacy of a therapeutic regimen designed for an individual patient with RA

## PATIENT PRESENTATION

### Chief Complaint

"I'm stiff and my joints are swollen."

### History of Present Illness

Ching Li is a 55-year-old postmenopausal woman presenting to the rheumatologist for evaluation and treatment of RA. CL presented to her primary care physician 3 months ago with complaints of symmetrical joint pain in her hands and feet and morning stiffness lasting more than an hour. She tried ibuprofen followed by naproxen for about 2 months with limited pain relief. During a follow-up visit with her primary care physician approximately 1 month ago, naproxen was discontinued and low-dose corticosteroids were initiated. The corticosteroids have helped joint discomfort partially, but have not had an impact on joint swelling. She reports significant difficulty with dressing (especially buttons, zippers, and tying her shoes) and meal preparation. She has experienced progressive morning stiffness, now lasting for 2–3 hours daily. She reports that she feels down, but does not understand why. Her husband passed away 3 years ago and, in her opinion, she dealt with her husband's passing immediately after his death.

### Past Medical History

Peptic ulcer disease diagnosed 7 months ago

Hypertension × 3 years

Blood transfusion following C-section in China 30 years ago

Menopause at age 50

### Family History

Father had CAD and died of MI at age 82. Mother died at age 70 from hepatocellular carcinoma. Her only brother has dyslipidemia and hypertension. Daughter is alive and well.

### Social History

CL, a homemaker, moved to the United States from China to live with her daughter 3 years ago after her husband died. She speaks Mandarin and English. Her husband was employed by an international brokerage firm prior to his death and she has health insurance/prescription coverage available as part of his employment benefits.

### Tobacco/Alcohol/Substance Use

(+) Tobacco 1 ppd × 40 years; (−) alcohol or illicit drug use

### Allergies/Intolerances/Adverse Drug Events

Trimethoprim/sulfamethoxazole—rash

### Medications (Current)

Hydrochlorothiazide 12.5 mg PO daily

Prednisone 5 mg PO daily in the morning

Lansoprazole 30 mg PO daily

Red yeast rice 1,200 mg PO twice daily

Kava kava 500 mg PO at bedtime

## Review of Systems

Generalized malaise and fatigue for 4 months; unintentional 10 lb (4.5 kg) weight loss over the past 3 months; (−) fevers, night sweats, adenopathy, dry eyes, oral ulcers, or skin rashes; morning cough productive of clear sputum, resolves 15–30 minutes after arising; (−) hemoptysis, chest pain, shortness of breath, exertional chest discomfort, abdominal pain, or diarrhea; initial difficulty falling asleep at night due to joint discomfort, but then awakens two to three times per night for unknown reasons; self-prescribed use of kava kava at bedtime decreases the nighttime awakening; (−) suicidal ideation

## Physical Examination

### ▶ General

Thin, middle-aged, Asian woman in obvious discomfort on shaking hands and arising from sitting

### ▶ Vital Signs

BP 146/88 mm Hg, P 72, RR 15, T 36.8°C

Weight 112.5 lb (51.1 kg)

Height 60 in. (152 cm)

Pain rated as 6/10

### ▶ Skin

(−) Rashes, lesions or evidence of vasculitis

### ▶ HEENT

(−) Conjunctival or sclera injection; (−) oral or nasal ulcers; mucus membranes moist

### ▶ Neck and Lymph Nodes

(−) Adenopathy, thyromegaly, or masses

### ▶ Chest

Prolonged expiratory phase bilaterally; (−) rales, rhonchi, wheezes, or rubs

### ▶ Breasts

(−) Nodules, masses, skin changes, or nipple discharge

### ▶ Cardiovascular

RRR; $S_4$ gallop present; (−) $S_3$ gallop or rubs

### ▶ Abdomen

Scaphoid and nontender; (−) masses, hepatomegaly, or splenomegaly

### ▶ Extremities

Small olecranon nodules bilaterally; 1+ synovitis and tenderness of the bilateral dorsal wrists; 2+ synovitis of the right metacarpophalangeal (MCP) joints and 1+ synovitis of the left MCP joints; 1+ synovitis and tenderness of the bilateral proximal interphalangeal joints (PIP) joints; 2+ synovitis and tenderness of the right metatarsophalangeal (MTP) joints and 1+ synovitis of the left MTP joints; (−) joint effusions.

### ▶ Genitourinary

Examination deferred

### ▶ Rectal

Normal sphincter tone; (−) masses; stool brown and (−) guaiac

### ▶ Laboratory Tests

#### Fasting Obtained 2 Weeks Ago

|  | Conventional Units | SI Units |
|---|---|---|
| Na | 140 mEq/L | 140 mmol/L |
| K | 4.2 mEq/L | 4.2 mmol/L |
| Cl | 99 mEq/L | 99 mmol/L |
| $CO_2$ | 24 mEq/L | 24 mmol/L |
| BUN | 12 mg/dL | 4.3 mmol/L |
| SCr | 0.8 mg/dL | 71 μmol/L |
| Glu | 106 mg/dL | 5.9 mmol/L |
| Ca | 9.2 mg/dL | 2.3 mmol/L |
| Mg | 1.8 mEq/L | 0.90 mmol/L |
| Phosphate | 3.6 mg/dL | 1.16 mmol/L |
| RF | 200 IU/mL | 200 kIU/L |
| Anti-CCP | 160 units | |
| C-reactive protein (CRP) | 3.2 mg/dL | 32 mg/L |
| Hgb | 12.2 g/dL | 122 g/L; 7.57 mmol/L |
| Hct | 36.8% | 0.368 |
| Platelets | $500 \times 10^3/\mu L$ | $500 \times 10^9/L$ |
| MCV | 90 μm$^3$ | 90 fL |
| WBC | $5.2 \times 10^3/mm^3$ | $5.2 \times 10^9/L$ |
| Albumin | 4 g/dL | 40 g/L |
| AST | 26 IU/L | 0.43 μkat/L |
| ALT | 32 IU/L | 0.53 μkat/L |
| Alk Phos | 120 mg/dL | 2 μKat/L |
| ESR | 52 mm/h | 14.5 μm/s |
| Total cholesterol | 247 mg/dL | 6.39 mmol/L |
| LDL-C | 162 mg/dL | 4.19 mmol/L |
| HDL-C | 28 mg/dL | 0.72 mmol/L |
| Triglycerides | 282 mg/dL | 3.19 mmol/L |

## Assessment

Fifty-five-year-old woman with signs, symptoms, and laboratory tests consistent with RA of moderate-to-high disease activity and poor prognostic factors

### Student Workup

**Missing Information?**

Evaluate: Patient Database

Drug Therapy Problems

Care Plan (by Problem)

## TARGETED QUESTIONS

1. On the basis of initial disease activity, which medications are appropriate for the treatment of RA in this patient?

   *Hint: See p. 1029 and 1032, Table 57-4 and Figure 57-1 in PPP*

2. What tests should be included in the prescreening workup prior to initiating therapy? What tests should be included in the long-term monitoring for the therapeutic regimen you are recommending?

   *Hint: See p. 1028 in PPP and Table 57-3*

3. Which comorbid conditions related to RA or its treatment must also be addressed for this patient?

   *Hint: See p. 1027 in PPP*

4. What is the most appropriate treatment for each comorbid condition?

   *Hint: See p. 1029 and 1032 in PPP*

5. What pharmacologic and nonpharmacologic measures should your patient education plan include?

   *Hint: See Table 57-4 in PPP*

## FOLLOW-UP

CL returns to the rheumatologist 3 months after initiation of DMARD (disease-modifying antirheumatic drug) and biologic therapy and indicates her pain is 1 on a 0 to 10 scale. She notes significant improvement in completing activities of daily living (dressing, bathing, and meal preparation for her family). Physical examination reveals global improvement in joint synovitis and swelling overall, with only trace synovitis of the right MCP joints. Small bilateral olecranon nodules are unchanged. X-rays of her hands and feet reveal periarticular osteopenia at the MCP and MTP joints, but no erosions. Significant laboratory values include ESR 20 mm/h (5.6 μm/s),

CRP 0.7 mg/dL (7 mg/L), AST 35 IU/L (0.58 μKat/L), ALT 40 IU/L (0.67 μKat/L), SCr 0.8 mg/dL (71 μmol/L), and glucose (fasting) 109 mg/dL (6.0 mmol/L).

6. On the basis of the disease activity at follow-up, what medication adjustments are appropriate for the treatment of RA in this patient?

   *Hint: See p. 1032 and Table 57-4 in PPP*

7. What tests should be included in the long-term monitoring for the therapeutic regimen you are recommending?

   *Hint: See p. 1032 in PPP and Table 57-4*

## ⟳ GLOBAL PERSPECTIVE

RA is a common chronic systemic autoimmune inflammatory disease with a prevalence of 1–2% across all populations. Women are affected more commonly than men, with a peak incidence in the fourth and fifth decades of life. Synovium is the primary site of inflammation and the condition typically progresses to a chronic state with substantial morbidity and disability. Comorbid diseases are common due to the ongoing inflammatory response with cardiovascular disease and infections representing the most common causes of death. Treatment of RA requires early assessment of disease activity with selection of disease-modifying and biologic agents in combination representing the gold standard of care.

## CASE SUMMARY

- Her current clinical picture is consistent with RA of moderate-to-high disease activity, and combination disease-modifying therapy with biologic therapy should be initiated.
- Initial treatment with methotrexate, etanercept, and prednisone improved her overall joint swelling, tenderness and disease activity. The focus going forward is a gradual reduction of prednisone with adjustments of methotrexate as needed to control disease progression.
- Initiation and ongoing treatment with immunosuppressive therapy requires continual clinical vigilance for medication side effects.
- RA is associated with a number of comorbid conditions, including cardiovascular disease, depression, and osteoporosis, all of which should be addressed.

**For more information on the care plan and facilitator's guide please visit http://www.mhpharmacotherapy.com.**

# 65 Osteoarthritis

Steven M. Smith        John G. Gums

Eric A. Dietrich

## CASE LEARNING OBJECTIVES

- Identify the risk factors associated with osteoarthritis (OA)
- Recognize the signs and symptoms of OA
- Formulate a nonpharmacologic plan for patients with OA
- Recommend a pharmacologic plan for patients with OA that considers individual patient factors
- Develop monitoring parameters to assess the effectiveness and adverse effects of pharmacotherapy for OA
- Deliver effective disease-state counseling, including lifestyle modifications and drug therapy, to facilitate effective and safe management of OA

## PATIENT PRESENTATION

### Chief Complaint

"My knees are starting to hurt more and more every time I climb stairs. I also fell last week at work because my right knee gave out."

### History of Present Illness

Bryce Johnson is a 68-year-old white male who presents to his primary care physician complaining of increasing bilateral knee pain over the past 4 months with recent joint instability, most notably in the right knee. His knee pain is frequently associated with climbing stairs. He also reports knee stiffness on waking, which lasts approximately 15–20 minutes and abates with ambulation. He has not previously sought care for his knee pain. On "bad" days, he reports taking acetaminophen 1,000 mg 2–3 times daily. Although this dose is generally inadequate to fully alleviate his pain, he is concerned about taking larger doses because of the recent news coverage of acetaminophen-induced liver toxicity. He has also been trying to lose weight using an over-the-counter product containing orlistat. He reports poor compliance with this medication due to diarrhea on numerous occasions. Lastly, he requests your advice on taking a product that a family member recommended, called Cosamin DS. He has been told that it prevents joint breakdown and is safer than painkillers.

### Past Medical History

Hypertension × 7 years

Hyperlipidemia × 5 years

Insomnia × 8 months

Diabetes mellitus type 2 × 4 years

Obesity

### Family History

Father died of MI at age 49.

### Social/Work History

Retired, former packaging plant floor manager for a mail-order company. Currently, a part-time volunteer for a local political campaign. Divorced; has 2 children, aged 35 and 37.

### Tobacco/Alcohol/Substance Use

Social drinker; (−) tobacco; 10 pack-year history, quit 18 years ago; (−) illicit drug use

### Allergy/Intolerance/Adverse Event History

NKDA

### Medications (Current)

Indapamide 2.5 mg PO once daily

Lisinopril 20 mg PO twice daily

Metformin/sitagliptin 1,000/50 mg PO twice daily

Rosuvastatin 10 mg PO once daily

Orlistat 60 mg PO 3 times daily with meals

Zolpidem 10 mg PO once daily at bedtime

Acetaminophen 1,000 mg PO q 8 h PRN pain

Os-Cal 500+D (calcium carbonate 500 mg/vitamin D 400 IU) PO q 12 h

Aspirin 81 mg PO once daily

Pantoprazole 40 mg PO once daily

## Review of Systems

Knee pain (right > left) and right knee instability, most noticeable on climbing stairs; decreased quadriceps and hamstring strength in right leg; impaired range of motion due to knee pain; (–) hip and right ankle pain; (–) joint swelling; (–) joint tenderness. Negative for fever. Self-monitored blood glucose averages in the 130–160s mg/dL (~7–9.5 mmol/L) on most days of the week; no visual disturbances. Five-pound (2.3 kg) weight loss in previous 4 weeks

## Physical Examination

### ▶ General

Pleasant, obese, elderly, white male in no acute distress

### ▶ Vital Signs

BP 122/80 mm Hg, P 76, RR 14, T 36.6°C (97.9°F)

Weight 268 lb (121.8 kg), BMI 37.4 kg/m$^2$, 5 lb (2.3 kg) weight loss in last 4 weeks

Height 71 in. (180.3 cm)

(+) Pain, 5/10

### ▶ Skin

Large bruise on lateral aspect of the right thigh; (–) lesions or rash

### ▶ HEENT

PERRL, EOMI; TMs normal appearing

### ▶ Chest

Clear to auscultation

### ▶ Cardiovascular

RRR, normal $S_1$, $S_2$; (–) $S_3$ or $S_4$; (–) shortness of breath

### ▶ Abdomen

Obese, soft, nontender, nondistended; (–) organomegaly; (+) bowel sounds

### ▶ Neurology

Grossly intact; deep tendon reflexes equal bilaterally; muscle strength 4/5 on extension and flexion of right and left knees, 5/5 for upper extremities; muscle tone normal; slight gait impairment secondary to knee pain; no focal deficits

### ▶ Extremities

Range of motion in left knee limited by pain; (–) hip, ankle pain; (–) swelling; (–) tenderness; (–) heat

## Laboratory Tests

### Fasting

|  | Conventional Units | SI Units |
| --- | --- | --- |
| Na | 144 mEq/L | 144 mmol/L |
| K | 5 mEq/L | 5 mmol/L |
| Cl | 105 mEq/L | 105 mmol/L |
| $CO_2$ | 26 mEq/L | 26 mmol/L |
| Ca | 8.9 mg/dL | 2.23 mmol/L |
| Mg | 2.1 mEq/L | 1.05 mmol/L |
| Phosphate | 3.5 mg/dL | 1.13 mmol/L |
| SCr | 1.1 mg/dL | 97 μmol/L |
| BUN | 9 mg/dL | 3.2 mmol/L |
| Glu | 113 mg/dL | 6.3 mmol/L |
| $A_{1c}$ | 6.6% | 0.066; 49 mmol/mol Hgb |
| CK | 41.4 IU/L | 0.69 μkat/L |
| Hgb | 12.8 g/dL | 128 g/L; 7.94 mmol/L |
| Hct | 44.3% | 0.443 |
| WBC | 8.4 × 10$^3$/mm$^3$ | 8.4 × 10$^9$/L |
| Albumin | 3.4 g/dL | 34 g/L |
| AST | 34 IU/L | 0.57 μkat/L |
| ALT | 37 IU/L | 0.62 μkat/L |
| Total cholesterol | 184 mg/dL | 4.76 mmol/L |
| LDL cholesterol | 116 mg/dL | 3.00 mmol/L |
| HDL cholesterol | 39 mg/dL | 1.01 mmol/L |
| Triglycerides | 145 mg/dL | 1.64 mmol/L |
| Uric acid | 6.1 mg/dL | 363 μmol/L |

## Assessment

Sixty-eight-year-old obese male with signs and symptoms consistent with OA of the knee (Figure 65-1).

### Student Workup

#### Missing Information?

**Evaluate:**   Patient Database

Drug Therapy Problems

Care Plan (by Problem)

**FIGURE 65-1.** Osteoarthritis of the knee. (Reproduced, with permission, from Usatine RP, Smith MA, Mayeaux Jr EJ, Chumley H, Tysinger J. The Color Atlas of Family Medicine. New York, McGraw-Hill, 2009, Fig 91-3.)

## TARGETED QUESTIONS

1. What signs and symptoms of OA does this patient have?

   *Hint: See p. 1043 in PPP*

2. What are the first-line treatment options for OA?

   *Hint: See pp. 1043–1048 in PPP and Figure 58-2*

3. Would this patient be a candidate for a COX-2 selective NSAID?

   *Hint: Consider current gastrointestinal and cardiovascular risk factors and concomitant medications when choosing between a nonselective NSAID and COX-2 selective agent. See pp. 1048–1049 in PPP and Table 58-3*

4. Would you recommend the use of glucosamine/ chondroitin for this patient?

   *Hint: Additional information with regard to allergies may be required before making this recommendation. See p. 1049 in PPP*

5. How would you counsel this patient on the expected benefits and risks of NSAID therapy?

   *Hint: See pp. 1047–1048 in PPP*

## FOLLOW-UP

The patient returns to the clinic after 3 months for routine follow-up. He reports decreased pain, but persistent joint instability in the right knee.

6. What nonpharmacologic strategies would you recommend for this patient to improve joint stability and reduce the risk of further joint deterioration?

   *Hint: See p. 1051 in PPP*

## ⚙ GLOBAL PERSPECTIVE

OA is the most common rheumatic disease worldwide; however, the prevalence of OA varies widely across geographic regions. Prevalence rates in Europe approximate those in North America and generally do not exceed 10%. In contrast, the prevalence in developing regions can range from 3% to 20%. These differences are probably more closely associated with differences in populations than geographic location because the development of OA is not predicated solely on environmental factors. For example, when compared with North American Caucasians, Asians exhibit higher rates of symptomatic knee OA, but lower rates of hip and hand OA. This finding may be attributable to the higher proportion of rural farmers and hard laborers in many Asian regions than in North America. Thus, the prevalence of OA in any region reflects population differences in age, lifestyle, genetics, and occupational history.

### CASE SUMMARY

- The overall clinical picture is consistent with OA of the right knee.
- Acetaminophen has been only modestly effective in treating his knee pain.
- Nonpharmacologic therapies should reduce further joint damage and improve joint stability.

**For more information on the care plan and facilitator's guide please visit http://www.mhpharmacotherapy.com.**

# 66 Gout and Hyperuricemia

William Joshua Guffey

## CASE LEARNING OBJECTIVES

- Recognize the major risk factors for developing gout
- Identify the goals of therapy for gout
- Select an appropriate drug to provide acute pain relief and reduce serum uric acid concentrations in patients with gout, and outline a plan for monitoring efficacy and toxicity
- Properly educate a patient on appropriate lifestyle modifications to help prevent gouty arthritis attacks

## PATIENT PRESENTATION

### Chief Complaint

"My feet throb when I walk or stand and my big toe is swollen."

### History of Present Illness

John Smith is a 62-year-old Caucasian male who presents to his primary care physician complaining of bilateral foot pain (L > R) and swelling of the first phalanx (hallux) of the left foot (Figure 66-1). The patient describes the pain as a constant throbbing sensation when standing or walking. Initially the patient thought the pain could have been from an ingrown toenail. He became more concerned when his other foot started to hurt and his left big toe started swelling with redness and warmth present. The pain has been present for approximately 2 weeks but has worsened over the past few days. He has tried to alleviate the pain through soaking his feet in a warm bath with Epsom salts, which provided minimal relief. He has no prior history of diabetes, and his fasting blood glucose level 3 months ago was 105 mg/dL (5.8 mmol/L).

### Past Medical History

Atrial fibrillation
HTN
Hyperlipidemia
Depression
Dyspepsia

### Family History

Father had type 2 diabetes mellitus and died from a stroke at age 72; mother is alive at age 82 with hypertension and osteoarthritis

### Social History

Married and lives with his wife of 40 years; has no children; works as a service mechanic at a local automobile dealership

### Tobacco/Alcohol/Substance Use

Drinks 3–4 beers weekly and may consume more in social situations; nonsmoker ×10 years; denies any illicit drug use

### Allergies/Intolerances/Adverse Drug Events

No known drug allergies

### Medications (Current)

Atenolol 50 mg PO daily for hypertension
Hydrochlorothiazide/lisinopril 12.5/20 mg PO daily for hypertension
Omeprazole 20 mg PO q AM
Sertraline 100 mg PO daily
Simvastatin 40 mg PO daily
Extended-release niacin 1,000 mg PO q hs
Warfarin 5 mg PO q PM
Ibuprofen 200 mg PO q 4–6 h PRN

**FIGURE 66-1.** Typical inflammatory changes of gout at first metatarsal phalangeal joint. (Adapted, with permission, from Usatine RP, Smith MA, Mayeaux Jr EJ, Chumley H, Tysinger J. The Color Atlas of Family Medicine. New York, McGraw-Hill, 2009, Fig 94-3.)

## Review of Systems

Frequent headaches relieved with over-the-counter pain reliever; denies any recent chest pain, shortness of breath, abdominal pain, unusual bruising or bleeding, or changes in bladder or bowel habits

## Physical Examination

### ▶ General

Obese, middle-aged, Caucasian male in acute distress

### ▶ Vital Signs

BP 140/84 mm Hg, P 99, RR 20, T 37.1°C, SpO$_2$ 98% (0.98)

Weight 276 lb (125.5 kg)

Height 73 in. (185.4 cm)

Reports pain score of 8/10

### ▶ Skin

Warm and dry to touch; (+) erythema and swelling of left foot

### ▶ HEENT

PERRLA, EOMI; (−) sinus tenderness; TMs appear normal

### ▶ Neck and Lymph Nodes

Unremarkable

### ▶ Chest

Clear to auscultation

### ▶ Breasts

Examination deferred

### ▶ Cardiovascular

RRR, normal S$_1$, S$_2$; (−) S$_3$ or S$_4$

### ▶ Abdomen

Obese; soft, nontender/nondistended; (−) organomegaly

### ▶ Neurology

Alert and oriented × 3; cranial nerves II to XII grossly intact; deep tendon reflexes normal

### ▶ Genitourinary

Examination deferred

### ▶ Rectal

Examination deferred

## Laboratory Tests

### Fasting Obtained Today

|  | Conventional Units | SI Units |
|---|---|---|
| Na | 136 mEq/L | 136 mmol/L |
| K | 4.9 mEq/L | 4.9 mmol/L |
| Cl | 97 mEq/L | 97 mmol/L |
| CO$_2$ | 27 mEq/L | 27 mmol/L |
| BUN | 15 mg/dL | 5.4 mmol/L |
| SCr | 1.1 mg/dL | 97 μmol/L |
| Glu | 109 mg/dL | 6 mmol/L |
| Ca | 9.7 mg/dL | 2.43 mmol/L |
| Uric acid | 10.9 mg/dL | 648 μmol/L |
| Hgb | 13.8 g/dL | 138 g/L; 8.57 mmol/L |
| Hct | 39.9% | 0.399 |
| RBC | 4.17 × 10$^6$/μL | 4.17 × 10$^{12}$/L |
| Platelets | 277 × 10$^3$/μL | 277 × 10$^9$/L |
| Westergren ESR | 26 mm/h | 7.2 μm/s |
| MCV | 95 μm$^3$ | 95 fL |
| WBC | 8.8 × 10$^3$/μL | 8.8 × 10$^9$/L |
| Neutrophils | 82% | 0.82 |
| Lymphocytes | 6% | 0.06 |
| Monocytes | 10% | 0.10 |
| Eosinophils | 1% | 0.01 |
| Basophils | 1% | 0.01 |
| Bands | 0% | 0 |
| INR | 2.8 | |
| Total cholesterol | 158 mg/dL | 4.09 mmol/L |
| LDL cholesterol | 66 mg/dL | 1.71 mmol/L |
| HDL cholesterol | 36 mg/dL | 0.93 mmol/L |
| Triglycerides | 280 mg/dL | 3.16 mmol/L |

## Assessment

Sixty-two-year-old man with signs, symptoms, and laboratory tests consistent with gout

### Student Workup

**Missing Information?**

**Evaluate:**    Patient Database

Drug Therapy Problems

Care Plan (by Problem)

## TARGETED QUESTIONS

1. What signs and symptoms of gout does the patient have?
   *Hint: See p. 1056 in PPP*

2. What risk factors for the development of gout are present in the patient?
   *Hint: See pp. 1055–1056 in PPP*

3. What are the possible treatment options in most patients suffering from an acute gout attack?
   *Hint: See pp. 1057–1058 in PPP*

4. What risks and adverse effects of therapy would you discuss with the patient?
   *Hint: See pp. 1061–1062 in PPP*

5. What lifestyle modification patient education points should be discussed with the patient regarding the prevention of future gout attacks?
   *Hint: See pp. 1058–1059 in PPP*

## FOLLOW-UP

Six months later, the patient returns to the clinic with an elevated uric acid level and recurrent acute gout attack.

6. What risks would persistent hyperuricemia and recurrent gout attacks pose to the patient?
   *Hint: See p. 1056 in PPP*

7. What would be an appropriate maintenance regimen for the prophylaxis of future gout attacks?
   *Hint: See pp. 1058–1061 in PPP*

8. What risks and adverse effects of therapy would you discuss with the patient?
   *Hint: See pp. 1061–1062 in PPP*

9. What would be an appropriate monitoring plan for the selected maintenance regimen?
   *Hint: See pp. 1061–1062 in PPP*

## ☼ GLOBAL PERSPECTIVE

Gout is the most common form of inflammatory arthritis in the United States and western Europe. It is a condition caused by an abnormality of uric acid metabolism, resulting in hyperuricemia. The findings from the Rochester Epidemiology Project have estimated the annual incidence of gout in the United States as 62 cases per 100,000 people. Over the past decade, the prevalence of gout in the United States has significantly increased due to several factors, including changes in diet, increased use of medications associated with the development of gout, increased rates of hypertension, dyslipidemias, metabolic syndrome, diabetes, and renal impairment, and an increase in the overall population life expectancy. Until recent years, there have been few new developments in therapeutic options for the management of gout. Despite the availability of these new options, these therapies are reserved only for those unresponsive to traditional treatments and can be costly to those who receive them.[1,2] To help decrease the incidence of gout and hyperuricemia, it is important for health care professionals to educate patients at risk for developing gout on the signs and symptoms of gout, potential drug interactions, and therapeutic lifestyle changes, including weight reduction and avoidance of foods high in purine content.

## REFERENCES

1. Weaver AL. Epidemiology of gout. Cleve Clin J Med 2008 75:S9–S12.
2. Neogi T. Gout. N Engl J Med 2011 364:443–452.

## CASE SUMMARY

- His current clinical picture is consistent with an acute gout attack, and appropriate pain management therapy should be initiated.

- Colchicine would be a reasonable initial therapy for this patient with a dose of 1.2 mg PO immediately followed by 0.6 mg PO 1 h later (1.8 mg/day) and then 0.6 mg PO 1–2 times daily until 24 h after gout attack has subsided.[2] The patient should be educated on appropriate use and potential gastrointestinal side effects.

- Lifestyle modifications, including weight reduction and avoidance of substances with high purine content, should also be implemented.

- Maintenance therapy may not be indicated at this time since this is not a recurrent attack and there is no known evidence of joint destruction or tophi present.

For more information on the care plan and facilitator's guide please visit http://www.mhpharmacotherapy.com.

# 67 Glaucoma

Jon P. Wietholter

## CASE LEARNING OBJECTIVES

- List the goals of treatment for patients with primary open-angle glaucoma
- Choose the most appropriate therapy using patient-specific data for open-angle glaucoma
- Develop a monitoring plan for patients on specific pharmacologic regimens
- Counsel patients about glaucoma, drug therapy options, ophthalmic administration techniques, and the importance of adherence to the prescribed regimen

## PATIENT PRESENTATION

### Chief Complaint

"My eyes are hurting and I feel like my vision is worsening. It has been worsening over the last few months and, now that I'm in the hospital, I'd like to have my eyes examined."

### History of Present Illness

Carrie Kindred is a 52-year-old female who was admitted to the hospital 6 days ago for suspected community-acquired pneumonia (CAP). She had complained of a progressively worsening cough with increased sputum production and a tough time catching her breath on admission. These symptoms have improved drastically and are no longer a concern for this patient. While doing the initial review of systems with the patient, the physician who admitted her to the hospital asked her about any other problems she was currently experiencing. The only other problem she described was a dull, aching pain in her eyes and a subjective feeling that she needs new glasses or contacts as her vision seems to be worsening and becoming blurrier every day. When asked about this vision loss, she claims to be less able to see things to her sides and that her peripheral vision seems to be the main aspect of her vision loss. Additionally, she has noticed that she seems to have blind spots in her visual field that were not there previously.

### Past Medical History

HTN diagnosed at age 43

AF diagnosed at age 47

COPD diagnosed last year

Insomnia, for the last 15 years

### Family History

Father is alive and well with only medical problem being CAD. Mother passed away from breast cancer at age 74. Her mother also had a history of glaucoma and type 2 DM. Three younger siblings have no medical issues, except for her brother who has type 2 DM and HTN.

### Social History

Works as a receptionist at a local dentist's office. Married for 30 years and lives with her husband. Has four children, aged 17, 22, 24, and 28.

### Tobacco/Alcohol/Substance Use

Has smoked 2 ppd cigarettes for 25 years. (−) Illicit drug use. Drinks three to five glasses of wine per week (usually a glass of wine with dinner).

### Allergies/Intolerances/Adverse Drug Events

Allergic to sulfamethoxazole/trimethoprim (anaphylaxis) and codeine (hives)

### Medications (Current)

Metoprolol tartrate 50 mg PO twice daily

Amlodipine 5 mg PO daily

Albuterol inhaler two puffs every 4 hours as needed

Tiotropium 18 mcg inhaled daily

Fluticasone/salmeterol 250/50 one inhalation twice daily

Amitriptyline 25 mg PO before bedtime

Warfarin 4 mg PO daily

Ceftriaxone 1,000 mg IV daily (day 6 of 7 for CAP)

Azithromycin 500 mg PO daily (day 6 of 7 for CAP)

## Physical Examination

### ▸ General

Patient in no acute distress. Sitting in bed without complaints other than that she is having trouble reading anything on the television.

### ▸ Vital Signs

BP 125/79 mm Hg, HR 81, RR 17, T 36.9°C, $O_2$ sat: 98% (0.98) on room air

Weight 130 lb (59 kg)

Height 67 in. (170 cm)

### ▸ Skin

Nothing acute; no acute rashes or lesions

### ▸ HEENT

EOMI; PERRLA; open anterior chamber angles noted; optic disc cupping noted; visual field testing reveals a paracentral scotoma; IOP 35 mm Hg (4.7 kPa); TMs appear normal; (−) sinus tenderness; remainder of examination (−)

### ▸ Neck and Lymph Nodes

(−) Examination; no thyroid nodules or lymphadenopathy present

### ▸ Chest

Minor wheezing and rhonchi present on auscultation

### ▸ Breasts

(−) Examination

### ▸ Cardiovascular

Rate irregularly irregular; no discernable regularity in rhythm but rate seems to be in the 80s

### ▸ Abdomen

Nontender; (−) organomegaly

### ▸ Neurology

Grossly intact; deep tendon reflexes normal

### ▸ Genitourinary

Deferred

### ▸ Rectal

Deferred

## Laboratory Tests

### Fasting Obtained with Morning Laboratory Draw at 5 AM

|  | Conventional Units | SI Units |
|---|---|---|
| Sodium | 138 mEq/L | 138 mmol/L |
| Potassium | 4.1 mEq/L | 4.1 mmol/L |
| Chloride | 105 mEq/L | 105 mmol/L |
| $CO_2$ | 24 mEq/L | 24 mmol/L |
| BUN | 8 mg/dL | 2.9 mmol/L |
| SCr | 1 mg/dL | 88 μmol/L |
| Glucose | 101 mg/dL | 5.6 mmol/L |
| Calcium | 8.9 mg/dL | 2.23 mmol/L |
| Magnesium | 2.1 mEq/L | 1.05 mmol/L |
| Phosphate | 3 mg/dL | 0.97 mmol/L |
| Albumin | 4.1 g/dL | 41 g/L |
| INR | 2.4 | |
| Hgb | 14.1 g/dL | 141 g/L; 8.75 mmol/L |
| Hct | 42.4% | 0.424 |
| WBC | $8 \times 10^3/mm^3$ | $8 \times 10^9/L$ |
| Platelets | $230 \times 10^3/mm^3$ | $230 \times 10^9/L$ |
| MCV | 83 μm³ | 83 fL |
| AST | 25 IU/L | 0.42 μkat/L |
| ALT | 27 IU/L | 0.45 μkat/L |
| Total bilirubin | 0.4 mg/dL | 6.8 μmol/L |
| Direct bilirubin | 0.1 mg/dL | 1.7 μmol/L |
| Alkaline phosphatase | 71 IU/L | 1.18 μkat/L |
| Prothrombin time | 23.9 s | |

### Pertinent Diagnostic Tests

Chest x-ray done this morning shows resolving pneumonia.

## Assessment

This is a hospitalized 52-year-old female with signs, symptoms, and physical examination consistent with uncontrolled primary open-angle glaucoma.

### Student Workup

#### Missing Information?

**Evaluate:**   Patient Database

Drug Therapy Problems

Pharmacotherapy Care Plan (by Problem)

Patient Education Needed

## TARGETED QUESTIONS

1. What signs and symptoms of open-angle glaucoma is this patient currently experiencing?

   *Hint: See p. 1081 in PPP*

2. What are the goal(s) of therapy in this patient?

   *Hint: See p. 1082 in PPP*

3. Does this patient have any concomitant disease states that could factor into the selection of a medication to treat her glaucoma and how could that alter your drug selection? Additionally, is this patient on any current medications that could worsen or exacerbate her glaucoma?

   *Hint: Think about what side effects each class of medications used for glaucoma can cause (see pp. 1086–1089 in PPP) and evaluate whether any of those side effects could be detrimental in any of her concomitant disease states contained in her PMH above. Additionally, this patient is on amitriptyline for her insomnia. This medication will have some unwanted anticholinergic side effects that could worsen or exacerbate her glaucoma. See p. 1089 in PPP*

4. What are appropriate first-line treatment options in this patient and what adverse effects should be monitored for with each possible treatment option?

   *Hint: See pp. 1086–1089 and Figure 61-4 in PPP*

5. If this patient was instead experiencing acute angle-closure glaucoma, how would the treatment plan differ from your original suggestions for this patient's primary open-angle glaucoma?

   *Hint: See p. 1083 and 1086 in PPP*

## FOLLOW-UP

Three weeks later, the patient reports to the outpatient clinic affiliated with your hospital for a follow-up appointment. She says that her vision seems to be improving (at least not worsening) since you started her on timolol 0.5% eye drops (1 drop to each eye twice daily). Her complaints at this point in time do not have to do with her eyes, but she claims that she has been really down in the dumps lately and that some days she feels so depressed that she will not leave the house. She also has had more trouble with shortness of breath since the timolol has been started. She is convinced that the timolol has caused all these symptoms.

6. What should you tell the patient in regard to her complaint and what would your therapeutic recommendation be in this patient?

*Hint: Review common adverse effects from ocular β-blocker therapy on p. 1086 in PPP. Additionally, think if there is a patient-counseling point that should be made regarding the administration of her timolol eye drops that could possibly improve her clinical picture and reduce side effects.*

## ☞ GLOBAL PERSPECTIVE

Glaucoma is a disease state that affects people of all races and nationalities. Although many different countries and cultures use medications and procedures similar to what are used in the United States, there are many practitioners around the world that will turn to acupuncture or Chinese herbal remedies to aid in the treatment of both primary open-angle glaucoma and primary angle-closure glaucoma. Traditional Chinese medicine teaches that glaucoma suggests that there is a liver–kidney yin deficiency with liver yang rising. Although this may seem complicated, the practice of traditional Chinese medicine has been around for centuries and can be used to appropriately place acupuncture needles or select the appropriate combination(s) of herbal remedies (e.g., Wen Dan Tang and You Gui Wan) for the clinical scenario.

## CASE SUMMARY

- Patient presentation is consistent with the diagnosis of primary open-angle glaucoma and should be appropriately treated.
- Appropriate first-line treatment options include an ocular β-blocker, a prostaglandin analog (AKA ocular hypotensive lipid), or brimonidine. Selection should be based on numerous factors including cost, concomitant disease states, and the patient's likelihood of compliance.
- Initial follow-up monitoring should take place at 2–4 weeks and adjustment of therapy should be based on improvement in IOP (initial goal is 20% lower than baseline).
- Care should be taken to not miss the diagnosis of acute angle-closure glaucoma as this is a medical emergency and should be surgically treated as soon as possible.

For more information on the care plan and facilitator's guide please visit http://www.mhpharmacotherapy.com.

# 68 Allergic Rhinitis

David A. Apgar

## PATIENT PRESENTATION

### Chief Complaint

"What can you recommend for my itchy, stuffy nose and sneezing?"

### History of Present Illness

Brenda Baresdale is a 27-year-old female who comes into your retail pharmacy seeking advice for the above complaints. Your history reveals the following information. She began having significant nasal allergy symptoms for the first time about 8 years ago after moving to the Southwest (Phoenix, AZ) from the Midwest (Zionsville, IN). Her nose is affected most, but there are some mouth, throat, chest, and even occasional eye symptoms. The congestion in the nasal passages is so bad that usually she can breathe only through her mouth. The nasal symptoms are characterized by watery discharge, sneezing, itch, and severe congestion. Sometimes she has "itchiness" in the roof of the mouth and back of the throat. Sometimes there is cough, which seems to be stimulated by nasal discharge "dripping down" the back of the throat. The cough is usually mild and nonproductive. When her other symptoms are at their worst, there is sometimes a sensation of "chest tightness." Also, sometimes both her eyes become itchy, red, and even have increased tearing. She cannot identify specific triggers for her symptoms other than seasons of the year. Her condition is the worst from about May through July. However, in most years, she also has problems during the period from mid-September through December. Actually, in the last few years, she even noticed symptoms at other times, although less frequently and less severely. When her symptoms start in May and mid-September, they occur only two to three times per week. However, after 2–3 weeks, they

increase in frequency to almost every day. She has horses, and cares for them every weekend, but her symptoms do not seem to be worse at those times. Sometimes her symptoms are worse when she spends a lot of time outdoors. However, she also notices that being in her kitchen can sometimes start her sneezing. She has tried several medications, some of which have helped. She began treating herself 4–5 years ago, with loratadine (Claritin), but that hardly helped at all. Next, she tried diphenhydramine, which did help, and she has continued that medication. The first few days she takes it, she notices sleepiness, but that "wears off" if she continues it for several days. She has tried decongestant nose sprays, usually oxymetazoline, in the past, especially when the stuffy nose was bad. It did help for a while. She continues to use it intermittently. She has tried a neti (or nettie) pot, but finds it messy, hard to use, and not particularly helpful. Because her father uses fluticasone propionate (Flonase), she tried that about 3 years ago. She thought it helped, so she got a prescription for it from her primary care physician (PCP) several years ago. She tries to start using it in early May and during the second week of September before her seasonal symptoms begin. She starts with one spray into each nostril twice a day. Although it still seems to help, she notices some vague "belly" pain and sometimes even loses her appetite. She has paid close attention to this, and thinks that these symptoms occur about 1 hour after using the spray. As a result, she usually uses the spray only once a day, most often at bedtime. With that regimen, the Flonase still helps some, and she hardly notices the stomach symptoms. On further questioning, she admits to skipping some doses of Flonase because she dislikes the bitter aftertaste. A large portion of the dose seems to run down the back of her throat. Also, it smells bad and sometimes even affects her ability to smell normally. The same PCP had her also try an albuterol inhaler for the sensation of chest tightness. She used this during one summer season a few years ago. She says it only made her feel nervous and jittery, but did not really help the chest tightness. Subsequently, her PCP had her try montelukast (Singulair) for the chest tightness. This seemed to work better than the albuterol, and it even seemed to help some of the nasal symptoms. She continues to use montelukast, one tablet daily, during the times when her symptoms are very bothersome. Except for the allergy symptoms specified above and the stomach symptoms that she attributes to the Flonase, she denies having other symptoms. She thinks that she needs more medication or something that will work better to control her symptoms, especially when they get worse.

## Past Medical History

AR × 8 years

UTI about 9 months ago

Acute sinusitis about 2½ years ago

No unusual childhood diseases, no other chronic illnesses, and no history of surgery

## Family History

Mother is alive and well, perimenopausal, but with no chronic diseases. Father is alive and well, with AR and asthma. She has no siblings. She knows nothing about the health status of other, more remote family.

## Social History

She is married, has no children, and is currently a full-time university student. She claims to have a "normal" diet. She has no formal exercise program. She denies being victimized by any type of abuse.

## Tobacco/Alcohol/Substance Use

Denies all tobacco use; drinks alcohol "socially, but not to excess"; denies illicit drug/substance use except for remote (9 years ago) and brief "experimentation" with marijuana.

## Allergies/Intolerances/Adverse Drug Reactions

Albuterol inhaler caused her to feel nervous and jittery.

Amoxicillin (diffuse, itchy, maculopapular skin rash during last few days of a 10-day course when used for sinus infection about 2½ years ago).

Ciprofloxacin (moderate-to-severe myalgias [both arms and shoulders] starting the last day of a 3-day course and continuing for 3 more days, about 9 months ago when used for treatment of a urine infection).

Fluticasone propionate (Flonase) seems to cause abdominal discomfort, and it tastes and smells bad, as mentioned in the HPI.

## Medications (Current)

Diphenhydramine 50-mg capsule PO up to 3 times a day PRN allergy symptoms

Montelukast 10 mg tablet PO once daily, but only PRN for sensation of chest tightness

Fluticasone propionate nasal solution—1 spray into both nostrils once or sometimes twice daily, at least during the time of her worst seasonal symptoms

Oxymetazoline nasal spray PRN severe nasal congestion

Acetaminophen 500 mg tablets—1–2 tablets PO up to four times daily, only PRN for aches, pains, or headache

Seasonal influenza vaccine (every year in the fall for at least the last 5 years) most recently given about 6 months ago

Denies other medications, including vitamins, dietary supplements, herbs, or other complementary and alternative remedies.

## Review of Systems

Admits to feeling quite tired some days, and has some trouble sleeping, mostly due to nasal congestion. The tiredness causes her to miss some social events associated with school. Although she rarely misses any classes, she often has trouble paying attention and taking notes during lectures.

Denies fever, facial pain, headache, or purulent nasal discharge.

Denies change in hearing, pain in ears, or discharge from ears.

Denies cough, but admits to occasional SOB or wheezing, but only when she has the "tightness in the chest" sensation.

Denies eyelids stuck shut in the mornings, purulent discharge from the eyes, changes in vision, or light sensitivity.

Admits to some abdominal discomfort and even anorexia, especially shortly after using Flonase during the day. Also admits to some heartburn, especially after big meals and sometimes at bedtime.

Denies dysuria, urinary frequency or urgency, and denies, fever, lower abdominal, back/flank pain, or bloody urine.

## Physical Examination

▶ *General*

Well-developed, well-nourished Caucasian female who appears her stated age. Responds appropriately to questions in well-phrased full sentences without breathlessness.

▶ *Vital Signs*

BP (left arm standing) 110/68 mm Hg and (right arm sitting) 114/66 mm Hg; P 64 and regular; RR 14; T 37.4°C

Weight 134.2 lb (61 kg)

Height 65 in. (165.1 cm)

Denies and has no indication of pain at the present time

### ► Skin

No obvious lesions seen with the patient fully clothed.

### ► HEENT

Conjunctivas are slightly injected, but there is no discharge in the eyes, no corneal lesions, and no discharge or matting on the eyelids; PERRLA; EOMI; fundi not examined.

Nasal examination (without instrumentation, except a small flashlight) reveals a somewhat red and swollen-appearing mucosa with some watery nasal discharge.

Deep palpation and/or percussion of the maxillary, frontal, and ethmoid sinuses cause no pain.

Mouth examination reveals normal oral mucosa, good dental hygiene, no malodorous breath, but some evidence of postnasal drip and a mildly irritated posterior oropharynx.

### ► Neck and Lymph Nodes

Neck examination is within normal limits, except for one small (2-mm) nontender, easily movable lymph node in the left submandibular area.

### ► Chest

Patient evaluated while fully clothed; respiratory excursions grossly normal; auscultation through blouse reveals no crackles or wheezes in posterior, lateral, and upper anterior lung fields.

### ► Breasts

Deferred

### ► Cardiovascular

Deferred

### ► Abdomen/Gastrointestinal–Hepatic

Deferred

### ► Neurology

Normal gait; normal facial movements during conversation; normal and appropriate responses to questions; remaining detail deferred.

### ► Extremities

No deformities evident; apparent full range of motion of all four limbs; no clubbing, cyanosis, or edema; radial and dorsalis pedis pulses normal bilaterally.

### ► Genitourinary

Deferred

### ► Rectal

Deferred

## Laboratory Tests

The patient has the following printout of *fasting* laboratory results from her last (and annual) visit with her PCP, about 2 months ago.

| | Conventional Units | SI Units |
|---|---|---|
| Na | 145 mEq/L | 145 mmol/L |
| K | 4.3 mEq/L | 4.3 mmol/L |
| Cl | 102 mEq/L | 102 mmol/L |
| $CO_2$ | 27 mEq/L | 27 mmol/L |
| BUN | 8 mg/dL | 2.9 mmol/L |
| SCr | 0.8 mg/dL | 71 µmol/L |
| Glu | 94 mg/dL | 5.2 mmol/L |
| Ca | 9.7 mg/dL | 2.43 mmol/L |
| Mg | 1.8 mEq/L | 0.90 mmol/L |
| Phosphate | 4.1 mg/dL | 1.32 mmol/L |
| Urinalysis | | |
| pH | 5.0 | |
| Specific gravity | 1.015 | |
| Protein | (–) | |
| Glucose | (–) | |
| Ketones | (–) | |
| RBC | None seen | |
| WBC | 0–2/hpf | |
| Nitrite | (–) | |
| Hgb | 13.2 g/dL | 132 g/L; 8.19 mmol/L |
| Hct | 40% | 0.40 |
| MCV | 87 µm$^3$ | 87 fL |
| Platelets | $230 \times 10^3$/mm$^3$ | $230 \times 10^9$/L |
| WBC | $6.2 \times 10^3$/mm$^3$ | $6.2 \times 10^9$/L |
| Total cholesterol | 157 mg/dL | 4.06 mmol/L |
| LDL cholesterol | 95 mg/dL | 2.46 mmol/L |
| HDL cholesterol | 52 mg/dL | 1.34 mmol/L |
| Albumin | 4.1 g/dL | 41 g/L |
| Alanine aminotransferase (ALT) | 32 IU/L | 0.53 µkat/L |
| Aspartate aminotransferase (AST) | 37 IU/L | 0.62 µkat/L |
| Alkaline phosphatase | 73 IU/L | 1.22 µkat/L |
| Bilirubin, total | 0.8 mg/dL | 13.7 µmol/L |

## Assessment

Twenty-seven-year-old female with AR, which is predominantly seasonal but probably has a perennial component (by traditional classification), and is moderate to severe and persistent by new ARIA (Allergic Rhinitis and its Impact on Asthma) classification, which is not optimally controlled on her current regimen. There may be complicating factors of inadequate adherence, asthma, and GERD. She has a history of UTI and sinusitis.

### Student Workup

**Missing Information?**

**Evaluate:**  Patient Database

Drug Therapy Problems

Care Plan (by Problem)

## TARGETED QUESTIONS

1. What additional information do you want to optimize your recommendations?

   *Hint: See Table 63-3 in PPP for allergen avoidance information*

2. What categories of medications are available to improve the control of her AR?

   *Hint: See Table 63-4 in PPP*

3. What categories of medications are most effective for management of the nasal congestion that is associated with AR?

   *Hint: See Table 63-10 in PPP*

4. What specific recommendations can you suggest to optimize her allergic rhinitis?

   *Hint: See Tables 63-5 through 63-9 and the associated text (First-Line Agents on pp. 1113–1116 and Adjunctive or Secondary-Choice Agents on pp. 1116–1119 in PPP)*

5  If your initial recommendations do not help, what alternatives remain?

   *Hint: See the considerations for referral in the Outcome Evaluation text on pp. 1121–1122 and the text on p. 1111 in PPP that relates to concurrence of AR and asthma*

## FOLLOW-UP

The same patient returns 6 months later. She is currently on a new regimen consisting of (1) appropriate use (≤3 days in a row) of intranasal decongestant (oxymetazoline) with supplemental as-needed intranasal antihistamine (olopatadine); (2) oral cetirizine taken as needed (in place of diphenhydramine); (3) mometasone intranasal corticosteroid (in place of fluticasone propionate) taken every day; (4) oral montelukast taken daily during her bad seasons; (5) ketotifen eye drops used as needed only for bloodshot, itchy, and watery eyes; and

(6) implementation of several environmental control measures (weekly laundering of bedclothes, treatment for elimination of cockroaches in her kitchen, and removal of cloth drapes in her bedroom). Her AR is quite well controlled. However, now she asks for a home pregnancy-test kit.

6. How will pregnancy change her symptoms and how might it change her medication regimen?

   *Hint: See text on p. 1120 in the Special Populations section of PPP*

## ☉ GLOBAL PERSPECTIVE

The main difference between AR in the United States compared with other parts of the world is the increasing incidence, especially in many developing countries. This increase is predominantly in the more urbanized regions of those developing countries. There is evidence that "westernization," especially urbanization, increases the risk and prevalence of AR (as well as some other chronic allergic diseases). This phenomenon is usually attributed to the increased air and environmental pollution that is often associated with westernization and industrialization. There may also be some contribution by the increasingly crowded living conditions often associated with urbanization. It is also said that immigrants from a rural area of a developing country may have an increased incidence of AR if they settle in an urbanized, westernized area of a developed country. Again, this is attributable to their being exposed to an increased number and probably amount of new pollutants and allergens. Complicating an evaluation of this is the fact that there is almost certainly an element of underdiagnosis of AR in developing countries. The basic approach to the management of AR is similar around the world. The only differences appear to be variable availability of certain specific medications in some classes of agents.

## CASE SUMMARY

- This patient's condition is mixed seasonal and perennial AR, or as classified by the alternative system, it is moderate-to-severe and persistent AR. By either classification system, her condition is inadequately controlled by her current regimen.

- She has the most common symptoms of AR (runny, itchy nose, sneezing, and nasal congestion [which is often the most bothersome and difficult to treat when it occurs]). She also has other symptoms (some eye symptoms [itchy, red, and watery eyes sometimes]), sleep disturbance, tiredness, "presenteeism" (difficulty taking notes during class lectures), and decreased quality of life (decreased socialization). Finally, she has some chest tightness, sometimes accompanied by SOB and wheezing.

- Several unanswered questions need clarification before an optimal regimen can be suggested. First, the detail of oxymetazoline usage must be determined. Second, a search for other identifiable triggers is appropriate. Third, when caring for any woman of childbearing age, it is always important to get a complete contraception and menstrual history. This may help with decisions concerning therapeutic management of that patient's medical conditions. Although it may be difficult, an attempt should be made to determine whether or not the current diphenhydramine is causing cognitive or performance problems.

- Depending on what is found out about the intranasal decongestant use (above), an intranasal antihistamine may be appropriate.

- A second-generation oral antihistamine should probably replace her diphenhydramine, as she may be having cognitive and performance degradation from the diphenhydramine without being aware of it.

- A replacement intranasal corticosteroid product should be considered to minimize side effects and thus optimize adherence and efficacy.

- Monitoring should consist of tracking the usual three components that apply to monitoring of any chronic medical problem that is treated with medications (i.e., control, compliance, complications). First, monitoring

should consist of keeping careful records of her symptoms (frequency, severity, duration) to establish the efficacy of the new regimen. Second, monitoring should include tracking of any adverse events from any component of her new regimen, especially those that have any negative impact on adherence. Third, the symptoms of any known complications (e.g., sinusitis, otitis media) or other problems known to be associated with AR (asthma) should be monitored.

- Failure of the new regimen should be a consideration for referral to her PCP and possibly to an allergist. The primary benefits of referral include ruling out asthma (and if present, also ruling out GERD), and ruling out sinusitis (because of her history of having at least one episode). If any of these problems are discovered, appropriate management can be implemented. Another possible benefit of referral is identification of specific allergens. If any are identified, it may be possible to improve avoidance techniques and/or possibly facilitate implementation of immunotherapy.

**For more information on the care plan and facilitator's guide please visit http://www.mhpharmacotherapy.com.**

# 69 Conjunctivitis

Michelle L. Hilaire    Jaime R. Hornecker

## CASE LEARNING OBJECTIVES

- Differentiate between the various ophthalmic disorders using patient-specific information
- Choose an appropriate treatment regimen for an ophthalmic disorder
- Discuss the product differences that direct the selection of ophthalmic medications
- Educate patients about ophthalmic disease states and appropriate drug and nondrug therapies

## PATIENT PRESENTATION

### Chief Complaint

"My eyes are so red and watery. It started 2 days ago in my right eye and now my left eye is just as bad. I want to wear sunglasses because the light is making them water more. I hate coming to the office so you know I think it's serious."

### History of Present Illness

Lena Petz is a 53-year-old woman who comes to see her physician because currently both of her eyes are red and watering (Figure 69-1). Two days ago, she noticed that her right eye was irritated and looked a little red, but she just figured that it was because she had been up late the previous night grading projects. She tried a couple drops of Visine but did not notice much difference. Yesterday, she noticed that she had to wipe away a watery discharge from her eye several times during the day. Today when she woke up, her left eye looked the same as the right. She thinks they look redder than yesterday and are watering more and now she is light sensitive. She mentions that a lot of the children in her classes have been coughing and sniffling and having watery eyes recently.

### Past Medical History

Osteopenia diagnosed 1 year ago

Type 2 DM diagnosed 2 years ago

HTN diagnosed 7 years ago

### Family History

Mother has osteoporosis and HTN, and is alive at age 78. Father had lung cancer and died at age 60. She has a brother and a sister, who both have HTN and hyperlipidemia.

### Social History

Married and lives with her husband of 32 years; has no children. Works as an art teacher at a local elementary school. Walks with husband 1 mile 3 days a week for exercise.

### Tobacco/Alcohol/Substance Use

Social drinker (one to two drinks per week)
(–) Tobacco or illicit drug use

### Allergies/Intolerances/Adverse Drug Events

Penicillin (breaks out in hives)

### Medications (Current)

Glucophage 500 mg PO q 12 h

Lisinopril 20 mg PO daily

Calcium carbonate 1,000 mg PO q 12 h

Alendronate 35 mg PO weekly

Vitamin D 1000 international units PO daily

Aspirin 81 mg PO daily

Ibuprofen 200 mg PO PRN headache

### Review of Systems

(+) Eye discharge and tearing in both eyes

(–) Double vision and blind spots

Occasional headaches relieved with nonaspirin pain reliever

### Physical Examination

▶ *General*

Well-developed, well-nourished, middle-aged, Caucasian female in no acute distress. Speech is clear and affect is appropriate.

**FIGURE 69-1.** Viral conjunctivitis. (Adapted, with permission, from Usatine RP, Smith MA, Mayeaux Jr EJ, Chumley H, Tysinger J. The Color Atlas of Family Medicine. New York, McGraw-Hill, 2009, Fig 15-1.)

► **Vital Signs**

BP 128/82 mm Hg, P 72, RR 15 (easy and nonlabored), T 36.9°C

Weight 155 lb (70 kg)

Height 66 in. (167.6 cm)

Denies pain

► **Skin**

Dry-appearing skin and scalp

(−) Rashes or lesions

► **HEENT**

Vision 20/40 in each eye with glasses

Both eyes—conjunctiva red and slightly swollen

PERRLA

EOMI

Ear canals without erythema, swelling, discharge, or cerumen

► **Neck and Lymph Nodes**

Physical examination of neck is unremarkable; (−) thyroid nodules; (−) lymphadenopathy; (−) carotid bruits

► **Chest**

Clear to auscultation bilaterally with no wheezing, rhonchi, or rales

► **Breasts**

Examination deferred

► **Cardiovascular**

RRR

Normal $S_1$, $S_2$

(−) $S_3$ or $S_4$

No murmurs, rubs, or gallops

► **Abdomen**

Nontender/nondistended

(−) Organomegaly

► **Neurology**

Cranial nerves II–XII intact

Deep tendon reflexes normal

No complaints of weakness, numbness, or loss of coordination

► **Genitourinary**

Examination deferred

► **Rectal**

Examination deferred

## Laboratory Tests

### Fasting Obtained 6 Months Ago

|  | Conventional Units | SI Units |
|---|---|---|
| Na | 138 mEq/L | 138 mmol/L |
| K | 4.2 mEq/L | 4.2 mmol/L |
| Cl | 104 mEq/L | 104 mmol/L |
| $CO_2$ | 26 mEq/L | 26 mmol/L |
| BUN | 15 mg/dL | 5.4 mmol/L |
| SCr | 0.68 mg/dL | 60 μmol/L |
| Ca | 9.4 mg/dL | 2.35 mmol/L |
| Mg | 1.6 mEq/L | 0.80 mmol/L |
| Phosphate | 3.1 mg/dL | 1 mmol/L |
| Hgb | 13.1 g/dL | 131 g/L; 8.13 mmol/L |
| Hct | 40.1% | 0.401 |
| WBC | $7.2 \times 10^3/mm^3$ | $7.2 \times 10^9/L$ |
| MCV | $89 mm^3$ | 89 fL |
| Albumin | 4.0 g/dL | 40 g/L |
| Hemoglobin $A_{1c}$ | 7.6% | 0.076; 60 mmol/mol Hgb |
| Glucose | 146 mg/dL | 8.1 mmol/L |
| Total cholesterol | 232 mg/dL | 6.00 mmol/L |
| Triglycerides | 335 mg/dL | 3.79 mmol/L |
| LDL cholesterol | 119 mg/dL | 3.08 mmol/L |
| HDL cholesterol | 46 mg/dL | 1.19 mmol/L |

## Assessment

Fifty-three-year-old woman with signs and symptoms consistent with viral conjunctivitis (pink eye)

### Student Workup

**Missing Information?**

**Evaluate:**   Patient Database

Drug Therapy Problems

Care Plan (by Problem)

## TARGETED QUESTIONS

1. What types of conjunctivitis exist?

   *Hint: See Figure 62-1 in PPP*

2. What is the primary cause of viral conjunctivitis?

   *Hint: See pp. 1096 and 1097 in PPP*

3. What pharmacologic therapy should be used to treat viral conjunctivitis?

   *Hint: See pp. 1097 and 1098 in PPP*

4. When should the patient see significant improvement in the viral conjunctivitis?

   *Hint: See p. 1098 in PPP*

## FOLLOW-UP

Three weeks later, the patient returns for follow-up. Her symptoms have resolved, but she notes that her husband is experiencing similar symptoms.

5. What actions, if any, would you take? What nonpharmacologic measures would you share with the patient?

   *Hint: See p. 1097 in PPP*

## GLOBAL PERSPECTIVE

Conjunctivitis is a worldwide ophthalmic disorder and viral conjunctivitis is one of the most common forms. This condition is very contagious and poses a significant health problem in schools and workplaces where touch contamination is poorly controlled. Poor living conditions can contribute to continuous cases of viral conjunctivitis as household items such as towels and pillows are shared. If the etiology of the conjunctivitis is not clear, the patient should be referred to an eye care practitioner.

## CASE SUMMARY

- Her current clinical picture is consistent with viral conjunctivitis. Although it is self-limiting, the patient needs to observe nonpharmacologic measures to avoid spreading conjunctivitis to others.
- Antibiotic medications should be avoided in viral infections.

For more information on the care plan and facilitator's guide please visit http://www.mhpharmacotherapy.com.

# 70 Psoriasis

Meghan K. Sullivan

## PATIENT PRESENTATION

### Chief Complaint

"I'm so itchy! This stuff just keeps on spreading! I don't know what to do!"

### History of Present Illness

Kathryn Leahy is a 32-year-old female who presents to her primary care provider complaining of severe itching, redness, and a psoriatic flare-up. She was diagnosed with psoriasis 4 years ago, and has experienced sporadic flare-ups during this time, the most recent being 4 months ago. She has been able to control her flare-ups over the years with a variety of creams and lotions. Most recently, she has been using betamethasone 1% cream and calcipotriol 50 mcg/g cream. Although this combination has worked well for her in the past, she is concerned that she is not seeing improvement in her current condition as rapidly as she had previously. The patient is also complaining of being both physically and emotionally drained, and having difficulties sleeping.

### Past Medical History

Psoriasis diagnosed 4 years ago

Melanoma diagnosed 2 years ago

Depression × 2 years

Anxiety × 6 weeks

Prediabetes × 6 months

### Family History

Mother is alive at the age of 62 with type 1 DM, had a psoriatic episode in her late forties but has since been in remission. Father is alive at age 63. He has had two melanoma removed over the past 15 years. She has 1 brother and 1 sister, both of whom are healthy.

### Social History

The patient is a lawyer at a prominent and established law firm, working to make partner in the next eighteen months. She is recently married, and is planning to stop her birth control in the coming months to start a family.

### Tobacco/Alcohol/Substance Use

Social drinker; (–) tobacco or illicit drug use

### Allergies/Intolerances/Adverse Drug Events

Sulfa antibiotics (rash as child)

Codeine (rash postop melanoma)

### Medications (Current)

Alprazolam 1 mg PO PRN anxiety

Betamethasone valerate 1% cream daily PRN treatment of psoriatic plaques

Calcipotriol 50 mcg/g cream daily PRN treatment of psoriatic plaques

Ibuprofen 200 mg and diphenhydramine citrate 38 mg PO PRN sleep

NuvaRing insert vaginally for 3 weeks and remove for 1 week

Sertraline 50 mg PO once daily

### Review of Systems

(+) Depression; (+) test anxiety; (+) difficulty sleeping, relieved with NSAID/antihistamine combination product; (+) multiple skin lesions/plaques, increased in the past 3 weeks; (+) pruritus.

## Physical Examination

### ▶ General

The patient appears to be distressed and depressed about lesions.

### ▶ Vital Signs

BP 104/70 mm Hg, P 72, RR 14, T 36.2°C

Weight 165 lb (75 kg)

Height 68 in. (173 cm)

Denies pain and complains of severe pruritus

### ▶ Skin

Lesions on scalp, chest, back, and elbows (Figure 70-1)

### ▶ HEENT

TMs normal; PERRLA

### ▶ Neck and Lymph Nodes

No masses

### ▶ Chest

Clear lung fields

### ▶ Breasts

Examination deferred

### ▶ Cardiovascular

RRR; no murmurs heard

### ▶ Abdomen

On inspection the abdomen was scaphoid, and without scars or lesions; by auscultation BS were present; palpation and percussion of the abdomen were not done

### ▶ Neurology

Motor strength 5/5 symmetrical

### ▶ Genitourinary

Examination deferred

### ▶ Rectal

Examination deferred

## Laboratory Tests

### Fasting Obtained During Appointment

|  | Conventional Units | SI Units |
|---|---|---|
| Na | 138 mEq/L | 138 mmol/L |
| K | 3.5 mEq/L | 3.5 mmol/L |
| Cl | 100 mEq/L | 100 mmol/L |
| HCO$_3$ | 24 mEq/L | 24 mmol/L |
| BUN | 18 mg/dL | 6.4 mmol/L |
| SCr | 0.9 mg/dL | 80 μmol/L |
| Glu | 115 mg/dL | 6.4 mmol/L |
| Ca | 9.4 mg/dL | 2.35 mmol/L |
| Mg | 1.4 mEq/L | 0.70 mmol/L |
| Phosphate | 3.5 mg/dL | 1.13 mmol/L |
| Hgb | 13.8 g/dL | 138 g/L; 8.57 mmol/L |
| Hematocrit | 40.1% | 0.401 |
| MCV | 88.2 μm$^3$ | 88.2 fL |
| WBC | 6.4 × 10$^3$/mm$^3$ | 6.4 × 10$^9$/L |
| Albumin | 3.8 g/dL | 38 g/L |
| AST | 14 IU/L | 0.23 μkat/L |
| ALT | 10 IU/L | 0.17 μkat/L |
| Total cholesterol | 150 mg/dL | 3.88 mmol/L |
| LDL cholesterol | 80 mg/dL | 2.07 mmol/L |
| HDL cholesterol | 50 mg/dL | 1.29 mmol/L |

**FIGURE 70-1.** Typical plaque psoriasis on elbow and arm. (Adapted, with permission, from Usatine RP, Smith MA, Mayeaux Jr EJ, Chumley H, Tysinger J. The Color Atlas of Family Medicine. New York, McGraw-Hill, 2009, Fig 145-1.)

## Assessment

Thirty-two-year-old female with signs/symptoms consistent with a moderate-to-severe psoriasis exacerbation

### Student Workup

#### Missing Information?

**Evaluate:** Patient Database
Drug Therapy Problems
Care Plan (by Problem)

## TARGETED QUESTIONS

1. What signs and symptoms of moderate-to-severe psoriasis does this patient possess?
   *Hint: See p. 1130 and Table 64-1 in PPP*

2. What risk factors are present that may have influenced the exacerbation of a flare-up?
   *Hint: See p. 1129 in PPP*

3. What nonpharmacologic treatment should be recommended to this patient?
   *Hint: See pp. 1131–1132 in PPP*

4. Why would the addition of systemic therapy be preferred in this patient rather than phototherapy?
   *Hint: See pp. 1134–1137 in PPP*

5. What risks and adverse events should be discussed with this patient in regard to the chosen therapy?
   *Hint: See pp. 1139 and 1140 in PPP*

## FOLLOW-UP

Four weeks later, the patient returns for follow-up. Improvement in her lesions is seen.

6. What actions will you take, if any, to enhance the therapeutic effect of this patient's current therapy? What additional steps will you take to ensure that she enters remission and experiences minimal flare-ups? In the future, what steps will need to be taken if the patient becomes pregnant? What therapeutic options will be available to her?
   *Hint: See p. 1139 in PPP*

## ⟳ GLOBAL PERSPECTIVE

Psoriasis is a common chronic inflammatory disease of the skin that is seen in people throughout the world. Incidence and prevalence of psoriasis continues to be studied on an ongoing basis. It is thought that psoriasis dates back to Biblical times as a common disorder is made mention of in the Bible. Throughout the years, the diagnosis of psoriasis has changed as more is learned about the disease. Several patterns have been identified in studies that have been conducted in patients suffering from psoriasis. However, these findings cannot always be deemed conclusive for the fact that many patients do not seek medical attention for the treatment of psoriasis. Observations that have been made include a greater incidence of psoriasis seen in patients living in regions further from the equator. Studies conducted in Australia show that people residing in southern Australia are more likely to experience psoriasis than those residing in northern Australia. The opposite is true for a study conducted in Norway, helping to prove the theory that those residing close to the equator are less likely to suffer from the disease. In terms of race, Caucasians have been found to have psoriasis more often than those of Asian or African descent. Lifestyle plays a large role in the incidence and prevalence of the disease as well. Individuals living in third-world countries are less likely to have psoriasis in comparison to developed countries where smoking, stress, and obesity are more prominent and have been shown to increase a person's risk for developing the disease.

## CASE SUMMARY

- The patient's current condition can be classified as moderate psoriasis.
- The current flare-up is most likely due to ongoing stress in the patient's life. Stress, depression, anxiety, and trouble sleeping are all culprits of this flare-up. Encouragement of nonpharmacologic stress-reducing activities should be recommended (i.e., hobbies, exercise, relaxation techniques).
- Current treatment with topical therapy is subpar. The addition of a biologic response modifier, alefacept, will be beneficial in this patient. Therapy needs to be monitored closely for side effects, and patient should be educated to notify the prescriber, should she become pregnant.
- Past medical history positive for melanoma is of concern in regard to therapeutic options; UV therapy should not be considered in this patient.

**For more information on the care plan and facilitator's guide please visit http://www.mhpharmacotherapy.com.**

# 71 Acne

Jean E. Cunningham

## CASE LEARNING OBJECTIVES

- Recognize the signs and symptoms of common skin disorders, such as acne, in a presenting patient
- Identify the goals of therapy for acne
- Develop an appropriate treatment and monitoring plan for acne, including nonpharmacologic and pharmacologic agents, on the basis of individual patient characteristics
- Select an appropriate product for acne disorders
- Properly educate a patient using acne treatment options

## PATIENT PRESENTATION

### Chief Complaint

"My son's acne medication is not working!"

### History of Present Illness

Jefferson Roberts is a shy 17-year-old male who is brought into your pharmacy by his mother, Luanne Roberts, complaining that the acne medication prescribed to him is just not working. On further questioning and examination, you find that the patient currently has several papules and pustules on his chin and cheeks, and you also notice a lot of small, depressed pits in the same area along with some excessively dry patches of skin. He has more closed comedones on his cheeks and forehead than open, with the majority of open comedones on his nose. His mother informs you that she watches the patient wash his face three times a day with soap and water, and reminds him constantly that dirty skin leads to "blackheads." The patient's mother admits to buying an "extraction tool" in which she uses to help "clean out the dirt and puss" in the patient's "zits." After looking at the patient's prescription history, you see that he has prescriptions from a local dermatologist. When questioned, you find out from the patient's mother that when he first started "breaking out" he was 13 years old, and tretinoin seemed to help. But in the past year, his acne has only worsened and she was hopeful his skin would further improve once his dermatologist added minocycline. However, she feels that these measures are not enough and wants to know what else they can do to clear up his skin. You hear the patient mumble something about wasting money on the soap that was advertised on television and also sense that he is very uncomfortable talking about his skin disorder.

## Past Medical History

Hospitalized 5 years ago due to a severe upper respiratory infection

## Family History

The patient is the youngest of three and his mother reports no one else in the family having so much trouble with acne.

## Social History

The patient is a varsity swimmer and wants to try out for the US Olympic Water Polo team. He lives at home with his mother and is currently a high school junior. Family recently returned from a skiing vacation in Colorado. He has always been positive and upbeat until a few months ago and has now become more withdrawn and distressed. He works during the summer for his uncle's landscaping company.

## Tobacco/Alcohol/Substance Use

Denies any and all use of tobacco, alcohol, or other substances

## Allergies/Intolerances/Adverse Drug Events

No known allergies

## Medications (Current)

Minocycline 100 mg PO once daily PRN acne

Tretinoin 0.01% gel—apply small amount q hs to clean, dry skin

Salicylic acid face wash—washes face with cleanser three times per day

Over the counter "vitamin for skin health"

## Review of Systems

Painful swelling and redness located on face and reports similar issues with upper back and chest; (+) papules, pustules, open and closed comedones, moderately painful lesions; (+) scarring; (+) dry skin; (+) hyperpigmentation; (−) nodules.

## Physical Examination

▶ *Vital Signs*

Weight 162 lb (74 kg)

Height 75 in. (190 cm)

Admits that swelling and inflammation are bothersome, but mostly embarrassing

▶ *Skin*

Red, flaky, swollen, and irritated skin; (+) papules and pustules on cheeks, chin, back, and chest; (+) closed comedones on cheeks and forehead; (+) open comedones on nose; (+) scarring and lesions; (−) nodules and conglobate (Figure 71-1)

▶ *HEENT*

Wears contacts; also has glasses that he will not wear in public

**FIGURE 71-1.**   Acne with scarring. (Adapted, with permission, from Usatine RP, Smith MA, Mayeaux Jr EJ, Chumley H, Tysinger J. The Color Atlas of Family Medicine. New York, McGraw-Hill, 2009, Fig 106-1.)

---

### Student Workup

#### Missing Information?

**Evaluate:**     Patient Database

Drug Therapy Problems

Care Plan (by Problem)

## Assessment

Seventeen-year-old male with signs, symptoms, and physical examination consistent with moderate acne

## TARGETED QUESTIONS

1. What signs and symptoms of moderate acne does the patient have?

   *Hint: See Table 65-1 in PPP*

2. For what type of acne is benzoyl peroxide the treatment of choice and why?

   *Hint: See pp. 1146–1147 in PPP*

3. What risks and adverse effects of topical and oral therapy would you discuss with the patient?

   *Hint: See Tables 65-2, 65-3, and 65-4 in PPP*

4. What are additional acne therapy options for the patient?

   *Hint: See Figure 65-3 in PPP*

5. Should the patient receive medical treatment for his psychologic distress associated with his acne?

   *Hint: The patient's moderate acne is generally a self-limiting condition that with proper care may reduce the appearance and severity of the acne. Since the patient has no other signs or symptoms of depression besides apparent discomfort and awkwardness, the risk of medications for depressed mood far outweigh the benefit for the time being. It would be reasonable to optimize current acne therapy and reassess the patient for signs of improvement before suggesting additional measures. See p. 1149 in PPP*

## FOLLOW-UP

6. How would your treatment recommendation change if the patient returned in a few weeks presenting with extensive papules, pustules, nodules, and further scarring?

   *Hint: See Figure 65-3 in PPP*

7. What if the patient returns in 8 months with improved skin and only has a few issues with the open and closed comedones?

   *Hint: See Figure 65-3 in PPP*

8. If the patient were to begin isotretinoin capsules 40 mg PO twice daily, what are some considerations/counseling tips you would want to review with him?

   *Hint: See Table 65-4 in PPP*

## ☼ GLOBAL PERSPECTIVE

Acne affects races and skin types differently and may present with different clinical manifestations depending on the affected patient. Although acne is considered the most common disease in the United States, it is also common in other countries, but in different forms. Cystic acne is commonly found in countries such as Spain, Italy, Iran, and other countries in the Mediterranean region. African Americans or people of other ethnicities can also develop a certain type of acne commonly associated with the use of oil or ointment-based hair pomades. Although the primary cause of acne depends on pathogenic factors, additional factors, whether culturally related or not, such as the use of occluding cosmetic and hair products, certain medications, disease states, and items worn directly against skin that obstruct skin pores can worsen acne and should be identified, discussed, and avoided if possible.

## CASE SUMMARY

- His current clinical picture is consistent with moderate papular pustular acne not responding to his current therapy, and alternative treatments should be initiated.

- Alternative pharmacologic therapy for moderate papular pustular acne includes the option to switch the patient to tretinoin (Retin-A Micro) 0.1% gel—apply small amount once daily at bedtime as it may be a less drying option.

- A change in oral antibiotic therapy can be considered depending on the current length of therapy and actual use pattern of the minocycline. Isotretinoin could also be considered based on his symptoms.

- A topical benzoyl peroxide lotion can be recommended over the counter for the patient, since it can further treat the acne. Also, provide a much-needed moisturizer and sunscreen to help decrease his skin redness and irritation.

For more information on the care plan and facilitator's guide please visit http://www.mhpharmacotherapy.com.

# 72 Atopic Dermatitis

Kim W. Benner

## CASE LEARNING OBJECTIVES

- Assess the signs and symptoms of common skin disorders in a presenting patient
- List the goals of treatment for patients with common skin disorders
- Select appropriate nonpharmacologic and pharmacologic treatment regimens to patients presenting with common skin disorders
- Identify the adverse effects that may result from pharmacologic agents used in the treatment of common skin disorders
- Develop a monitoring plan that will assess the safety and efficacy of the overall disease management of common skin disorders

## PATIENT PRESENTATION

### Chief Complaint

"This rash seems to be getting worse and it itches so bad that I cannot sleep at night."

### History of Present Illness

Emily Evan is a 17-year-old female who presents to the dermatologist complaining of a rash on her hands and face that is getting worse. In these areas, the rash appears as pruritic, thickened plaques. A similar rash has recently appeared in the folds of her arms and legs; however, these pruritic areas also include erythematous papules and vesicles. A family friend who is a nurse recommended a nonprescription topical corticosteroid (hydrocortisone). The patient recalls having a similar rash as a child that responded to the hydrocortisone, so she has tried it sporadically over the last several months. In addition, in her childhood, she suffered food allergies to peanuts, eggs, and milk, but eventually outgrew this allergy and can tolerate these foods now. The rash, however, seems to come and go with the seasons and her stress level. She is currently having trouble in school and with her boyfriend; she is also trying to find a college despite her lack of funds and poor grades. She frequently wears tight-fitting clothes, makeup, and perfume.

### Past Medical History

Food allergies to peanuts, eggs, and milk as a young child, now resolved.

Allergic rhinitis since age 6

### Family History

Both parents are alive. Father currently has asthma and mother has a history of allergic rhinitis. She has two younger sisters, one of which has asthma.

### Social/Work History

Currently, she is a "C" student in high school and is not involved in extracurricular activities. She claims to have a boyfriend in college who likes to "spend a lot of time with her." She was employed part-time at a local fast-food restaurant but quit due to decreasing grades and to spend more time with her boyfriend.

### Tobacco/Alcohol/Substance Abuse

Denies any routine use, but does admit to occasional alcohol use when around her friends. Admits her boyfriend smokes constantly.

### Allergies/Intolerances/Adverse Drug Events

None known at this time; seems to tolerate peanuts, eggs, and milk, but seldom eats them due to her childhood allergy

### Medications (Current)

Hydrocortisone acetate cream, applies to rash on arms, hands, face, and legs PRN rash/itch

Fluticasone nasal spray, one spray in each nostril 2 times a day, admits noncompliance

Yasmin 1 PO each day, questionable compliance

## Review of Systems

(+) Dry skin all over. Thick plaques on hands and face. Fossa of legs and arms have erythematous lesions. No complaints of muscle or joint pain. Complains of being tired due to stress of school and boyfriend, and that she is up all night scratching her rash.

## Physical Examination

### ▶ General

Tired and stressed teenager who appears anxious and depressed, yet in no acute distress

### ▶ Vital Signs

BP 104/65 mm Hg, P 72, RR 13, T 36.3°C

Weight 115 lb (52.3 kg)

Height 64 in. (163 cm)

### ▶ Skin

Generally dry all over; (+) thick fibrotic plaques with lichenification on hands and face. Pruritic, erythematous papules and vesicles on antecubital and popliteal fossa of arms and legs (Figure 72-1). She also has markings on her skin due to tight-fitting clothes.

### ▶ HEENT

PERRLA, EOMI, nares moist with mucus; Dennie-Morgan lines present

**FIGURE 72-1.** Severe chronic atopic dermatitis. (Adapted, with permission, from Usatine RP, Smith MA, Mayeaux Jr EJ, Chumley H, Tysinger J. The Color Atlas of Family Medicine. New York, McGraw-Hill, 2009, Fig 139-10.)

### ▶ Neck and Lymph Nodes

Not significant

### ▶ Chest

CTA bilaterally

### ▶ Breasts

Normally developed female teenage breasts; the patient denies performing monthly breast examination.

### ▶ Cardiovascular

RRR; no m/r/g

### ▶ Abdomen

Not tender, not distended; (+) BS; (−) organomegaly

### ▶ Neurology

Grossly intact; A&O × 3; CNs intact

### ▶ Genitourinary

Patient menstruating

### ▶ Rectal

Deferred

## Laboratory Tests

|  | Conventional Units | SI Units |
|---|---|---|
| Na | 141 mEq/L | 141 mmol/L |
| K | 3.8 mEq/L | 3.8 mmol/L |
| Cl | 102 mEq/L | 102 mmol/L |
| $CO_2$ | 24 mEq/L | 24 mmol/L |
| BUN | 10 mg/dL | 3.6 mmol/L |
| SCr | 0.6 mg/dL | 53 mmol/L |
| Glu | 92 mg/dL | 5.1 mmol/L |
| Ca | 9.1 mg/dL | 2.28 mmol/L |
| Mg | 1.9 mEq/L | 0.95 mmol/L |
| Phosphate | 3.6 mg/dL | 1.16 mmol/L |
| Hgb | 11.9 g/dL | 119 g/L; 7.39 mmol/L |
| Hct | 36% | 0.36 |
| WBC | $10.9 \times 10^3/mm^3$ | $10.9 \times 10^9/L$ |
| Eosinophils | 9% | 0.09 |
| MCV | $81 \mu m^3$ | 81 fL |
| IgE | 400 IU/mL | 400 kIU/L |

## Assessment

Seventeen-year-old female with signs and symptoms consistent with atopic dermatitis (AD)

**Missing Information?**

Evaluate:        Patient Database

                 Drug Therapy Problems

                 Care Plan (by Problem)

## TARGETED QUESTIONS

1.  What signs and symptoms of AD does the patient have? Are the lesions acute, subacute, or chronic?

    *Hint: See pp. 1151–1152 in PPP*

2.  What significant findings in EE's history contribute to the development of her AD?

    *Hint: Her history of food allergies, allergic rhinitis and positive family history of asthma all are consistent with atopy and thus development of atopic dermatitis.*

3.  What nonpharmacologic therapy can you recommend for AD?

    *Hint: See p. 1152 in PPP*

4.  Is a topical corticosteroid the treatment of choice for her? If so, what potency of steroid should be utilized?

    *Hint: See Table 65-6 in PPP*

5.  What are the second-line options available for the acute control of AD?

    *Hint: See pp. 1152 and 1154 in PPP*

6.  What adjunct therapy is needed for the more erythematous lesions on her arms and legs?

    *Hint: Skin in AD is often colonized with bacteria.*

## FOLLOW-UP

Three weeks later, the patient returns for a follow-up and states that after using the prescribed initial therapy, her lesions are only moderately improved. She had begun to notice some "skin thinning" and discoloration in the areas of steroid use. She is interested in trying something other than topical steroids.

7.  What therapy is available for long-term maintenance therapy or refractory cases?

    *Hint: See pp. 1153 and 1154 in PPP*

8.  What can you recommend to help decrease the itching and help her sleep?

    *Hint: See p. 1154 and Table 65-7 in PPP*

## ⟲ GLOBAL PERSPECTIVE

Atopic dermatitis is a common skin disorder that is often associated with triggers such as food allergies. The incidence of food allergies can differ around the world due to variations in diets. For example, rice allergies occur more often in Asia where rice is a major component of Asian diet, whereas corn allergies may be more prevalent inside the United States since corn derivatives are commonplace in the US (and Canadian) diet. The most common allergies in many countries include milk, eggs, peanuts, tree nuts, fish, shellfish, soy, wheat, and sesame. Seed allergies, especially sesame, have been reported to be increasing in many countries. The United States has the FDA to mandate appropriate labeling for possible allergens in the food supply; third-world countries may not have safeguards in place for consumers to take note of possible triggers. Often exposure to extreme hot or cold temperature can be a cause of an exacerbation, so inhabitants of such environments worldwide may suffer exacerbations more (or less) often.

## CASE SUMMARY

* Her current skin problem is consistent with AD on her hands and face. Since she is uncontrolled on low-potency corticosteroids (first-line therapy), a stronger cortico steroid may be utilized on the arm and leg lesions. However, due to the patient experiencing intolerable side effects, alternative therapy includes topical calcineurin inhibitors.

* Often nonpharmacologic measures and avoidance of triggers can decrease the severity of AD.

* Bacterial colonization often occurs with chronic lesions and can be exacerbated by the constant scratching. Topical and/or oral antibiotics may be beneficial.

For more information on the care plan and facilitator's guide please visit http://www.mhpharmacotherapy.com.

# 73 Iron Deficiency Anemia

Colleen Clark Dula        Teri L. West

## CASE LEARNING OBJECTIVES

- Identify the common causes of anemia
- Describe the common signs and symptoms of anemia
- Discuss the appropriate diagnostic evaluation to determine the type of anemia and guide therapeutic decisions
- State the desired therapeutic outcomes for patients with anemia
- Compare and contrast the various oral and parenteral iron preparations
- Recommend a specific treatment regimen for anemia considering the underlying cause of anemia and patient-specific variables
- Develop a plan to monitor the outcomes of anemia pharmacotherapy

## PATIENT PRESENTATION

### Chief Complaint

"I'm tired all the time, I just feel exhausted."

### History of Present Illness

Neeraja Singh is a 30-year-old woman who presents to her primary care physician (PCP) complaining of fatigue that has continued to worsen over the past several months. She began an exercise regimen a few months ago after she was told this would help her blood pressure, but has been unable to stick to her routine lately because she has just been too tired and weak. She states that she checks her blood pressure once or twice a week and it usually runs in the 120–130s/80s mm Hg. She follows a traditional Indian diet; vegetables and rice are a large part of her diet and she does not eat meat.

### Past Medical History

GERD

HTN × 1 year

### Family History

Mother deceased at age 52 of breast cancer and father alive at age 65 with HTN and type 2 DM. She has 2 older brothers with HTN, both alive and well.

### Social History

She is married for 2 years and lives with her husband; they currently have no children but would like to begin trying soon. She works full time as a receptionist at a dental clinic.

### Tobacco/Alcohol/Substance Use

Denies alcohol, tobacco, or illicit drug use

### Allergies/Intolerances/Adverse Drug Events

Codeine (stomach upset)

### Medications (Current)

Omeprazole 20 mg PO every morning

Lisinopril 10 mg PO once daily

### Review of Systems

(+) Fatigue; HA around periods; no CP or SOB; 28-day cycles, menses approximately 5–6 days (5 pads/day), LMP 14 days ago; denies any recent episodes of bleeding, including no hematochezia, melena, epistaxis, or hematuria

### Physical Examination

▶ *General*

WDWN Indian woman in NAD, who appears her stated age

▶ *Vital Signs*

BP 134/88 mm Hg, P 80, RR 14, T 37°C

Weight 152 lb (69.1 kg)

Height 61 in. (155 cm)

▶ *Skin*

Dry skin

▶ *HEENT*

PERRLA, EOMI; pale conjunctivas; normal funduscopic examination; no retinopathy; TMs intact; oropharynx clear

▶ *Neck and Lymph Nodes*

No thyromegaly, lymphadenopathy, or JVD

▶ *Chest*

CTA bilaterally

▶ *Breasts*

No masses or discharge

▶ *Cardiovascular*

RRR; normal $S_1$, $S_2$; w/o $S_3$ and $S_4$

▶ *Abdomen*

Normal bowel sounds, soft, not tender/not distended, no masses

▶ *Neurology*

A&O × 3; deep tendon reflexes normal

▶ *Genitourinary*

Examination deferred

▶ *Rectal*

(−) Stool guaiac

## Laboratory Tests

### Obtained Today

|       | Conventional Units       | SI Units        |
| ----- | ------------------------ | --------------- |
| Na    | 135 mEq/L                | 135 mmol/L      |
| K     | 4.2 mEq/L                | 4.2 mmol/L      |
| Cl    | 105 mEq/L                | 105 mmol/L      |
| $CO_2$ | 23 mEq/L                | 23 mmol/L       |
| BUN   | 8 mg/dL                  | 2.9 mmol/L      |
| SCr   | 0.75 mg/dL               | 66 μmol/L       |
| Glu   | 90 mg/dL                 | 5 mmol/L        |
| Ca    | 9 mg/dL                  | 2.25 mmol/L     |
| AST   | 23 IU/L                  | 0.38 μkat/L     |
| ALT   | 20 IU/L                  | 0.33 μkat/L     |

| Albumin  | 4 g/dL                  | 40 g/L                  |
| -------- | ----------------------- | ----------------------- |
| TSH      | 3.76 μIU/mL             | 3.76 mIU/L              |
| Hgb      | 8 g/dL                  | 80 g/L; 4.97 mmol/L     |
| Hct      | 26.3%                   | 0.263                   |
| WBC      | $6.1 \times 10^3/mm^3$  | $6.1 \times 10^9/L$     |
| RBC      | $3.95 \times 10^6/\mu L$ | $3.95 \times 10^{12}/L$ |
| MCV      | $66 \ \mu m^3$          | 66 fL                   |
| MCHC     | 30.6 g/dL               | 306 g/L                 |
| RDW      | 21.7%                   | 0.217                   |
| Iron     | 8 mcg/dL                | 1.4 μmol/L              |
| TIBC     | 493 mcg/dL              | 88.2 μmol/L             |
| TSAT     | 2%                      | 0.02                    |
| Ferritin | 1 ng/mL                 | 1 mcg/L                 |

### *Peripheral Blood Smear*

Microcytic, hypochromic RBCs

## Assessment

Thirty-year-old woman with signs, symptoms, and laboratory tests consistent with iron deficiency anemia

### Student Workup

**Missing Information?**

**Evaluate:**   Patient Database

Drug Therapy Problems

Care Plan (by Problem)

## TARGETED QUESTIONS

1. What signs, symptoms, and laboratory values are consistent with iron deficiency anemia in this patient?
   *Hint: See pp. 1160–1162 and Table 66-2 in PPP*

2. What are the potential causes of iron deficiency anemia?
   *Hint: See pp. 1160–1161 in PPP*

3. What iron replacement treatment options are available for this patient?
   *Hint: See pp. 1163–1165 and Table 66-4 and Table 66-5 in PPP*

4. What risks and adverse effects of therapy would you discuss with this patient?
   *Hint: See pp. 1163–1165 in PPP*

5. Would you recommend a transfusion in this patient? If so why or why not?
   *Hint: See p. 1162 in PPP*

## FOLLOW-UP

The patient tolerates the therapy well, and her Hgb and Hct stabilized over the first few weeks of therapy. At her 6-month follow-up, her laboratory tests showed that her iron stores returned to normal, so her PCP stopped the iron supplement. She was also started on a prenatal vitamin by her OB-GYN as she and her husband were actively trying to conceive.

One year later, the patient returns to your clinic with persistent fatigue and weakness. Her OB-GYN restarted the oral iron supplements 2 months ago suspecting anemia, and laboratory tests confirmed iron deficiency anemia at that time (Hgb 8.8 g/dL [88 g/L; 5.46 mmol/L], Hct 26.3% [0.263], MCV 77 $\mu m^3$ [77 fL], ferritin 4 ng/mL [4 mcg/L]). She informs you today that she is expecting twins and is about 28 weeks along in her pregnancy. She has had significant morning sickness and frequent vomiting throughout her entire pregnancy. She has tried several oral iron supplements, including ferrous sulfate, ferrous gluconate, and an OTC polysaccharide-iron complex. Today's laboratory test results include Hgb 9.1g/dL (91 g/L; 5.65 mmol/L) and Hct 29.7% (0.297).

6. What are the potential reasons that she is not responding to oral iron therapy? What suggestions or changes would you make today?

   *Hint: See pp. 1166–1168 in PPP*

## 🌐 GLOBAL PERSPECTIVE

Iron deficiency anemia is one of the most prevalent micronutrient deficiencies in the world and contributes to the global burden of disease. It has been estimated to affect 2 billion people in the world and is associated with approximately one-fifth of perinatal deaths and approximately one-tenth of maternal deaths in developing countries. In children living with iron deficiency anemia, the disease can lead to retarded physical and mental development. In adults, iron deficiency anemia can reduce aerobic capacity and work productivity of entire populations, resulting in serious economic consequences to a developing nation.

Many people around the world are at a high risk for iron deficiency anemia, including those individuals with blood loss from parasitic infections such as hookworms, ascaris, and schistosomiasis. Others at high risk are individuals with acute or chronic infections of malaria, cancers, tuberculosis, and HIV. Additional precipitators of iron deficiency anemia may include reduced iron intake in the diet. Iron absorption can be further reduced as a result of diets high in nonheme sources, such as plants and supplementation, when combined with foods that inhibit absorption, such as phytates (bran), phenolics (coffee and tea), or calcium (dairy) compounds.

Women are at a high risk for iron deficiency anemia, particularly those who have experienced a pregnancy with multiple babies or more than one pregnancy. Women who are pregnant have higher iron demands due to blood volume expansion and subsequent increases in RBCs and Hgb production, and growth of the fetus, placenta, and maternal tissues. During the second and third trimester, there is a threefold increase in the demand for iron. Unlike many countries in the world, iron deficiency anemia in the United States has declined over the past decade because of the availability of iron-fortified foods, increased iron supplementation, increased vitamin C, and the use of contraception to decrease the incidence of pregnancy.

## CASE SUMMARY

- Her current signs, symptoms, and laboratory values are consistent with iron deficiency anemia, and iron replacement therapy should be initiated.
- Oral iron therapy should be initiated with a total daily dose of 150–200 mg of elemental iron in divided doses.

**For more information on the care plan and facilitator's guide please visit http://www.mhpharmacotherapy.com.**

# 74 Vitamin B$_{12}$ Deficiency

Janice L. Stumpf

## CASE LEARNING OBJECTIVES

- Identify common causes of anemia
- Describe common signs and symptoms of anemia
- Describe diagnostic evaluation required to determine the etiology of anemia
- Explain the optimal use of vitamin B$_{12}$ in patients with macrocytic anemia
- Recommend a treatment regimen for anemia considering the underlying cause and patient-specific variables
- Develop a plan to monitor the outcomes of anemia pharmacotherapy

## PATIENT PRESENTATION

### Chief Complaint

"I think I have another UTI. I've really been tired out recently. It's been busy at work."

### History of Present Illness

Ellie Harbison is a 28-year-old white female who presents to her physician with complaints of increased frequency and pain on urination over the past 2 days. She also notes a lack of energy. For the past 1–2 months, she has begun taking naps in the early evening, after work. In addition, she used to run 5–6 miles each morning, but has stopped recently because her legs feel weak after just a few blocks.

### Past Medical History

History of UTI × 10 years—last 2 years ago

Appendectomy 4 years ago

Gravida 1, para 1

### Family History

Mother with breast cancer, otherwise healthy. Father with HTN. No siblings.

### Social History

Vegan since age 13 years—no meat, poultry, fish, eggs, or dairy products eaten. Married with 18-month old daughter. Manager of a department store.

### Tobacco/Alcohol/Substance Use

Occasional alcohol (one to two glasses of red wine two to three times monthly); no tobacco; no illicit drugs

### Allergies/Intolerances/Adverse Drug Events

Penicillin—rash

### Medications (Current)

Calcium carbonate 650 mg PO once daily, when she remembers

Ibuprofen 400 mg PO PRN menstrual cramps

### Review of Systems

Fatigue; weakness during exercise; sore, tender tongue, making eating difficult; increased frequency and pain with urination × 2 days, but no flank pain or blood in the urine; menstrual cramps relieved with ibuprofen; dry skin; fingernails break easily

### Physical Examination

▶ *General*

Petite, thin, white female who appears pale and somewhat uncomfortable

▶ *Vital Signs*

BP 110/65 mm Hg, P 90, RR 16, T 38.2°C (100.8°F)

Weight 103 lb (46.8 kg)

Height 63 in. (160 cm)

Acute genitourinary pain only

▶ **Skin**

Pale, dry skin noted

▶ **HEENT**

PERRLA; glossitis: tongue smooth and red

▶ **Neck and Lymph Nodes**

Thyroid normal size; no lymphadenopathy noted

▶ **Chest**

Clear to auscultation

▶ **Breasts**

Normal breast examination

▶ **Cardiovascular**

RRR; normal $S_1$, $S_2$; (–) $S_3$ or $S_4$

▶ **Abdomen**

Not tender; no distention; no rebound

▶ **Neurology**

Grossly intact; normal deep tendon reflexes and sensory examination; some muscle weakness noted

▶ **Extremities**

Cold extremities; fingernails short and brittle

▶ **Genitourinary**

Normal female genitalia; no vaginal discharge noted

▶ **Rectal**

Examination deferred

## Laboratory and Diagnostic Tests

|  | Conventional Units | SI Units |
|---|---|---|
| Na | 138 mEq/L | 138 mmol/L |
| K | 3.6 mEq/L | 3.6 mmol/L |
| Cl | 110 mEq/L | 110 mmol/L |
| $CO_2$ | 22 mEq/L | 22 mmol/L |
| BUN | 9.8 mg/dL | 3.5 mmol/L |
| SCr | 0.6 mg/dL | 53 μmol/L |
| Glu (non-fasting) | 160 mg/dL | 8.9 mmol/L |
| Ca | 9.0 mg/dL | 2.25 mmol/L |
| Phosphate | 3.4 mg/dL | 1.10 mmol/L |
| Albumin | 3.5 g/dL | 35 g/L |
| WBC | $12 \times 10^3/mm^3$ | $12 \times 10^9/L$ |

| Hgb | 10.8 g/dL | 108 g/L; 6.70 mmol/L |
|---|---|---|
| Hct | 31.4% | 0.314 |
| RBC | $3.04 \times 10^6/\mu L$ | $3.04 \times 10^{12}/L$ |
| MCV | 102.2 μm³ | 102.2 fL |
| MCH | 31.8 pg/cell | |
| MCHC | 34.4 g/dL | 344 g/L |
| RDW | 14.5% | 0.145 |
| Plasma folate | 10.6 ng/mL | 24 nmol/L |
| Vitamin $B_{12}$ | 158 pg/mL | 117 pmol/L |

Urinalysis

| Color | Normal | |
|---|---|---|
| Appearance | Cloudy | |
| pH | 6.4 | |
| Specific gravity | 1.025 | |
| Protein | 100 mg/dL | 1 g/L |
| RBC | 250 erythrocytes/μL | |
| Leukocyte esterase | 25 leukocytes/μL | |
| Nitrite | (+) | |

## Urine Gram Stain and Culture

$>10^5$ CFU/mL ($>10^8$ CFU/L) Gram-negative rods; identification and susceptibilities pending

## Assessment

Pleasant, febrile 28-year-old vegan female with history of urinary tract infections, who presents with symptoms of urinary tract infection as well as complaints of recent fatigue, muscle weakness, and tongue tenderness, likely related to anemia

### Student Workup

**Missing Information?**

**Evaluate:**      Patient Database

Drug Therapy Problems

Care Plan (by Problem)

## TARGETED QUESTIONS

1. With what signs and symptoms of anemia does the patient present?

   *Hint: See p. 1162 and Table 66-2 in PPP*

2. What is the likely etiology of the patient's anemia?

   *Hint: See pp. 1160–1161 and Table 66-3, and Figure 66-3 in PPP*

3. How should the patient's anemia be treated?

   *Hint: See pp. 1166–1167 in PPP*

4. What parameters should be monitored after treatment is initiated?

   *Hint: See pp. 1168 and 1169 in PPP*

## FOLLOW-UP

The patient returns to the clinic 6 months later, happily reporting that she is now 18 weeks pregnant. She continues on a regimen of cyanocobalamin 1,000 mcg intramuscularly once monthly. Her Hgb and Hct levels are within the normal range and she has no symptoms of anemia; however, her serum cyanocobalamin concentration is again low.

5. What may account for the low serum cyanocobalamin concentration?

   *Hint: The patient's pregnancy may be increasing her vitamin B$_{12}$ requirements, leading to early signs of deficiency. In addition, high doses of folic acid can correct the macrocytic anemia associated with vitamin B$_{12}$ deficiency, so she should be questioned regarding the use of folate supplements. However, in light of her adherence to parenteral cyanocobalamin maintenance therapy and lack of clinical symptoms and laboratory measures consistent with anemia, it is unlikely that the patient is again deficient in vitamin B$_{12}$. Instead, low serum vitamin B$_{12}$ concentrations unrelated to anemia have been described during pregnancy. In vitamin B$_{12}$–deficient states, serum methylmalonic acid and homocysteine concentrations will be increased. Results of these determinations may therefore allow differentiation between pregnancy-related decreases in serum cyanocobalamin concentrations and true deficiency. See pp. 1165–1166 in PPP*

## 🌏 GLOBAL PERSPECTIVE

Macrocytic anemia caused by micronutrient deficiencies occurs worldwide in those suffering from malnutrition. Vitamin B$_{12}$ is available from a variety of animal sources, including meat, fish, poultry, eggs, and dairy products; however, populations without ready access to these foods and who instead rely on plant sources for the majority of their calorie intake may develop deficiencies. Malabsorption of vitamin B$_{12}$ is more often the cause of deficiency in advanced nations, in which dietary ingestion is generally sufficient. According to the 2007–2008 National Health and Nutrition Examination Survey (NHANES), the mean intake of vitamin B$_{12}$ for the United States population is 5.2 mcg/d, which is well above the 2.4-mcg recommended daily allowance for adults. Yet vitamin B$_{12}$ deficiency affects between 1.5% and 15% of the United States population. Malabsorption of vitamin B$_{12}$ is especially common in older people due to atrophic gastritis and subsequent reduced levels of gastric acid secretion, but it is also noted following gastric surgical procedures, in those with GI disorders such as Crohn's and celiac disease, and in patients with pernicious anemia. In addition, prolonged acid suppression therapy has been recognized as a cause of decreased vitamin B$_{12}$ absorption, although the clinical significance of this finding is debated.

In addition to macrocytic anemia, permanent neurologic damage may result if vitamin B$_{12}$ deficiency is not corrected. Although cognitive decline has been reported in vitamin B$_{12}$–deficient patients, supplementation in nondeficient patients with dementia or Alzheimer's disease has not improved cognitive function. A link between low vitamin B$_{12}$ concentrations and cardiovascular disease has also been suggested due to the effects of the nutrient on homocysteine metabolism. Elevated homocysteine concentrations are associated with an increased risk of stroke and coronary heart disease and are noted in vitamin B$_{12}$–deficient states. Despite reductions in homocysteine levels following administration of vitamin and mineral supplements that included vitamin B$_{12}$, differences in cardiovascular outcomes following long-term use of vitamin B$_{12}$ have not been documented. To date, data from large clinical trials do not support the use of vitamin B$_{12}$ supplements to protect against cardiovascular events.

## CASE SUMMARY

- The patient's clinical picture is consistent with vitamin B$_{12}$ deficiency anemia resulting from inadequate dietary intake.
- Therapy with vitamin B$_{12}$ should be initiated, with parenteral therapy more reliably correcting the deficiency than oral therapy.
- Clinical symptoms should improve within days of vitamin B$_{12}$ supplementation. A CBC and serum cyanocobalamin concentrations should be obtained in 1 month to evaluate the efficacy of therapy.

For more information on the care plan and facilitator's guide please visit http://www.mhpharmacotherapy.com.

# 75 Folic Acid Deficiency

Janice L. Stumpf

## CASE LEARNING OBJECTIVES

- Identify common causes of anemia
- Describe common signs and symptoms of anemia
- Discuss diagnostic evaluation required to determine the etiology of anemia
- Explain the optimal use of folic acid in patients with macrocytic anemia
- Recommend a specific treatment regimen for anemia considering the underlying cause and patient-specific variables
- Develop a plan to monitor the outcomes of anemia pharmacotherapy

## PATIENT PRESENTATION

### Chief Complaint

"Why am I here? I need to go home now. You can't keep me here."

### History of Present Illness

Charles Logan is a 68-year-old thin, white male brought to the emergency department by paramedics after being found unconscious on the grounds of a local church. He is now awake, but somewhat confused. He appears to be mildly hypothermic and dehydrated. He is known to the ED medical staff as a homeless veteran with a history of schizophrenia and alcoholism.

### Past Medical History

Alcoholism × 45 years

Schizophrenia

Nonadherent with drug therapy

### Family History

Unknown

### Social History

Vietnam veteran. Homeless (long-term). Well known to local social agencies. Sister lives in town; no other family members.

### Tobacco/Alcohol/Substance Use

Currently smokes 1 to 2 ppd × 50 years. Alcohol—up to two-fifths Southern Comfort per day. No illicit drug use reported.

### Allergies/Intolerances/Adverse Drug Events

Reports allergies to all antipsychotic medications—"make him lose control of his mind"

### Medications (Current)

Risperidone 6 mg PO once daily (not adherent)

Calcium carbonate PRN stomach pain

### Review of Systems

Hears voices, usually of his mother. Complains of cold extremities and tingling in his hands and feet. Occasional stomach pains that he relieves with calcium carbonate.

### Physical Examination

#### ▶ General

Thin, pale white male exhibiting some confusion about whereabouts. A&O × 2, to person and time only

#### ▶ Vital Signs

BP 126/76 mm Hg, P 86, RR 18, T 34.4°C (36.6°C after 1 h)

Weight 135.6 lb (61.6 kg)

Height 70 in. (178 cm)

"Fingertips hurt"

#### ▶ Skin

Pale, especially extremities. Dry and thickened, showing signs of exposure to winter temperatures. No obvious signs of frostbite

▶ *HEENT*

PERRLA

▶ *Neck and Lymph Nodes*

Normal

▶ *Chest*

Decreased breath sounds. Slight wheezing

▶ *Cardiovascular*

RRR; normal $S_1$, $S_2$; (–) $S_3$ or $S_4$

▶ *Abdomen*

Not tender; no distention; no rebound

▶ *Neurology*

Deep tendon reflexes intact. Decreased sharp touch sensation in feet and hands

▶ *Extremities*

Cold to touch; palpable pulses

▶ *Genitourinary/Rectal*

Prostate somewhat enlarged

## Laboratory and Diagnostic Tests

|  | Conventional Units | SI Units |
|---|---|---|
| Na | 145 mEq/L | 145 mmol/L |
| K | 3.9 mEq/L | 3.9 mmol/L |
| Cl | 102 mEq/L | 102 mmol/L |
| $CO_2$ | 31 mEq/L | 31 mmol/L |
| BUN | 24 mg/dL | 8.6 mmol/L |
| SCr | 1.5 mg/dL | 133 μmol/L |
| Glu | 80 mg/dL | 4.4 mmol/L |
| Ca | 8.8 mg/dL | 2.20 mmol/L |
| Phosphate | 2.4 mg/dL | 0.78 mmol/L |
| Albumin | 2.8 g/dL | 28 g/L |
| AST | 40 IU/L | 0.67 μkat/L |
| ALT | 60 IU/L | 1 μkat/L |
| Alk phos | 70 IU/L | 1.17 μkat/L |
| Bilirubin | 1.2 mg/dL | 20.5 μmol/L |
| WBC | $9 \times 10^3/mm^3$ | $9 \times 10^9/L$ |
| Hgb | 10.5 g/dL | 105 g/L; 6.52 mmol/L |
| Hct | 30.2% | 0.302 |
| Plt | $154 \times 10^3/\mu L$ | $154 \times 10^9/L$ |
| RBC | $2.97 \times 10^6/\mu L$ | $2.97 \times 10^{12}/L$ |
| MCV | 101.7 μm³ | 101.7 fL |
| MCH | 28.2 pg/cell | |
| MCHC | 34.7 g/dL | 347 g/L |
| RDW | 24% | 0.240 |
| Plasma folate | 2.8 ng/mL | 6.3 nmol/L |
| Vitamin $B_{12}$ | 280 pg/mL | 207 pmol/L |
| Blood alcohol | 120 mg/dL | 26 mmol/L |
| Hemoccult | (–) | |

## Assessment

Confused 68-year-old male with history of schizophrenia and alcoholism, who now presents s/p loss of consciousness with mild hypothermia, dehydration, and anemia

### Student Workup

**Missing Information?**

Evaluate:     Patient Database

Drug Therapy Problems

Care Plan (by Problem)

## TARGETED QUESTIONS

1. What signs and symptoms of anemia does the patient have?

   *Hint: See pp. 1161–1162 and Table 66-2 in PPP*

2. What is the likely cause of the patient's anemia?

   *Hint: See pp. 1160–1161 in PPP*

3. How should the patient's anemia be managed?

   *Hint: See pp. 1165–1166 and Table 66-3 in PPP*

4. How soon after initiating the therapy should the anemia resolve?

   *Hint: See p. 1168 in PPP*

## FOLLOW-UP

The patient is admitted to the hospital and a thorough workup performed to evaluate the cause of his loss of consciousness. A CT scan reveals a recent head injury, and abnormal results are documented on an EEG. The neurologist recommends initiation of phenytoin therapy to prevent seizures.

5. What impact may folic acid supplementation have on the patient's anticonvulsant therapy?

   *Hint: There is a drug interaction between folic acid and phenytoin. Although the mechanism is not well understood, folic acid may decrease serum phenytoin concentrations by 15–50% and may also reduce its therapeutic efficacy. Higher phenytoin doses may therefore be required to achieve therapeutic concentrations. Phenytoin concentrations should be monitored closely during folic acid therapy and after folate supplementation is discontinued and the phenytoin dose adjusted as appropriate. In addition, folic acid concentrations may be decreased following long-term phenytoin administration, perhaps due to effects on absorption. Use of an alternative anticonvulsant for the patient while folic acid supplementation is required should be considered.*

## ☉ GLOBAL PERSPECTIVE

Because folic acid deficiency develops in all populations in which malnutrition is apparent, macrocytic anemia is a global health concern. Anemia affects an estimated 1.62 billion individuals, nearly 25% of the world's population. The primary cause of anemia worldwide is iron deficiency, although mixed anemias resulting from concurrent deficiencies in folic acid and vitamin $B_{12}$ may also be noted.

Because of the association between low folic acid levels during pregnancy and neural tube birth defects, in 1998, the FDA mandated addition of folic acid to many grain products, including bread, pasta, and cereals. Foods in several other countries, including Australia, Canada, and Chile, are also fortified with folic acid. The folate food fortification program as well as increased awareness regarding the need for prenatal folic acid supplementation has reduced the incidence of neural tube defects by 30–50%. Low folate diets have also been associated with an increased risk of breast, pancreatic, and colon cancer. However, folic acid supplementation is not known to prevent particular cancers. In fact, some recent data show that high serum folate concentrations may actually increase the risk of cancer. In addition, low dietary ingestion of folic acid has been associated with an increase in the risk of coronary events, perhaps due to increases in homocysteine concentrations. Homocysteine is an amino acid that, when increased, has been associated with CHD and strokes. Supplementation with folic acid appears to reduce homocysteine levels to normal. Studies are under way to determine if folic acid supplementation reduces the risk of CV events.

## CASE SUMMARY

- The patient's clinical picture is consistent with macrocytic anemia due to folic acid deficiency.
- Therapy with folic acid 1 mg PO daily should be initiated.
- Clinical symptoms should improve within days of initiating folic acid supplementation. CBC and plasma folate concentrations should be obtained in 2 months to assess response to therapy.

**For more information on the care plan and facilitator's guide please visit http://www.mhpharmacotherapy.com.**

# 76 Sickle Cell Disease

Tracy M. Hagemann

## PATIENT PRESENTATION

### Chief Complaint

"I had a mosquito bite on my leg that really bothered me so I scratched it until it got angry looking and now it is all red and swollen. My leg really hurts, and my home pain medications are not helping. My pain is 6 out of 10 right now. I've noticed that I am not going to the bathroom as much as I used to. I really feel lousy."

### History of Present Illness

Jacob Adams is an 18-year-old male with sickle cell disease, who has been admitted to the hospital with cellulitis of the lower right leg, pain and an acute decrease in urine output with a weight gain of 2 kg during the past 2 weeks. He is maintained on a chronic transfusion program secondary to sickle cell related stroke as a child. He claims to be "mostly adherent" to his physician appointments every month, but between school and work, he has missed two appointments within the past 6 months. He states that he takes his medications daily as prescribed and rarely misses doses. He had not taken his pain medication in several months before yesterday. He denies any feelings of dizziness or lightheadedness, but does feel fatigue. He also mentions that prior to admission his urine has been a dark yellow/brown color.

### Past Medical History

Sickle cell anemia (HbSS)

Stroke at age 4 years; walks with a limp on the right side

*Streptoccus pneumoniae* sepsis at age 3 and 12 years

Chronic transfusions monthly × 13 years

Cholecystectomy

### Family History

Father had SCD, died at age 42 from complications of renal failure and myocardial infarction. Mother is alive at age 34 and has SCT, type II diabetes, obesity and history of renal stones. Sister is alive at 22 and has SCT, is pre-diabetic, with a history of renal impairment.

### Social History

He is a junior in high school and works part-time at a local steakhouse where he often eats. Has his own car and drives himself to school and work.

### Tobacco/Alcohol/Substance Use

Social drinker (3–4 beers on weekends only); (–) tobacco or illicit drug use.

### Allergies/Intolerances/Adverse Drug Events

Documented allergy to erythromycin (hives).

### Medications (Current)

Penicillin VK potassium 125 mg PO BID

Hydrocodone/acetaminophen 7.5/500 mg 1 tablet every 6 hours PRN pain

Deferasirox 3.5 g PO daily in the morning before breakfast

Acetaminophen 500 mg PRN

Ibuprofen 600 mg PO every 8 hours PRN

Ranitidine 150 mg PO BID

## Review of Systems

Occasional sickle cell-related pain relieved with acetaminophen and hydrocodone/acetaminophen and ibuprofen. (–) tinnitus, vertigo, dizziness, lightheadedness; (+) fatigue. Slightly yellow sclera.

## Physical Examination

### ▸ General

Well-appearing, muscular, young African American male in some distress

### ▸ Vital Signs

BP 122/69 mm Hg, P 65, RR 18, T 39.5°C, Pain 6/10

Weight 176 lb (79.8 kg)

Height 69 in. (175 cm)

### ▸ HEENT

PERRLA; atraumatic; normocephalic; no lymphadenopathy; Slightly yellow sclera.

### ▸ Chest

Clear to auscultation

### ▸ Cardiovascular

RRR, no m/g/r

### ▸ Abdomen

Not tender/not distended; palpable liver

### ▸ Extremities

Erythematous, excoriated 5 cm area on lower right leg. Area is warm to the touch and painful to patient.

### ▸ Genitourinary

Examination deferred

### ▸ Rectal

Examination deferred

## Laboratory Tests

### Current

|  | Conventional Units | SI Units |
|---|---|---|
| Na | 145 mEq/L | 145 mmol/L |
| K | 4.9 mEq/L | 4.9 mmol/L |
| BUN | 55 mg/dL | 19.6 mmol/L |
| Creatinine | 3 mg/dL | 265 μmol/L |
| AST | 37 IU/L | 0.62 μkat/L |
| ALT | 44 IU/L | 0.73 μkat/L |
| Bilirubin | 1.2 mg/dL | 20.5 μmol/L |
| Hgb | 10.1 g/dL | 101 g/L or 6.26 mmol/L |
| Hct | 34% | 0.34 fraction |
| WBC | 11.5 × 10³/ mm³ | 11.5 × 10⁹/L |
| Serum ferritin | 623 ng/mL | 623 mcg/L |

### Two Months Ago

|  | Conventional Units | SI Units |
|---|---|---|
| Na | 138 mEq/L | 138 mmol/L |
| K | 4.2 mEq/L | 4.2 mmol/L |
| BUN | 17 mg/dL | 6.1 mmol/L |
| Creatinine | 1.1 mg/dL | 97 μmol/L |
| AST | 35 IU/L | 0.58 μkat/L |
| ALT | 46 IU/L | 0.77 μkat/L |
| Alk phos | | |
| Bilirubin | 1.3 mg/dL | 22.2 μmol/L |
| Hgb | 10.8 g/dL | 108 g/L or 6.7 mmol/L |
| Hct | 36% | 0.36 fraction |
| WBC | 9.3 × 10³/ mm³ | 9.3 × 10⁹/L |
| Serum ferritin | 751 ng/mL | 751 mcg/L |

Chest x-ray: Clear with no evidence of acute chest syndrome or infiltrates

## Assessment

Seventeen-year old male with lower extremity cellulitis and acute renal impairment. SCD managed on chronic transfusion therapy with resulting iron overload. He has a history of complications from his SCD.

## Student Workup

### Missing Information?

**Evaluate:**     Patient Database
                  Drug Therapy Problems
                  Care Plan (by Problem)

## TARGETED QUESTIONS

1. What sickle cell-related complications does the patient have?
   *HINT: See pp. 1199–1204 and Table 68-5 in PPP*

2. What modifications should be made to his drug therapy management plans?
   *HINT: See Table 68-3 in PPP*

3. How should the patient's therapeutic plan be monitored?
   *HINT: See p. 1205 and Tables 68-1 68-2 and 68-3 in PPP*

## FOLLOW-UP

Four months later JA has completely recovered from his cellulitis and currently has no reported pain. His BUN and serum creatinine are 22 mg/dL (7.9 mmol/L) and 1.4 mg/dL (124 μmol/L), respectively. Current serum ferritin is 1,050 ng/mL (1050 mcg/L).

4. What changes do you recommend to his medication regimen today?

    *HINT: See pp. 1193–1200 in PPP*

5. When would you recommend re-institution of his chelation therapy and how should the dose be initiated?

    *HINT: See pp. 1198–1199 in PPP*

6. How often should his renal function be monitored?

    *HINT: See Table 68-5 in PPP*

## ☼ GLOBAL PERSPECTIVE

Sickle cell disease is an inherited group of red blood cell disorders that affects millions worldwide and is most common among those whose ancestry includes sub-Saharan Africa, regions in the Western Hemisphere (South America, the Caribbean, and Central America), Saudi Arabia, India, and Mediterranean countries such as Turkey. Because of population migration, SCD is present in most countries. SCD is a significant cause of morbidity and mortality. The World Health Organization estimates that SCD contributes to 5% of the deaths of children younger than 5 years of age in some African countries.[1] Many young adults with SCD are at risk for premature death. Each year more than 300,000 babies with severe forms of SCD are born worldwide, with the majority in low- and middle-income countries. The most cost-effective strategy for reducing the burden of SCD worldwide is to utilize disease management with prevention programs, such as genetic counseling. Barriers include inequitable access to health services, lack of research initiatives, and lack of awareness of the international community of the global burden of SCD and related disorders.

## REFERENCE

1. World Health Organization. http://www.who.int/mediacentre/factsheets/fs308/en/index.html. Accessed April 21, 2013.

## CASE SUMMARY

- The patient needs an antibiotic for treatment of cellulitis. However, he has acute renal impairment, so dose adjustment should be made.

- Because of his acute renal impairment, adjustments to his chelation therapy and other medications are warranted. His dose of deferasirox is more than 40 mg/kg/dose and his ferritin level is near the threshold for chelation, so a temporary cessation of chelation therapy may be considered. Monitoring and follow up to assess and track resolution of renal impairment is crucial, especially as he will need to continue his chronic transfusion program.

- Lifestyle considerations should be evaluated, not just for his SCD but also in light of his renal impairment.

**For more information on the care plan and facilitator's guide please visit http://www.mhpharmacotherapy.com.**

# 77 Bacterial Meningitis

April Miller Quidley    P. Brandon Bookstaver

## CASE LEARNING OBJECTIVES

- Describe the signs, symptoms, and clinical presentation of CNS infections
- List the most common pathogens causing CNS infections, and identify risk factors for infection with each pathogen
- State the goals of therapy for CNS infections
- Design appropriate empiric antimicrobial regimens for patients suspected of having CNS infections caused by any of the following pathogens: *Neisseria meningitidis*, *Haemophilus influenzae*, *Listeria* spp., group B *Streptococcus* spp., Gram-negative bacillary organisms, and herpes simplex encephalitis
- Identify the candidates for vaccines and other prophylactic therapies to prevent CNS infections

## PATIENT PRESENTATION

### Chief Complaint

The patient is currently unresponsive. Her history is from medical records and nursing staff at long-term care facility, who report somnolence and "talking out of her head."

### History of Present Illness

Ruth Johnson is a 67-year-old female resident of a local assisted-living facility, who presents to the ED with a 3-day history of worsening confusion and somnolence. Prior to her delirium, she also complained of headache and stiff neck. None of her friends/contacts at the nursing home have reported any signs or symptoms of illness, but her 10-year-old grandson who visited last week was recently diagnosed with pneumonia. She has a history of seizure disorder and one of her friends reported that she may have had some seizure-like activity yesterday.

### Past Medical History

Type 2 DM diagnosed 1 year ago

Stroke at age 60, no residual neurologic deficits except seizure disorder

Seizure disorder following stroke

Depression diagnosed at age 62 following the death of her husband

### Family History

Father had CAD, deceased from MI at age 72. Mother had diabetes and osteoporosis and died of "old age." She had one brother who was killed in an accident at age 16.

### Social/Work History

The patient moved to assisted-living facility with her husband following stroke at age 60. Staff reports that she is independent in her ADLs, including taking her medications, and is quite active. She has 2 children, aged 45 and 40, and 5 grandchildren. She is a retired homemaker.

### Tobacco/Alcohol/Substance Abuse

Unable to assess due to the patient's mental status; no known tobacco or illicit drug use.

### Allergies/Intolerances/Adverse Event History

Morphine (itching)

### Medications

▶ *Inpatient*

Naloxone 2 mg IV × 1 administered on arrival (no response)

Flumazenil 0.2 mg IV × 1 administered on arrival (no response)

0.9% sodium chloride IV at 125 mL/h

▸ **Home**

Aspirin 81 mg PO daily

Phenytoin ER 300 mg PO at bedtime

Sertraline 50 mg PO daily in the morning

Diphenhydramine 25 mg PO at bedtime

## Review of Systems

Unable to obtain secondary to the patient's condition

## Physical Examination

▸ **General**

Unresponsive, ill-appearing elderly female in acute distress

▸ **Vital Signs**

BP 88/62 mm Hg, P 122, RR 20, T 38.8°C

Weight 140 lb (63.6 kg)

Height 65 in. (165 cm)

Unable to report pain

▸ **Skin**

Reduced skin turgor

▸ **HEENT**

PERRLA; TMs grossly normal

▸ **Neck and Lymph Nodes**

(+) Nuchal rigidity; (−) Kernig's sign; (−) Brudzinski's sign

▸ **Chest**

Clear to auscultation bilaterally

▸ **Breasts**

Examination deferred

▸ **Cardiovascular**

Sinus tachycardia

▸ **Abdomen**

Nontender; nondistended; no organomegaly

▸ **Neurology**

Normal DTRs; (+) corneal, gag, and cough reflexes

▸ **Genitourinary**

Examination deferred

▸ **Rectal**

Examination deferred

## Laboratory and Diagnostic Tests

### Obtained in ED

|  | Conventional Units | SI Units |
|---|---|---|
| Na | 140 mEq/L | 140 mmol/L |
| K | 3.9 mEq/L | 3.9 mmol/L |
| Cl | 100 mEq/L | 100 mmol/L |
| $CO_2$ | 21 mEq/L | 21 mmol/L |
| BUN | 20 mg/dL | 7.1 mmol/L |
| SCr | 1.2 mg/dL | 106 μmol/L |
| Glu | 220 mg/dL | 12.2 mmol/L |
| Ca | 9.6 mg/dL | 2.40 mmol/L |
| Mg | 2 mEq/L | 1 mmol/L |
| Phosphate | 3.5 mg/dL | 1.13 mmol/L |
| Hgb | 12.5 g/dL | 125 g/L; 7.76 mmol/L |
| Hct | 37.5% | 0.375 |
| WBC | $15.7 \times 10^3/mm^3$ | $15.7 \times 10^9/L$ |
| Plt | $220 \times 10^3/mm^3$ | $220 \times 10^9/L$ |
| Albumin | 3.8 g/dL | 38 g/L |
| Phenytoin | 6 mg/L | 24 μmol/L |
| CSF Studies |  |  |
| WBC | $6.3 \times 10^3/mm^3$ | $6.3 \times 10^9/L$ |
| WBC differential |  |  |
| Monos | 12% | 0.12 |
| PMNs | 80% | 0.80 |
| Lymphs | 8% | 0.08 |
| Protein | 120 mg/dL | 1,200 mg/L |
| Glu | 66 mg/dL | 3.7 mmol/L |

## Cultures

*Blood cultures × 2:* Pending

*CSF opening pressure:* 26 mm Hg

*CSF Gram stain:* Gram-positive diplococci

## Radiology

▸ **CT Scan of Head**

No acute abnormalities

## Assessment

Sixty-seven-year-old female with signs, symptoms, and laboratory/diagnostic tests consistent with bacterial meningitis

---

**Student Workup**

**Missing Information?**

Evaluate:    Patient Database

Drug Therapy Problems

Care Plan (by Problem)

## TARGETED QUESTIONS

1. Which symptoms in this patient's history suggest the diagnosis of bacterial meningitis?

   *Hint: See p. 1227 in PPP*

2. What do this patient's CSF findings indicate?

   *Hint: See Table 70-2 in PPP*

3. What in this patient's history may indicate the causative organism of bacterial meningitis?

   *Hint: See Table 70-1 in PPP*

4. Why should empiric antibiotic therapy in bacterial meningitis include broad-spectrum coverage with more than one agent?

   *Hint: See pp. 1228–1229 in PPP*

5. What route(s) of antibiotic administration is (are) appropriate in bacterial meningitis?

   *Hint: See pp. 1228–1229 in PPP*

6. What vaccination(s) should be administered to help prevent invasive *Streptococcus pneumoniae* meningitis?

   *Hint: See p. 1224 in PPP*

## FOLLOW-UP

Twenty-four hours later, CSF cultures return and are positive for *S. pneumoniae*. The patient continues to receive empiric antibiotics (as recommended in your Care Plan).

7. Should your antibiotic regimen be altered? If so, how? Also, what (if any) prophylaxis would you recommend for this patient's contacts?

   *Hint: See p. 1236 and Table 70-3 in PPP*

## ☾ GLOBAL PERSPECTIVE

Worldwide, approximately 1.2 million cases of bacterial meningitis occur annually and result in 135,000 deaths. Vaccination has changed the microbiology and predominant causative organisms in the United States. Both *Haemophilus influenzae* and pneumococcal vaccination have decreased the incidence of infections secondary to these organisms in the United States. Due to limited vaccine availability and cost in developing countries, the incidence of disease secondary to these organisms has not decreased significantly. Likewise, polio and mumps vaccination in the United States has virtually eliminated these organisms as a cause of viral encephalitis. However, these remain important causative agents to consider in developing countries.

## CASE SUMMARY

- The patient's clinical picture is consistent with a severe case of bacterial meningitis. Prompt initiation of broad-spectrum antimicrobial therapy is essential to ensure optimal patient outcomes.

- Initial broad-spectrum therapy should include agents such as a third-generation cephalosporin (ceftriaxone 2 g IV q 12 h), vancomycin dosed to target trough concentrations of 15–20 mg/L (10–14 μmol/L), and ampicillin 2 g IV q 4 h.

- Using culture and susceptibility data, the regimen can be narrowed to target-specific pathogens.

**For more information on the care plan and facilitator's guide please visit http://www.mhpharmacotherapy.com.**

# 78 Community-Acquired Pneumonia

Diane M. Cappelletty      David M. Jacobs

Shelley A. Klochan

## CASE LEARNING OBJECTIVES

- Recognize the signs and symptoms of mild and moderate-to-severe pneumonia
- Identify the goals of therapy for pneumonia
- Develop an appropriate empiric treatment and monitoring plan for pneumonia on the basis of individual patient characteristics
- Properly educate patients taking their antibiotic therapy
- Discuss the role of vaccination in pneumonia

## PATIENT PRESENTATION

### Chief Complaint

"For the last 2 days I have been more and more short of breath, even occurring at rest. I have also been coughing and the color of the secretions is now green."

### History of Present Illness

Cindy Milner is a 65-year-old woman who presents to the emergency department complaining of increasing SOB and increasing coughing. She has had a fever for the last 24 hours. She has some mild-to-moderate chest discomfort, but denies any sharp pains or heaviness in her chest.

### Past Medical History

COPD × 15 years

DM × 20 years

HTN × 10 years

### Family History

Father died in a car accident at age 50. Mother had diabetes, HTN, and CRF, and died at age 56. She has 1 sister who has diabetes and HTN.

### Social History

She lives with her husband and has no children. She works as a legal secretary.

### Tobacco/Alcohol/Substance Use

Social drinker; + tobacco history 1 ppd × 30 years, quit 5 years ago, no illicit drug use

### Allergies/Intolerances/Adverse Drug Events

Penicillin

Sulfamethoxazole

### Medications (Current)

Lisinopril 20 mg PO daily

Insulin glargine 40 units subcutaneous daily

Insulin aspart  subcutaneous sliding scale

Fluticasone/salmeterol DPI 250 mcg/50 mcg 1 inhalation twice daily

Albuterol 1–2 puffs every 4–6 hours as needed for SOB

Acetaminophen 500 mg PO as needed for headache

## Review of Systems

Occasional headaches relieved with acetaminophen; occasional tinnitus; (–) vertigo; (–) history of seizures, syncope, or loss of consciousness; mild pain/discomfort in her chest/abdomen; SOB; (–) nausea, vomiting, or diarrhea.

## Physical Examination

### ► General

Breathing fast, with increased work of breathing, appears in moderate-to severe respiratory distress

### ► Vital Signs

BP 88/58 mm Hg, P 100, RR 30, T 38.8°C, pulse oximetry 89% (0.89) on room air

Weight 223 lb (101.4 kg)

Height 65 in. (165 cm)

### ► Skin

Normal; (–) rashes or lesions

### ► HEENT

PERRLA, EOMI; trace periorbital edema; (–) sinus tenderness; TMs appear normal

### ► Neck and Lymph Nodes

Negative for lymphadenopathy

### ► Chest

Wheezing bilaterally, worse on the left side; decreased breath sounds over the lower left lobe.

### ► Cardiovascular

RRR; normal $S_1$, $S_2$; (–) $S_3$ or $S_4$

### ► Abdomen

Not tender, not distended

### ► Neurology

Grossly intact; deep tendon reflexes normal

### ► Radiologic Studies

Chest x-ray: left lower lobe infiltrate (Figure 78-1)

### ► Sputum Culture

Pending; Gram stain: moderate WBCs, rare squamous epithelial cells, no organisms seen

### ► Blood Culture

Pending

**FIGURE 78-1.** Consolidation in the left lower lobe. (Reproduced, with permission, from Usatine RP, Smith MA, Mayeaux Jr EJ, Chumley H, Tysinger J. The Color Atlas of Family Medicine. New York, McGraw-Hill, 2009, Fig 51-3.)

## Laboratory Tests

|  | Conventional Units | SI Units |
|---|---|---|
| Na | 142 mEq/L | 142 mmol/L |
| K | 4.1 mEq/L | 4.1 mmol/L |
| Cl | 100 mEq/L | 100 mmol/L |
| $CO_2$ | 24 mEq/L | 24 mmol/L |
| BUN | 15 mg/dL | 5.4 mmol/L |
| SCr | 1.4 mg/dL | 124 μmol/L |
| Glu | 308 mg/dL | 17.1 mmol/L |
| Ca | 8.4 mg/dL | 2.10 mmol/L |
| Mg | 1.8 mEq/L | 0.90 mmol/L |
| Phosphate | 4.95 mg/dL | 1.60 mmol/L |
| WBC | $13.4 \times 10^3/mm^3$ | $13.4 \times 10^9/L$ |
| WBC differential |  |  |
| Neutrophils | 72% | 0.72 |
| Lymphocytes | 20% | 0.20 |
| Monocytes | 6% | 0.06 |
| Bands | 2% | 0.02 |
| RBC | $3.6 \times 10^6/mm^3$ | $3.6 \times 10^{12}/L$ |
| Hgb | 11.5 g/dL | 115 g/L; 7.14 mmol/L |
| Hct | 33.9% | 0.339 |

| MCV | 87 μm$^3$ | 87 fL |
| MCH | 28 pg | |
| Platelets | 380 × 10$^3$/mm$^3$ | 380 × 10$^9$/L |

## Assessment

Sixty-five-year-old woman with signs, symptoms, and laboratory tests consistent with severe community-acquired pneumonia

### Student Workup

#### Missing Information?

**Evaluate:**  Patient Database
Drug Therapy Problems
Care Plan (by Problem)

## TARGETED QUESTIONS

1. What signs, symptoms, and diagnostic tests support the diagnosis of pneumonia in the patient?
   *Hint: Please see pp. 1246–1247 in PPP*

2. What are the organisms that most likely cause pneumonia and what resistance issues are associated with these organisms?
   *Hint: Please see p. 1244 in PPP*

3. What patient factors need to be considered prior to selecting an empiric treatment regimen?
   *Hint: Please see pp. 1248–1249 in PPP*

4. What therapeutic regimen would you select (including the duration of therapy)?
   *Hint: Please see pp. 1249–1254 in PPP*

5. How would you monitor the patient?
   *Hint: Please see p. 1254 in PPP*

6. What risks and adverse effects of therapy would you discuss with the patient?
   *Hint: See p. 1254 in PPP*

7. Should the patient be vaccinated, and if so, what vaccinations should she receive?
   *Hint: See pp. 1254–1255 in PPP*

## FOLLOW-UP

8. What would happen to the therapeutic regimen or monitoring for each of the following situations:
   What if the patient had risk factors for pseudomonas or MRSA?
   *Hint: See pp. 1249–1254 in PPP*

   What if the patient's β-lactam allergy was a rash?
   *Hint: See pp. 1249–1254 in PPP*

   What if the patient had a condition that required warfarin therapy?
   *Hint: See pp. 1249–1254 in PPP*

## ⟳ GLOBAL PERSPECTIVE

Viral pneumonia (specifically influenza) is of much greater concern for global spread causing pandemics than is bacterial pneumonia. Not all patients infected with influenza develop pneumonia, but those that do have a greater mortality risk than those without pneumonia. Vaccination against influenza can prevent the disease or minimize symptomatology if the disease is contracted. The polysaccharide vaccine against *Streptococcus pneumoniae* covers 85–90% of the isolates responsible for causing disease in human beings. A conjugated pneumococcal vaccine was recently approved for adults 50 years of age and older, which may provide an improved immune response.

## CASE SUMMARY

- Her clinical picture is consistent with severe community-acquired pneumonia, and antimicrobial and oxygen therapy should be initiated.
- She is allergic to penicillin (anaphylaxis) and sulfa drugs (rash).
- Her age and history of diabetes puts her at increased risk of infection; she should receive the pneumococcal vaccine once and the influenza vaccine yearly.

For more information on the care plan and facilitator's guide please visit http://www.mhpharmacotherapy.com.

# 79 Influenza

Heather L. VandenBussche

## CASE LEARNING OBJECTIVES

- Identify the clinical signs and symptoms associated with influenza
- Develop an appropriate treatment plan for influenza using patient-specific information
- Create a monitoring plan for a patient with influenza using patient-specific information
- Educate patients about influenza and vaccination

## PATIENT PRESENTATION

### Chief Complaint

"My son has a fever, headache, and a cough. I'm worried he might need antibiotics."

### History of Present Illness

Matthew Jackson is a 9-year-old boy who presents with his father to the pediatrician with complaints of fever, headache, and cough for 3 days. He began feeling ill 3 days ago when he developed a fever of 102.6°F (39.2°C) and chills. He has had an intermittent headache for 2 days that is worse when he coughs. His cough is nonproductive and dry. He is more tired than usual and he has not been eating or drinking as much as usual. His fever has been constant over the past 3 days, spiking to 103.5°F (39.7°C) yesterday, but it is responsive to "cold medicine." He also complains of achy muscles in his legs and wants to remain in bed most of the time. His father wants to know if his son needs antibiotic treatment and why Echinacea is not working.

### Past Medical History

Exercise-induced asthma diagnosed 2 years ago

Sinusitis at age 4 and 6 years

Febrile seizure at age 2 years

### Family History

Father's family has strong history of diabetes, heart disease, and lung cancer. Father has HTN and seasonal allergic rhinitis. Mother is deceased but was healthy.

### Social History

The patient lives with father and a 3-year-old sister. Father smokes cigarettes in the house and car. Sister is healthy.

The patient is in fourth grade at private elementary school. No pets at home.

### Allergies/Intolerances/Adverse Drug Events

Amoxicillin—(rash)

### Medications (Current)

Children's Triaminic Multi-Symptom Fever (acetaminophen 160 mg/5 mL; chlorpheniramine 1 mg/5 mL; dextromethorphan 7.5 mg/5 mL) 10 mL q 6 h as needed

*Echinacea purpurea* 180 mg daily

Albuterol MDI one puff as needed

### Review of Systems

(+) Fatigue, fever, headache, chills; (−) rhinorrhea, nasal congestion, sneezing, neck stiffness, or ear pain; (+) intermittent dry cough; (−) difficulty breathing or wheezing; (+) reduced appetite; (−) abdominal pain, vomiting, constipation, or diarrhea; (+) reduction in urinary frequency

### Physical Examination

▶ *General*

Generally well-appearing, mixed-race boy in no acute distress

▶ *Vital Signs*

BP 84/58 mm Hg, P 116, RR 18, T 101.1°F (38.4°C)

Weight 87.8 lb (39.9 kg)

Height 56.7 in. (144 cm)

Pain: 4/10 on numeric scale

▶ *Skin*

No rashes or bruises; 1-cm-long abrasion on left forearm

► *HEENT*

(–) Sinus or facial tenderness; PERRLA, EOMI; (–) conjunctivitis; left TM slightly erythematous, but with landmarks present and no effusion noted; right TM obscured with cerumen; nares patent with moist nasal mucosa; oral mucus membranes moist

► *Neck and Lymph Nodes*

(–) Neck stiffness or pain; neck supple; bilateral shotty anterior cervical lymphadenopathy

► *Chest*

Good air entry bilaterally; (–) crackles or wheezes heard

► *Cardiovascular*

Slightly tachycardic, but regular rhythm, normal $S_1$, $S_2$; (–) $S_3$ or $S_4$

► *Abdomen*

Positive bowel sounds; not tender or distended; (–) organomegaly or masses

► *Neurology*

Grossly intact; deep tendon reflexes normal; no focal deficits noted

► *Extremities*

No swelling or edema noted

► *Genitourinary*

Examination deferred

► *Rectal*

Examination deferred

## Laboratory Tests

Nasopharyngeal swab positive for influenza A virus

## Assessment

Nine-year-old boy with signs and symptoms consistent with influenza

### Student Workup

**Missing Information?**

Evaluate:    Patient Database

                Drug Therapy Problems

                Care Plan (by Problem)

## TARGETED QUESTIONS

1. What signs and symptoms of influenza does this patient have?

   *Hint: Symptoms of influenza are similar to those of the common cold (fatigue, headache, cough, fever), but it is typical to have higher fevers and muscle aches with influenza. See p. 1273 in PPP*

2. What treatments could be considered for this patient?

   *Hint: Symptomatic therapy is recommended. Antiviral therapy is not likely to affect the course of influenza after more than 48 hours of the onset of illness. See pp. 1251, 1274 and Table 72-6 in PPP*

3. What counseling points would you discuss with this patient's father?

   *Hint: Many of the same principles that pertain to the common cold also apply to influenza. See pp. 1274–1276 in PPP*

4. Is this patient a candidate for influenza vaccine?

   *Hint: See pp. 1473–1474 in PPP*

## FOLLOW-UP

5. What if this patient was 3 years old instead of 9 years old?

   *Hint: See pp. 1274–1275, 1474 in PPP*

6. What if this patient had evidence of pneumonia at the time of presentation?

   *Hint: See pp. 1248–1254 in PPP*

7. What if this patient had a severe egg allergy?

   *Hint: See pp. 1472–1473 and Table 86-1 in PPP*

## ☉ GLOBAL PERSPECTIVE

The global impact of influenza on morbidity and mortality is notable with more than 1 million deaths occurring annually. Influenza infection rates peak in cold winter months in temperate climates, but there is a high background rate of infection in tropical climates where epidemics also occur at certain times of the year. Poor outcome is associated with secondary bacterial infections or infection with certain strains of influenza (e.g., the recent H5N1 or avian influenza). Similar to the United States, morbidity and mortality is higher in the age extremes and those with certain chronic illnesses. Vaccination can limit the spread of infection, but it is not as effective in preventing illness in the elderly. Limited resources in developing countries limit the impact of vaccination on the spread of influenza. Educational efforts should focus on hand hygiene, isolation of those who are ill, and other infection control measures where possible.

## CASE SUMMARY

- His current clinical picture is consistent with influenza infection.

- Supportive treatment is recommended for fever or pain; single-ingredient acetaminophen or ibuprofen is an appropriate choice. Other medications are not indicated at this time.

- He is a candidate for influenza vaccination once the acute stage of his illness is over, if he has not had one this year, and it is still influenza season. He should receive injectable influenza vaccine before each influenza season because of his underlying asthma; influenza vaccine is also indicated annually because of his age.

**For more information on the care plan and facilitator's guide please visit http://www.mhpharmacotherapy.com.**

# 80 Upper Respiratory Infection

Heather L. VandenBussche

## CASE LEARNING OBJECTIVES

- Identify the clinical signs and symptoms associated with streptococcal pharyngitis and acute otitis media (AOM)
- List the treatment goals for streptococcal pharyngitis and AOM
- Develop an appropriate treatment plan using patient-specific data
- Create a monitoring plan for a patient with streptococcal pharyngitis and AOM using patient-specific data
- Educate patients about upper respiratory tract infections and proper use of antibiotic therapy

## PATIENT PRESENTATION

### Chief Complaint

"My daughter has a head cold and fever. She needs antibiotics so she can go back to school tomorrow."

### History of Present Illness

Jasmine Henderson is a 5-year-old girl who presents with her mother to the pediatrician with complaints of fatigue, nasal congestion, reduced appetite, fever, and ear and throat pain on swallowing. The patient began feeling tired 4 days ago and developed mild nasal congestion 1 day later. Her mother reports that the patient's appetite has diminished over the past couple of days. She complained of ear and throat pain on swallowing water this morning and she was sent home from school this morning with a fever of 102.4°F (39.1°C). Her mother has been giving her a nonprescription cold medication for the past 2 days, but it has not helped alleviate her symptoms. She is requesting antibiotics so that the patient can return to school tomorrow, and she wants to know what other nonprescription medicines she can give to her to relieve her symptoms.

### Past Medical History

Perennial allergic rhinitis (cat dander, dust mites) diagnosed last year

Mild intermittent asthma diagnosed 2 years ago

Atopic dermatitis diagnosed 6 months ago

Iron-deficiency anemia diagnosed 6 months ago

Prior episodes of otitis media (ages 14 months and 3 years)

Upper respiratory tract infections three to five times each year

### Family History

Father has atopic dermatitis, hypercholesterolemia, and seasonal allergies. Mother has perennial allergic rhinitis and exercise-induced asthma. She has a 7-year-old sister and a 2-year-old brother, who are healthy.

### Social History

Lives with mother, father, sister, and brother. Both parents work outside of the home. Has 2 pets (cat, goldfish). Attends kindergarten at public elementary school. No recent travel.

### Allergies/Intolerances/Adverse Drug Events

Erythromycin—abdominal pain and diarrhea

### Medications (Current)

Loratadine 5 mg PO q 24 h PRN allergy symptoms

Albuterol 2.5 mg solution for nebulization twice daily and q 6 h PRN wheezing

Hydrocortisone 1% ointment once daily to affected area(s)

Children's Tylenol Plus Cold (acetaminophen 160 mg/5 mL; chlorpheniramine 1 mg/5 mL; phenylephrine 2.5 mg/5 mL) 5 mL PO q 6 h PRN

Ferrous sulfate 150 mg/2 mL PO q 12 h

## Review of Systems

(+) Fatigue, fever, headache, nasal congestion, throat and left ear pain; (+) hearing difficulty on left side; (–) conjunctivitis, rhinorrhea, sneezing, neck stiffness, or dizziness; (+) intermittent dry cough; (–) wheezing; (+) abdominal pain and reduced appetite; (–) nausea, vomiting, constipation, or diarrhea; (–) change in urinary frequency; (+) scaly itchy skin on left and right shins.

## Physical Examination

### ▶ General

Ill-appearing and slightly irritable young Caucasian female in no acute distress

### ▶ Vital Signs

BP 90/60 mm Hg, P 120, RR 24, T 101.8°F (38.8°C)

Weight 41.5 lb (18.9 kg)

Height 44.5 in. (113 cm)

Pain score: 6/10 on Faces scale

### ▶ Skin

Slightly pale skin; scaly areas on left and right distal lower extremities; no skin breakdown or discharge

### ▶ HEENT

(–) Sinus or facial tenderness; PERRLA, EOMI; (–) conjunctivitis; (+) erythematous left TM with bulging and limited mobility; (+) fluid behind right TM, but no erythema and normal mobility; (–) otorrhea; (+) inflamed nasal mucosa with no discharge; bilateral tonsillar hypertrophy with erythema and white exudates; foul-smelling breath; mucus membranes moist

### ▶ Neck and Lymph Nodes

(+) Bilateral tender cervical lymphadenopathy; (–) neck stiffness or pain

### ▶ Chest

Mild bilateral expiratory wheezes heard intermittently

### ▶ Cardiovascular

RRR, normal $S_1$, $S_2$; (–) $S_3$ or $S_4$

### ▶ Abdomen

Not tender or distended; (–) organomegaly

### ▶ Neurology

Grossly intact; deep tendon reflexes normal

### ▶ Extremities

No swelling or edema noted

### ▶ Genitourinary

Examination deferred

### ▶ Rectal

Examination deferred

## Laboratory Tests

(+) Rapid streptococcal antigen from throat swab

## Assessment

Five-year-old girl with signs, symptoms, and laboratory tests consistent with streptococcal pharyngitis and AOM

### Student Workup

**Missing Information?**

| Evaluate: | Patient Database |
| | Drug Therapy Problems |
| | Care Plan (by Problem) |

## TARGETED QUESTIONS

1. What signs and symptoms of streptococcal pharyngitis does this patient have?

   *Hint: See p. 1273 in PPP*

2. What signs and symptoms of AOM does this patient have?

   *Hint: See p. 1261 in PPP*

3. Why is amoxicillin the treatment of choice for this patient?

   *Hint: See pp. 1262–1263 and 1271, and Figures 72-1, 72-2, and 72-5, and Tables 72-2 and 72-5 in PPP*

4. What counseling points regarding antibiotic treatment would you discuss with this patient's mother?

   *Hint: See pp. 1265, 1272, and 1273, and Table 72-2 in PPP*

5. What adjunctive treatments could be considered for this patient?

   *Hint: A viral upper respiratory tract infection may have preceded AOM and streptococcal pharyngitis in this patient. Nonprescription medication use should be limited in young children with viral upper respiratory tract infections. See pp. 1263 and 1274 and Figure 72-6 in PPP*

## FOLLOW-UP

Three days later, the patient and her mother return to the pediatrician because the patient developed a rash. It is a pruritic, maculopapular rash on her trunk that is spreading to her groin and upper legs. Reported medication adherence is 100% and her last reported dose of amoxicillin was at 8 AM today. Her throat and ear pain have resolved and she has been afebrile for about 36 hours. However, she has bilateral middle ear effusions present at this time.

6. What actions, if any, would you take?

> *Hint: See pp. 1262–1265, Figure 72-2, and Tables 72-2 and 72-5 in PPP*

## ⟳ GLOBAL PERSPECTIVE

Group A streptococcus is a common contributor to global morbidity and mortality. Developing countries have significantly higher rates of streptococcal pharyngitis, rheumatic fever, heart disease, and poststreptococcal glomerulonephritis that lead to chronic cardiac and renal disease and their associated mortality in children and young adults. Antibiotics may not be readily available in less developed countries to treat infected patients in order to minimize the spread of infection and complications. Educational efforts should focus on reducing transmission of infection and use of secondary prophylaxis for rheumatic fever and heart disease.

AOM is a common childhood infection worldwide with an increased incidence in high-risk populations, such as American and Canadian Indians, Inuit, and aboriginal Australians. Complications such as mastoiditis and hearing impairment are more common in these high-risk groups, in children with lower socioeconomic status or who live in crowded conditions, and in developing countries. Geographic differences in bacterial causes of AOM, microbial resistance patterns, and access to pneumococcal conjugate vaccines can affect treatment choices that are based on likely etiologies of middle ear infections. Watchful waiting may be an appropriate option for most children in the developed world, but it requires access to medical follow-up care. Risk factor reduction is an important educational target for developing countries and other high-risk groups that may lack access to modern medical care.

## CASE SUMMARY

- Her current clinical picture is consistent with streptococcal pharyngitis and AOM, and antibiotic therapy with amoxicillin should be initiated. Amoxicillin is active against *Streptococcus pyogenes, Streptococcus pneumoniae,* and *Haemophilus influenzae.*

- An amoxicillin dose of 800 mg twice daily is reasonable (85 mg/kg/d) for treating AOM potentially caused by penicillin-resistant *S. pneumoniae.*

- Nonprescription medications such as single-ingredient acetaminophen or ibuprofen could be considered for pain and fever control; other nonprescription medications should be discouraged because of a lack of data supporting their safety and efficacy in young children.

**For more information on the care plan and facilitator's guide please visit http://www.mhpharmacotherapy.com.**

# 81 Cellulitis

Christy M. Weiland

## CASE LEARNING OBJECTIVES

- Recognize the signs and symptoms of skin and skin-structure infections
- Understand the significant laboratory and imaging tests that should be performed to assist in the diagnosis and treatment of cellulitis
- Develop an appropriate treatment regimen for cellulitis
- Determine the appropriate monitoring parameters to evaluate therapeutic response to treatment of cellulitis

## PATIENT PRESENTATION

### Chief Complaint

"My leg has been hurting for the last few days and now it is red."

### History of Present Illness

Richard Rogers is a 54-year-old male who presents to his primary care provider complaining of a painful leg that has become red within the last day (Figure 81-1). Last week, he was hiking with his son and they both ended up with multiple lower and upper extremity abrasions secondary to tree brush. The abrasions have mostly healed, but he noticed his left calf became painful 2 days ago and now today it has become erythematous. He is worried that it may be related to a tick since he removed one from his dog the day of the hike. He denies any fever, chills, nausea, or vomiting.

### Past Medical History

Peripheral artery disease (diagnosed 2 years ago)

s/p lower extremity stent (6.5 months ago)

Diastolic heart failure (ejection fraction 60% [0.60] measured 10 months ago)

Hyperlipidemia (diagnosed 10 years ago, last lipid panel 3 years ago)

HTN (diagnosed 13 years ago, controlled on medications)

### Family History

Father deceased at the age of 70 years secondary to an MI. Mother is alive at the age of 82 years with hypothyroidism, HTN, and history of breast cancer. The patient is negative for thrombolic disorders.

### Social/Work History

The patient lives with his wife of 34 years. He has 3 adult children. He works as a lawyer.

### Tobacco/Alcohol/Substance Use

The patient has a "few beers on the weekends." He smokes ½ ppd × 35 years. He denies illicit drug use.

### Allergy/Intolerance/Adverse Event History

Codeine (unknown reaction)

### Medication History

Clopidogrel 75 mg PO daily

Simvastatin 20 mg PO daily

Lisinopril/HCTZ 20/12.5 mg PO daily

Aspirin 81 mg PO daily

Naproxen 550 mg PO every 12 hours PRN pain

### Review of Systems

(−) Fever, chills, nausea, or vomiting. Left calf has reproducible pain and erythema; pain and symptoms have been present for 2 days and lesions occurred last week; decreased perfusion to lower extremities secondary to peripheral artery disease and current smoking.

### Physical Examination

#### ▶ General

Well-nourished, middle-aged, white male who appears in no acute distress

**FIGURE 81-1.**   Cellulitis of leg after minor abrasion. (Adapted, with permission, from Usatine RP, Smith MA, Mayeaux Jr EJ, Chumley H, Tysinger J. The Color Atlas of Family Medicine. New York, McGraw-Hill, 2009, Fig 114-6.)

▶ **Vital Signs**

BP 134/86 mm Hg, P 71 bpm, RR 18, T 38.7°C

Weight 240 lb (109 kg)

Height 72 in. (183 cm)

▶ **Skin**

Intact with healed abrasions noted under extremities; moist

▶ **HEENT**

Moist mucous membranes. Oropharynx is pink and moist. Pupils are equal, round, and reactive to light.

▶ **Chest**

Dull to percussion at the base bilaterally

▶ **Cardiovascular**

RRR; no murmurs, rubs, or gallops

▶ **Abdomen**

Soft, nontender, not distended

▶ **Neurology**

CNs grossly intact; moves all extremities well

▶ **Extremities**

Left calf has some erythema that is slightly tender with touch consistent with a previous lesion. It is slightly warmer than the right calf. He does have a full range of motion. No crepitation, no bulla, no petechia or purpura. Multiple healed abrasions on lower extremities.

▶ **Genitourinary**

Examination deferred

## Laboratory and Other Diagnostic Tests

|  | Conventional Units | SI Units |
|---|---|---|
| Na | 136 mEq/L | 136 mmol/L |
| K | 4.1 mEq/L | 4.1 mmol/L |
| Cl | 103 mEq/L | 103 mmol/L |
| $CO_2$ | 24 mEq/L | 24 mmol/L |
| BUN | 9 mg/dL | 3.2 mmol/L |
| SCr | 0.91 mg/dL | 80 μmol/L |
| Glu | 161 mg/dL | 8.9 mmol/L |
| Hgb | 14.5 g/dL | 145 g/L; 9.00 mmol/L |
| Hct | 43.5% | 0.435 |
| WBC | $13 \times 10^3/mm^3$ | $13 \times 10^9/L$ |
| Bands | 12% | 0.12 |
| Eosinophils | 0% | 0.00 |
| Albumin | 4 g/dL | 40 g/L |
| D-dimer | 175 ng/mL | 175 mcg/L |
| CRP | 26 mg/dL | 260 mg/L |
| Total cholesterol | 180 mg/dL | 4.65 mmol/L |
| LDL | 93 mg/dL | 2.40 mmol/L |
| HDL | 19 mg/dL | 0.49 mmol/L |
| Triglycerides | 130 mg/dL | 1.47 mmol/L |

## Blood Culture

Pending

## Assessment

Fifty-four-year-old male with left lower extremity cellulitis

## TARGETED QUESTIONS

1. What signs, symptoms, and laboratory data support that this patient has an infection?

   *Hint: Infections normally present with a source where organisms can enter the area such as broken skin barriers. Symptoms can present as both localized to the area of infection and systemic, so you would want to consider both. A CRP can be useful in this setting as it is a marker of acute inflammatory changes. CRP will show a rise within 4–6 hours of the onset of inflammation. CRP is very sensitive to inflammation, but has very low specificity. See Table 73-2 in PPP*

2. What laboratory data rule out other possible cause of this patient's symptoms?

   *Hint: With pain specifically in a leg with a patient who is predisposed to a thrombosis process (peripheral artery disease), a DVT should be considered. A plasma D-dimer is a fibrin product generated by the action of plasmin on cross-linked fibrin molecules indicating that a clot has formed. It has a high sensitivity, but low specificity therefore helpful in ruling out disease. The negative D-dimer rules out a DVT.*

3. What disease states does this patient have that predispose and complicate the cellulitis?

*Hint: Peripheral artery disease leads to a decrease in the blood flow and perfusion to the extremities including arms and legs. With decreased blood flow the patient becomes predisposed to infection. Once a patient does have an infection, it makes it more difficult to treat since drug concentrations will be lower due to the decreased blood supply. In addition, smoking delays wound healing, leading to an increase in infection where the skin loses its integrity. See p. 1282 in PPP.*

4. How would you classify this patient's cellulitis?

*Hint: See p. 1282 in PPP*

5. How would this patient benefit from smoking cessation?

*Hint: Smoking decreases the blood flow by constricting arteries. Smoking cessation would not help this infection, but would provide benefit if he has a future infection, which he is at a high risk for secondary to peripheral artery disease. Smoking cessation would also benefit his hyperlipidemia, HTN, and diastolic heart failure. These effects can start to reverse in just 2 months of cessation.*

## FOLLOW-UP

After starting the patient on amoxicillin/clavulanate 875 mg PO every 12 hours for 10 days, 3 days later, the susceptibilities from the culture are received and are as follows:

### Blood Culture Final Result (MRSA recovered from 2/2 bottles)

| Drug | Interpretation | MIC (mcg/mL or mg/L) |
|---|---|---|
| Oxacillin | Resistant | $\geq 4$ |
| Linezolid | Susceptible | 2 |
| Vancomycin | Susceptible | 1 |
| Trimethoprim/ sulfamethoxazole | Susceptible | $\leq 0.5/9.5$ |
| Amoxicillin/clavulanate | Resistant | $\geq 4/2$ |

After talking with the patient, his left leg has not improved, although it does not seem to be getting worse per the patient: the inflammation, temperature, and pain are the same.

6. Is this patient's infection being treated appropriately? Please explain your answer. If this patient is being treated inappropriately, what medication would you recommend on the basis of the new information? How long would the medication be continued for?

*Hint: When organisms are susceptible to many drug therapies, other factors should be taken into consideration, including allergies, simplicity of regimen (i.e., once-a-day vs. four-times-a-day medication), route of administration, side-effect profile of medication, and lastly cost. If an organism is resistant to an antibiotic, the patient should receive the full-recommended duration of therapy with the appropriate antibiotic since the patient was not on the appropriate therapy previously. See pp. 1283–1284 in PPP*

## ⚘ GLOBAL PERSPECTIVE

The organisms associated with cellulitis are consistent across the world, with *S. aureus* being the most common; however, the frequency of cellulitis and the type of *S. aureus* varies for travelers abroad. It has been noted that the second most common diagnosis in returned travelers from international travel with skin problems is soft-tissue bacterial infections including cellulitis.[1] Bacterial skin infections are more common in those returning from sub-Saharan Africa or Southeast Asia, and hot spots identified by the GeoSentinel Network, including Madagascar, Kenya, Philippines, Sri Lanka, South Africa, and Thailand. The tropical conditions, including heat and humidity, make organisms such as MRSA and Pantone–Valentine leukocidin toxin-associated *S. aureus* much more common. Travelers are at increased risk of Pantone–Valentine leukocidin strains of *S. aureus* infections, which are correlated with more severe tissue destruction. It is thought that the increased risk is due to the use of doxycycline that may select for it as well as reduced hygiene

## REFERENCE

1. O'Brien BM. A practical approach to common skin problems in returning travelers. Travel Med Infect Dis 2009 7:125–146.

### CASE SUMMARY

- The patient's clinical presentation is typical for cellulitis with a recent wound, pain at site, and erythema.
- The majority of cellulitis infections are linked to Gram-positive organisms; however, due to comorbidities such as peripheral artery disease and smoking, the infection is at risk for containing Gram-positive and/or Gram-negative organisms.
- Both peripheral artery disease and smoking will delay the healing of lesions by decreasing the blood flow.

**For more information on the care plan and facilitator's guide please visit http://www.mhpharmacotherapy.com.**

# 82 Diabetic Foot Infection

Christy M. Weiland

## CASE LEARNING OBJECTIVES

- Assess the signs and symptoms of diabetic foot infections
- List the goals of treatment for patients with diabetic foot infections
- Select appropriate nonpharmacologic and pharmacologic treatment regimens for patients presenting with diabetic foot infections
- Identify adverse effects that may result from pharmacologic agents used in the treatment of diabetic foot infections
- Develop a monitoring plan that will assess the safety and efficacy of the overall disease management of diabetic foot infections

## PATIENT PRESENTATION

### Chief Complaint

"I cannot handle the pain in my foot anymore, I need a pain medication."

### History of Present Illness

Ted Read is a 34-year-old male with type 1 DM who presents to the emergency department complaining of pain from an ulcer on the sole of his right foot. He reports having an ulcer in the past, but it healed after he borrowed a cream (unknown by the patient) from his friend. He has been using the same cream on this ulcer for the past week with no relief. He works in construction, so he needs to be on his feet all day, and today he could not handle the pain anymore. The ulcer started about 2 weeks ago. He thinks there was a rock in his shoe for an entire work day that started it. The pain has continuously worsened. He reports not regularly checking his feet. He is worried that this will affect his job since he is concerned about getting laid off.

### Past Medical History

Type 1 DM diagnosed at the age 6
History of one foot ulcer reported by the patient

### Family History

Father is alive at age 56 with a history of suicide ideation. Mother is alive at age 54 with a history of hypothyroidism, HTN, and Addison's disease. He has 2 siblings who live locally. Medical history unknown.

### Social/Work History

Single; has a child of age 4 years; works in construction; lately, reports an increase in stress due to concerns of getting laid off.

### Tobacco/Alcohol/Substance Use

He admits to a few beers a night and maybe a little more on the weekends; no illicit drug use; he smokes cigarettes socially.

### Allergy/Intolerance/Adverse Event History

Sulfa: Rash

### Medication History

Insulin glargine injects 32 units subcutaneously at bedtime

Insulin lispro injects insulin according to carbohydrate intake and as needed prior to meals

Acetaminophen as needed

Ibuprofen 400 mg PO as needed for aches and pains

Hydrocodone/acetaminophen 5/500 mg PO as needed (he borrows from a friend occasionally; recently, due to the pain he has borrowed quite a bit)

Cream unknown, borrowed from a friend

### Review of Systems

(+) Occasional pain mostly aches which he takes ibuprofen and acetaminophen for unknown doses. He also borrows hydrocodone/acetaminophen occasionally. Frequency of use has increased as pain has increased. (+) Right foot secondary to ulcer; (+) fever, (−) nausea, vomiting, chills, or SOB.

## Physical Examination

### ▶ General

The patient is a well-nourished individual, who is A&O × 4 and in minimal distress.

### ▶ Vital Signs

BP 132/92 mm Hg, P 84 bpm, RR 16, T 38.9°C

Weight 180 lb (82 kg)

Height 72 in. (183 cm)

Pain 7/10

### ▶ Skin

Moist, cold to touch, intact except right foot as noted below

### ▶ HEENT

Pupils rounds and reactive to light; extraocular muscles intact; no pharyngeal erythema or edema

### ▶ Chest

(−) Chest pain; lungs are clear to auscultation bilaterally without wheezes, rhonchi, or rales

### ▶ Cardiovascular

Regular rate and rhythm without $S_3$, $S_4$, or murmurs

### ▶ Abdomen

Positive bowel sounds, soft, nontender, and nondistended

### ▶ Neurology

CNs II–XII grossly intact; 5/5 muscle strength bilaterally; negative sensation at 4 of 10 touch points with monofilament examination

### ▶ Extremities

No lower extremity edema except around lesion. Extensive ulcer on the heel of the right foot (about 1 in. [2.5 cm] × 2 in. [5.1 cm]). Skin erythematous around the ulcer and spreading 2.5 in. (6.4 cm). Drainage of foul-smelling fluid on pressure. Lesion does not probe to bone.

## Laboratory and Other Diagnostic Tests

|        | Conventional Units | SI Units |
|--------|--------------------|----------|
| Na     | 132 mEq/L          | 132 mmol/L |
| K      | 3.3 mEq/L          | 3.3 mmol/L |
| Cl     | 100 mEq/L          | 100 mmol/L |
| $CO_2$ | 23 mEq/L           | 23 mmol/L |
| BUN    | 20 mg/dL           | 7.1 mmol/L |
| SCr    | 0.9 mg/dL          | 80 μmol/L |
| Glu    | 412 mg/dL          | 22.9 mmol/L |
| Hgb    | 14 g/dL            | 140 g/L; 8.69 mmol/L |
| Hct    | 42%                | 0.42 |
| WBC    | $17 \times 10^3/mm^3$ | $17 \times 10^9/L$ |
| Bands  | 11%                | 0.11 |
| Platelets | $312 \times 10^3/mm^3$ | $312 \times 10^9/L$ |
| Albumin | 3.5 g/dL          | 35 g/L |
| AST    | 45 IU/L            | 0.75 μkat/L |
| ALT    | 33 IU/L            | 0.55 μkat/L |
| CRP    | 12.1 mg/dL         | 121 mg/L |
| $HbA_{1c}$ | 10.2%          | 0.102; 88 mmol/mol Hgb |

## Cultures

*Tissue:* Pending

*Blood × 2:* Pending

## Radiology

Foot x-ray: no evidence of osteomyelitis is seen on the plain x-ray film of the right foot

## Assessment

A 34-year-old male with uncontrolled type 1 DM with an infected foot ulcer

## TARGETED QUESTIONS

1. What signs, symptoms, and laboratory data support the patient's diagnosis of infection?

   *Hint: See pp. 1287 and 1288 in PPP*

2. What is the classification of the patient's diabetic foot infection? Please explain your answer.

   *Hint: See p. 1288 and Table 73-5 in PPP*

3. Once the patient is treated, what are preventative measures that can reduce reoccurrence?

   *Hint: See p. 1288 in PPP*

4. What would be the most appropriate empiric antimicrobial regimen for this patient? Please include dose, route, frequency, and duration. Please explain the rationale.

   *Hint: Anaerobic organisms are commonly malodorous or foul smelling. See pp. 1289–1290 and Table 73-6 in PPP*

## FOLLOW-UP

The patient was initiated on piperacillin/tazobactam and vancomycin. The patient has been afebrile for 48 hours. The foot has decreased erythema. His WBC has decreased to $9 \times 10^3/mm^3$ ($9 \times 10^9/L$) with 3% (0.03) band neutrophils.

Two days later, the following culture and susceptibilities were reported:

- **Blood culture:** Negative (pending)
- **Tissue culture:** *Pseudomonas aeruginosa* from 2 of 2 bottles

| Drug | Interpretation | MIC (mcg/mL or mg/L) |
|------|----------------|----------------------|
| Levofloxacin | Susceptible | ≤2 |
| Ceftazidime | Resistant | 10 |
| Piperacillin/tazobactam | Susceptible | 16/4 |

5. On the basis of the above culture, susceptibilities, and the patient's clinical picture, would changing antibiotic therapy be appropriate? Please explain. If yes, what would be an appropriate therapy, including drug, dose, route, frequency, and duration?

> *Hint: Once the patient is afebrile for 24–48 hours and hemodynamically stable, it is appropriate to change the therapy from intravenous to by mouth. In addition, when able, narrow the spectrum of antibiotic therapy on the basis of the culture and susceptibilities to decrease the incidence of antibiotic resistance and side effects to the patient, including risk of Clostridium difficile.*

## ☉ GLOBAL PERSPECTIVE

Diabetic foot infections are a global burden, resulting in major debilitating complications with severe morbidity and possible amputations across the globe; developing countries as compared to developed countries have additional barriers to overcome. Peripheral neuropathy in populations with type 2 DM tends to be higher in developing countries, which leads to a higher incidence of foot ulcerations. It has been estimated in India to be as high as 27.5%, in Tanzania to be 28.1%, and in Sudan to be 37% of all patients with type 2 DM.[1] One of the most important factors leading to an increase in diabetic foot infections is the lack of proper footwear, which has been noted in most developing countries. Other contributing factors include lack of proper education on diabetes, lack of proper hygiene, lack of health insurance, and cultural beliefs to surgical interventions.[2] In India and many parts of Africa, the sociocultural practice is to walk barefoot; in Africa, it has been estimated that 70% of patients with diabetes have inadequate glycemic control; and in Africa, patients are reluctant to participate in any minor surgical intervention due to cultural beliefs, which is thought to contribute to an increase in mortality of diabetic foot.

## REFERENCES

1. Ramachandra A. Specific problems of the diabetic foot in developing countries. Diabetes Metab Res Rev 2004 20(suppl 1):S19–S22.
2. Lipsky BA, Berendt AR, Cornia PB, et al. Infectious Diseases Society of American Clinical Practice Guideline for the Diagnosis and Treatment of Diabetic Foot Infections. Clin Infect Dis 2012 54:1679–1684.

## CASE SUMMARY

- The patient's clinical presentation was a typical diabetic foot infection consistent with inflamed foot ulceration and elevated blood sugars.
- Diabetic foot infections are generally polymicrobial and require empiric broad-spectrum antibiotics for adequate organism coverage.
- Foot care maintenance, including daily foot inspection, is an essential part of maintaining healthy diabetic feet.

For more information on the care plan and facilitator's guide please visit http://www.mhpharmacotherapy.com.

# 83 Infective Endocarditis

Ronda L. Akins        Katie E. Barber

## CASE LEARNING OBJECTIVES

- Recognize the signs and symptoms of infective endocarditis (IE)
- Understand the pertinent laboratory and imaging tests that should be performed to assist in the diagnosis, treatment, and monitoring of IE
- Identify the initial and long-term goals of therapy for IE
- Develop an appropriate treatment regimen, including length of treatment, for this particular patient on the basis of organism characteristics and treatment guidelines for IE
- Determine appropriate monitoring parameters to evaluate response of the IE therapy
- Understand which patients need prophylactic therapy and what therapy is appropriate for the prevention of IE

## PATIENT PRESENTATION

### Chief Complaint

"I've had a fever off and on for the past 2 weeks. My leg hurts and is swollen. I just don't feel very good, my body aches and I am tired all the time."

### History of Present Illness

LB is a 38-year-old Caucasian man who presents to the emergency department with complaints of intermittent high fever (103–104°F [39.4–40.0°C]), chills, malaise, myalgias, and arthralgias for the past 2 weeks, as well as lower right leg erythema and edema for the past 3–4 weeks. He has been treated numerous times for recurrent cellulitis over the area of a previous gunshot wound (GSW) with evidence of injection drug use noted in the same area. Over the past year, he has been admitted to the hospital three times with right leg cellulitis (last admission was 2 months ago). He has been treated in the past with cefazolin, vancomycin, and trimethoprim/sulfamethoxazole. The area of cellulitis extends down from the groin to midthigh. The patient reports that the last intravenous drug abuse (IVDA) was 4 weeks ago. He has chronic leg pain due to the GSW and takes tramadol, Lortab, and Percocet for pain control. He states that the pain has increased over the past month, and he has been taking more medication to control the pain.

### Past Medical History

GSW 8 years ago (right upper leg/groin area)

Recurrent cellulitis over the past 3–4 years (CA-MRSA + in the past)

HTN

Dyslipidemia × 3 years

Hepatitis B

### Family History

Father and mother are both alive. Father is 55 years and has a history of COPD and dyslipidemia. Mother is 52 years and has no significant past medical history. He has 2 younger siblings: one sister aged 24 years and 1 brother aged 21 years; both are healthy.

### Social History

He was married but divorced after being incarcerated for selling illicit drugs. He has 1 child, aged 14 years, but does not have any contact. He was in prison for 6 years, but was released about 1½ years ago. He lives with his girlfriend at the present time and is unemployed.

### Tobacco/Alcohol/Substance Use

Admits to a 10-year history of injective drug use (reports heroin and cocaine use). Denies any use of alcohol. Admits to tobacco use (1 ppd × 18 years)

## Allergies/Intolerances/Adverse Drug Events

Penicillin—unknown reaction

## Medications (Current)

Simvastatin 20 mg PO q hs

Atenolol 100 mg PO bid

Citalopram 40 mg PO q day

Gabapentin 300 mg PO tid

Tramadol 50 to 100 mg PO q 6 h

Hydrocodone/acetaminophen 10/500 mg PO q 4 to 6 h PRN pain

Oxycodone/acetaminophen 7.5/325 mg PO q 6 h PRN severe pain

Acetaminophen PO PRN fever × 2 weeks

## Review of Systems

Significant right leg pain due to previous GSW, some relief with pain medications (tramadol, Lortab, and Percocet); recurrent cellulitis in right leg/groin area; no other significant medical problems

## Physical Examination

### ▸ General

Ill-appearing, Caucasian man in mild-to-moderate distress

### ▸ Vital Signs

BP 145/90 mm Hg, P 120, RR 22, T 39.6°C

Weight 148.2 lb (67.4 kg)

Height 71 in. (180 cm)

Complains of significant right leg pain extending up into the groin

### ▸ Skin

Pale appearing with numerous areas of scarred and leathery skin secondary to IVDA; (+) petechial rash on trunk, multiple lesions, and track marks on right leg and groin

### ▸ HEENT

PERRLA, EOMI; no scleral icterus, (+) petechia on palate, dry mucus membranes, no exudates noted in throat

### ▸ Neck and Lymph Nodes

Supple; (−) lymphadenopathy

### ▸ Chest

Clear to auscultation bilaterally

### ▸ Cardiovascular

RRR, (+) murmur noted (newly identified)

### ▸ Abdomen

Soft, nondistended, nontender; (+) bowel sounds; (−) organomegaly

### ▸ Neurology

AAO × 3; (−) focal or sensory deficit noted

### ▸ Extremities

Significant edema in right leg; pulses are 2+ and equal bilaterally. No clubbing or cyanosis noted. Splinter hemorrhages noted on left, middle, and ring fingers

## Laboratory Tests

### On Admission

|  | Conventional Units | SI Units |
|---|---|---|
| Na | 132 mEq/L | 132 mmol/L |
| K | 3.9 mEq/L | 3.9 mmol/L |
| Cl | 102 mEq/L | 102 mmol/L |
| $CO_2$ | 26 mEq/L | 26 mmol/L |
| BUN | 34 mg/dL | 12.1 mmol/L |
| SCr | 1.6 mg/dL | 141 μmol/L |
| Glu | 122 mg/dL | 6.8 mmol/L |
| Albumin | 2.9 g/dL | 29 g/L |
| RBC | $3.14 \times 10^6/mm^3$ | $3.14 \times 10^{12}/L$ |
| Hgb | 8.8 g/dL | 88 g/L; 5.46 mmol/L |
| Hct | 27.8% | 0.278 |
| Platelets | $184 \times 10^3/mm^3$ | $184 \times 10^9/L$ |
| WBC | $19.6 \times 10^3/mm^3$ | $19.6 \times 10^9/L$ |
| Neutrophils | 78% | 0.78 |
| Bands | 14% | 0.14 |
| Lymphocytes | 7% | 0.07 |
| Monocytes | 1% | 0.01 |
| Eosinophils | 0% | 0.00 |
| Basophils | 0% | 0.00 |

## Cultures

Blood cultures taken on admission; results pending

## Assessment

A 38-year-old man with signs, symptoms, and laboratory tests consistent with right leg cellulitis and suspected bacteremia/endocarditis

## Plan

Admit the patient to hospital, begin broad-spectrum antibiotics, and perform additional tests to evaluate for IE

## AFTER HOSPITAL ADMISSION

### Cultures

*Day 2:* Gram stain of blood cultures × 2 taken at admission show Gram-positive cocci in clusters.

*Day 3:* Blood cultures × 2 show *Staphylococcus aureus*; susceptibilities pending.

*Day 4:* Right leg abscess aspirate grows *S. aureus*; susceptibilities pending.

*Day 5:* Culture sensitivities (see Table 83-1).

*Day 17:* Gram stain of blood cultures × 2 show Gram-positive cocci in clusters.

*Day 18:* Blood cultures show *S. aureus*; susceptibilities pending.

*Day 19:* Culture susceptibilities (see Table 83-1).

*Day 26:* Blood cultures × 2 are negative.

### Imaging

*Day 3:* CT of the right groin showed a 3 × 4 cm (1.2 × 1.6 in.) abscess. Surgery drains abscess and sends aspirate for culture.

*Day 4:* TTE showed possible small vegetation; poor visualization of the valves; results inconclusive.

*Day 20:* TEE shows large vegetation (1.9 × 3.8 cm [0.75 × 1.5 in.]) on the posterior leaflet of the tricuspid valve.

### Pertinent Labs

#### During Hospitalization

|  | Conventional Units | SI Units |
| --- | --- | --- |
| Day 7: |  |  |
| SCr | 1.8 mg/dL | 159 µmol/L |
| WBC | 15.5 × 10³/mm³ | 15.5 × 10⁹/L |
| Day 12: |  |  |
| SCr | 2.4 mg/dL | 212 µmol/L |
| WBC | 16.2 × 10³/mm³ | 16.2 × 10⁹/L |
| Day 22: |  |  |
| SCr | 1.9 mg/dL | 168 µmol/L |
| WBC | 14.3 × 10³/mm³ | 14.3 × 10⁹/L |
| Day 30: |  |  |
| SCr | 1.3 mg/dL | 115 µmol/L |
| WBC | 10.7 × 10³/mm³ | 10.7 × 10³/mm³ |

**TABLE 83-1. CULTURE AND SUSCEPTIBILITY**

|  | Blood Culture—Aerobic and Anaerobic Bottles (Arm—Left) Specimen # B31126 06/12/2012 16:24 | Blood Culture—Aerobic and Anaerobic Bottles (Right Internal Jugular Triple-Lumen Catheter) Specimen # B31278 06/12/2012 18:45 | Abscess Fluid Right Groin—Aerobic and Anaerobic Bottle Note: Patient on Vancomycin Specimen # X48002 06/14/2012 10:18 | Blood Culture—Aerobic and Anaerobic Bottles (Arm—Left Peripherally Inserted Center Catheter, PICC; Arm—Right) Note: Patient on Vancomycin Specimen # B42151; B42189 06/29/2012 21:52; 21:55 |
| --- | --- | --- | --- | --- |
| Gram stain | Gram-positive cocci in clusters | Gram-positive cocci in clusters | Gram-positive cocci in clusters | Gram-positive cocci in clusters |
| Organism | *S. aureus* MIC (mcg/mL; mg/L) | *S. aureus* MIC (mcg/mL; mg/L) | *S. aureus* MIC (mcg/mL; mg/L) | *S. aureus* MIC (mcg/mL; mg/L) |
| Clindamycin | >4 (R) | >4 (R) | >4 (R) | >4 (R) |
| Daptomycin | 0.5 (S) | 0.5 (S) | 0.5 (S) | 1.0 (S) |
| Erythromycin | >4 (R) | >4 (R) | >4 (R) | >4 (R) |
| Gentamicin | >8 (R) | >8 (R) | >8 (R) | >8 (R) |
| Moxifloxacin | >4 (R) | >4 (R) | >4 (R) | >4 (R) |
| Linezolid | 1 (S) | 1 (S) | 2 (S) | 2 (S) |
| Oxacillin | >2 (R) | >2 (R) | >2 (R) | >2 (R) |
| Penicillin | >8 (R) | >8 (R) | >8 (R) | >8 (R) |
| Rifampin | ≤1 (S) | ≤1 (S) | ≤1 (S) | ≤1 (S) |
| Quinupristin/ dalfopristin | ≤0.25 (S) | ≤0.25 (S) | 0.50 (S) | 0.50 (S) |
| Tetracycline | ≤1 (S) | ≤1 (S) | ≤1 (S) | ≤1 (S) |
| Trimethoprim/ sulfamethoxazole | ≤0.5/9.5 (S) | ≤0.5/9.5 (S) | ≤0.5/9.5 (S) | ≤0.5/9.5 (S) |
| Vancomycin | 1 (S) | 1 (S) | 2 (S) | 2 (S) |

S = susceptible, I = intermediate, R = resistant

## Treatment in Hospital

The patient was placed on vancomycin 1,000 mg IV q 12 h and gentamicin 150 mg IV q 8 h for broad coverage of common organisms of IE and right upper leg cellulitis/abscess. He continues to have intermittent febrile episodes (spikes up to 38.8°C [101.8°F]) despite therapy. On hospital day 12, peaks and troughs were drawn for both vancomycin and gentamicin, and results were as follows: vancomycin, peak 41.6 mcg/mL (41.6 mg/L; 28.7 μmol/L; 11:40) and trough 15.3 mcg/mL (15.3 mg/L; 10.6 μmol/L; 08:15); gentamicin, peak 12.2 mcg/mL (12.2 mg/L; 25.5 μmol/L; 17:30) and trough 4.8 mcg/mL (4.8 mg/L; 10.0 μmol/L; 15:20). At this time, gentamicin was discontinued and vancomycin was held for one dose and then restarted at the same dose. On hospital day 16, the patient became SOB with complaints of a dry cough and chest pain. A chest x-ray revealed bilateral lower infiltrates, which were believed to be septic pulmonary emboli. He had repeat blood cultures on hospital day 17, which grew *S. aureus* (see Table 83-1). Antimicrobial therapy was reassessed on the basis of the patient's clinical deterioration (large vegetation on TEE), development of IE complications (septic emboli), and continued positive cultures showing increased MICs. At this time (day 20), vancomycin was discontinued and daptomycin 300 mg q 24 h was started.

### Student Workup

**Missing Information?**

| | |
|---|---|
| **Evaluate:** | Patient Database |
| | Drug Therapy Problems/Monitoring Issues |
| | Care Plan (by Problem) |

## TARGETED QUESTIONS

1. What signs and symptoms of IE does this patient have? Categorize by modified Duke classifications as major or minor criteria and specify what "type" of clinical diagnosis is appropriate for this patient.

   *Hint: See p. 1298 and Table 74-2 in PPP*

2. Is it appropriate to start vancomycin as empiric therapy in this patient?

   *Hint: See pp. 1301, 1302, and 1304, Table 74-1 in PPP*

3. Is synergistic therapy with gentamicin appropriate in this patient?

   *Hint: See pp. 1303–1308 in PPP*

4. What should you recommend after reviewing this patient's vancomycin and gentamicin levels?

   *Hint: See Tables 74-4 and 74-6 (footnotes) in PPP, and see the following articles:*

Rybak MJ, Lomaestro BM, Rotschafer JC, Moellering RC, Craig WA, Billeter M, Dalovisio JR, Levine DP. Therapeutic monitoring of vancomycin in adults—summary of consensus recommendations from the American Society of Health-System Pharmacists, the Infectious Diseases Society of America, and the Society of Infectious Diseases Pharmacists. Pharmacotherapy 2009 29:1275–1279.

Liu C, Bayer A, Cosgrove SE, et al. Clinical practice guidelines by the Infectious Diseases Society of America for the treatment of methicillin-resistant *Staphylococcus aureus* infections in adults and children: executive summary. Clin Infect Dis 2011 52:285–292.

5. What concerns develop with the empiric therapy during the initial hospital course of this patient?

   *Hint: See pp. 1302–1308 and Tables 74-5 and 74-7 in PPP*

6. Is it appropriate to change therapy?

   *Hint: Pay particular attention to Table 83-1 and see the following articles:*

Rybak MJ, Lomaestro BM, Rotschafer JC, Moellering RC, Craig WA, Billeter M, Dalovisio JR, Levine DP. Therapeutic monitoring of vancomycin in adults—summary of consensus recommendations from the American Society of Health-System Pharmacists, the Infectious Diseases Society of America, and the Society of Infectious Diseases Pharmacists. Pharmacotherapy 2009 29:1275–1279.

Liu C, Bayer A, Cosgrove SE, et al. Clinical practice guidelines by the Infectious Diseases Society of America for the treatment of methicillin-resistant *Staphylococcus aureus* infections in adults and children: executive summary. Clin Infect Dis 2011 52:285–292.

Holland TL, Fowler Jr, VG. Vancomycin minimum inhibitory concentration and outcome in patients with *Staphylococcus aureus* bacteremia: pearl or Pellet? J Infect Dis 2011 204:329–331.

7. Is daptomycin an appropriate alternative therapy?

   *Hint: See pp. 1301–1308 in PPP, and see the following article:*

Fowler V, Boucher HW, Corey GR, et al. Daptomycin versus standard therapy for bacteremia and IE caused by *Staphylococcus aureus*. N Engl J Med 2006 355:653–665.

8. Are there any concerns with concurrent drug therapy and daptomycin?

   *Hint: See Table 74-7 in PPP, and the Cubicin package insert pp. 10 and 11 (http://www.cubicin.com/pdf/PrescribingInformation.pdf), and see the following articles:*

Fowler V, Boucher HW, Corey GR, et al. Daptomycin versus standard therapy for bacteremia and IE caused by *Staphylococcus aureus*. N Engl J Med 2006 355:653–665.

Parra-Ruiz J, Duenas-Gutierrez C, et al. Safety analysis of high dose daptomycin in patients with concomitant statin therapy. Eur J Clin Microbiol Infect Dis 2012 31:1771–1774.

9. How long this patient should be treated?

   *Hint: See Table 74-4 in PPP. In addition, take into account that the patient had a positive culture on day 18 with worsening symptoms when therapy was changed.*

10. How should this patient be monitored for resolution of infection/adverse drug effects? Include additional tests, procedures, etc.

    *Hint: See pp. 1310–1311 and Table 74-7 in PPP*

11. Should this patient receive IE prophylactic therapy for future invasive dental procedures? Include reason and regimen as appropriate.

    *Hint: See pp. 1309–1310 in Table 74-8 in PPP*

## CLINICAL COURSE

During the first 2 weeks of therapy, the patient showed some initial improvement. The WBC decreased but then began to show an increase and the patient continued to have intermittent febrile episodes. Over these 2 weeks, the right upper leg cellulitis resolved but not cured. The right groin abscess remained visible on repeat CT, but was smaller in size. During week 3, the patient's renal function declined and drug levels for vancomycin and gentamicin were drawn, showing abnormal levels. Dosage recommendations were made by the pharmacokinetic pharmacy service. After the patient deteriorated clinically, experienced a complication of IE (pulmonary septic emboli), and had positive repeat blood cultures with increased MICs, therapy was changed to daptomycin. Over the next week, the patient's bacteremia resolved, right upper leg cellulitis resolved, and the right groin abscess was healing. The patient reported that he was feeling much better and had no complaints. The medicine team recommended continuing therapy for the appropriate length of treatment for his IE.

## GLOBAL PERSPECTIVE

IE is an infection typically involving the heart valves and nearby endocardial tissue. This disease state often has an aggressive clinical course with numerous complications and high mortality rates. Incidence of IE appears to be similar throughout developed countries. Patients have various clinical presentations, ranging from subtle illness to severe sepsis with multiple complications. Certain patients (IVDA, diabetics, elderly) have an increased risk of having less common and/or resistant organisms. Regardless of patient type, IE can be difficult to diagnose and treat. The patient must be carefully monitored throughout treatment for disease complications, therapeutic or toxic drug levels (as appropriate), drug interactions, and clinical improvement (both laboratory results and patient response). Patient follow-up is critical in ensuring that a cure has been achieved and that no adverse events have occurred.

## CASE SUMMARY

- His clinical presentation is consistent with IE requiring appropriate antibiotic therapy.
- Vancomycin therapy on the basis of organism and susceptibilities is appropriate per IE treatment guidelines.
- Worsening clinical picture and susceptibilities require reassessment of therapy.

For more information on the care plan and facilitator's guide please visit http://www.mhpharmacotherapy.com.

# 84 Tuberculosis

Rocsanna Namdar

## CASE LEARNING OBJECTIVES

- Identify the risk factors for developing active tuberculosis (TB) disease
- Design a therapeutic plan for active TB disease in an immunocompetent and immunocompromised patient
- Assess the effectiveness of therapy in patients being treated for TB
- Design an appropriate regimen for the treatment of latent TB infection

## PATIENT PRESENTATION

### Chief Complaint

"I have had a cough for a month. Two nights ago I woke up with a sharp pain in my chest and I coughed up some blood."

### History of Present Illness

HS is a 52-year-old Hispanic female who presents to the emergency department with complaints of cough, productive of small amounts of yellow sputum within the last month. She has experienced increasing fatigue, occasional SOB on exertion, and mild, nonpleuritic, substernal chest discomfort. She has had periodic night sweats; last night her temperature was 38.9°C. Two nights ago, she noticed streaks of bright-red blood in her sputum without any particular odor or taste. The only medication she has taken is an over-the-counter cough preparation. Three months ago, the patient presented to a free clinic with fatigue, increased urinary frequency, and headaches. Evaluation revealed a diagnosis of type 2 diabetes and stage I HTN. A purified protein derivative (ppd) test, required for work clearance, was placed. She was noted to have a positive ppd test, but because her chest x-ray showed no active disease, she was cleared to work.

### Past Medical History

HTN diagnosed 3 months ago

Type 2 DM diagnosed 3 months ago

Depression diagnosed 9 months ago

Immunized with BCG

### Family History

Mother (age 77 years) is in good health. Sisters (ages 49 and 56 years) have HTN. Her father in Mexico died of lung disease 4 years ago at age 72 years. Her husband died of colon cancer 2 years ago.

### Social History

The patient immigrated to the United States from Mexico 1 year ago. She lives with her son and his family. She has 2 daughters who still live in Mexico and has visited them on several occasions during the past year. She has recently started working at a day care.

### Tobacco/Alcohol/Substance Use

Social drinker; (−) tobacco or illicit drug use

### Allergies/Intolerances/Adverse Drug Events

Penicillin (rash)

### Medications (Current)

Lisinopril 20 mg PO daily

Metformin 500 mg PO twice daily

Sertraline 50 mg PO daily

Calcium carbonate 1,000 mg PO daily

Ibuprofen PRN pain

Alprazolam 2 mg PRN

### Review of Systems

The patient reports a more-than-9 lb (4-kg) weight loss over the past 2 months. She also complains of fever, body aches, intermittent chest pain associated with cough, SOB, and intermittent cough productive of sputum and blood. She states that she has had improvement in urinary frequency since starting metformin.

### Physical Examination

▶ **General**

Pleasant, slightly overweight Hispanic female in no acute distress

▶ *Vital Signs*

BP 144/92 mm Hg, P 82, RR 18, T 37.9°C (100.2°F)

Weight 160 lb (72.7 kg)

Height 61 in. (155 cm)

▶ *HEENT*

PERRLA, EOMI; pharynx: slightly inflamed, no exudate

▶ *Neck and Lymph Nodes*

Few small 2–3-mm nontender, freely movable lymph nodes in left anterior cervical and axial area

▶ *Chest*

Configuration and expansion symmetrical. Tactile fremitus, percussion symmetrical bilaterally. Breath sounds and vocal fremitus are normal. A few posttussive rales are noted at the left apex posteriorly.

▶ *Cardiovascular*

RRR, normal $S_1$, $S_2$

▶ *Abdomen*

Not tender/not distended; (–) organomegaly

▶ *Neurology*

Grossly intact; deep tendon reflexes normal

▶ *Genitourinary*

Examination deferred

▶ *Rectal*

Examination deferred

▶ *Skin Test Results*

PPD (tuberculin) 16 mm (0.63 in.) at 48 hours

▶ *Chest X-Ray*

Bilateral upper lobe infiltrates with well-defined cavitating lesion of the left apex (Figure 84-1)

## Laboratory Tests

### On Admission

|  | Conventional Units | SI Units |
|---|---|---|
| Na | 139 mEq/L | 139 mmol/L |
| K | 3.9 mEq/L | 3.9 mmol/L |
| Cl | 98 mEq/L | 98 mmol/L |
| $CO_2$ | 26 mEq/L | 26 mmol/L |
| BUN | 20 mg/dL | 7.1 mmol/L |
| SCr | 0.7 mg/dL | 62 μmol/L |
| Glu | 153 mg/dL | 8.5 mmol/L |

**FIGURE 84-1.**  Left upper lobe with cavitation. (Reproduced, with permission, from Miller WT Jr. Diagnostic Thoracic Imaging. New York, McGraw-Hill, 2006.)

| AST | 55 IU/L | 0.92 μkat/L |
|---|---|---|
| ALT | 61 IU/L | 1.02 μkat/L |
| Total bilirubin | 1 mg/dL | 17.1 μmol/L |
| $HbA_{1c}$ | 7.2% | 0.072 (55 mmol/ mol Hgb) |

| Urinalysis | | |
|---|---|---|
| Protein | Trace | |
| Microalbumin | <30 mg/24 h | |
| Glucose | (–) | |
| Ketone | (–) | |
| Sputum culture | Normal respiratory flora | |
| Acid-fast bacilli smear | (+) | |
| Hgb | 13.5 g/dL | 135 g/L; 8.38 mmol/L |
| Hct | 40% | 0.40 |
| WBC | $10.6 \times 10^3/mm^3$ | $10.6 \times 10^9/L$ |
| PMN | 62% | 0.62 |
| Lymphocytes | 34% | 0.34 |
| Monocytes | 5% | 0.05 |
| RBC | $4.6 \times 10^6/mm^3$ | $4.6 \times 10^{12}/L$ |

## Assessment

A 52-year-old woman with signs, symptoms, and laboratory tests consistent with active TB.

**Student Workup**

**Missing Information?**

Evaluate:     Patient Database

              Drug Therapy Problems

              Care Plan (by Problem)

## TARGETED QUESTIONS

1. What groups are at highest risk for developing TB?

   *Hint: See p. 1316 in PPP*

2. How does vaccination with BCG (Bacille Calmette Guerin) affect TST (Tuberculin Skin Test) and IGRA (Interferon Gamma Release Assay) test results?

   *Hint: See pp. 1318–1319 in PPP*

3. In patients with laboratory-confirmed drug-susceptible active pulmonary *Mycobacterium tuberculosis* (MTB), what are the standard medication(s) and duration of treatment? How would this differ if the patient were HIV positive?

   *Hint: See Table 75-3 in PPP*

4. The patient's liver function tests are slightly elevated. Why is this important and does it change the management of her TB infection?

   *Hint: See pp. 1323 and 1325 in PPP*

5. How is therapeutic efficacy assessed in the treatment of TB?

   *Hint: See pp. 1325 and 1326 in PPP*

## FOLLOW-UP

Four weeks later, the patient returns for follow-up. Her sputum cultures are positive for AFB and the organism is identified as *M. tuberculosis* resistant to isoniazid (INH).

6. How does this information change your recommended drug combination and duration of drug therapy?

   *Hint: See pp. 1320–1322 in PPP*

7. How should the close contacts of this patient be treated?

   *Hint: See Table 75-2 in PPP*

## ⟳ GLOBAL PERSPECTIVE

TB remains a leading infectious killer globally. Approximately 2 billion people are infected by *M. tuberculosis*, and roughly 2 million people die from active TB each year despite the fact that it is curable.[1] India, China, Indonesia, Nigeria, and South Africa have the highest number of reported incident cases worldwide. Africa accounts for approximately 80% of the HIV-positive TB cases. HIV is the most important risk factor for active TB, especially among people 25–44 years of age. The countries with the highest incidence of multi drug-resistant TB (MDR-TB) are India, China, and Russia. MDR-TB is defined as resistance to at least INH and rifampin (RIF). Extremely MDRTB (XDR-TB) is MDR-TB that is also resistant to any fluoroquinolone, and at least 1 of 3 injectable second-line drugs. MDR- and XDR-TB pose a serious threat to TB control. Other challenges in TB treatment worldwide include lack of qualified human resources, poor infection control, development of new drugs, limitations of available treatment options, insufficient laboratory capacity, and weak surveillance systems.[2] Directly observed therapy (DOT) and therapeutic drug monitoring are ways to optimize therapy. DOT programs have been expanded across the world to ensure that patients with TB can have access to optimal care.

## REFERENCES

1. World Health Organization. Global tuberculosis control. http://www.who.int/tb/publications/global_report/en/index.html. Accessed October 3, 2012.

2. World Health Organization. The global plan to stop TB 2011-2015. http://www.who.int/tb/strategy/en/. Accessed October 3, 2012.

## CASE SUMMARY

- This patient's current clinical picture is consistent with pulmonary TB, and therapy should be initiated.

- Initial treatment with INH, RIF, PZA, and EMB is recommended. However, after susceptibility test results, the treatment regimen must be revised.

- Liver function tests should be monitored due to drug toxicity and preexisting enzyme elevations.

- Close contacts should be treated with RIF because of INH-resistant strain in the patient.

**For more information on the care plan and facilitator's guide please visit http://www.mhpharmacotherapy.com.**

# 85 Clostridium difficile— Associated Diarrhea

Jeremiah J. Duby        Monica A. Donnelley
Brett H. Heintz

## CASE LEARNING OBJECTIVES

- Identify the signs and symptoms of *Clostridium difficile*–associated diarrhea (CDAD)
- List the risk factors for CDAD
- Select an appropriate treatment and monitoring plan for antimicrobial therapy
- Consider the role of adjunctive agents and supportive care

## PATIENT PRESENTATION

### Chief Complaint

"Please give me something for this cramping, diarrhea, and nausea."

### History of Present Illness

Shannon Rasmussen is a 69-year-old woman who is brought to the emergency department for a 3-day history of diffuse abdominal pain, fever/chills, frequent, voluminous, foul-smelling stools, and lethargy. Her husband reports that "she has not been able to keep anything down" since her recent discharge and has had 5–10 profuse, watery bowel movements per day. The patient was in her usual state of health until 1 week ago when she developed severe, acute abdominal pain. She was admitted at that time with a small bowel obstruction and received an urgent exploratory laparotomy with resection. Her postoperative course was complicated by a polymicrobial intra-abdominal abscess. She was empirically treated with cefepime and clindamycin, which was changed to ampicillin–sulbactam on the basis of the culture/susceptibility results. She was discharged on amoxicillin–clavulanate to complete a 14-day course.

### Past Medical History

Type 2 DM
HTN
OA

### Family History

Father died of bone cancer at age 66 years. Mother died of MI at age 72 years.

### Social History

Married and lives with her husband, aged 65 years.

### Tobacco/Alcohol/Substance Use

Social drinker (1–2 glasses of wine daily); (–) tobacco or illicit drug use

### Allergies/Intolerances/Adverse Drug Events

"Sulfa drugs" cause a rash.

### Medications (Current)

Metformin 500 mg PO twice daily

Metoprolol 50 mg PO twice daily

Lisinopril 40 mg PO at bedtime

Ibuprofen 200–400 mg PO q 3–4 h as needed

Amoxicillin–clavulanate 875/125 mg PO twice daily (day 13/14)

Loperamide 4 mg PO followed by 2 mg after each loose stool (max 16 mg/day)

Esomeprazole 40 mg PO twice daily (husband's prescription)

### Review of Systems

In addition to her symptoms noted in the *History of Present Illness* section, the patient reports that her husband gave her some of his prescription-strength esomeprazole for her abdominal pain; however, it did not help. Also, the patient states that she thinks she has lost several pounds over the last month, "since this all began and that the pain in all around her belly is sharp."

## Physical Examination

### ▶ General

Elderly woman in acute distress

### ▶ Vital Signs

BP 85/40 mm Hg, HR 120, RR 22, T 38.4°C

Weight 150 lb (68.2 kg)

Height 66 in. (167.6 cm)

Abdominal pain 6/10

### ▶ Skin

Dry and warm with poor turgor

### ▶ HEENT

PERRLA, EOMI; trace of periorbital edema; (–) sinus tenderness; TMs appear normal

### ▶ Neck and Lymph Nodes

Supple. No JVD or palpable lymph nodes

### ▶ Chest

Clear to auscultation. Shallow/rapid breathing

### ▶ Breasts

Examination deferred

### ▶ Cardiovascular

Sinus tachycardia, normal $S_1$, $S_2$; (–) $S_3$ or $S_4$

### ▶ Abdomen

Abdomen is positive for guarding, tender, and distended. Pain is sharp but diffuse, and it is exacerbated by pressure and movement. Diminished bowel sounds. Recent midline incision is noted.

### ▶ Neurology

Oriented times 2/4. Grossly apathetic and lethargic. Deep tendon reflexes normal

### ▶ Genitourinary

Examination deferred

### ▶ Rectal

Negative guaiac

## Laboratory Tests

### On Admission

|  | Conventional Units | SI Units |
|---|---|---|
| Na | 160 mEq/L | 160 mmol/L |
| K | 5.2 mEq/L | 5.2 mmol/L |
| Cl | 100 mEq/L | 100 mmol/L |
| $CO_2$ | 16 mEq/L | 16 mmol/L |
| BUN | 42 mg/dL | 15 mmol/L |
| SCr | 1.7 mg/dL | 150 μmol/L |
| Glu | 180 mg/dL | 10 mmol/L |
| Ca | 8 mg/dL | 2 mmol/L |
| Mg | 2 mEq/L | 1 mmol/L |
| Phosphate | 4.6 mg/dL | 1.49 mmol/L |
| Hgb | 9.7 g/dL | 97 g/L; 6.02 mmol/L |
| Hct | 29% | 0.29 |
| WBC | $52 \times 10^3/mm^3$ | $52 \times 10^9/L$ |
| MCV | $80 \ \mu m^3$ | 80 fL |
| Albumin | 3 g/dL | 30 g/L |
| Stool sample | Positive for *C. difficile* toxins A/B | |
| ABG | | |
| pH | 7.31 | |
| $PaO_2$ | 32 mm Hg | 4.3 kPa |
| $PaCO_2$ | 94 mm Hg | 12.5 kPa |

## Procedures

CT of the abdomen indicates postoperative changes, including a profound ileus and acute dilation of the colon suggestive of toxic megacolon, but reveals complete resolution of the previous abscess.

Sigmoidoscopic examination indicates diffuse erythematous colitis characterized by yellow plaques in distal colon.

## Assessment

69-year-old woman with signs, symptoms, and laboratory tests consistent with severe CDAD and complications that require direct transfer to the ICU.

## Student Workup

### Missing Information?

Evaluate:     Patient Database

Drug Therapy Problems

Care Plan (by Problem)

## TARGETED QUESTIONS

1. What signs and symptoms of CDAD does the patient have?

   *Hint: See p. 1338 in PPP*

2. What are the patient's risk factors for CDAD?

   *Hint: See p. 1337 in PPP*

3. How would you classify this patient's episode of CDAD?

   *Hint: See pp. 1337–1338 in PPP*

4. What antimicrobial agents are active against *C. difficile*?

   *Hint: See pp. 1337–1338 in PPP*

5. What antimicrobial agent(s) are most appropriate for the patient? (Please include dose, route, frequency, and duration of therapy.)

   *Hint: See pp. 1337–1338 in PPP*

6. List other pharmacologic and nonpharmacologic changes to the patient's therapy that may improve her outcome?

   *Hint: See pp. 1337–1338 in PPP*

7. What clinical and laboratory endpoints should be used to monitor the patient's progress?

   *Hint: See pp. 1337–1339 in PPP*

## FOLLOW-UP

The patient presents to the outpatient surgery clinic 8 weeks after successful treatment and discharge with symptoms that she describes as "exactly the same but much milder" compared to those from her previous presentation.

8. How would you characterize another episode of CDAD in the patient? What is the most appropriate antimicrobial therapy at this time? What recommendations can you provide the patient to prevent future episodes?

   *Hint: See pp. 1337–1338 in PPP*

9. What is the role of probiotics in preventing recurrence of CDAD?

   *Hint: See pp. 1337–1338 in PPP*

## GLOBAL PERSPECTIVE

Several outbreaks of *C. difficile* have been associated with highly virulent strain (NAP1/027) across the world, specifically first recognized in Canada and United Kingdom in 2003.[1] Since this time, several other outbreaks have been associated with this strain of *C. difficile* with high toxin production. Oral vancomycin therapy is currently recommended for severe *C. difficile* infection, but many patients may require surgical intervention. The availability of oral vancomycin therapy is limited in certain countries and the IV formulation of vancomycin administered orally is often prescribed.

## REFERENCE

1. Cohen SH, Gerding DN, Johnson S, et al. Clinical practice guidelines for *Clostridium difficile* infection in adults: 2010 update by the Society of Healthcare Epidemiology of America (SHEA) and the Infectious Diseases Society of America (IDSA). Infect Control Hosp Epidemiol 2010 31:431–455.

## CASE SUMMARY

- Her current clinical picture is consistent with severe, complicated *C. difficile* disease, and appropriate antimicrobial therapy should be initiated.

- Oral vancomycin therapy would be a reasonable initial therapy for this patient with a dose of 500 mg PO q 6 h in addition to metronidazole 500 mg IV q 8 h. The patient should be educated on appropriate use and potential GI side effects.

- Since the patient has evidence of toxic megacolon and evidence of ileus, she may require the addition of vancomycin as a retention enema and/or surgical intervention to remove the affected bowel.

For more information on the care plan and facilitator's guide please visit http://www.mhpharmacotherapy.com.

# 86 Intra-Abdominal Infection

Sarah M. Adriance          Monica A. Donnelley

Brian L. Erstad

## CASE LEARNING OBJECTIVES

- Recognize the clinical presentation of a secondary intra-abdominal infection involving abscess
- Identify the microorganisms typically involved in secondary intra-abdominal infections
- Develop an appropriate treatment and monitoring plan for a secondary intra-abdominal infection on the basis of specific patient characteristics
- Recommend the most appropriate drug and nondrug interventions to treat a secondary intra-abdominal infection

## PATIENT PRESENTATION

### Chief Complaint

"I feel sick. My stomach hurts, especially right by my belly button. I have been running a fever for two days."

### History of Present Illness

John Romans is a 34-year-old male who presents to the emergency department complaining of acute onset of severe abdominal pain, localized in the periumbilical region. The patient states that his persistent fever and a localized region of pain in his abdomen are new symptoms for him. His oral intake has decreased over the past week due to the pain. He has a past medical history significant for Crohn's disease, which was diagnosed 15 years ago. Currently, he receives infliximab infusions for his Crohn's disease. Methotrexate was prescribed in the past, but was not tolerated. In the past, intermittent high-dose corticosteroid tapers have been used for disease exacerbations with success. His last flare was 1 month ago. Past surgical history includes a colostomy performed 12 years ago with no subsequent complications.

### Past Medical History

Crohn's disease (ileocolonic) diagnosed 15 years ago
Colostomy placement 12 years ago

### Family History

Father died at age 36 from colon cancer. Paternal grandmother suffers from osteoporosis.

### Social History

Works for a local nonprofit organization. No recent travel history outside the United States.

### Tobacco/Alcohol/Substance Use

(−) Alcohol; (−) tobacco or illicit drug use

### Allergies/Intolerances/Adverse Drug Events

No known medication allergies

### Medications (Current)

Infliximab 760 mg IV q 8 wk

### Review of Systems

Malaise and fever for a couple of days despite use of acetaminophen; abdomen tender right of umbilicus with palpable mass that has developed over past few days; abdomen pain increases with eating; (−) significant weight loss, but states that he has lost a couple of pounds this past week; (−) hematochezia; patient reports increase in colostomy output during last week; no history of fistula or abscess formation.

### Physical Examination

▶ **General**

Ill-appearing, diaphoretic Caucasian male in moderate acute distress

▶ **Vital Signs**

BP 108/43 mm Hg, P 101, RR 22, T 39.1°C

Weight 167 lb (76 kg)

Height 70 in. (177.8 cm)

Abdominal pain 8/10

▶ *Skin*

(−) Rash, ulcerations, or other skin lesions

▶ *HEENT*

PERRLA, EOMI

▶ *Neck and Lymph Nodes*

Supple; (−) lymphadenopathy

▶ *Chest*

Clear to auscultation

▶ *Cardiovascular*

RRR, normal $S_1$, $S_2$; (−) $S_3$ or $S_4$

▶ *Abdomen*

(+) Bowel sounds; (−) distension; small palpable mass present just right of umbilicus; tender with mild guarding to palpitation

▶ *Neurology*

Grossly intact; deep tendon reflexes normal

▶ *Colorectal*

(+) Colostomy; stoma is normal, appearing pink in color and moist

▶ *Microbiologic Data*

Blood cultures pending

▶ *Imaging*

Abdominal CT shows evidence of abdominal wall abscess arising from terminal ileum.

## Laboratory Tests

▶ *On Admission*

|  | Conventional Units | SI Units |
|---|---|---|
| Na | 140 mEq/L | 140 mmol/L |
| K | 3.9 mEq/L | 3.9 mmol/L |
| Cl | 101 mEq/L | 101 mmol/L |
| $CO_2$ | 22 mEq/L | 22 mmol/L |
| BUN | 10 mg/dL | 3.6 mmol/L |
| SCr | 0.9 mg/dL | 80 μmol/L |
| Glu | 102 mg/dL | 5.7 mmol/L |
| Ca | 9.2 mg/dL | 2.30 mmol/L |
| Mg | 1.8 mEq/L | 0.90 mmol/L |

| Phosphate | 4.2 mg/dL | 1.36 mmol/L |
|---|---|---|
| Hgb | 14.2 g/dL | 142 g/L; 8.81 mmol/L |
| Hct | 39.3% | 0.393 |
| WBC | $15 \times 10^3/mm^3$ | $15 \times 10^9/L$ |
| Albumin | 3.1 g/dL | 31 g/L |
| Prealbumin | 10 mg/dL | 100 mg/L |

## Assessment

A 34-year-old male with signs, symptoms, and clinical evidence of an intra-abdominal infection secondary to an anterior abdominal wall abscess attributable to the underlying Crohn's disease

---

### Student Workup

**Missing Information?**

**Evaluate:**    Patient Database

Drug Therapy Problems

Care Plan (by Problem)

---

## TARGETED QUESTIONS

1. What characteristics of the patient's case are consistent with a secondary intra-abdominal infection?

   *Hint: See pp. 1347 and 1348 in PPP*

2. On the basis of the patient's history and presentation, should empiric antibiotic treatment cover for a monomicrobial or polymicrobial infection?

   *Hint: See pp. 1349 and 1350 in PPP*

3. What are the likely pathogens on the basis of the patient's site of infection and underlying disease process?

   *Hint: See Table 77-1 in PPP*

4. What intervention is foremost in the management of an intra-abdominal abscess?

   *Hint: See p. 1349 in PPP*

## FOLLOW-UP

Abdominal wall abscess was accessible via percutaneous CT-guided drainage, which was carried out on day 2 of admission. On discharge, IV antimicrobial therapy was continued and radiologic-evaluation follow-up was scheduled at the end of therapy.

5. For how long should the patient be treated? What are some other aspects of care that should be addressed in the patient?

   *Hint: See pp. 1350–1354 in PPP*

## 🌐 GLOBAL PERSPECTIVE

Crohn's disease is becoming increasingly common across the world, but there is a higher incidence in industrialized northern countries, potentially due to environmental factors. Additionally, a bimodal age distribution has been shown in certain European countries and the United States. Of these patients with Crohn's disease, up to 30% may experience an intra-abdominal or pelvic abscess during the course of their illness. Abscess formation in Crohn's disease arises from deep fissuring ulceration associated with the transmural nature of the inflammatory process of Crohn's disease. Surgical drainage followed by resection of the bowel disease was once conventional therapy in these patients; however, current management involves percutaneous drainage with interventional radiologic techniques if the abscess is accessible. Appropriate nutrition and consideration of potential complications such as osteoporosis, which can occur due to malabsorption or long-term corticosteroid therapy, are also important aspects of care.

## CASE SUMMARY

- The patient's current clinical picture is consistent with a secondary intra-abdominal infection in which management should focus primarily on infection source control with abscess drainage.

- Appropriate empiric antibiotic therapy should cover typical organisms inhabiting area, including enteric Gram-negative bacilli and anaerobic pathogens.

- De-escalation of antibiotic therapy should be initiated when a pathogen(s) is identified to avoid overuse of broad-spectrum antibiotics, although anaerobic coverage should be continued regardless of growth on cultures.

**For more information on the care plan and facilitator's guide please visit http://www.mhpharmacotherapy.com.**

# 87 Uncomplicated Urinary Tract Infection

Kathryn R. Matthias

## CASE LEARNING OBJECTIVES

- Recognize the common signs and symptoms of uncomplicated urinary tract infections
- Describe factors that may affect empiric therapy for uncomplicated urinary tract infections
- Develop an appropriate plan for treatment of an uncomplicated urinary tract infection
- Evaluate factors that may decrease risk of recurrent urinary tract infections

## PATIENT PRESENTATION

### Chief Complaint

"I have to go to the bathroom more often and it is getting really annoying."

### History of Present Illness

Elizabeth Wilson is a 26-year-old woman who presents to the emergency department with complaints of increased urinary urgency over the past 4 days. The patient reports that she had been diagnosed with a urinary tract infection at the age of 14 years but has had no other urinary tract issues since that time. The patient states that she heard cranberry juice may help with urinary tract infections (UTIs) and has drank about 10 cups of cranberry juice over the past couple days but her urinary urgency symptoms seem to be getting worse.

### Past Medical History

UTI at age 14 years (treated with trimethoprim–sulfamethoxazole)

History of generalized tonic–clonic seizures (last reported seizure 3.5 years ago)

Hypothyroidism

Seasonal allergies

### Family History

Mother and father are both alive. Father is 49 and has a history of HTN. Mother is also 49 and has a history of hypothyroidism.

### Social History

Patient works currently as a waitress at a local sandwich cafe but does not have health insurance. She is currently single and broke up with her previous boyfriend 2 weeks ago. She denies smoking, alcohol, and intravenous drug abuse.

### Allergies/Intolerances/Adverse Drug Events

Penicillin (unknown reaction)

Valproic acid (rash)

### Medications

Cetirizine 10 mg PO daily PRN seasonal allergies

Levothyroxine 50 mcg PO daily

Phenytoin extended-release 300 mg PO daily

### Review of Systems

Denies chest pain, SOB, abdominal pain; (+) Dysuria; (+) increase in urinary frequency or urgency (every 1–3 hours during the past 2 days)

### Physical Examination

▶ *General*

Well appearing, obese 26-year-old Caucasian woman in no acute distress

▶ **Vital Signs**

BP 122/78 mm Hg, P 72, RR 16, T 38.5°C

Weight 175 lb (80 kg)

Height 61 in. (155 cm)

▶ **Skin**

Dry appearing skin; (–) rashes or lesions

▶ **HEENT**

PERRLA, EOMI; (–) sinus tenderness; TMs appear normal

▶ **Neck and Lymph Nodes**

Thyroid gland symmetrical; (–) nodules; (–) lymphadenopathy

▶ **Chest**

Clear to auscultation

▶ **Cardiovascular**

RRR, normal $S_1$, $S_2$; (–) $S_3$ or $S_4$

▶ **Abdomen**

Not tender; not distended; (–) organomegaly

▶ **Neurology**

Grossly intact; DTRs normal

▶ **Genitourinary**

Normal external genitalia; (–) vaginal discharge; no costovertebral angle tenderness

▶ **Rectal**

No hemorrhoids

## Laboratory Tests

### Urine Cultures

(+) Gram-negative rods—final results pending

|  | Conventional Units | SI Units |
|---|---|---|
| Na | 138 mEq/L | 138 mmol/L |
| K | 4.5 mEq/L | 4.5 mmol/L |
| Cl | 104 mEq/L | 104 mmol/L |
| $CO_2$ | 22 mEq/L | 22 mmol/L |
| BUN | 5 mg/dL | 1.8 mmol/L |
| SCr | 0.6 mg/dL | 53 μmol/L |
| Glu | 70 mg/dL | 3.9 mmol/L |
| WBC | $13.5 \times 10^3$/mm³ | $13.5 \times 10^9$/L |
| TSH | 1.3 μIU/mL | 1.3 mIU/L |

| Phenytoin | 12.1 mg/L | 47.9 μmol/L |
|---|---|---|
| Urinalysis | Urine is yellow, cloudy | |
| pH | 5.2 | |
| Specific gravity | 1.023 | |
| WBC | 28 cells/mm³ | $28 \times 10^6$/L |
| RBC | 3 cells/mm³ | $3 \times 10^6$/L |
| Protein | Trace | |
| Glucose | (–) | |
| Ketones | (–) | |
| Blood | (–) | |
| Nitrite | (–) | |

## Assessment

Twenty-six-year-old woman with s/s and laboratory tests consistent with an uncomplicated UTI

### Student Workup

**Missing Information?**

**Evaluate:** Patient Database

Drug Therapy Problems

Care Plan (by Problem)

## TARGETED QUESTIONS

1. What signs and symptoms of an uncomplicated UTI does the patient have?

   *Hint: See pp. 1372 and 1374 in PPP*

2. What risk factors does the patient have for uncomplicated UTIs?

   *Hint: See p. 1373 in PPP*

3. What treatment options including duration of therapy should be considered in this patient?

   *Hint: See p. 1377 and Tables 79-2 and 79-3 in PPP*

4. What risks and adverse effects of therapy should be discussed with the patient?

   *Hint: Remember to evaluate potential drug–drug interactions with patient's current medication and treatment options. Consider any missing laboratory tests that should be potentially performed prior to start of therapy. See p. 1378 and Table 79-4 in PPP*

5. How would you counsel this patient on the expected benefits of "cranberry juice"?

   *Hint: Is there any proven benefit of cranberry juice for treatment of UTIs. See p. 1374 in PPP*

## FOLLOW-UP

One day later, the patient's urine culture and sensitivity results are reported:

Urine culture: *Escherichia coli*

| Drug | Interpretation | MIC (mcg/mL or mg/L) |
|---|---|---|
| Ampicillin | Susceptible | 4 |
| Ampicillin-sulbactam | Susceptible | ≤8/4 |
| Amoxicillin-clavulanic acid | Susceptible | ≤8/4 |
| Cefazolin | Susceptible | ≤8 |
| Ciprofloxacin | Susceptible | 0.5 |
| Gentamicin | Resistant | >8 |
| Imipenem | Susceptible | ≤0.25 |
| Levofloxacin | Susceptible | ≤2 |
| Nitrofurantoin | Susceptible | ≤32 |
| Tetracycline | Susceptible | ≤4 |
| Trimethoprim/ sulfamethoxazole | Resistant | ≥8/152 |

6. Based on the above culture and susceptibility results along with the patient's clinical status, how would you change the patient's UTI therapy?

   *Hint: See p. 1379 in the Patient Care and Monitoring section in PPP*

## 🌀 GLOBAL PERSPECTIVE

Approximately 130 million to 175 million cases of uncomplicated cystitis due to *E. coli* occur in premenopausal women worldwide every year.[1] In the United States, these infections have been associated with over $1 billion direct (2003 dollars) in health care costs per year plus indirect costs due to an average of 2 restricted-activity days.

Although *E. coli* urinary isolate resistance rates to ampicillin and trimethoprim–sulfamethoxazole have increased over the past couple of decades worldwide based on surveillance reports, fluoroquinolone resistance rates (specifically ciprofloxacin and levofloxacin) have also increased significantly in Europe and Canada in the past decade. Development of such resistance has limited empiric treatment options in certain patient populations.[2,3]

## REFERENCES

1. Russo TA, Johnson JR. Medical and economic impact of extraintestinal infections due to *Escherichia coli*: Focus on an increasingly important endemic problem. Microbes Infect 2003 5:449–456.
2. Oteo J, Pérez-Vázquez M, Campos J. Extended-spectrum beta-lactamase producing *Escherichia coli*: changing epidemiology and clinical impact. Curr Opin Infect Dis 2010 23:320–326.
3. Johnson JR, Johnston B, Calbots C, et al. *Escherichia coli* sequence type ST131 as the major cause of serious multidrug-resistant *E. coli* infections in the United States. Clin Infect Dis 2010 51:286–294.

## CASE SUMMARY

- The patient's signs and symptoms are consistent with an uncomplicated urinary tract infection.
- Although there are several options for empiric uncomplicated urinary tract infection therapy, patient-specific factors including drug allergies, renal function, potential drug–drug interactions, and teratogenicity potential should be evaluated prior to antibiotic selection.
- The patient should be counseled on potential adverse effects of antibiotic therapy.

**For more information on the care plan and facilitator's guide please visit http://www.mhpharmacotherapy.com.**

# 88 Complicated Urinary Tract Infection

Kathryn R. Matthias     John J. Radosevich

## CASE LEARNING OBJECTIVES

- Recognize the common signs and symptoms of complicated urinary tract infections (UTIs)
- Describe factors that may affect empiric therapy for complicated UTIs
- Develop an appropriate plan for treatment of a complicated UTI
- Evaluate factors that may decrease risk of recurrent complicated UTIs

## PATIENT PRESENTATION

### Chief Complaint (from Patient's Wife)

"He is not acting like himself ... he seems really confused."

### History of Present Illness

Joseph Jones is a 74-year-old resident of an assisted-living facility who is transferred to ABC Medical Center due to altered mental status. Initial differential diagnosis includes bacteremia, sepsis from a urinary source, UTI, or meningitis. On the basis of diagnostic studies including a chest x-ray and CT scan along with laboratory data, it is determined that the patient's altered mental status is due to a complicated UTI and dehydration from acute N/V. The patient is started on ciprofloxacin 200 mg IV q12h.

### Past Medical History

History of acute kidney injury, resolved 6 months ago

HTN

### Past Surgical History

Kidney abscess (intrarenal), s/p drainage with pigtail catheter 6 months ago

Right knee surgery in 1974

### Family History

Mother died at the age of 68 and had a past medical history significant for HTN and type 2 diabetes mellitus. Father died at the age of 72 and had a past medical history significant for COPD. Patient has 2 children and 5 grandchildren, none with any significant medical history.

### Social History

Patient and his wife are currently residents of an assisted-living facility. They moved to this facility 4 years ago after his wife's hip replacement. As per the patient's wife, he does not smoke or drink alcohol.

### Allergies/Intolerances/Adverse Drug Events

NKDA

### Medications

Fluoxetine 10 mg PO daily

Esomeprazole 40 mg PO daily

### Review of Systems

(+) Fever; (+) vomiting; (−) eye changes; (−) complaints of chest pain or shortness of breath

### Physical Examination

▶ General

Acutely ill male with decreased level of consciousness who is sleepy but arousable and able to answer yes and no questions

▶ Vital Signs

BP 102/56 mm Hg, P 108, RR 24, T 38.3°C, saturation 100% (1.0) on a nonrebreather mask

Weight 154 lb (70 kg)

Height 69 in. (175 cm)

▶ *Skin*

Dry appearing skin; (−) rashes or lesions

▶ *HEENT*

PERRLA, EOMI, head normocephalic, mucous membranes dry

▶ *Neck and Lymph Nodes*

(−) Nodules; (−) lymphadenopathy

▶ *Chest*

Clear to auscultation bilaterally

▶ *Cardiovascular*

RRR, normal $S_1$, $S_2$; no murmurs

▶ *Abdomen*

Not tender; not distended; (+) bowel sounds

▶ *Neurology*

Patient will open eyes to gentle stimulus; he is able to follow commands and move extremities

▶ *Genitourinary*

Normal external genitalia

▶ *Rectal*

No hemorrhoids

## Laboratory Tests

|  | Conventional Units | SI Units |
|---|---|---|
| Na | 142 mEq/L | 142 mmol/L |
| K | 4.7 mEq/L | 4.7 mmol/L |
| Cl | 108 mEq/L | 108 mmol/L |
| $CO_2$ | 19 mEq/L | 19 mmol/L |
| BUN | 28 mg/dL | 10 mmol/L |
| SCr | 2.4 mg/dL | 212 µmol/L |
| Glu | 140 mg/dL | 7.8 mmol/L |
| Ca | 9.7 mg/dL | 2.43 mmol/L |
| WBC | $3.9 \times 10^3$/mm³ | $3.9 \times 10^9$/L |
| Neutrophils | 78% | 0.78 |
| Bands | 11% | 0.11 |
| Hgb | 12.1 g/dL | 121 g/L; 7.51 mmol/L |
| HCT | 36.9% | 0.369 |
| Platelets | $192 \times 10^3$/mm³ | $192 \times 10^9$/L |
| Urinalysis | Urine is yellow, cloudy |  |
| pH | 5.50 |  |
| Specific gravity | 1.012 |  |

| WBC | > 150 cells/mm³ | $> 150 \times 10^6$/L |
|---|---|---|
| RBC | 48 cells/mm³ | $48 \times 10^6$/L |
| Protein | (+) |  |
| Glucose | (−) |  |
| Ketones | (−) |  |
| Blood | Moderate |  |
| Nitrite | (+) |  |
| Casts | (−) |  |
| Urine toxicology | (−) |  |

### Blood Cultures

(−) No growth

Urine cultures (obtained after placement of a foley catheter):

*Klebsiella pneumoniae* (>100,000 colonies/mL [$>100 \times 10^6$/L])— extended spectrum β-lactamase (ESBL) producing

| Drug | Interpretation | MIC (mcg/mL or mg/L) |
|---|---|---|
| Amikacin | Susceptible | 16 |
| Ampicillin | Resistant | ≥32 |
| Cefepime | Susceptible | 8 |
| Ceftriaxone | Resistant | ≥8 |
| Cephazolin | Resistant | ≥64 |
| Ciprofloxacin | Resistant | ≥4 |
| Gentamicin | Resistant | ≥ 4 |
| Levofloxacin | Resistant | ≥8 |
| Imipenem | Susceptible | ≤1 |
| Meropenem | Susceptible | 1 |
| Nitrofurantoin | Susceptible | ≤32 |
| Piperacillin/tazobactam | Resistant | ≥128/4 |
| Trimethoprim/ sulfamethoxazole | Resistant | ≥16/304 |

### Assessment

Seventy-four-year-old man with s/s and laboratory tests consistent with a complicated UTI

## Student Workup

### Missing Information?

**Evaluate:** Patient Database

Drug Therapy Problems

Care Plan (by Problem)

## TARGETED QUESTIONS

1. What characteristics does the patient have of a complicated UTI?

   *Hint: See pp. 1372 and 1374 in PPP*

2. What risk factors does the patient have for complicated UTI?

   *Hint: See p. 1373 in PPP*

3. On day 2, the patient serum creatinine has decreased to 1.8 mg/dL (159 μmol/L). On the basis of the patient's urine culture and clinical factors, what changes do you recommend to the patient's UTI therapy?

   *Hint: See p. 1377 and Tables 79-2 and 79-3 in PPP*

4. How should the patient be monitored for resolution of infection and ADEs?

   *Hint: See p. 1379 and Table 79-4 in PPP*

5. How long should the patient's UTI therapy be continued?

   *Hint: See p. 1377 and Tables 79-2 and 79-3 in PPP*

## FOLLOW-UP

The patient's UTI symptoms improved and he was discharged from the hospital 4 days after admission. He received his UTI therapy as prescribed through a home health program at his assisted-living facility. Unfortunately, 2 months later he fell and fractured his left hip. An indwelling urinary catheter was inserted and 2 weeks later a urine culture is obtained when the catheter was being exchanged. The culture grew *Enterococcus* species (10,000–100,000 colonies/mL [$10 \times 10^6$–$100 \times 10^6$/L]) and *Candida glabrata* (10,000–50,000 colonies/mL [$10 \times 10^6$–$50 \times 10^6$/L]). The urine sample has a pH 5.50, specific gravity 1.008, WBC 8 cells/mm$^3$ ($8 \times 10^6$/L), RBC 12 cells/mm$^3$ ($12 \times 10^6$/L), protein (+), glucose (–), ketones (–), and nitrite (–).

6. What would be the appropriate therapy for the patient?

   *Hint: See p. 1377 and Tables 79-2 and 79-3 in PPP*

## ☉ GLOBAL PERSPECTIVE

Worldwide the most common cause of nosocomial infection is associated with the use of urinary catheters that lead to UTIs.[1,2] Patients with an indwelling catheter have an estimated daily 5% incidence of UTIs. Therefore, the best way to avoid catheter-associated UTIs is to remove the catheter when no longer indicated as soon as possible based on the patient's clinical status. In addition, catheter-associated UTI has been estimated to cost more than 4 times the cost of symptomatic UTI in a patient without a catheter.[3]

## REFERENCES

1. Hooton TM, Bradley SF, Cardenas DD, et al. Diagnosis, prevention, and treatment of catheter-associated urinary tract infection in adults: 2009 International Clinical Practice Guidelines from the Infectious Diseases Society of America. Clin Infect Dis 2010 50:625–663.
2. Gould CV, Umscheid CA, Agarwal RK, et al. Healthcare Infection Control Practices Advisory Committee: guideline for prevention of catheter-associated urinary tract infections, 2009. www.cdc.gov/hicpac/cauti/001_cauti.html. Accessed April 17, 2013.
3. Saint S. Clinical and economic consequences of nosocomial catheter-related bacteriuria. Am J Infect Control 2000 28:68–75.

## CASE SUMMARY

- The patient's signs and symptoms are consistent with a complicated UTI.
- Although the majority of UTIs are caused by *E. coli*, non-*E. coli* causes are more common in patients with complicated UTIs, patients with recurrent UTIs, and nosocomial UTIs.
- Recommended duration of therapy is usually longer for complicated UTIs and catheter-associated UTIs compared with uncomplicated UTIs.

For more information on the care plan and facilitator's guide please visit http://www.mhpharmacotherapy.com.

## CASE LEARNING OBJECTIVES

- Analyze the behavioral considerations and assess the importance of contraception with regard to the contributing factors
- Apply the "expedited partner treatment" method when recommending treatment
- Identify the patient populations that are epidemiologically affected
- Identify the clinical signs and symptoms associated with tertiary syphilis
- Select an appropriate therapy for the management of syphilitic meningitis
- Develop an appropriate treatment and monitoring plan for the management of syphilitic meningitis

## PATIENT SUMMARY

### Chief Complaint

"I have been feeling very dizzy and have had a severe headache since last night."

### History of Present Illness

A 35-year-old Hispanic female presents to her physician with complaints of a severe headache accompanied by vomiting and dizziness that has been present for 2 days.

### Past Medical History

Syphilis × 3 years

Depression × 5 years

GERD × 1 year

HIV × 1 month

HTN × 2 years

Recurrent yeast infections

### Family History

Father had colon cancer and died at the age of 55. Mother is alive at age 65, with a history of alcoholism and depression. She has two sisters who are alive and healthy.

### Social History

The patient came to the United States from Mexico at the age of 13. She is fluent in both English and Spanish. Currently, she is married and lives with her husband of 5 years; she has one child of age 3. She works at a retail clothing store.

### Tobacco/Alcohol/Substance Abuse

Smokes 1 ppd × 15 years; (−) alcohol; (−) illicit drug use

### Allergies/Intolerances/Adverse Drug Events

Penicillin (anaphylaxis)

### Medications (Current)

Venlafaxine 150 mg PO q 24 h

Yaz 1 tablet PO q 24 h

Lisinopril 40 mg PO q 24 h

Efavirenz 600 mg PO q 24 h at bedtime

Emtricitabine/tenofovir PO q 24 h

St. John's Wort 1 tablet PO daily

Acetaminophen 500 mg PO q 4 h PRN headache

### Medications (Past)

Doxycycline 100 mg PO q 12 h × 14 days for the treatment of syphilis

Miconazole (Monistat-7)

Tioconazole (Vagistat 1)

Fluconazole 150 mg PO × two tablets

### Review of Systems

Headache, not relieved with nonaspirin pain reliever; (−) tinnitus; (+) vertigo; (+) infection; (+) Kernig's sign; (+) Brudzinski's sign; (+) cervical rigidity; (+) photophobia; (−) history of seizures, syncope, or loss of consciousness; A&O × 3; (−) rash; (−) petechiae; (+) hyperpigmentation of palms.

## Physical Examination

### ▶ General

Ill-appearing adult female in acute distress

### ▶ Vital Signs

BP 166/96, P 88, RR 16, T 40°C

Weight 180 lb (82 kg)

Height 60 in. (152 cm)

### ▶ Skin

(−) Rashes; (−) lesions

### ▶ HEENT

PERRLA; EOMI; (−) hemorrhages or papilledema

### ▶ Neck

(+) Cervical rigidity; (−) lymphadenopathy

### ▶ Neurology

(+) Kernig's sign; (+) Brudzinski's sign; A&O × 3

### ▶ Chest

Clear to auscultation

### ▶ Breast

Examination deferred

### ▶ Abdomen

Soft, nontender, nondistended

### ▶ Genitourinary

Examination deferred

### ▶ Rectal

Examination deferred

## Laboratory Tests

|  | Conventional Units | SI Units |
|---|---|---|
| Na | 141 mEq/L | 141 mmol/L |
| K | 4.5 mEq/L | 4.5 mmol/L |
| Cl | 103 mEq/L | 103 mmol/L |
| BUN | 9 mg/dL | 3.2 mmol/L |
| SCr | 0.9 mg/dL | 80 mmol/L |
| Glucose | 99 mg/dL | 5.5 mmol/L |
| Hgb | 13.5 g/dL | 135 g/L; 8.38 mmol/L |
| Hct | 41.2% | 0.412 |
| WBC | $3.5 \times 10^3$/mm³ | $3.5 \times 10^9$/L |
| Lymphocytes | 46.1% | 0.461 |
| Monocytes | 16.5% | 0.165 |
| Eosinophils | 4.2% | 0.042 |
| Basophils | 1% | 0.01 |
| Neutrophils | 32.2% | 0.322 |
| ANC | $1.1 \times 10^3$/mm³ | $1.1 \times 10^9$/L |
| HIV RNA | Nondetectable | |
| CD4 | 360 cells/mm³ | $360 \times 10^6$/L |

## Blood Cultures

No growth

## CSF Findings

|  | Conventional Units | SI Units |
|---|---|---|
| WBC | 100 cells/mm³ | $100 \times 10^6$/L |
| Protein | 68 mg/dL | 680 mg/L |
| Glucose | 35 mg/dL | 1.9 mmol/L |
| Gram stain | Negative | |
| VDRL | 1:32 | |

## Assessment

A 35-year-old female with signs, symptoms, and laboratory tests consistent with syphilitic meningitis

### Student Workup

**Missing Information?**

**Evaluate:**   Patient Database

Drug Therapy Problems

Care Plan (by Problem)

## TARGETED QUESTIONS

1. What is the causative agent associated with syphilis?

   *Hint: See p. 1385 in PPP*

2. What are the clinical signs and symptoms associated with neurosyphilis?

   *Hint: Please refer to CDC Guidelines (2010), Sexually Transmitted Diseases Treatment Guidelines, at http://www.cdc.gov/ std/treatment/2010/genital-ulcers.htm#mansexpart3*

3. Which form of penicillin is recommended for the management of neurosyphilis?

   *Hint: See p. 1389 in PPP*

4. Should the patient's husband be treated for syphilis?

   *Hint: Please refer to CDC Guidelines (2010), Sexually Transmitted Diseases Treatment Guidelines, at http://www.cdc.gov/ std/treatment/2010/genital-ulcers.htm#mansexpart*

5. What monitoring parameters should be implemented in the patient and what are our goals of therapy?

   *Hint: See pp. 1389–1390 in PPP*

## FOLLOW-UP

After having a conversation with the physician, JR's spouse agrees to be tested for syphilis and his VDRL titer returns as 1:32.

6. Her husband shows CSF pleocytosis, what is the recommended therapy?

   *Hint: See pp. 1388–1389 in PPP*

7. Penicillin is recommended for him, what formulation is used? Justify your answer.

   *Hint: See pp. 1388–1389 in PPP*

8. An individual is allergic to penicillin, what would be the appropriate procedure for performing penicillin desensitization?

   *Hint: See pp. 1388–1389 in PPP*

## ☼ GLOBAL PERSPECTIVE

STDs present a major public health concern in both industrialized and developing countries. However, since different countries have different types and levels of reporting systems of STD statistics, it is thought that many reports substantially underestimate the number of new STD cases because of social stigma and other factors prevent people from seeking health care. A WHO report published in 2001 provides estimates of the extent of the world's STD epidemics as they were in 1999, and as of early 2007, there were no more recent international estimates. Syphilis is a bacterial infection that is usually sexually transmitted, but may also be passed from an infected mother to an unborn child. It is a curable STD, which if left untreated, can eventually lead to irreversible damage to the heart and nervous system. An estimated 12.22 million cases of syphilis occurred worldwide in 1999, with an increase in incidence in Eastern Europe and Central Asia, Sub-Saharan Africa, Latin America, and the Caribbean. STDs are a major global cause of acute illness, infertility, long-term disability, and death, with severe medical and psychologic consequences for millions of men, women, and children. The WHO states that, "In developing countries, STDs and their complications are amongst the top five disease categories for which adults seek health care. In women of childbearing age, STDs are second only to maternal factors as causes of disease and death."[1] Many STDs can be treated and cured relatively easily and cheaply if diagnosed early enough. To combat these epidemics, patients must have access to testing and treatment facilities and become more educated about prevention of STDs.

## REFERENCE

1. World Health Organization. Global prevalence and incidence of selected curable sexually transmitted infections overview and estimates. 2001. Accessed at http://www.who.int/hiv/pub/sti/who_hiv_aids_2001.02.pdf on April 17, 2013.

## CASE SUMMARY

- The patient with a history of syphilis is treated previously with doxycycline.
- Her current clinical presentation is consistent with syphilitic meningitis, and appropriate antibiotic therapy should be initiated.
- The patient may need to undergo desensitization due to her history of penicillin allergy.

**For more information on the care plan and facilitator's guide please visit http://www.mhpharmacotherapy.com.**

# 90 Gonorrhea, Chlamydia, and Herpes Simplex

David E. Nix          Patty Ghazvini

Velliyur V. Viswesh

## CASE LEARNING OBJECTIVES

- Recognize the signs and symptoms of gonorrhea, chlamydia, and type 2 herpes simplex
- Identify the pertinent diagnostic techniques and goals of therapy
- Develop an appropriate treatment and monitoring plan for the infection(s)
- Select an appropriate pharmacologic agent to treat the infection(s)
- Educate the patient regarding the administration of medications and the importance of self-care

## PATIENT PRESENTATION

### Chief Complaint

"I have been having pain when I urinate. I tried an over-the-counter drug, but it didn't help. I just can't take it anymore. And please don't forget to refill all of my narcotics. Last time, the nurse only called in one of them."

### History of Present Illness

Carmen Rodriguez is a 47-year-old Latin American female who regularly visits the local community health center for a myriad of health reasons, with the latest visit revolving around complaints of a purulent, vaginal discharge and pain on urination. After self-testing with an OTC urinary tract infection testing kit and detecting a positive result, she subsequently began orally taking phenazopyridine for 4 days with minimal relief. She admits that her dysuric symptoms commenced approximately 10 days prior and have worsened over the past 2 days. Additionally, she admits to observing a cluster of small, painful, itchy bumps in her vaginal area. When asked by the clinician to describe her recent sexual history, she acknowledged that she does not have a steady boyfriend and that she currently engages in frequent sexual activity with 2 men, one of which she traveled to Hawaii with last week for vacation. Finally, as she requested a refill on her narcotics and her BP, cholesterol, and diabetic medications, she divulged that she felt "tingling" in her hands and feet and that she has been constipated for 3 days although she has been taking docusate sodium for 2 consecutive days.

### Past Medical History

HTN diagnosed 7 years ago

Type 2 DM diagnosed 5 years ago

Hyperlipidemia diagnosed 1 year ago

Back pain from car accident that occurred 3 months ago

### Family History

The patient's father had CAD and died of an MI at age 70. Her mother is alive at age 64 with HTN, diabetes, and osteoporosis. She has 2 sisters, one of whom was recently diagnosed with diabetes.

### Social History

The patient migrated to the United States at age 16 from Mexico. She speaks fluent Spanish and English, and is a single mother, who lives alone with one son, age 20, from a previous marriage. As a result of the recession, her original job as a receptionist for a car dealership was terminated 4 months ago. She was recently hired (3 weeks prior to her visit) as a receptionist for a prominent law firm.

### Tobacco/Alcohol/Substance Abuse

Social drinker; (−) tobacco or illicit drug use

### Allergies/Intolerances/Adverse Drug Events

Tetracycline (rash as a child)

Propoxyphene (rash)

## Medications

Glyburide 2.5 mg PO q AM

HCTZ 12.5 mg PO q AM

Amlodipine 2.5 mg PO q AM

Atorvastatin 40 mg PO q AM

Calcium carbonate one to two tablets PO q 8–12 h PRN

Docusate sodium 100 mg PO q AM

Hydrocodone 7.5 mg/acetaminophen 750 mg 1–2 tablets PO q 4–6 h PRN pain

Oxycodone 5 mg/acetaminophen 500 mg 2 tablets PO q 4–6 h PRN severe pain

Acetaminophen 325 mg 1–2 capsules PO q 4–6 h PRN pain

## Review of Systems

Occasional headaches relieved by acetaminophen; (–) fever; (–) tinnitus and vertigo; increased urinary frequency with pain; (+) bowel distention on palpation; (–) history of seizures, syncope, or loss of consciousness; reports "tingling" in the extremities; (–) muscle pain; dry mucus membranes; deep and rapid breathing.

## Physical Examination

### ▶ General

Overweight, middle-aged, Latin American woman in no acute distress

### ▶ Vital Signs

BP 150/97 mm Hg, P 74, RR 22, T 37.2°C (99.0°F)

Weight 215 lb (97.7 kg)

Height 66 in. (168 cm)

### ▶ Skin

Skin slightly dry; (–) rash or lesions

### ▶ HEENT

PERRLA; EOMI; TMs appear normal

### ▶ Neck and Lymph Nodes

Thyroid gland smooth and symmetrical; (–) thyroid nodules; (+) lymphadenopathy

### ▶ Chest

Clear to auscultation

### ▶ Breasts

Examination deferred

### ▶ Cardiovascular

RRR, normal $S_1$, $S_2$; (–) $S_3$ or $S_4$

### ▶ Abdomen

Non-tender/distended; (–) organomegaly

### ▶ Neurology

Grossly intact; deep tendon reflexes normal

### ▶ Genitourinary

Cluster of vesicles; (+) vaginal discharge

### ▶ Rectal

Examination deferred

## Laboratory Tests

### Fasting Obtained 3 Months Ago

|  | Conventional Units | SI Units |
|---|---|---|
| Na | 139 mEq/L | 139 mmol/L |
| K | 4.4 mEq/L | 4.4 mmol/L |
| Cl | 103 mEq/L | 103 mmol/L |
| $CO_2$ | 22 mEq/L | 22 mmol/L |
| BUN | 12 mg/dL | 4.3 mmol/L |
| SCr | 0.9 mg/dL | 80 mmol/L |
| Glu | 135 mg/dL | 7.5 mmol/L |
| Ca | 10.1 mg/dL | 2.53 mmol/L |
| Mg | 1.7 mEq/L | 0.85 mmol/L |
| Phosphate | 3.7 mg/dL | 1.20 mmol/L |
| pH (arterial) | 7.38 | |
| Hgb | 13 g/dL | 130 g/L; 8.07 mmol/L |
| Hct | 41% | 0.41 |
| WBC | $4.1 \times 10^3/mm^3$ | $4.1 \times 10^9/L$ |
| MCV | 89 um$^3$ | 89 fL |
| Albumin | 3.9 g/dL | 39 g/L |
| Total cholesterol | 183 mg/dL | 4.73 mmol/L |
| LDL cholesterol | 91 mg/dL | 2.35 mmol/L |
| HDL cholesterol | 36 mg/dL | 0.93 mmol/L |
| AST | 45 IU/L | 0.75 μkat/L |
| ALT | 51 IU/L | 0.85 μkat/L |
| $HbA_{1c}$ | 6.9% | 0.069 (52 mmol/mol Hgb) |

### Fasting Obtained Yesterday

|  | Conventional Units | SI Units |
|---|---|---|
| Na | 135 mEq/L | 135 mmol/L |
| K | 3.5 mEq/L | 3.5 mmol/L |
| Cl | 107 mEq/L | 107 mmol/L |
| $CO_2$ | 23 mEq/L | 23 mmol/L |
| BUN | 40 mg/dL | 14.3 mmol/L |
| SCr | 1.3 mg/dL | 115 mmol/L |

| | | |
|---|---|---|
| Glu | 180 mg/dL | 10 mmol/L |
| Ca | 10.1 mg/dL | 2.53 mmol/L |
| Mg | 1.8 mEq/L | 0.90 mmol/L |
| Phosphate | 3.8 mg/dL | 1.23 mmol/L |
| pH (arterial) | 7.41 | |
| Urinalysis | (+) ketones | |
| Hgb | 14 g/dL | 140 g/L; 8.69 mmol/L |
| Hct | 42% | 0.42 |
| WBC | $10.7 \times 10^3/mm^3$ | $10.7 \times 10^9/L$ |
| MCV | $88 \, \mu m^3$ | 88 fL |
| Albumin | 3.7 g/dL | 37 g/L |
| Total cholesterol | 185 mg/dL | 4.78 mmol/L |
| LDL cholesterol | 92 mg/dL | 2.38 mmol/L |
| HDL cholesterol | 34 mg/dL | 0.88 mmol/L |
| AST | 120 IU/L | 2.00 µkat/L |
| ALT | 130 IU/L | 2.17 µkat/L |
| HbA$_{1c}$ | 10% | 0.10 |

▶ *Urine Culture*

Gram stain shows many Gram-negative diplococci (some intracellular). *Chlamydia trachomatis* and *Neisseria gonorrhoeae* nucleic acid identification testing ordered for confirmation.

## Assessment

A 47-year-old woman with signs and symptoms consistent with a gonococcal infection.

Further, the patient has constipation and uncontrolled HTN and diabetes.

### Student Workup

**Missing Information?**

**Evaluate:**    Patient Database

Drug Therapy Problems

Care Plan (by Problem)

## TARGETED QUESTIONS

1. What are the signs and symptoms of a gonococcal infection?

   *Hint: See p. 1383 in PPP*

2. Are there any other possible infections besides gonorrhea?

   *Hint: See p. 1383 in PPP*

3. When infected with gonorrhea, what is the probability of a coinfection?

   *Hint: See p. 1383 in PPP*

4. What would be the recommended drug therapy for gonococcal infections in patients with anaphylaxis to cephalosporins?

   *Hint: See p.1384 in PPP*

5. Should treatment be provided for her partner?

   *Hint: See p.1383–1384 in PPP*

6. What is the etiology of the elevated hepatic enzymes?

   *Hint: Liver enzymes may be elevated for a variety of reasons. Since the patient's past medical history is inconsistent with hepatic damage, a medication-induced elevation of liver enzymes is a reasonable suspicion. Testing for Hepatitis B and C should be considered. See p. 1384 in PPP*

## FOLLOW-UP

Twelve weeks later, the patient returns for a follow-up. Although reevaluation of her infection is not required, it is vital to express the importance of altering her sexual behaviors and reiterate the importance of practicing preventive measures (e.g., condoms, spermicides) and to determine whether her partners have received treatment. Essential to this process is an interaction between the patient and a knowledgeable, yet patient-friendly, clinician.

7. How can this be accomplished?

   *Hint: See p.1398–1399 in PPP*

Finally, the clinician and the patient must gain control of her HTN and diabetes by promoting a healthy diet, exercise, and continuous self-monitoring; effectively altering her medications to achieve optimal BP and glucose measurements; and scheduling the patient for education classes on diabetes.

## ⟳ GLOBAL PERSPECTIVE

Globally, new cases of STDs amenable to antimicrobial treatment amount to approximately 340 million per year. Evidence supports the need for better control of gonorrhea, especially with the emergence of fluoroquinolone-resistant strains of *N. gonorrhoeae*. Such strains have been documented in several other countries, including Australia, China, India, Korea, and New Zealand. Another notable concern is the appearance of diminished gonococcal susceptibility to the third-generation cephalosporins, of which cefixime and ceftriaxone are commonly prescribed as effective options. In the United States, cefixime is no longer recommended as a first-line treatment without follow-up test of cure. Once 5% resistance or more to an antibiotic is recognized, the WHO recommends that the antibiotic be removed from the treatment recommendations for gonorrhea. Diminished susceptibility of *N. gonorrhoeae* to drugs of choice has been attributed to the overuse and misuse of antibiotics in a nonregulated environment. Although instituting change may be complex, global integration of treatment measures may be more feasible than continuing to rely on antibiotics as the primary mechanism of control.

## CASE SUMMARY

- Her clinical picture is consistent with a gonococcal infection and with herpes simplex type 2. Patient counseling and effective treatment measures are necessary. In addition to covering the primary organisms, treatment should also cover *Chlamydia trachomatis,* which is commonly present as a co-infection.

- Ceftriaxone 250 mg IM and azithromycin 1 g PO as a one-time dose is reasonable for the coverage of gonorrhea and chlamydia. Fluoroquinolones and oral cefixime are no longer recommended by the CDC guidelines for the treatment of gonococcal infections.

- Valacyclovir 1 g orally once daily for 7 days is appropriate for the initial treatment of herpes simplex.

- Expedited partner treatment should be instituted in this case.

**For more information on the care plan and facilitator's guide please visit http://www.mhpharmacotherapy.com.**

# 91 Acute Osteomyelitis

Melinda M. Neuhauser     Susan L. Pendland

## CASE LEARNING OBJECTIVES

- Identify the goals of therapy for acute osteomyelitis
- Identify the clinical signs, symptoms, laboratory, and imaging tests in the diagnosis and therapeutic monitoring of acute osteomyelitis
- Develop an appropriate treatment and monitoring plan for acute osteomyelitis
- Educate the patient regarding disease state and drug therapy

## PATIENT PRESENTATION

### Chief Complaint

"I have severe pain in my left arm, which was broken in a car accident last week. I've taken a few pain pills since then, but now it really hurts. Maybe I need a stronger pain pill."

### History of Present Illness

SC is a 19-year-old Caucasian male who presented to the emergency department complaining of severe pain in his left upper arm. He was involved in a car accident 7 days ago and had an open fracture of the left proximal humerus. At that time, he was admitted to the hospital for surgery. He received pre- and postoperative cefazolin, and was discharged after overnight observation on an oral antibiotic and PRN pain medications. At the time of discharge, the patient showed no signs of infection and required only occasional hydrocodone/acetaminophen for pain. He was scheduled for a follow-up office visit with the orthopedic surgeon in 1 week.

### Past Medical History

Asthma, diagnosed in childhood
Allergic rhinitis, diagnosed in childhood

### Family History

Father is 46 years old with type 2 DM and HTN, whereas mother is 43 years old with asthma. He has a younger sister in high school. Both sets of grandparents are alive.

### Social History

The patient graduated from high school and currently attends community college. He lives with his parents and maintains a part-time job at a movie theater. His health insurance is covered under his father's insurance plan.

### Tobacco/Alcohol/Substance Use

Occasionally drinks beer; denies tobacco and illicit drug use

### Allergies/Intolerance/Adverse Drug Events

Benadryl causes him to be "jittery."

### Medications (Current)

Cephalexin 500 mg 1 capsule PO q 6 h for 7 days

Ibuprofen 400 mg 1 tablet PO q 6 h PRN mild-to-moderate arm pain

Hydrocodone/acetaminophen 5/325 mg 1 tablet PO q 4 h PRN severe arm pain

Fluticasone/salmeterol 250/50 mcg 1 puff twice daily

Albuterol 1–2 puffs q 4 h PRN wheezing (needs refill)

Loratadine 10 mg 1 tablet PO once daily

Fluticasone intranasal spray 2 puffs each nostril once daily PRN allergies

Acetaminophen 325 mg 1–2 tablets PO PRN headaches

The views expressed in this article are those of the authors and do not necessarily reflect the position or policy of the Department of Veterans Affairs or the United States government.

## Review of Systems

The patient experiences frequent headaches usually relieved with acetaminophen, although he admits that he also uses some "sinus medication" that his grandparents bought at a supermarket; he reports that his breathing is fine now, although he has had several hospital visits for asthma in the past year, for which he received steroids and nebulizer treatments. He has noticed that his breathing and allergies worsen when he spends a lot of time with his friends who smoke. He thought his arm had been getting better and attributed the recent severe pain to not keeping the arm immobile after going back to work.

## Physical Examination

▶ *General*

Young adult male with arm in sling and experiencing acute pain in recently fractured arm

▶ *Vital Signs*

BP 117/76 mm Hg, P 85, RR 16, T 37.9°C

Weight 162.8 lb (74 kg)

Height 69 in. (175.3 cm)

Reports acute pain in fractured arm (pain 6/10)

▶ *Skin*

Swelling and erythema around the surgical wound

▶ *HEENT*

Swollen nasal mucosa; rhinorrhea

▶ *Neck and Lymph Nodes*

(−) Lymphadenopathy

▶ *Chest*

Mild expiratory wheezing on auscultation

▶ *Cardiovascular*

RRR, normal $S_1$, $S_2$; (−) $S_3$ or $S_4$

▶ *Abdomen*

Not tender/not distended

▶ *Neurology*

Grossly intact; deep tendon reflexes normal

▶ *Genitourinary*

Examination deferred

▶ *Rectal*

Examination deferred

## Laboratory Tests

### Obtained Today in Emergency Department

|  | Conventional Units | SI Units |
|---|---|---|
| Na | 141 mEq/L | 141 mmol/L |
| K | 3.9 mEq/L | 3.9 mmol/L |
| Cl | 101 mEq/L | 101 mmol/L |
| $CO_2$ | 25 mEq/L | 25 mmol/L |
| BUN | 5 mg/dL | 1.8 mmol/L |
| SCr | 0.5 mg/dL | 44 μmol/L |
| Glu | 105 mg/dL | 5.8 mmol/L |
| Hgb | 15 g/dL | 150 g/L; 9.31 mmol/L |
| Hct | 43.7% | 0.437 |
| WBC | $12.1 \times 10^3/mm^3$ | $12.1 \times 10^9/L$ |
| ESR | 119 mm/h | 33.1 μm/s |
| CRP | 68 mg/dL | 680 mg/L |

## Microbiology

*Blood culture (× 2):* Pending

*Bone biopsy:* Gram stain shows Gram-positive cocci in clusters; culture pending

## Imaging

▶ *Magnetic resonance imaging (MRI)*

Positive for increased uptake in left proximal humerus

## Assessment

An 18-year-old male with signs, symptoms, and laboratory and imaging tests consistent with acute osteomyelitis

---

**Student Workup**

**Missing Information?**

**Evaluate:**  Patient Database

Drug Therapy Problems

Care Plan (by Problem)

---

## TARGETED QUESTIONS

1. What antimicrobial agent(s), dosage regimen, and monitoring would you recommend for this patient?

   *Hint: See pp. 1405–1407 in PPP*

2. What duration of antimicrobial therapy do you anticipate for this patient?

   *Hint: See p. 1405 in PPP*

3. Is this patient an appropriate candidate for step-down oral therapy?

   *Hint: See p. 1405 in PPP*

4. What counseling topics would you discuss with this patient?

   *Hint: See p. 1408 in PPP*

## FOLLOW-UP

The patient was started on an IV antimicrobial regimen through an outpatient infusion center. The bone aspirate grew *Staphylococcus aureus* (resistant to penicillin, oxacillin, cefazolin, clindamycin, erythromycin; sensitive to vancomycin, tetracycline, trimethoprim/sulfamethoxazole). Blood cultures were negative with no growth × 5 days. Following 1 week of therapy, he reports only minimal pain associated with extension of the arm that is necessary with certain daily functions (e.g., getting dressed). Laboratory tests were drawn yesterday.

Please answer the following question with the assumption that the patient was started on IV vancomycin twice daily through an outpatient infusion center:

5. What, if any, modifications would you recommend regarding this patient's drug therapy if the vancomycin steady-state trough concentration was 10.5 mcg/mL (7.2 µmol/L)? Assume that renal function is stable, and a slight decline in ESR and CRP was observed following 1 week of IV therapy.

   *Hint: See p. 1407 and Table 81-2 in PPP*

Please answer the following question with the assumption that the patient successfully completed 4 weeks of IV antibiotic therapy:

6. The physician is considering completing the course of treatment with oral therapy. What oral antimicrobial agents(s) would you recommend for this patient?

   *Hint: See p. 1405 and Table 81-1 in PPP*

## ⟳ GLOBAL PERSPECTIVE

Acute osteomyelitis affects patients, particularly pediatrics, throughout the world. In developing countries, the diagnosis of acute osteomyelitis may be more challenging with limited access to advanced imaging studies (e.g., MRI). Antimicrobial therapy may differ globally on the basis of local or regional susceptibility patterns, access to hospitals or infusion centers, drug availability and cost.

## CASE SUMMARY

- His clinical picture and diagnostic tests are consistent with acute osteomyelitis secondary to direct trauma.
- IV antimicrobial therapy should be initiated on the basis of suspected etiologic organism(s) with definitive therapy per microbiology culture and susceptibilities results.
- An optimal dosage regimen should be utilized to obtain drug concentrations at the site of infection as well as effectiveness and safety parameters should be monitored to guide therapy.

For more information on the care plan and facilitator's guide please visit http://www.mhpharmacotherapy.com.

# 92 Sepsis

Sara A. Stahle          Brian L. Erstad

## CASE LEARNING OBJECTIVES

- Recognize the signs and symptoms of systemic inflammatory response syndrome (SIRS), sepsis, and severe sepsis
- Identify the initial goals of therapy for the treatment of patients with sepsis
- Devise an appropriate initial treatment plan, including fluid resuscitation and antibiotics, on the basis of patient characteristics and circumstances surrounding the patient's presentation
- Formulate a monitoring plan for the initial treatment while considering chosen therapies
- Determine the appropriateness of additional pharmacologic therapies for sepsis, including vasoactive agents and corticosteroids, as well as adjunctive therapies

## PATIENT PRESENTATION

### Chief Complaint

"My father is confused and not responding to me. He looks pale and fatigued."

### History of Present Illness

James Stallings is an 84-year-old male who was brought to the emergency department via emergency medical services (EMS) after his daughter found him sitting on the floor of his kitchen. She visits him at home twice a week to help him with his medications and other chores around the house, but he is normally very independent in his ADL despite having a stroke within the past year. She says that he has some small memory deficits post-stroke, but his current mental status is much more altered than his baseline. The last time she checked on him was 3 days ago when she took him to his primary care physician (PCP) for evaluation of a respiratory infection and an INR check. At that time, he was prescribed a course of antibiotics. She believes that he is compliant with his medications since she puts them in a pillbox for him and the medications are always gone when she returns. The EMS medic reports that the patient was hypotensive on arrival with SBPs in the 90s mm Hg and was subsequently given a 500-mL bolus of 0.9% sodium chloride en route to the emergency department. The medic also states that the patient would only intermittently answer questions, and was not aware of his current situation.

### Past Medical History

BPH × 7 years
Type 2 DM × 9 months
HTN × 35 years

AF × 2 years
Cerebral vascular accident diagnosed 7 months ago
Depression × 4 years

### Family History

Father died of a CVA at age 89. Mother died of bladder cancer at age 90. He has 2 brothers, one of which died at age 65 due to lung cancer and one alive at age 89 with a medical history that includes HTN, AF, and Parkinson's disease. He has 2 daughters, who are both alive and healthy.

### Social History

Retired US Air Force and commercial airline pilot. Has lived alone since his wife passed away at age 80 due to colon cancer. Has 2 daughters, ages 57 and 54, 5 grandchildren, and 2 great-grandchildren.

### Tobacco/Alcohol/Substance Use

Remote smoking history when he was in the US Air Force (approximately 50–60 years ago). Drinks an occasional beer socially. No history of illicit substance use

### Allergies/Intolerances/Adverse Drug Events

Codeine (nausea)
Ramipril (cough)

### Medications (Current)

Metformin 850 mg PO bid
Losartan 25 mg PO daily

Metoprolol succinate 50 mg PO daily

Sertraline 100 mg PO daily

Finasteride 5 mg PO daily

Terazosin 5 mg PO q hs

Warfarin 5 mg PO on Monday, Wednesday, and Friday;
   7.5 mg PO on Tuesday, Thursday, Saturday, and Sunday

Doxycycline 100 mg PO BID (prescribed 3 days ago by PCP)

## Review of Systems

Unable to obtain secondary to the patient's current neurologic status. APACHE II score is 27. Glasgow Coma Score is 11.

## Physical Examination

### ▶ General

Ill-appearing, elderly Caucasian male who is minimally responsive and communicative

### ▶ Vital Signs

BP 82/54 mm Hg, P 129, RR 26, T 39.5°C

Weight 172 lb (78 kg)

Height 70 in. (178cm)

### ▶ Skin

Cold; (–) erythema; (–) rash

### ▶ HEENT

Scleral icterus; dry mucus membranes; pinpoint pupils

### ▶ Neck and Lymph Nodes

Minimal JVD; no nodules; minimal lymphadenopathy

### ▶ Chest

Decreased breath sounds; wheezes and crackles bilaterally

### ▶ Cardiovascular

Sinus tachycardia; (–) M/R/G; (–) bruits; (+) femoral and pedal pulses

### ▶ Abdomen

Nontender, nondistended; (–) hepatosplenomegaly; (–) ascites

### ▶ Neurology

Unresponsive; obtunded

### ▶ Genitourinary

Mildly enlarged prostate

### ▶ Rectal

Decreased tone; (–) bright red blood per rectum (BRBPR)

## Laboratory Tests

|  | Conventional Units | SI Units |
|---|---|---|
| Na | 134 mEq/L | 134 mmol/L |
| K | 4.9 mEq/L | 4.9 mmol/L |
| Cl | 108 mEq/L | 108 mmol/L |
| $CO_2$ | 18 mEq/L | 18 mmol/L |
| BUN | 45 mg/dL | 16.1 mmol/L |
| SCr | 2.6 mg/dL | 230 μmol/L |
| Glucose | 205 mg/dL | 11.4 mmol/L |
| Ca | 7.7 mg/dL | 1.93 mmol/L |
| Mg | 2.2 mEq/L | 1.10 mmol/L |
| Phosphate | 2.4 mg/dL | 0.78 mmol/L |
| ABG |  |  |
| pH | 7.26 |  |
| $pCO_2$ | 25 mm Hg | 3.3 kPa |
| $pO_2$ | 90 mm Hg | 12.0 kPa |
| Hgb | 11.2 g/dL | 112 g/dL; 6.95 mmol/L |
| Hct | 35.4% | 0.354 |
| WBC | $19.8 \times 10^3/\mu L$ | $19.8 \times 10^9/L$ |
| Platelets | $303 \times 10^3/\mu L$ | $303 \times 10^9/L$ |
| PT | 37.5 s |  |
| INR | 3.6 |  |

## Assessment

An 84-year-old man with vital signs, physical examination, and laboratory tests consistent with sepsis

---

**Student Workup**

**Missing Information?**

**Evaluate:**    Patient Database

Drug Therapy Problems

Care Plan (by Problem)

---

## TARGETED QUESTIONS

1. What signs and symptoms of sepsis does this patient have?

   *Hint: See p. 1413 in PPP*

2. What potential pathogens should empiric antimicrobial therapy cover?

   *Hint: See Table 82-2 and p. 1412 in PPP*

3. What initial choice of IV fluids would be appropriate for this patient?

   *Hint: See p. 1416 in PPP*

4. What monitoring parameters should be utilized to determine if this patient is responding to initial therapy?

   *Hint: See pp. 1415–1417 in PPP*

5. Which vasoactive agent(s) would be an appropriate choice in this patient and why?

   *Hint: See p. 1420 in PPP*

## FOLLOW-UP

After receiving numerous fluid boluses with IV crystalloid therapy, as well as initiation of norepinephrine (current rate is 15 mcg/min) and vasopressin (current rate is 0.04 units/min), the patient remains hypotensive and tachycardic (BP 87/60 mm Hg; HR 130). The patient is now intubated and his mental status has not improved. Cultures have been sent to the laboratory and are pending. The medical resident asks you if any other therapy can be initiated in this patient.

6. Provide rationale for initiating steroids in this patient and devise an appropriate regimen.

   *Hint: See pp. 1420–1421 in PPP*

## GLOBAL PERSPECTIVE

Global treatment of sepsis and septic shock has been a topic of particular interest as of late with the prevalence of sepsis and the varying clinical approach to treatment. Initial results from the PROGRESS registry, which was designed to collect data that describe the management and outcomes of severe sepsis worldwide, detail the variability in mortality rate and use of treatment modalities.[1] Of participating countries and institutions, the highest overall hospital mortality rate was seen in Brazil (67.4%), whereas the lowest hospital mortality rate was seen in Australia (32.6%). Use of standard therapies such as antibiotics, mechanical ventilation, fluid resuscitation, and vasopressors was relatively consistent across participating institutions. There was relatively high usage of anticoagulants for venous thromboembolism prophylaxis, an increasing use of low-dose steroids, and a low usage of drotrecogin alfa (no longer marketed in the US) overall. Marked differences were seen in the choice of adjunctive therapies in specific countries, such as increased parenteral nutrition utilization in Germany and increased use of albumin for fluid resuscitation in Australia, India, and Malaysia. Initiation of programs such as PROGRESS will hopefully increase the global awareness of sepsis, provide data regarding the treatment and outcomes associated with sepsis, and contribute to improved outcomes in the treatment of patients with sepsis worldwide.

## REFERENCE

1. Beale R, Reinhart K, Brunkhorst FM, Dobb G, Levy M, Martin G, et al. Promoting global research excellence in severe sepsis (PROGRESS): lessons from an international sepsis registry. Infection 2009 37:222–232.

## CASE SUMMARY

- The patient's acute clinical picture is consistent with sepsis, likely due to an infectious process.
- Initial treatment of sepsis should include aggressive IV fluid resuscitation with crystalloids and/or colloids, as well as broad-spectrum antibiotic therapy targeted toward suspected sources of infection.
- Vasoactive agents should be initiated if initial fluid resuscitation is inadequate to reach a sufficient MAP.
- Adrenal insufficiency should be suspected in patients with an inadequate response to fluid resuscitation and vasopressor therapy, which should prompt initiation of hydrocortisone therapy.

For more information on the care plan and facilitator's guide please visit http://www.mhpharmacotherapy.com.

# 93 Dermatophytosis

Lauren S. Schlesselman

## CASE LEARNING OBJECTIVES

- Recognize the signs and symptoms of tinea pedis and tinea cruris
- Identify the goals of therapy for tinea pedis and tinea cruris
- Develop an appropriate treatment and monitoring plan for tinea pedis and tinea cruris on the basis of individual patient characteristics
- Select an appropriate product for tinea pedis and tinea cruris therapy
- Properly educate a patient receiving tinea pedis and tinea cruris therapy

## PATIENT PRESENTATION

### Chief Complaint

"I have an itchy rash in my groin area. It looks like little red rings. By the way, I don't know if it is related but I have something similar on my feet … but I can't imagine why my feet and jock area would have the same rash. I have been rubbing petroleum jelly on the area, thinking that it might be chafing."

### History of Present Illness

Edward Jacoby is a 26-year-old man who presents to the physician's clinic complaining of severe inguinal itching and soreness, accompanied by a red ring-shaped rash. Thinking that the rash may be due to chafing, he has been applying petroleum jelly to the area. He is an otherwise healthy male who has never been to the clinic before today. Other than petroleum jelly for prevention of chafing, he has not tried any over-the-counter products for the rash. He also expresses concern about the presence of a similar red, itchy rash on his feet.

### Past Medical History

No significant medical history

### Family History

Father is alive at age 50 with no significant medical history. Mother is alive at age 48 and has HTN. He has 1 sister who is 24 years old with no significant medical history.

### Social History

Single and lives with a roommate; has no children. Employed as a physical trainer at a local gym.

### Tobacco/Alcohol/Substance Use

Denies alcohol, tobacco, or illicit drug use

### Allergies/Intolerances/Adverse Drug Events

No known drug allergies

### Medications

No current oral medications

Petroleum jelly to groin area PRN

### Review of Systems

▶ **General**

Healthy and fit-appearing, Caucasian man in no acute distress

▶ **Vital Signs**

BP 115/65 mm Hg, P 60, RR 12, T 36.2°C

Weight 180 lb (81.8kg)

Height 72 in. (183 cm)

Denies pain

▶ **Skin**

Follicular papules and pustules on medial thigh and inguinal folds; fissures and maceration present between toes

▶ **HEENT**

PERRLA, EOMI; (−) sinus tenderness; TMs appear normal

▶ **Neck and Lymph Nodes**

Thyroid gland symmetrical; (−) nodules; (−) lymphadenopathy; (−) carotid bruits

▶ *Chest*

Clear to auscultation

▶ *Cardiovascular*

RRR, normal $S_1$, $S_2$; (−) $S_3$ or $S_4$

▶ *Abdomen*

Not tender; not distended; (−) organomegaly

▶ *Neurology*

Grossly intact; deep tendon reflexes normal

▶ *Genitourinary*

Follicular papules and pustules on medial thigh and inguinal folds

▶ *Rectal*

Examination deferred

## Laboratory Tests

|  | Conventional Units | SI Units |
|---|---|---|
| Na | 140 mEq/L | 140 mmol/L |
| K | 3.7 mEq/L | 3.7 mmol/L |
| Cl | 98 mEq/L | 98 mmol/L |
| $CO_2$ | 24 mEq/L | 24 mmol/L |
| BUN | 12 mg/dL | 4.3 mmol/L |
| SCr | 0.7 mg/dL | 62 mmol/L |
| Glu | 105 mg/dL | 5.8 mmol/L |

## Assessment

A 26-year-old man with signs and symptoms consistent with tinea pedis and tinea cruris

### Student Workup

**Missing Information?**

**Evaluate:**     Patient Database

Drug Therapy Problems

Care Plan (by Problem)

## TARGETED QUESTIONS

1. What signs and symptoms of tinea pedia and tinea cruris does the patient have?

    *Hint: See p. 1433 and Table 83-5 in PPP*

2. What treatment options are available for treating tinea pedis and tinea cruris?

    *Hint: See p. 1435 and Table 83-6 in PPP*

3. What risk factors does the patient have for tinea pedia and tinea cruris?

    *Hint: See p. 1435 and Table 83-5 in PPP*

4. What adverse effects of therapy would you discuss with the patient?

    *Hint: See p. 1437 in PPP*

## FOLLOW-UP

5. What nonpharmacologic treatment options should be recommended to the patient?

    *Hint: See p. 1435 in PPP*

6. Would the treatment plan change if the infection site was significantly inflamed and macerated?

    *Hint: See pp. 1435–1436 and Table 83-6 in PPP*

7. How would hyperkeratosis of the site alter the treatment plan?

    *Hint: See pp. 1435–1436 and Table 83-6 in PPP*

### ⊙ GLOBAL PERSPECTIVE

Mycotic infections of the skin, hair, and nails are superficial fungal infections in which the pathogen remains within the keratinous layers. These infections, typically named for the affected body part, are commonly referred to as ringworm due to the characteristic circular lesions, although they can vary from rings to scales to lesions. Tinea infections are second only to acne in frequency of reported skin disease. They are primarily caused by dermatophytes such as *Trichophyton*, *Microsporum*, and *Epidermophyton* species.

### CASE SUMMARY

- His current clinical picture is consistent with tinea pedis and tinea cruris. Antifungal therapy should be initiated.

- For the treatment of tinea pedis, clotrimazole, tolnaftate, or terbinafine cream applied 1–2 times daily for 4 weeks is recommended.

- For the treatment of tinea cruris, clotrimazole or terbinafine cream or solution applied 1–2 times daily for 2 weeks is recommended.

- Treatment should be continued at least 1 week after resolution of symptoms.

- Systemic therapy should be reserved for refractory cases or widespread lesions.

For more information on the care plan and facilitator's guide please visit http://www.mhpharmacotherapy.com.

# 94 Candida Vaginitis

Lauren S. Schlesselman

## CASE LEARNING OBJECTIVES

- Recognize the signs and symptoms of vaginal candidiasis
- Identify the goals of therapy for vaginal candidiasis
- Develop an appropriate treatment and monitoring plan for vaginal candidiasis on the basis of individual patient characteristics
- Select an appropriate product for vaginal candidiasis therapy
- Properly educate a patient receiving vaginal candidiasis therapy

## PATIENT PRESENTATION

### Chief Complaint

"My private area is really itchy and sore. I think I have another one of those infections."

### History of Present Illness

Lilly Hayes is a 39-year-old woman who presents to the physician's clinic complaining of severe vaginal itching and soreness, accompanied by a thick vaginal discharge. Her first visit to the clinic was 4 days earlier for an *Escherichia coli* UTI. For the UTI, she was prescribed ciprofloxacin 250 mg twice daily for 3 days. After initiating the antibiotic therapy, the patient noted the development of the vaginal discharge, followed by vaginal itching and soreness. Although records are not currently available from her previous physician, the patient reports a history of recurrent vaginal candidiasis, including five episodes in the last year (excluding this episode). She expresses frustration with the repeated infections, especially since she cannot afford over-the-counter medications and therefore must make time to go to the physician's office to get a prescription medication that is covered on her assistance plan.

### Past Medical History

Type 2 DM, diagnosed 5 years ago
Obesity
Dysmenorrhea, diagnosed 10 years ago
h/o UTI, diagnosed 4 days ago

### Family History

Father is alive at age 65 with no significant medical history. Mother had DM, dyslipidemia, CAD, and died of complications due to DM at age 60. She has one sister who is 44 and has type 2 DM.

### Social History

Single and lives with her sister; has no children. Has been unemployed for 5 years

### Tobacco/Alcohol/Substance Use

Drinks 1–2 beers on the weekend; (–) tobacco or illicit drug use

### Allergies/Intolerances/Adverse Drug Events

No known drug allergies

### Medications (Current)

Glipizide 5 mg PO q 24 h
Metformin 850 mg PO q 24 h
Ortho Tri-Cyclen LO PO q 24 h

### Review of Systems

▶ *General*

Well-appearing, obese Caucasian woman in no acute distress

▶ **Vital Signs**

BP 124/69 mm Hg, P 68, RR 14, T 36.2°C (97.2°F)

Weight 175 lb (80 kg)

Height 66 in. (168 cm)

Denies pain

▶ **Skin**

Dry-appearing skin; (−) rashes or lesions

▶ **HEENT**

PERRLA, EOMI; (−) sinus tenderness; TMs appear normal

▶ **Neck and Lymph Nodes**

Thyroid gland symmetrical; (−) nodules; (−) lymphadenopathy; (−) carotid bruits

▶ **Chest**

Clear to auscultation

▶ **Breast**

Examination deferred

▶ **Cardiovascular**

RRR, normal $S_1$, $S_2$; (−) $S_3$ or $S_4$

▶ **Abdomen**

Not tender; not distended; (−) organomegaly

▶ **Neurology**

Grossly intact; deep tendon reflexes normal

▶ **Genitourinary**

White exudate on internal genitalia and cervix; (+) thick, curd-like discharge

▶ **Rectal**

Examination deferred

## Laboratory Tests

|  | Conventional Units | SI Units |
|---|---|---|
| Na | 140 mEq/L | 140 mmol/L |
| K | 3.7 mEq/L | 3.7 mmol/L |
| Cl | 98 mEq/L | 98 mmol/L |
| $CO_2$ | 24 mEq/L | 24 mmol/L |
| BUN | 12 mg/dL | 4.3 mmol/L |
| SCr | 1.2 mg/dL | 106 μmol/L |
| Glu | 175 mg/dL | 9.7 mmol/L |
| Vaginal smear | (+) *Candida albicans* | |

**FIGURE 94-1.** Wet mount with KOH of *Candida albicans* in a woman with candida vaginitis. (Reproduced, with permission, from Usatine RP, Smith MA, Mayeaux Jr EJ, Chumley H, Tysinger J. The Color Atlas of Family Medicine. New York, McGraw-Hill, 2009, Fig 79-3.)

## Assessment

A 39-year-old woman with signs, symptoms, and laboratory tests consistent with vulvovaginal candidiasis (Figure 94-1).

### Student Workup

**Missing Information?**

| Evaluate: | Patient Database |
|---|---|
| | Drug Therapy Problems |
| | Care Plan (by Problem) |

## TARGETED QUESTIONS

1. What signs and symptoms of vaginal candidiasis does the patient have?

   *Hint: See p. 1426 in PPP*

2. What treatment options are available for treating vaginal candidiasis?

   *Hint: See pp. 1427–1428 and Table 83-2 in PPP*

3. What risk factors does the patient have for vaginal candidiasis?

   *Hint: See p. 1426 and Table 83-1 in PPP*

4. What risks and adverse effects of therapy would you discuss with the patient?

   *Hint: See p. 1428 in PPP*

5. Is the patient a candidate for suppressive therapy and why?

   *Hint: See p. 1428 and Table 83-3 in PPP*

## FOLLOW-UP

Six months later, the patient tells her primary care physician that she is trying to conceive a child. However, she is concerned about the treatment of vaginal candidiasis if she becomes pregnant.

6. What treatment options would be recommended if the patient was pregnant?

   *Hint: See p. 1429 in PPP*

7. Would the treatment plan for the acute infection be changed if the patient was taking theophylline?

   *Hint: See pp. 1427–1428 in PPP*

8. What treatment plan for suppressive therapy should be changed if the patient was taking warfarin?

   *Hint: See pp. 1427–1428 and Table 83-3 in PPP*

## ☽ GLOBAL PERSPECTIVE

Vulvovaginal candidiasis is a common form of vaginitis with *C. albicans* accounting for more than 90% of cases across the world. Nearly 50% of women will experience one or more episodes by the age of 25 years. Uncontrolled diabetes, antibiotic use, hormonal contraceptives, obesity, pregnancy, and debilitation are all risk factors for developing candidiasis, which do vary across the world. Recurrent candidiasis, defined as four or more infections per year, occurring in less than 5% of women, is distinguishable from a persistent infection by the presence of a symptom-free interval between infections.

## CASE SUMMARY

- Her current clinical picture is consistent with vaginal candidiasis, and antifungal therapy should be initiated.
- A single dose of fluconazole 150 mg orally is recommended. The dose can be repeated in 3 days.
- The patient is unable to afford over-the-counter antifungal agents, but fluconazole would be covered by her insurance.
- Suppressive therapy of weekly fluconazole should be considered due to her history of recurrent candidiasis.

For more information on the care plan and facilitator's guide please visit http://www.mhpharmacotherapy.com.

# 95 Invasive Fungal Infection

Russell E. Lewis

## CASE LEARNING OBJECTIVES

- Recognize the host risk factors that predispose patients to invasive fungal infections
- Identify the common patterns of antifungal resistance that affect the selection and dosing of antifungal therapy
- Develop an appropriate treatment and monitoring plan for the management of invasive candidiasis
- Compare and contrast the relative strengths and weaknesses of current systemic antifungal agents for the empiric treatment of an invasive fungal pathogen
- Properly educate patients on potential drug interactions and adverse effects of triazole antifungal agents

## PATIENT PRESENTATION

### Chief Complaint

"Patient in the intensive care unit has persistent fever despite broad-spectrum antibiotic therapy."

### History of Present Illness

Steven Johnson is a 49-year-old male who presented to the emergency department 5 days ago with a history of worsening diffuse abdominal pain and vomiting. During the workup in the emergency department, a contrast-enhanced CT scan of the abdomen was ordered that showed inflammation and necrosis involving less than 15% of the pancreas. The patient was started on IV fluids, meropenem 1 g q 8 h plus vancomycin 1 g q 12 h. The patient underwent an exploratory abdominal laparotomy, which revealed inflammation of the common bile and stones in the gallbladder requiring cholecystectomy. The patient was subsequently transferred to the surgical ICU for postsurgical care where he remained in a guarded condition and extubated, but has developed a new fever in the last 24 hours on broad-spectrum antibiotic therapy.

### Past Medical History

HTN

Hyperlipidemia

### Family History

Father had CAD and died of an MI at age 56. Mother is alive at age 70 with type 2 DM and osteoporosis.

### Social History

Construction worker in Chicago. No recent travel or unusual exposures. Married and lives with wife of 18 years, has 2 kids, ages 12 and 15, and 2 pet dogs.

### Tobacco/Alcohol Substance Abuse

Social drinker; occasional cigars; (−) illicit drug use

### Allergies/Intolerances/Adverse Drug Events

None

### Medications (Current)

Meropenem 1 g IV q 8 h

Vancomycin 1 g IV q 12 h

Normal saline, IV, 50 mL/h

Fentanyl 75 mcg/h IV

Lorazepam 0.05 mg/kg/h IV

Tube feeds q 6 h via Dobhoff catheter as tolerated

Pantoprazole 40 mg IV daily

HCTZ 25 mg PO daily (on hold)

Atorvastatin 40 mg PO daily (on hold)

Acetaminophen 500 mg PO q 6 h PRN

Diphenhydramine 50 mg PO q 4–6 h PRN

Docusate sodium liquid 100 mg PO twice daily

## Review of Systems

The patient is somewhat difficult to arouse and appears to be developing a nonconfluent rash across the chest and upper back.

## Physical Examination

### ▶ General

Somewhat ill-appearing, difficult-to-arouse male in late forties with extremities that are cool to touch. The patient is not intubated.

### ▶ Vital Signs

BP 108/76 mm Hg, P 88, RR 17, T 38.4°C

Weight 218 lb (99 kg)

Height 69 in. (175 cm)

### ▶ Skin

Decreased skin turgor. Peripherally inserted central catheter (PICC) site is not indurated or inflamed. A light diffuse morbilliform rash evident on the upper chest that is spreading on the arms, neck, and back. Rash has slowly developed over the last 48 hours to involve the back. Surgical sites are clean and dressed without signs of erythema or pus.

### ▶ HEENT

PERRLA, EOMI; (–) sinus tenderness; TMs appear normal; mucus membranes dry

### ▶ Neck and Lymph Nodes

(–) Evidence of lymphadenopathy; (–) thyroid nodules; (–) carotid bruits

### ▶ Chest

Dullness to percussion in lower right and left bases; (–) wheezes; (+) crackles heard bilaterally during inspiration

### ▶ Cardiovascular

RRR, normal $S_1$, $S_2$; (–) $S_3$ or $S_4$

### ▶ Abdomen

Tender, not distended

### ▶ Neurology

The patient moderately sedated and not well oriented to person, place, or time

### ▶ Genitourinary

Foley catheter present

### ▶ Rectal

Examination deferred

## Laboratory Tests

|  | Conventional Units | SI Units |
| --- | --- | --- |
| Na | 138 mEq/L | 138 mmol/L |
| K | 3.6 mEq/L | 3.6 mmol/L |
| Cl | 101 mEq/L | 101 mmol/L |
| $CO_2$ | 23 mEq/L | 23 mmol/L |
| BUN | 23 mg/dL | 8.2 mmol/L |
| SCr | 1.5 mg/dL | 133 μmol/L |
| Glu | 122 mg/dL | 6.8 mmol/L |
| Ca | 9.4 mg/dL | 2.35 mmol/L |
| Mg | 1.2 mEq/L | 0.60 mmol/L |
| Phos | 3.3 mg/dL | 1.07 mmol/L |
| Albumin | 3.8 g/dL | 38 g/L |
| AST | 77 IU/L | 1.28 μkat/L |
| ALT | 92 IU/L | 1.53 μkat/L |
| ALP | 250 IU/L | 4.17 μkat/L |
| Total bilirubin | 2.6 mg/dL | 44.5 μmol/L |
| Hgb | 11 g/dL | 110 g/L; 6.83 mmol/L |
| Hct | 58% | 0.58 |
| WBC | $13.5 \times 10^3/mm^3$ | $13.5 \times 10^9/L$ |
| Segs | 50% | 0.50 |
| Bands | 8% | 0.08 |
| Lymphocytes | 28% | 0.28 |
| Monocytes | 6% | 0.06 |
| Eosinophils | 8% | 0.08 |
| Platelets | $290 \times 10^3/mm^3$ | $290 \times 10^9/L$ |

## Culture Results

*Blood:* (–) No growth

*Urine:* (+) Yeast

*Wound Swab:* (+) Coagulase-negative Gram-positive cocci

*Urinalysis:* Na 15 mEq/L (15 mmol/L); Osmolality 500 mOsmol/kg (500 mmol/kg); Hyaline casts; WBC (–); RBC (–); Protein (–)

## Assessment

A 49-year-old male s/p abdominal laparotomy with fever on broad-spectrum antibiotic therapy (suspected fungal infection), hypotension, and renal insufficiency with a possible drug hypersensitivity reaction.

## Student Workup

### Missing Information?

| Evaluate: | Patient Database |
| --- | --- |
|  | Drug Therapy Problems |
|  | Care Plan (by Problem) |

## TARGETED QUESTIONS

1. What are the patient's risk factors for developing an opportunistic mycosis? Which fungal pathogen is most likely?

   *Hint: See p. 1446 in PPP*

2. In the absence of definitive microbiologic data, what antifungal therapy should be started in this patient?

   *Hint: See pp. 1148–1450 and Table 84-4 in PPP*

3. If blood cultures acquired the following day come back positive for a germ-tube-negative yeast, how would this influence the selection of the antifungal agent?

   *Hint: See pp. 1148–1450 in PPP*

4. Is the (+) yeast culture from the urine indicative of true infection or colonization in this patient?

   *Hint: Review results of the urinalysis and see p. 1447 in PPP*

5. What is the most likely explanation of this patient's rash?

   *Hint: Review the CBC with differential*

## FOLLOW-UP

Three days after starting the antifungal therapy, the patient has defervesced, and renal function is improving. Fluconazole susceptibility test results for the yeast isolated from the blood (*Candida glabrata*) show an MIC of 64 mcg/mL (64 mg/L), which is considered resistant to fluconazole. The attending physician asks you if the patient can be transitioned from intravenous antifungal therapy to voriconazole oral solution to complete the treatment course for candidemia.

6. What is your recommendation?

   *Hint: See pp. 1448–1450 in PPP*

## � GLOBAL PERSPECTIVE

*Candida* species are the third to fourth most commonly isolated bloodstream pathogens in hospitalized patients associated with crude mortality rates approaching 30–40%.

Like many opportunistic invasive fungal pathogens, invasive candidiasis can be difficult to diagnose early. Therefore, early suspicion of infection in patients with multiple risk factors for infection (e.g., central venous catheters, broad-spectrum antibiotic therapy, recent intra-abdominal surgery, colonization with *Candida* at multiple sites) should prompt empiric treatment during the diagnostic workup, as delays in the initiation of appropriate antifungal therapy have been associated with increased patient mortality. Antifungal therapy selection is determined by local epidemiology (i.e., prevalence of *C. glabrata* and *C. krusei* in the institution), previous antifungal exposures, and underlying comorbidities of the host. For most patients, initial therapy with either appropriately dosed IV fluconazole (lower risk patient, *C. glabrata* or *C. krusei* unlikely) or an echinocandin antifungal (higher risk) is recommended until pathogen identification and clinical response can be assessed.

## CASE SUMMARY

- The patient's clinical picture is consistent with invasive candidiasis with developing sepsis, requiring immediate empiric antifungal therapy.

- Because the patient is at relatively higher risk (possible early sepsis, renal dysfunction), initial therapy with an echinocandin would be appropriate (i.e., intravenous caspofungin 70 mg on day 1 and then 50 mg/d thereafter). The patient should receive at least 2 weeks of therapy and have the PICC line replaced.

- Because the patient has a fluconazole-resistant *C. glabrata*, he should not be considered as a candidate for step-down (oral) fluconazole therapy.

For more information on the care plan and facilitator's guide please visit http://www.mhpharmacotherapy.com.

# 96 Pediatric Immunization

Hanna Phan          Lynn C. Nelson

## CASE LEARNING OBJECTIVES

- Evaluate pediatric immunization records and identify missing immunizations
- Recognize appropriate contraindications for holding immunizations until a subsequent visit
- Develop an appropriate plan for vaccine catch-up including selection of appropriate vaccine products for pediatric immunizations
- Properly educate caregivers regarding premedication, adverse effects of vaccines, and vaccine controversies, such as autism

## PATIENT PRESENTATION

### Chief Complaint

"Lately my son has been fussy and doesn't sleep very well. His forehead was warm to touch last night and I am concerned that he may be coming down with something."

### History of Present Illness

Kyle Smith is an 18-month-old male toddler who was brought into his pediatrician's office (use today's visit as 08/01/2012) by his mother. The mother notes that her son has been irritable and demonstrates difficulty sleeping over the past few days. Additionally, she reports that he has been eating less with meals over the past few days and has been tugging on his right ear for the past day or so and has become increasingly fussy. His mother has no other complaints at this time.

### Past Medical History

Normal spontaneous vaginal delivery (NSVD) at 37 weeks' gestation. No hospitalizations or complications since birth.

### Social History

The patient lives at home with mother and father. He attends day care during the weekdays as both parents work full time. Siblings include a 4-year-old sister who also attends day care as well as preschool.

### Allergies/Intolerances/Adverse Drug Events

Green gelatin ("itching" per mother)

### Medications (Current)

Acetaminophen infant drops 130 mg PO q 6 h PRN fever, last dose given at 21:00 last night

### Immunizations

Please see attached immunization record for this patient.

Per mother, the patient has not experienced any adverse reactions with immunizations except for some mild erythema with the Pediarix vaccine.

### Review of Systems

Positive for fever and decreased appetite; negative for rashes, bruises, recent trauma, or accidental falls; negative for discharge from the eyes or ear pulling; negative for nausea, vomiting, or changes in bowel or urinary patterns; positive for decreased oral intake; negative for lethargy

### Physical Examination

▸ *General*

Irritable and fussy 18-month-old male in no acute distress

▸ *Vital Signs*

BP 100/55 mm Hg, P 95, RR 24, T 37°C

Weight 28 lb (12.7 kg)

Height 33 in. (84 cm)

**IMMUNIZATION RECORD**

**Birthdate:** 1/1/2011

| Vaccine | Product Name | Date Given | Route and Site | Vaccinator Signature/Initials |
|---|---|---|---|---|
| Hepatitis B | Recombivax HB | 1/1/2011 | IM RT | A.R. |
| | Pediarix | 3/5/2011 | IM RT | B.C. |
| | Pediarix | 5/16/2011 | IM LT | A.B. |
| | Pediarix | 7/23/2011 | IM LT | A.B. |
| Diphtheria, tetanus, pertussis | Pediarix | 3/5/2011 | IM RT | B.C. |
| | Pediarix | 5/16/2011 | IM LT | A.B. |
| | Pediarix | 7/23/2011 | IM LT | A.B. |
| *Haemophilus influenzae* type b | PedvaxHIB | 3/5/2011 | IM LT | B.C. |
| | PedvaxHIB | 5/16/2011 | IM RT | A.B. |
| | PedvaxHIB | 3/5/2012 | IM LT | P.T. |
| Polio | Pediarix | 3/5/2011 | IM RT | B.C. |
| | Pediarix | 5/16/2011 | IM LT | A.B. |
| | Pediarix | 7/23/2011 | IM LT | A.B. |
| Pneumococcal | Prevnar | 3/5/2011 | IM LT | B.C. |
| | Prevnar | 5/16/2011 | IM LT | A.B. |
| | Prevnar | 7/23/2011 | IM RT | A.B. |
| | Prevnar | 1/5/2012 | IM RT | P.T. |
| Rotavirus | Rotarix | 3/5/2011 | PO | B.C. |
| | Rotarix | 5/16/2011 | PO | A.B. |
| Measles, mumps, rubella | ProQuad | 1/5/2012 | SC LT | P.T. |
| Varicella | ProQuad | 1/5/2012 | SC LT | P.T. |
| Hepatitis A | | | | |
| Meningococcal | | | | |
| Influenza | | | | |

IM, intramuscular; SC, subcutaneous; PO, oral; LT, left thigh; RT, right thigh.

Adapted from the Immunization Action Coalition Vaccine Administration Record for Children and Teens. http://www.immunize.org/catg.d/p2022.pdf.

▶ **Skin**

No abnormalities noted; normal skin turgor

▶ **HEENT**

PERRLA, EOMI; moist mucous membranes (MMM); slight erythema of the tympanic membrane on right side. No bulging or limitation in mobility of the tympanic membrane.

▶ **Neck and Lymph Nodes**

(−) Lymphadenopathy

▶ **Chest**

Clear to auscultation

▶ **Cardiovascular**

RRR, normal $S_1$, $S_2$; (−) $S_3$ or $S_4$

▶ **Abdomen**

Not tender/not distended; (−) organomegaly

▶ **Neurology**

Grossly intact; deep tendon reflexes normal

▶ **Genitourinary**

Examination deferred

▶ **Rectal**

Examination deferred

## Laboratory Tests

### Obtained During Routine Clinic Visit on 1/5/2012

|  | Conventional Units | SI Units |
|---|---|---|
| Na | 140 mEq/L | 140 mmol/L |
| K | 4.1 mEq/L | 4.1 mmol/L |
| Cl | 105 mEq/L | 105 mmol/L |
| $CO_2$ | 23 mEq/L | 23 mmol/L |
| BUN | 5 mg/dL | 1.8 mmol/L |
| SCr | 0.3 mg/dL | 27 μmol/L |
| Glu | 70 mg/dL | 3.9 mmol/L |
| Ca | 9.7 mg/dL | 2.43 mmol/L |
| Mg | 1.8 mEq/L | 0.90 mmol/L |
| Phosphate | 4.5 mg/dL | 1.45 mmol/L |
| Hgb | 12.2 g/dL | 122 g/L; 7.57 mmol/L |
| Hct | 36.7% | 0.367 |
| WBC | $15.2 \times 10^3/mm^3$ | $15.2 \times 10^9/L$ |
| MCV | 74 μm³ | 74 fL |
| Albumin | 4.2 g/dL | 42 g/L |

## Assessment

An 18-month-old male with signs and symptoms consistent with AOM of the right ear. Pharmacist to review immunization record.

### Student Workup

**Missing Information?**

Evaluate:    Patient Database
             Drug Therapy Problems
             Care Plan (by Problem)

## TARGETED QUESTIONS

1. What signs and symptoms would the physician evaluate to determine if KS should receive immunizations today?

   *Hint: See Guide to Vaccine Contraindications and Precautions (by the CDC), http://www.cdc.gov/vaccines/recs/vac-admin/contraindications.htm -or- http://www.cdc.gov/vaccines/recs/vac-admin/downloads/contraindications-guide-508.pdf*

2. What adverse effects should the mother be educated about regarding KS's immunizations?

   *Hint: See pp. 1477 and 1478 in PPP*

3. What combination vaccines were used for KS's immunizations based on review of his record and what vaccines are contained in these combination products?

   *Hint: See pp. 1470–1477 in PPP*

4. What would you educate the mother about in regard to thimerosal and vaccines?

   *Hint: See p. 1478 in PPP*

5. Which of KS's missing vaccines is/are likely to cause body temperature elevation?

   *Hint: See pp. 1470–1477 in PPP*

## FOLLOW-UP

KS and his mother return to the clinic for a routine checkup a couple months later that year in October. KS is well developed, not in distress, no present illnesses. The pediatrician asks you what vaccine(s) he should receive.

6. Which vaccine(s) should be given and why?

   *Hint: See pp. 1470–1477 and Table 86-2 in PPP*

## GLOBAL PERSPECTIVE

Immunization of children remains a significant public health concern internationally. According to the World Health Organization (WHO), immunizations do not reach every child worldwide, resulting in an estimated 1.5 million deaths from diseases preventable by vaccines recommended by the WHO. Up to 30% of deaths amongst infant and children worldwide are attributable to vaccine preventable diseases such as pneumococcal disease, rotavirus, and pertussis.[1] Due to growing immunization programs, improved access to clean water, improved nutrition, and sanitary living conditions by public health organizations, such as the WHO, the number of children dying every year has fallen below 10 million.[2] Optimal outreach of immunizations to the world's children is faced with challenges in financial support, logistics of organizing national and local public health groups, and support of caregivers regarding the importance of immunization for individual and community health.

## REFERENCES

1. World Health Organization. http://www.who.int/immunization_monitoring/Global_Immunization_Data.pdf Accessed May 25, 2012.
2. WHO, UNICEF, World Bank. State of the World's Vaccines and Immunization, 3rd ed. Geneva, World Health Organization, 2009. http://whqlibdoc.who.int/publications/2009/9789241563864_eng.pdf. Accessed March 7, 2010.

## CASE SUMMARY

- KS presents to the clinic with AOM of his right ear and will likely receive antibiotic therapy.

- KS is in no acute distress and has a history of possible low-grade fever based on tactile observation by his mother, treated with acetaminophen.

- Patients should be reviewed for missing scheduled or recommended immunizations on each visit to the primary care provider as each visit is an opportunity to maintain adherence to the recommended immunization schedule by the Advisory Committee on Immunization Practices within the CDC.

- The decision to vaccinate KS should be based on which vaccines may be missing and clinical judgment of the patient's current clinical status and ability to receive immunizations today.

For more information on the care plan and facilitator's guide please visit http://www.mhpharmacotherapy.com.

# 97 Adult Immunization

Kathryn R. Matthias          Joshua C. Caraccio

## CASE LEARNING OBJECTIVES

- Evaluate adult immunization records and identify missing recommended vaccinations based on patient's age, comorbid conditions, risk factors, and time since previous vaccinations
- Recognize appropriate contraindications and precautions for administration of immunizations in adult patients
- Develop an appropriate plan for vaccine catch-up including an evaluation of which vaccines can be administered at the same time
- Describe appropriate patient education for potential benefits and adverse reactions of vaccines

## PATIENT PRESENTATION

### Chief Complaint

"I was told to see my physician after being discharged from the local hospital. I was admitted to the hospital for 4 days because I broke my arm after a bad car accident."

### History of Present Illness

Eric Jones is a 23-year-old college student who was a restrained driver in a MVA 7 days ago on December 2, 2012. He was not ejected from the car and had no loss of consciousness. In the ED, he was found to have a left mid-shaft humerus fracture and spleen laceration. He was taken emergently to the operating room and a splenectomy was performed due to uncontrollable bleeding. The rest of his hospital stay was uneventful but he was told to see his primary care physician (PCP) after discharge for follow-up and to make an appointment with an orthopedic specialist for his humerus fracture. During his initial visit to his PCP, his physician asks the clinic's pharmacist to review his immunization history.

### Past Medical History

Migraines diagnosed 5 years ago
  Left humerus fracture 7 days ago

### Past Surgical History

Splenectomy 7 days ago

### Family History

Mother and father are both alive. Father is 52 and has a history of T2DM. Mother is 48 and has no significant past medical history. He has no siblings.

### Social History

Patient is currently a third year college student (psychology major) and lives off-campus in an apartment with his girlfriend and 2 other roommates. He has two healthy indoor-only cats. He denies smoking and IV drug use. He drinks alcohol socially (3–4 beers per week).

### Allergies/Intolerances/Adverse Drug Events

NKDA

### Medications (Current—No Medications Prior to Car Accident)

Acetaminophen 650 mg PO q 4 h PRN musculoskeletal pain

Docusate 100 mg PO q 12 h

Famotidine 20 mg PO q 12 h

Oxycodone (oral solution) 5–10 mg PO q 4 h PRN pain

### Immunizations

Most recent photocopy from 06/20/2011 of immunization record in patient's medical chart at clinic:

## IMMUNIZATION RECORD

**Name: Eric P. Jones**

**Birthdate: 2/8/1989**

| Vaccine | Date Given | Vaccinator Signature/ Initials |
|---|---|---|
| Hepatitis B | 8/15/1998 | F.G. |
| | 9/21/1998 | F.G. |
| | 2/17/1999 | F.G. |
| Diphtheria, tetanus, pertussis | 3/9/1989 | S.M. |
| | 4/20/1989 | S.M. |
| | 8/10/1989 | S.M. |
| | 8/15/1990 | S.M. |
| | 4/8/1993 | F.G. |
| Diphtheria and tetanus | 7/29/2000 | F.G. |
| Tetanus, diphtheria, pertussis | 9/15/2009 | H.J. |
| Polio | 3/9/1989 | S.M. |
| | 4/20/1989 | S.M. |
| | 8/10/1989 | S.M. |
| | 8/15/1990 | S.M. |
| | 4/8/1993 | F.G. |
| Pneumococcal | 3/9/1989 | S.M. |
| | 4/20/1989 | S.M. |
| | 8/15/1990 | S.M. |
| Measles, mumps, rubella | 6/20/1990 | S.M. |
| | 1/30/2000 | F.G. |
| Varicella | 1/5/1998 | F.G. |
| | 4/10/1998 | F.G. |
| Influenza [LAIV (live attenuated influenza vaccine)] | 9/15/2008 | P.M. |
| | 10/24/2009 | S.C. |

As per the patient's discharge paperwork from the hospital, he received a diphtheria, tetanus, pertussis (Tdap) vaccination on 12/2/2012. No other administered vaccinations were listed. The patient states that he got his annual influenza vaccine that was administered into his "nose rather than a shot" last month at a Flu Clinic on his college campus. He does not remember the exact date and did not bring an immunization record with him to clinic today but thinks it was mid-November.

## Review of Systems

Mild left arm pain; arm is in a sling. Minor abrasions over flank, arms, and face.

## Physical Examination

### ▸ General

Twenty-two-year-old Caucasian man in no acute distress

### ▸ Vital Signs

BP 126/74 mm Hg, P 88, RR 18, T 37.1°C

Weight 162 lb (73.6 kg)

Height 71 in. (180 cm)

Pain 2/10 (left arm)

### ▸ Skin

Multiple healing abrasions over flank, arms, and face. Three healing 2-inch (5-cm) surgical wounds on abdomen from splenectomy with no signs of infection.

### ▸ HEENT

PERRLA, EOMI

### ▸ Neck and Lymph Nodes

(−) Lymphadenopathy

### ▸ Chest

Clear to auscultation

### ▸ Cardiovascular

RRR, normal $S_1$, $S_2$; (−) $S_3$ or $S_4$

### ▸ Abdomen

Slight tenderness around surgical wound site but is not indurated, warm, or red

### ▸ Neurology

Grossly intact; DTRs normal

### ▸ Genitourinary

Examination deferred

### ▸ Rectal

Examination deferred

## Laboratory Tests

### Obtained 4 Days Ago

| | Conventional Units | SI Units |
|---|---|---|
| Na | 135 mEq/L | 135 mmol/L |
| K | 4.3 mEq/L | 4.3 mmol/L |
| Cl | 102 mEq/L | 102 mmol/L |
| $CO_2$ | 25 mEq/L | 25 mmol/L |
| BUN | 5 mg/dL | 1.8 mmol/L |
| SCr | 0.6 mg/dL | 53 μmol/L |
| Glu | 105 mg/dL | 5.8 mmol/L |
| Ca | 9.7 mg/dL | 2.43 mmol/L |
| Hgb | 13.9 g/dL | 139 g/L; 8.63 mmol/L |
| HCT | 39.7% | 0.397 |

| MCV | 95 µm³ | 95 fL |
| Platelets | 253 × 10³/mm³ | 253 × 10⁹/L |
| WBC | 6.8 × 10³/mm³ | 6.8 × 10⁹/L |

## Assessment

Twenty-three-year-old man in no acute distress with left humerus fracture and splenectomy 7 days ago after a MVA. Pharmacist to review immunization record.

### Student Workup

**Missing Information?**

**Evaluate:**   Patient Database
Drug Therapy Problems
Care Plan (by Problem)

## TARGETED QUESTIONS

1. Which comorbid conditions and lifestyle risk factors put the patient at higher risk of infection that can be prevented by vaccination?

   *Hint: See pp. 1477–1479 in PPP*

   *Hint: See guide to Vaccine-Preventable Adult Diseases (by the CDC), http://www.cdc.gov/vaccines/vpd-vac/adult-vpd.htm*

2. Why and when should adult asplenia patients receive additional vaccines beyond the recommended adult immunization schedule?

   *Hint: See pp. 1470–1477 in PPP*

   *Hint: See Adult Immunization Schedule (by the CDC), http://www.cdc.gov/vaccines/recs/schedules/adult-schedule.htm*

3. Does the patient have any comorbid conditions that would contraindicate him from receiving live or inactivated vaccinations today?

   *Hint: See pp. 1478 and 1479 in PPP*

   *Hint: See Guide to Vaccine Contraindications and Precautions (by the CDC), http://www.cdc.gov/vaccines/recs/vac-admin/contraindications.htm or http://www.cdc.gov/vaccines/recs/vac-admin/downloads/contraindications-guide-508.pdf*

4. Which recommended vaccinations are missing from the patient's immunization record and when should they be administered?

   *Hint: See Adult Immunization Schedule (by the CDC), http://www.cdc.gov/vaccines/recs/schedules/adult-schedule.htm*

5. What are the common and serious potential adverse effects of recommended vaccines determined in question 4?

   *Hint: See pp. 1477 and 1478 and Table 86-2 in PPP*

## FOLLOW-UP

EJ receives all immunizations as per the pharmacist and physician recommendations. He returns to his PCP 9 months later for his annual checkup. He had no further complications related to the motor vehicle accident and his left arm healed well. His physician asks the clinic pharmacist to evaluate his immunization record for any missing vaccinations.

6. Which vaccine(s) should be recommended and why?

   *Hint: See pp. 1470–1477 in PPP*

   *Hint: See Adult Immunization Schedule (by the CDC), http://www.cdc.gov/vaccines/recs/schedules/adult-schedule.htm.*

## 🌐 GLOBAL PERSPECTIVE

An annual review of immunizations reports from countries and territories from across the world is conducted by the World Health Organization (WHO) and United Nations Children's Fund (UNICEF).[1] Although global rates of certain immunizations have increased dramatically over the past 30 years, many vaccines on the United States' Immunization Schedule are not yet recommended in other countries' national immunization schedules. Although the United States and other industrialized countries have estimated vaccinated target populations (by antigen) above 90% based on childhood recommended immunization schedule, missed opportunities to vaccinate adult patients often occur. In a case-cohort study of two large tertiary medical centers in Australia only 2.3% of patients had their vaccination status for influenza or pneumococcal determined during a hospital visit.[2] In another study of adult patients who developed invasive pneumococcal disease, it was determined that 92% of these patients had at least one missed opportunity for vaccination such as a hospital, emergency department, or primary care visit in the 2 years prior to infection.[3] Due to high rates of missed opportunities to vaccinate, the Advisory Committee on Immunization Practices through the Centers for Disease Control and Prevention (CDC) has recommended the use of institution protocols for standing order immunization programs for administration of vaccines by nurses or pharmacists to decrease rates of eligible, unvaccinated patients.[4]

## REFERENCES

1. World Health Organization: Immunization surveillance, assessment and monitoring. http://www.who.int/immunization_monitoring/data/en/. Accessed February 10, 2010.
2. Skull SA, Andrews RM, Byrnes GB, et al. Missed opportunities to vaccinate a cohort of hospitalized elderly with pneumococcal and influenza vaccines. Vaccine 2007 25:5146–5154.
3. Kyaw MH, Greene CM, Schaffner W, et al. Adults with invasive pneumococcal disease: Missed opportunities for vaccination. Am J Prev Med 2006 31:286–292.

4. Centers for Disease Control and Prevention. Use of standing orders programs to increase adult vaccination rates. MMWR 2000 49:15–26.

## CASE SUMMARY

- EJ presents to his PCP 7 days after a motor vehicle accident and splenectomy. Despite receiving diphtheria/tetanus/pertussis vaccination while admitted to a local hospital, additional immunizations were missed during the hospital admission.

- EJ is in no acute distress but certain medical conditions and lifestyle put him at higher risk of certain infections that could be prevented by vaccination.

- EJ should receive his missing immunizations as per the recommended adult immunization schedule by the ACIP within the CDC.

- EJ should be counseled on potential adverse effects of recommended vaccines.

For more information on the care plan and facilitator's guide please visit http://www.mhpharmacotherapy.com.

# 98 HIV Infection

Amanda H. Corbett    Colin I. Sheffield

## CASE LEARNING OBJECTIVES

- Identify the typical and atypical signs and symptoms of acute and chronic human immunodeficiency virus (HIV) infection
- Identify the desired therapeutic outcomes for patients with HIV infection
- Recommend appropriate first-line pharmacotherapy interventions for patients with HIV infection
- Describe the components of a monitoring plan to assess the effectiveness and adverse effects of pharmacotherapy for HIV infection
- Educate patients about the disease state, appropriate lifestyle modifications, and drug therapy required for effective treatment

## PATIENT PRESENTATION

### Chief Complaint
"I am ready to start medications."

### History of Present Illness
Kim Jones is a 35-year-old African American female recently diagnosed with HIV after presenting with *Pneumocystis jiroveci* pneumonia. *P. jiroveci* pneumonia was diagnosed 1 month ago when she presented to the hospital with increased weight loss, SOB, insomnia, nonproductive cough, and unremarkable chest x-ray. During her hospitalization, antiretroviral therapy was discussed but the patient was not ready to start taking it yet. She also had no insurance or way to pay for her medications at the time.

### Past Medical History
*P. jiroveci* pneumonia (PJP) diagnosed 1 month ago
Depression × 5 years
HTN × 5 years

### Family History
She has not seen her father in more than 15 years and her mother is alive with a history of stroke and HTN.

### Social/Work History
She is currently unemployed and lives with her mother.

### Tobacco/Alcohol/Substance Use
Smokes 2 ppd; drinks about 10–12 drinks a week; former crack/cocaine use, but clean for 6 months

### Allergy/Intolerance/Adverse Drug Events
Sulfur drugs

### Medication (Current)
Dapsone 100 mg PO q 24 h
Azithromycin 1,200 mg PO weekly
Enalapril 10 mg PO q 24 h
Bupropion XL 150 mg PO q 24 h

### Review of Systems
(+) Weight loss; decreased appetite; (+) insomnia; (−) SOB; chest pain

### Physical Examination

▶ *General*

Well-appearing African American woman in no acute distress

▶ *Vital Signs*

BP 130/86 mm Hg, P 72, RR 13, T 36.4°C
Weight 130 lb (59 kg)
Height 65 in. (165.1 cm)
No pain

▶ **Skin**

Supple; (−) rashes

▶ **HEENT**

PERRLA; no evidence of retinopathy. Oropharynx, no evidence of thrush

▶ **Neck and Lymph Nodes**

Neck supple; no lymphadenopathy

▶ **Chest**

Clear to auscultation bilaterally

▶ **Breasts**

Breast nontender and (−) nodules

▶ **Cardiovascular**

RRR, normal $S_1$, $S_2$; (−) murmurs, rubs, or gallops

▶ **Abdomen**

Not tender/not distended; (−) organomegaly

▶ **Neurology**

Grossly intact; deep tendon reflexes normal

▶ **Extremities**

Thin, dry upper and lower extremities with no edema

▶ **Genitourinary**

Examination deferred

▶ **Rectal**

Examination deferred

## Laboratory Tests

### Fasting Obtained 2 Weeks Ago in Hospital

|  | Conventional Units | SI Units |
|---|---|---|
| Na | 137 mEq/L | 137 mmol/L |
| K | 4 mEq/L | 4 mmol/L |
| Cl | 101 mEq/L | 101 mmol/L |
| $CO_2$ | 25 mEq/L | 25 mmol/L |
| BUN | 12 mg/dL | 4.3 mmol/L |
| SCr | 0.9 mg/dL | 80 μmol/L |
| Glucose | 85 mg/dL | 4.7 mmol/L |
| Hgb | 14 g/dL | 140 g/L; 8.69 mmol/L |
| Hct | 38% | 0.38 |

| WBC | $4.4 \times 10^3/mm^3$ | $4.4 \times 10^9/L$ |
|---|---|---|
| Absolute lymphocyte count (ALC) | $0.9 \times 10^3/mm^3$ | $0.9 \times 10^9/L$ |
| ANC | $2.9 \times 10^3/mm^3$ | $2.9 \times 10^9/L$ |
| Platelets | $425 \times 10^3/mm^3$ | $425 \times 10^9/L$ |
| HIV RNA | 23,000 copies/mL | $23 \times 10^6$ copies /L |
| CD4⁺ T-cell count | 35 cells/mm³ | $0.035 \times 10^9/L$ |
| HIV genotype | Wild-type virus | |

## Assessment

A thirty-five-year-old woman with diagnosis of HIV in clinic ready to start her new antiretroviral regimen. She was initially prescribed as her first regimen tenofovir 300 mg/emtricitabine 200 mg by mouth once a day + atazanavir 300 mg by mouth once a day + ritonavir 100 mg by mouth once a day.

---

**Student Workup**

**Missing Information?**

**Evaluate:**    Patient Database

Drug Therapy Problems

Care Plan (by Problem)

---

## TARGETED QUESTIONS

1. What signs and symptoms (typical or atypical) of HIV infection does this patient have?

   *Hint: See pp. 1484 and 1485 in PPP*

2. What monitoring goals (treatment and adverse effects of medications) should be discussed with this patient?

   *Hint: See p. 1506 and Tables 87-2, 87-5 and 87-6 in PPP*

3. What medication(s) could be causing side effects that would preclude her from taking her regimen properly?

   *Hint: See Table 87-5 in PPP*

4. What risks and adverse effects of using efavirenz on this patient would you discuss with the patient and/or provider?

   *Hint: Teratogenicity with women of childbearing age and this patient's history of depression. See Table 87-5 in PPP*

5. In choosing a protease inhibitor (PI) for this patient, would using darunavir be a prudent choice? Why or why not?

   *Hint: This drug has a sulfa base, and with this patient's history of a sulfa allergy, there would be risk of allergic reaction to these medications. See Table 87-5 in PPP*

## FOLLOW-UP

She went to her local pharmacy 2 months after starting new antiretrovirals requesting refills for all her medications. The pharmacist noted that she was also purchasing a pregnancy test, St. John's Wort, and omeprazole. The pharmacist contacted the clinic provider and pharmacist, informed them of the patient's purchases, and stated that the patient was late on her refills last month. Her HIV RNA 2 weeks after starting medications decreased by 1 log copy/mL (23,000–2,000 copies/mL [$23 \times 10^6$ copies/L-$2 \times 10^6$ copies/L]). She reported side effects of stomach upset and some nausea.

6. What discussions of sexual behavior should be addressed in this patient, and if this patient becomes pregnant, what considerations must occur so that the baby can be taken to full term?

   *Hint: There should be discussions of contraceptive use and the effect of antiretrovirals on oral contraceptives and barrier protection. Discussions of risk of transmission of HIV between partners with unprotected sex and making sure that the mother is virologically suppressed and taking her regimen during pregnancy is also important. See p. 1499 in PPP*

7. What drug–drug interactions must be evaluated with the patient and how could the pharmacist intervene by counseling the patient and discussing with the provider?

   *Hint: St. John's Wort can significantly decrease concentrations of protease inhibitors (including atazanavir/ritonavir). The patient should be advised not to use St. John's Wort. Also, if she is still having uncontrolled depression, as suggested by purchasing St. John's Wort, her antidepressant therapy should be evaluated. In addition, omeprazole can interact with certain antiretrovirals including atazanavir so this should be discussed with her provider prior to taking any acid suppression agents (i.e., see Table 87-5 in PPP).*

8. What discussions should the pharmacist have concerning adherence with her current regimen and goals of treatment?

   *Hint: A discussion should take place concerning the importance of not missing doses and intervening with the patient to find out why she is missing doses (late refills). An initial VL of 23,000 copies/mL ($23 \times 10^6$ copies/L) and 2 months of therapy should result in an undetectable (<50 copies/mL[$<50 \times 10^3$ copies/L]) HIV RNA. See p. 1506 in PPP*

## ⟳ GLOBAL PERSPECTIVE

HIV infection is a global pandemic that affects the entire population. Access to care in resource-poor countries is much limited compared with those treated in the United States and other industrialized countries. Most resource-poor countries follow World Health Organization (WHO) guidelines with country-specific antiretroviral therapy recommendations. Many countries rely on generic antiretrovirals that are still under the US Food and Drug Administration patent or funding from countries, including the United States, through programs such as the US President's Emergency Plan for AIDS Relief. Pharmaceutical industry also provides resources for countries. Not only are therapies limited, but often only first-line therapy is available, with second-line therapy less readily available. Criterion for when to treat is also variable and typically delayed until CD4+ T-cell counts are lower than what is recommended in the US Department of Health and Human Services guidelines.

## CASE SUMMARY

- This is an HIV-infected patient that meets criteria for starting antiretrovirals, and combination HAART should be started.
- Multiple first-line therapies are available; however, the combination of tenofovir/emtricitabine 300/200 mg once daily + atazanavir 300 mg once daily + ritonavir 100 mg once daily is an acceptable choice for this patient.
- Continued adherence consultations with this patient are needed and should be reinforced by the pharmacist at each visit to the clinic and her local pharmacy.

**For more information on the care plan and facilitator's guide please visit http://www.mhpharmacotherapy.com.**

# 99 Breast Cancer

Christopher J. Campen    Leona Downey

## PATIENT PRESENTATION

### Chief Complaint

"I noticed a lump on my breast. It doesn't hurt, but I am worried it might be cancer."

### History of Present Illness

Cindy Thomas is a 56-year-old premenopausal woman who presents to her primary care physician (PCP) complaining of a new breast lump. She noticed this while trying on new clothes a week ago. There does not appear to be any pain associated with the lump. She last had a mammography 3 years ago, which showed no evidence of breast cancer.

### Past Medical History

Depression diagnosed 14 years ago
HTN diagnosed 12 years ago

### Family History

Her mother was diagnosed with early breast cancer at age 64. She underwent a total mastectomy followed by adjuvant chemotherapy and is currently free of cancer at age 78. Her father is currently in excellent health. She currently has no children.

### Social History

She is married to her husband of 34 years. She has lived outside of San Francisco for nearly all of her life. She is the head of a small IT company and works 60–80 hours per week.

### Tobacco/Alcohol/Substance Use

Past history of smoking for 6 years. Uses alcohol; 4–6 hard alcoholic drinks/wk. No illicit drug use

### Allergies/Intolerances/Adverse Drug Events

No known drug allergies

### Medications (Current)

Fluoxetine 40 mg PO q 24 h
HCTZ 12.5 mg PO q 24 h
Lisinopril 10 mg PO q 24 h
MVI 1 tablet PO daily

### Review of Systems

Slightly distressed female with new-onset painless breast lump. No complaints of pain, soreness, or fatigue at this time

### Physical Examination

▶ *General*

Slightly overweight woman in no acute distress

▶ *Vital Signs*

BP 152/96 mm Hg, P 78, RR 12, T 36.3°C
Weight 182 lb (82.7 kg)
Height 66 in. (168 cm)
Denies pain (pain 0/10)

▸ **Skin**

No suspicious lesions

▸ **HEENT**

PERRLA, EOMI

▸ **Lymph Nodes**

No palpable cervical, axillary, or clavicular adenopathy

▸ **Breasts**

*Right*: No masses or tenderness noted. Nipple everted. No abnormalities

*Left*: Breast lump approximately 5 cm palpable at the one o'clock position about 3 cm from the nipple. No nipple abnormalities or skin changes

▸ **Lungs**

Clear to auscultation and percussion. Good diaphragmatic movement

▸ **Cardiovascular**

RRR with normal $S_1$, $S_2$. Carotids without bruits

▸ **Abdomen**

Soft and nontender without hepatosplenomegaly or masses. Normal bowel sounds

▸ **Extremities**

No pedal edema

▸ **Neurology**

Grossly intact; reflexes normal

▸ **Psychiatric**

Mental status oriented × 4. Mood affect: slightly absent affect

## Laboratory Tests

|  | Conventional Units | SI Units |
|---|---|---|
| Na | 138 mEq/L | 138 mmol/L |
| K | 3.9 mEq/L | 3.9 mmol/L |
| Cl | 101 mEq/L | 101 mmol/L |
| $CO_2$ | 23 mEq/L | 23 mmol/L |
| BUN | 12 mg/dL | 4.3 mmol/L |
| SCr | 0.8 mg/dL | 71 μmol/L |
| Glu | 110 mg/dL | 6.1 mmol/L |
| Ca | 9.2 mg/dL | 2.30 mmol/L |
| Mg | 2 mEq/L | 1 mmol/L |
| Phosphate | 4 mg/dL | 1.29 mmol/L |
| Hgb | 13.3 g/dL | 133 g/L; 8.26 mmol/L |
| Hct | 39.3% | 0.393 |
| WBC | $7.6 \times 10^3/mm^3$ | $7.6 \times 10^9/L$ |
| Platelet | $340 \times 10^3/mm^3$ | $340 \times 10^9/L$ |
| Albumin | 4.1 g/dL | 41 g/L |
| Total bilirubin | 0.8 mg/dL | 13.7 μmol/L |
| Direct bilirubin | 0.2 mg/dL | 3.4 μmol/L |
| AST | 23 IU/L | 0.38 μkat/L |
| ALT | 40 IU/L | 0.67 μkat/L |
| Alkaline phosphatase | 76 IU/L | 1.27 μkat/L |
| ER | + (95%) | |
| PR | Slightly + (45%) | |
| HER2 | + (3+ out of 3+) via immunohistochemistry (IHC) | |

Radiology (see Figure 99-1)

MRI results

Tumor size   5.3 × 2.8 × 3.7 cm

Two lymph nodes appear positive in the ipsilateral axillary region

**FIGURE 99-1.** A screening mammogram with a significant mass with spiculations. (Reproduced, with permission, from Usatine RP, Smith MA, Mayeaux Jr EJ, Chumley H, Tysinger J. The Color Atlas of Family Medicine. New York, McGraw-Hill, 2009, Fig 89-3.)

Pathology

- Pathology results after left total mastectomy, see assessment below
- Invasive ductal carcinoma
- Tumor size 5.3 cm at maximum dimension
- Estrogen receptor (ER)/progesterone receptor (PR)+; HER2/neu+; no distant metastases seen
- Diagnosed with T3N1M0 disease

## Assessment

A 56-year-old premenopausal woman presents with new-onset breast cancer. She first undergoes a left total mastectomy with axillary lymph node dissection and is diagnosed with T3N1M0 breast cancer. The physician decides to initiate adjuvant chemotherapy with doxorubicin/cyclophosphamide (AC) for four cycles followed by paclitaxel (T) and trastuzumab (Herceptin) weekly for 12 weeks. This will be followed by trastuzumab for 1 year and tamoxifen for a minimum of 5 years. For the prevention of nausea/vomiting, she will be given ondansetron and dexamethasone, prior to AC, and prochlorperazine for breakthrough nausea/vomiting.

### Student Workup

**Missing Information?**

**Evaluate:**     Patient Database

Drug Therapy Problems

Care Plan (by Problem)

## TARGETED QUESTIONS

1. What are the common early signs and symptoms of breast cancer?

   *Hint: See p. 1544 in PPP*

2. What stage is this patient diagnosed as?

   *Hint: See p. 1546 and Table 89-3 in PPP*

3. Discuss the positive and negative prognostic factors for this patient.

   *Hint: See p. 1546 in PPP*

4. Compare and contrast the use of adjuvant or neoadjuvant chemotherapy for this patient.

   *Hint: See pp. 1547–1553 in PPP*

5. What are some of the common toxicities and counseling points for anthracyclines, alkylating agents, and taxanes?

   *Hint: See Table 89-7 in PPP*

6. What are the counseling points for patients taking tamoxifen?

   *Hint: See Table 89-9 in PPP*

## FOLLOW-UP

Three weeks later, the patient returns for the second course of doxorubicin and cyclophosphamide. She complains of significant nausea/vomiting lasting approximately 4 days following the first course, and is very fearful of this occurring again.

7. What are the patient-specific risk factors for nausea/vomiting, and what are the risks of uncontrolled nausea? What antiemetic options are available for the prevention of anticipatory, acute, and delayed nausea/vomiting in this patient?

   *Hint: See Table 90-5 in PPP*

## ⟳ GLOBAL PERSPECTIVE

Breast cancer is the number one cause of cancer-related deaths in women globally. In many underdeveloped countries, infectious diseases are the primary threat, making cancer a low priority for resources. Unfortunately, a lack of screening and prevention results in significant resources required to manage patients that more often present with late-stage or advanced disease. The most effective strategy is to develop programs that will result in early diagnosis and intervention. The use of local-regional treatment and systemic therapy depends on the level of resources available, and is often region and country specific.

## CASE SUMMARY

- The patient was diagnosed with locally advanced breast cancer, and multimodal therapy consisting of surgery, radiotherapy, and systemic therapy is indicated.
- The initial systemic chemotherapy regimen is appropriate given her diagnosis. Consider her pathology results when choosing additional endocrine and biologic therapy.

For more information on the care plan and facilitator's guide please visit http://www.mhpharmacotherapy.com.

# 100 Colorectal Cancer

Patrick J. Medina        Emily B. Borders

## PATIENT PRESENTATION

### Chief Complaint

"I've been tired for the past 3 months and have this pain in my stomach that is getting worse. Today I noticed some blood in my stool and got scared. I'm not sure what is going on."

### History of Present Illness

John Braxton is a 62-year-old Caucasian male who presented to his primary care physician with generalized fatigue for 3 months, abdominal pain, and new blood in his stool. Over-the-counter famotidine had been recommended for the abdominal pain, and provided no relief. He also reports that he has not been able to eat like he normally does due to "feeling full all the time" and constipation. A CBC revealed microcytic anemia and iron profile was consistent with iron deficiency. Fecal occult blood test was positive. Colonoscopy demonstrated a 5-cm (2-inch) frond-like, nonobstructing, villous lesion arising from the descending colon. Biopsies were positive for low-grade, moderately differentiated adenocarcinoma. Tumor marker carcinoembryonic antigen (CEA) was 80 ng/mL (80 mcg/L; normal 0–5 ng/mL [0–5 mcg/L]). There was no evidence of metastatic disease on staging CT scans. Pathology revealed 1.8-in. (4.5-cm), low-grade, moderately differentiated adenocarcinoma invading into the muscularis propria. Twenty-four lymph nodes were removed and four were positive for malignancy. The final diagnosis was stage 3 colorectal cancer. Postoperatively, CEA decreased to <0.1 ng/mL (<0.1 mcg/L). He underwent surgical resection with clear margins and is being evaluated 4 weeks later in your clinic for adjuvant treatment regimens.

### Past Medical History

HTN
Hypercholesterolemia

### Past Surgical History

Left-sided hemicolectomy for the colon mass

### Family History

Mother deceased at age 75 with MI. Father deceased at age 60 with colorectal cancer diagnosed at the age of 58. Sister diagnosed with breast cancer at the age of 52; no additional family history of cancer in family per the patient's report.

### Social History

The patient is a lifelong resident of the state of Florida. He currently works as a piano teacher. He is married and has two children.

### Tobacco/Alcohol/Substance Use

The patient has been a lifetime nonsmoker, drinks alcohol socially, and denies any drug use.

### Allergies/Intolerances/Adverse Drug Events

Not known

### Medications (Current)

Atenolol 50 mg PO q 24 h
Atorvastatin 10 mg PO q 24 h

Famotidine 20 mg PO PRN abdominal pain

Hydrocodone/acetaminophen 5/325 mg PO PRN pain

## Review of Systems

Abdominal pain/constipation with minor relief with famotidine; the patient has moderate postsurgical pain relieved with as-needed hydrocodone/acetaminophen. He denies any other symptoms, and additional review of symptoms is negative.

## Physical Examination

### ▸ General

Thinly built, well-dressed, white male in no acute distress

### ▸ Vital Signs

BP 104/74 mm Hg, P 64, RR 13, T 36.4°C

Weight 165.3 lb (75.1 kg)

Height 69 in. (175 cm)

Mild abdominal and postsurgical pain

### ▸ Skin

Normal color with good turgor; (–) lesions or pigments noted

### ▸ HEENT

PERRLA; (–) pallor, icterus; oropharynx clear

### ▸ Neck

Supple; no jugular venous distention; no significant lymphadenopathy

### ▸ Respiratory

Clear to auscultation

### ▸ Cardiovascular

RRR; no murmurs

### ▸ Abdomen

Soft; tender on palpation; ostomy site clean; normal BS; (–) organomegaly

### ▸ Extremities

(–) Edema, cyanosis, clubbing

### ▸ Neurology

AAO × 3; CNs grossly intact; no focal deficits noted

### ▸ Rectal

Stool is guaiac (+).

## Laboratory Tests

### Fasting Obtained 5 Days Ago (status post surgery 4 weeks ago)

|  | Conventional Units | SI Units |
|---|---|---|
| Na | 146 mEq/L | 146 mmol/L |
| K | 3.9 mEq/L | 3.9 mmol/L |
| Cl | 106 mEq/L | 106 mmol/L |
| $CO_2$ | 24 mEq/L | 24 mmol/L |
| BUN | 18 mg/dL | 6.4 mmol/L |
| SCr | 0.9 mg/dL | 80 μmol/L |
| Glu | 117 mg/dL | 6.5 mmol/L |
| Ca | 8.8 mg/dL | 2.20 mmol/L |
| Mg | 1.9 mEq/L | 0.95 mmol/L |
| WBC | $6 \times 10^3/mm^3$ | $6 \times 10^9/L$ |
| Hgb | 13.4 g/dL | 134 g/L; 8.32 mmol/L |
| Hct | 38.2% | 0.382 |
| Platelets | $295 \times 10^3/mm^3$ | $295 \times 10^9/L$ |
| Albumin | 3.1 g/dL | 31 g/L |
| Total cholesterol | 192 mg/dL | 4.97 mmol/L |
| LDL cholesterol | 140 mg/dL | 3.62 mmol/L |
| HDL cholesterol | 32 mg/dL | 0.84 mmol/L |
| Total bilirubin | 1.1 mg/dL | 18.8 μmol/L |
| CEA | 0.4 ng/mL | 0.4 mcg/L |

## Assessment

A 62-year-old male with signs, symptoms, and pathology results diagnostic of stage 3 colorectal cancer

### Student Workup

**Missing Information?**

| Evaluate: | Patient Database |
|---|---|
|  | Drug Therapy Problems |
|  | Care Plan (by Problem) |

## TARGETED QUESTIONS

1. What are the signs and symptoms this patient has for colorectal cancer?

   *Hint: See p. 1588 in PPP*

2. What risk factors did this patient have for the development of colorectal cancer?

   *Hint See pp. 1548 and 1549 in PPP*

3. Why does this patient require adjuvant therapy?

   *Hint: See pp. 1588 and 1589 in PPP*

4. Why is FOLFOX the recommended regimen in this patient?

   *Hint: See p. 1591 in PPP*

5. What risk factors and adverse effects of therapy would you discuss with this patient?

   *Hint: See pp. 1591 and 1598 in PPP; may also refer to individual chemotherapy summaries in Chapter 91 of PPP*

## FOLLOW-UP

The patient has been receiving the FOLFOX regimen for 4 months (8 cycles) with minimal adverse effects. During routine follow-up prior to his ninth cycle, he discusses a slight tingling in his fingers and toes.

6. What is most likely causing this problem? What actions, if any, would you take?

   *Hint: See pp. 1591–1598 in PPP*

## ☼ GLOBAL PERSPECTIVE

Colorectal cancer is one of the most common cancers worldwide. The rate of colorectal cancer is highest in industrialized countries such as the United States as well as many countries in Europe. Industrialized countries tend to have diets high in fat that partially explains the increased incidence, though other dietary and genetic factors play a role in its development. Early stage colorectal cancer (stages 1–3) is curable with either surgery alone or surgery in combination with chemotherapy. Most patients receive 6 months of adjuvant chemotherapy following surgical resection of the tumor. Metastatic disease (stage 4) is currently incurable though patients can live 2 or more years. The initial treatment for most patients is the same, though some of the chemotherapy agents (e.g., 5-fluorouracil, irinotecan) have pharmacogenomic factors, while others have tumor mutations (e.g., cetuximab and panitumumab) that partially determine their efficacy and toxicity.

## CASE SUMMARY

- The patient is diagnosed with stage 3 colorectal cancer requiring adjuvant chemotherapy.
- The initial regimen of FOLFOX is a reasonable choice, with 6 months of therapy recommended.
- Cumulative toxicities of the chemotherapy regimen should be evaluated at each clinic visit.

For more information on the care plan and facilitator's guide please visit http://www.mhpharmacotherapy.com.

# 101 Acute Lymphocytic Leukemia

Nancy H. Heideman    Richard L. Heideman

## CASE LEARNING OBJECTIVES

- Recognize the major prognostic factors in childhood pre–B-cell acute lymphocytic leukemia
- Identify the treatment-related complications associated with the therapy for acute lymphocytic leukemia
- Identify the role of thiopurine methyltransferase metabolism with respect to 6-mercaptopurine toxicity
- Develop a plan to evaluate the patient's current problems and determine if they are related to his ability to metabolize 6-mercaptopurine and select an appropriate new dose for this patient
- Describe the late effects of chemotherapy related to the treatment of acute lymphocytic leukemia

## PATIENT PRESENTATION

### Chief Complaint (Mother's)

"My son keeps having repeated episodes of infection and low blood counts. He needs to be transfused more often than the other patients I know who are on the same protocol."

### History of Present Illness

MC is a 12-year-old Hispanic male who was diagnosed with pre–B-cell acute lymphoblastic leukemia (ALL) at age 11. His presenting WBC count was $7.5 \times 10^3/\text{mm}^3$ ($7.5 \times 10^9/\text{L}$) with 80% leukemic cells. He had no testicular disease and his cerebrospinal fluid showed no leukemic cells. Cytogenetic evaluation of his leukemic cells showed random chromosomal loss and gain. Tumor-cell ploidy showed a DNA content of 1.15. He had a prompt response to induction therapy with a morphologic remission at day 8. His end-of-induction minimal residual disease (MRD) was low. He recently completed his final "delayed intensification" treatment module and began "maintenance" treatment 5 months ago. Since the start of maintenance, he has had two admissions for fever of 101.3°F (38.5°C) and ANC of 250–300/ $\text{mm}^3$ ($0.25$–$0.30 \times 10^9/\text{L}$), each lasting 7 days. Both episodes were associated with negative blood cultures. On each occasion, his maintenance chemotherapy [daily oral 6-mercaptopurine (6MP) and weekly oral methotrexate] was stopped until his ANC was above 500/$\text{mm}^3$ ($0.50 \times 10^9/\text{L}$), and he was afebrile for 48 hours.

### Past Medical History

Full-term infant, uncomplicated birth, and neonatal history

ALL s/p chemotherapy; history of 1 previous admission for fever and neutropenia during the delayed intensification

phase of treatment. He has received 2 prior platelet transfusions, one each during induction and delayed intensification phases of treatment. He has received 3 prior RBC transfusions, the last of which was greater than 3 months ago

Completely up-to-date on childhood immunizations for his age up to the time of his diagnosis for ALL

### Family History

Noncontributory

### Social/Work History

The patient is currently in seventh grade at an elementary school in a disadvantaged neighborhood where the first language of many residents is Spanish. He is a good student, and his parents were involved in his school and community in a positive way. There are two additional siblings in the home: a 6-year-old sister in kindergarten and a 9-year-old brother in fifth grade. All the children and parents are bilingual; even so, the parents are more comfortable in and prefer Spanish for oral and written communication.

### Tobacco/Alcohol/Substance Use

Noncontributory

### Allergies/Intolerances/Adverse Drug Events

None known

### Medications (Current)

6MP 100 mg/m$^2$ PO daily

Methotrexate 33.75 mg/m$^2$ PO once weekly

Vincristine 2 mg/m² IV once monthly

Dexamethasone 4 mg PO bid 5 days each month

Docusate 50 mg at bedtime PRN constipation

## Review of Systems

The patient has chronic and troublesome constipation, assumed to be related to vincristine. This is moderated by the administration of docusate at bedtime, but never completely resolves. He was discharged from the inpatient service 2 weeks ago for a culture-negative episode of fever and neutropenia, for which he received 3 days of IV cefepime. He has had no recent fevers and has resumed his oral 6MP and methotrexate after being off these agents for almost 2 weeks. He does complain that his hips are increasingly "sore" over the last 4–6 weeks and he takes acetaminophen as often as six times a day for these symptoms. There are no other systemic symptoms.

## Physical Examination

### ▶ General

Well appearing in no acute distress

### ▶ Vital Signs

BP 98/56 mm Hg, P 75, RR 18, T 99.7°F (37.6°C)

Weight 94.6 lb (43 kg)

Height 59 in. (150 cm)

Pain 6/10

### ▶ Skin

Warm, soft, supple, without rash

### ▶ HEENT

Partial alopecia; other within normal limits

### ▶ Neck and Lymph Nodes

No palpable adenopathy; no palpable thyroid gland

### ▶ Chest

Clear to auscultation; port site in right upper chest clean, dry, and intact

### ▶ Cardiovascular

Normal sinus rate and rhythm; good capillary refill; no murmurs appreciated

### ▶ Abdomen

Nontender, nondistended, palpable stool in left lower quadrant. Liver and spleen are not palpable.

### ▶ Extremities

Range of motion normal. No deformities noted. Some tenderness associated with extremes of motion and weight bearing, particularly on the right side. Some nonquantifiable discomfort associated with deep palpation at hip joint.

### ▶ Neurology

Loss of deep tendon reflexes at knees and somewhat flat-footed gait. Other within normal limits.

### ▶ Genitourinary

Unremarkable; testes normal size and texture for age

### ▶ Rectal

Small, healing perirectal tear with mild and perilesional erythema. No discharge or fluctuance.

## Laboratory Tests

|  | Conventional Units | SI Units |
|---|---|---|
| Na | 137 mEq/L | 137 mmol/L |
| K | 4.2 mEq/L | 4.2 mmol/L |
| BUN | 9 mg/dL | 3.2 mmol/L |
| SCr | 0.35 mg/dL | 31 μmol/L |
| Mg | 1.9 mEq/L | 0.95 mmol/L |
| Phosphate | 3.8 mg/dL | 1.23 mmol/L |
| AST | 51 IU/L | 0.85 μkat/L |
| ALT | 44 IU/L | 0.73 μkat/L |
| Total bilirubin | 0.9 mg/dL | 15.4 μmol/L |
| Direct bilirubin | 0.45 mg/dL | 7.7 μmol/L |
| Hgb | 11.8 g/dL | 118 g/L; 7.32 mmol/L |
| Hct | 34% | 0.34 |
| WBC | $1.2 \times 10^3/mm^3$ | $1.2 \times 10^9/L$ |
| ANC | 675/mm³ | $0.675 \times 10^9/L$ |
| MCV | 85 μm³ | 85 fL |
| Platelet count | 98,000/mm³ | $98 \times 10^9/L$ |

### ▶ Urinalysis

Pale color

Specific gravity 1.010

No RBCs or WBCs seen

Nitrate negative

### ▶ Radiology

X-ray of hips shows some sclerosis of both femoral heads and partial collapse on the right.

## Assessment

A 12-year-old boy with acute pre–B-cell ALL in the maintenance phase of treatment with two recent episodes of fever and neutropenia and a current somewhat low ANC. The history and current laboratory tests suggest repeated episodes of excessive hematologic toxicity. He additionally has chronic constipation that causes periodic rectal pain despite laxative use. Further, he complains of pain in both hips, which has been increasing in severity over the last 4–6 weeks.

## Student Workup

### Missing Information?

Evaluate:    Patient Database

Drug Therapy Problems

Care Plan (by Problem)

## TARGETED QUESTIONS

1. Evaluate the prognostic factors for ALL and evaluate the patient's potential risk for relapse.

   *Hint: See pp. 1656 and 1657 in PPP*

2. What do the patient's current CBC and prior problems with fever and neutropenia suggest with respect to potential drug toxicity?

   *Hint: See Table 95-9 and p. 1657 in PPP*

3. What additional testing should be considered to determine if there is an underlying problem in drug metabolism?

   *Hint: See Table 95-9 in PPP*

4. Is there a potential role for interviewing the patient's mother/father through a Spanish interpreter?

   *Hint: See patient/family's preferred language in "Social/Work History" for this case*

5. Are there any medications missing from the patient's treatment profile?

   *Hint: See pp. 1667–1668 in PPP*

6. What is the likely cause of the patient's bilateral hip pain?

   *Hint: See p. 1658 in PPP*

## FOLLOW-UP

The patient returns at 2 and 4 weeks after a 90% dose reduction in 6MP dose was started. His WBC counts at these points were 2.3 and $3.0 \times 10^3/mm^3$ (2.3 and $3.0 \times 10^9/L$), respectively, with corresponding ANCs of 1,600 and 2,000/$mm^3$ (1.6 and $2.0 \times 10^9/L$). At 3 months after the initial dose reduction, the WBC count is $4.8 \times 10^3/mm^3$ ($4.8 \times 10^9/L$), the ANC is 3,000/$mm^3$ ($3.0 \times 10^9/L$), and the patient has a normal hemoglobin, hematocrit, and platelet count.

7. What does this potentially say about you are the degree of your dose reduction?

   *Hint: The WBC and ANC recovery are consistent with a thiopurine methyltransferase (TPMT) genotype associated with diminished drug inactivation. The initial 90% dose reductions may have been too much and the latest*

*laboratory values suggest insufficient drug activity. Another possibility is that the family/patient have been giving even less 6MP because they were worried about toxicity. Check for compliance and consider adjusting the 6MP dose to 50% of the original dose. A 90% reduction is done only for patients with TPMT alleles with very diminished activity; 50% reductions are done in those with intermediate enzyme activity. After starting an additional drug for Pneumocystis jiroveci pneumonia (PJP) prophylaxis, the patient developed a pruritic, maculopapular rash over his chest and extremities.*

8. What drug is the most likely cause for this problem and what recommendations would you make regarding a change in therapy?

   *Hint: The most common agent used for PJP prophylaxis and the medication missing from the patient's profile is trimethoprim/sulfamethoxazole (TMP/SMX). Most patients tolerate this drug well; however, some develop an allergy to the drug, which is most typically a maculopapular rash. The drug should be discontinued. The patient's chart and records should also be labeled as "TMP/SMX and sulfa allergic." Because of the patient's age, he is a good candidate for monthly inhaled pentamidine as a substitute.*

## 🌍 GLOBAL PERSPECTIVE

Risk assessment (for relapse) is important in the treatment of ALL, and virtually all other malignancies. Knowing this allows for appropriate risk (toxicity of treatment) and reward (diminished risk of relapse) to be determined and thus the selection of a protocol with appropriate treatment intensity. Hematologic toxicity is common in patients receiving chemotherapy. Excessive toxicity may suggest an underlying problem with drug metabolism, clearance, or an incorrect dose. Likewise, the lack of expected myelosuppression may be an indicator of insufficient or absent doses. The etiologic distinction between drug interactions, incorrect dosing by the patient or family, or individual drug metabolic capacity can be difficult to determine, especially with oral medications. 6MP bioavailability is affected by the time of day the drug is given as well as the proximity to food and dairy products. Further, older children and adolescents may "game" their caretakers by not taking their medications ("cupping" their pills in their hand or holding them in their mouth without swallowing them and only later to dispose of them) or by only occasionally taking their medications. In addition, there is also great potential for misunderstanding the dose and schedule of administration among patients and families whose primary language is different than that of the prescriber; frequent questioning confirming the dose and timing is needed to assure compliance. It should also be kept in mind that, at times, the caretaker might change from the parent to a grandparent or other person during times when medications are due. The understanding and willingness of these persons to give the dose can be another source of problems. Related to this are cultural beliefs; other caretakers may possess beliefs contrary to the parents' and conventional medical advice. This can make them reluctant to give what they consider "toxic" medications and/or add the use of traditional remedies that have the potential to affect drug absorption, metabolism, and toxicity. Drug metabolism problems are the least frequent cause of toxicity than the other reasons noted above, and for the same reason, often the last to be considered as a cause for toxicity. For 6MP in particular, and other maintenance drugs for ALL, monitoring the WBC and ANC is an effective way to spot problems. Virtually all patients began treatment at a dose that assumes that they are among the 90% or more of patients who have normal drug-metabolizing activity. In these patients, excessive toxicity is rare, and monitoring WBC and ANC to make empiric and protocol-specific changes to the dose is effective and easy. In patients who show early and excessive toxicity, the likelihood of drug metabolism issues is heightened. In the absence of pretreatment genotyping for alleles associated with altered metabolism (a reasonable, but controversial, issue), these patients are best investigated with the use of 6MP metabolites and a determination of TPMT genotype. Both of these can be easily obtained from a patient's RBCs. However, the RBCs should not represent transfused cells; a minimum of 2–3 months since the last RBC transfusion is necessary to obtain reliable results.

## CASE SUMMARY

- The patient's clinical findings at diagnosis put him into a particular "risk" category for relapse.

- He has generally done well with aggressive therapy until the time he began daily 6MP and weekly methotrexate during his "maintenance" phase of treatment. His recent course and laboratory results are consistent with 6MP toxicity. This could be from potential overdosing as a result of poor provider/patient communication or inheritance of a polymorphism that limits drug metabolism and results in excessive levels of active metabolites. Given his "risk" category, his recent clinical course and laboratory results may warrant modification of the current treatment.

- A significant alteration in his 6MP dose was made that appears to have markedly diminished the patient's toxic episodes. However, his WBC and ANC seem to suggest that the dose reduction may have been too much or that some other problem has developed. A search for these problems and potential adjustments to the patient's dose may be needed to improve his antileukemic therapy and prevent relapse. Some critical tests and patient/family interviews are needed to determine what should be done next.

**For more information on the care plan and facilitator's guide please visit http://www.mhpharmacotherapy.com.**

# 102  Parenteral Nutrition

Michael D. Kraft          Melissa R. Pleva
Imad F. Btaiche

## CASE LEARNING OBJECTIVES

- List the appropriate indications for the use of parenteral nutrition (PN)
- List the elements of a nutrition assessment and factors considered in assessing a patient's nutritional status and nutritional requirements
- Develop a plan to design, initiate, and adjust a PN formulation using patient-specific factors
- Describe the etiology and risk factors for the refeeding syndrome
- Design a plan to monitor and correct fluid, electrolyte, vitamin, and trace-element abnormalities in patients receiving PN
- Design a plan to monitor and assess the efficacy and safety of PN therapy

## PATIENT PRESENTATION

### Chief Complaint

"I've had an upset stomach and pain which has been getting worse for about 10 days, and I started vomiting about 3 days ago. I can't keep any food or liquids down."

### History of Present Illness

Alex Rocker is a 46-year-old man with a history of morbid obesity s/p Roux-en-Y gastric bypass surgery in February 2010 for morbid obesity, who was admitted to the hospital 5 days ago on November 2, 2012, with abdominal pain, nausea, vomiting, and inability to tolerate oral intake. His postoperative course was complicated by anastomotic leak, peritonitis, sepsis, and high-output enterocutaneous (EC) fistula. He was initially placed nothing per os (NPO) with home PN and wound care for 6 months, and afterward underwent surgery for EC fistula takedown and small bowel resection with primary anastomosis. The patient has also had recurrent partial and total small bowel obstructions due to adhesions and had 2 other surgeries (exploratory laparotomies) for lysis of adhesions (in May 2011 and September 2012). Since his initial gastric bypass surgery, the patient lost approximately 100 lb (~46 kg) of his original pregastric bypass weight of 295 lb (134 kg). For the past 10 days before presentation to

the emergency department, he has had worsening nausea and abdominal pain that initially developed after eating a meal and appeared to get worse after eating. The abdominal pain gradually worsened, was associated with vomiting for the past 3 days, and he could not keep any food or liquids down. He described his symptoms as similar to the last time he had a bowel obstruction, but they now seem worse.

The patient was subsequently admitted to the GI surgery service for further management. Initially, he was managed conservatively by placing a NG tube for gastric fluid suctioning and bowel decompression, was placed NPO, and started on IV fluids for hydration. After 2 days of conservative management, the patient did not show any signs of improvement of his GI symptoms. A CT scan with oral contrast was done and demonstrated a complete small bowel obstruction. The surgical team decided on observing the patient and continuing conservative management for about a week until the patient's symptoms would resolve or otherwise would necessitate surgical intervention. Because the patient has had poor nutritional intake for about 12 days since the beginning of his symptoms, is currently NPO, has a complete bowel obstruction, and has had significant chronic weight loss since his gastric bypass surgery, he had a peripherally inserted central catheter (PICC) placed for PN therapy to be initiated.

PN therapy was initiated and then advanced to full nutritional goal on the second day. On the third day of PN therapy, the patient developed some confusion, and his biochemical workup showed multiple serum electrolyte abnormalities.

## Past Medical History

Type 2 DM × 5 years
  Morbid obesity for "most of his life" per patient

## Past Surgical History

Gastric bypass surgery (Roux-en-Y procedure) in February 2010
  Exploratory laparotomies and lysis of adhesions in May 2011 and September 2012

## Family History

Remarkable for obesity and type 2 DM (mother and father), HTN (mother and father), and hyperlipidemia (father)

## Social History

Married, lives with his wife

## Tobacco/Alcohol/Substance Abuse

Drinks alcohol occasionally/socially; no history of smoking

## Allergies/Intolerances/Adverse Drug Events

No known drug allergies

## Medications (Current)

Heparin 5,000 units subcutaneous tid

Pantoprazole 40 mg IV daily

Bisacodyl 10 mg suppository per rectum daily PRN constipation

Morphine sulfate 2–4 mg IV q 4 h PRN pain

Prochlorperazine 10 mg IV q 6 h PRN nausea

Regular insulin q 6 h, dosage per capillary blood glucose measurements

## Medications Prior to Admission

Glipizide XL 10 mg PO daily

Metformin XR 1,000 mg PO daily

## Review of Systems

Subjectively reporting ongoing abdominal pain, nausea, vomiting, no appetite. Also complains of dry mouth, feels thirsty, and abdomen feels bloated. (+) Dry mucus membranes. Denies fever, chills, or other pain.

## Physical Examination

### ▶ General

Middle-aged, slightly overweight African American man, uncomfortable because of abdominal pain, nausea, and vomiting

### ▶ Vital Signs

BP 134/84 mm Hg, P 92, RR 17, T 37.6°C

Weight 194 lb (88 kg)

Height 69 in. (175 cm)

Per patient, weight in 2009 prior to gastric bypass surgery 295 lb (~134 kg); weight in January 2012 reported to be 220 lb (100 kg)

Patient reports abdominal pain rated as 4–6/10, some relief with morphine and prochlorperazine

### ▶ Skin

Dry

### ▶ HEENT

PERRLA, EOMI, anicteric sclerae, mucus membranes dry

### ▶ Chest

Clear to auscultation bilaterally

### ▶ Cardiovascular

RRR; no murmurs, rubs, or gallops

### ▶ Abdomen

(+) Distention, hypoactive/absent bowel sounds, diffuse tenderness throughout all quadrants

### ▶ Neurology

A&O × 3; CNs II to XII intact

### ▶ Extremities

(−) Cyanosis, good pulse

### ▶ Genitourinary

Examination deferred

### ▶ Rectum

Examination deferred

## Laboratory Tests

### On Admission

| | Conventional Units | SI Units |
|---|---|---|
| Na | 138 mEq/L | 138 mmol/L |
| K | 3.6 mEq/L | 3.6 mmol/L |
| Cl | 94 mEq/L | 94 mmol/L |
| $CO_2$ | 28 mEq/L | 28 mmol/L |
| BUN | 12 mg/dL | 4.3 mmol/L |
| SCr | 0.5 mg/dL | 44 μmol/L |
| Ca | 7.6 mg/dL | 1.90 mmol/L |
| Mg | 1.7 mEq/L | 0.85 mmol/L |
| Phos | 3.1 mg/dL | 1 mmol/L |

| Glu | 152 mg/dL | 8.4 mmol/L |
| Hgb | 14.1 g/dL | 141 g/L; 8.75 mmol/L |
| Hct | 41.7% | 0.417 |
| Platelet | $348 \times 10^3/mm^3$ | $348 \times 10^9/L$ |
| WBC | $7.4 \times 10^3/mm^3$ | $7.4 \times 10^9/L$ |
| AST | 17 IU/L | 0.28 µkat/L |
| ALT | 21 IU/L | 0.35 µkat/L |
| Alk phos | 31 IU/L | 0.52 µkat/L |
| Total bilirubin | 0.6 mg/dL | 10.3 µmol/L |
| Alb | 2.4 g/dL | 24 g/L |
| Total protein | 5.6 g/dL | 56 g/L |

### On Hospital Day 5 (day 3 of PN)

|  | Conventional Units | SI Units |
| --- | --- | --- |
| Na | 135 mEq/L | 135 mmol/L |
| K | 2.9 mEq/L | 2.9 mmol/L |
| Cl | 92 mEq/L | 92 mmol/L |
| $CO_2$ | 38 mEq/L | 38 mmol/L |
| BUN | 19 mg/dL | 6.8 mmol/L |
| SCr | 0.6 mg/dL | 53 µmol/L |
| Glu | 207 mg/dL | 11.5 mmol/L |
| Ca | 7.1 mg/dL | 1.78 mmol/L |
| Mg | 1.2 mEq/L | 0.60 mmol/L |
| Phos | 1.9 mg/dL | 0.61 mmol/L |
| Hgb | 13.2 g/dL | 132 g/L; 8.19 mmol/L |
| Hct | 38.4% | 0.384 |
| Platelet | $297 \times 10^3/mm^3$ | $297 \times 10^9/L$ |
| WBC | $8.9 \times 10^3/mm^3$ | $8.9 \times 10^9/L$ |
| AST | 18 IU/L | 0.30 µkat/L |
| ALT | 19 IU/L | 0.32 µkat/L |
| Alk phos | 34 IU/L | 0.57 µkat/L |
| Total bilirubin | 0.9 mg/dL | 15.4 µmol/L |
| Alb | 2.1 g/dL | 21 g/L |
| Total protein | 5.2 g/dL | 52 g/L |

#### ▶ Radiology

CT scan with oral contrast demonstrates a complete small bowel obstruction

### Assessment

This is a 46-year-old man with a history of morbid obesity and type 2 DM, who is s/p Roux-en-Y gastric bypass surgery, gradual weight loss of approximately 100 lb (~46 kg) over the past 32 months, and weight loss of approximately 26 lb (~12 kg) since January; he was admitted to the hospital with abdominal pain and nausea for 10 days and vomiting for 3 days. The results of his abdominal CT scan and his symptoms are consistent with recurrent complete small

bowel obstruction. Given the patient's medical and surgical history, the attending surgeon did not believe the patient was an optimal candidate for immediate surgery and decided to continue conservative management by keeping the patient NPO, continue with an NG tube to suction, supportive care, symptomatic treatment, and PN for nutrition support. After 3 days of PN, the patient developed signs and symptoms consistent with refeeding syndrome.

### Student Workup

**Missing Information?**

**Evaluate:**    Patient Database
Drug Therapy Problems
Care Plan (by Problem)

## TARGETED QUESTIONS

1. Why is this patient at risk for refeeding syndrome?

   *Hint: See pp. 1772–1773 and reference 45 in Chapter 100 in PPP*

2. Does this patient have an appropriate indication for PN therapy?

   *Hint: See p. 1756, Table 100-1, and references 1 and 2 in Chapter 100 in PPP*

3. What signs, symptoms, and laboratory abnormalities does this patient have that are consistent with refeeding syndrome?

   *Hint: See pp. 1772–1773 and reference 45 in Chapter 100 in PPP*

4. What steps would you take to treat refeeding syndrome in this patient?

   *Hint: See pp. 1772–1773 and reference 45 in Chapter 100 in PPP*

5. Given that this patient has a complete small bowel obstruction and is NPO, what treatment would you recommend for his hyperglycemia? What target range for serum glucose concentrations would you recommend?

   *Hint: See pp. 1769–1770 and references 32–35 in Chapter 100 in PPP*

6. Is this patient receiving any medications that do not have an appropriate indication?

## FOLLOW-UP

The surgical team takes your recommendations, and the patient's symptoms and electrolyte abnormalities have resolved. His bowel obstruction has still not resolved, and the team wants to continue PN therapy. You found that the patient was receiving the following IV fluids: 5% dextrose and 0.45% sodium chloride in water ($D_5W$ ½ NS) at 80 mL/h prior to PN and then decreased to 20 mL/h when PN was started. He was also receiving the following PN prescription at goal (day 2 of PN):

Two-in-one PN formulation (intravenous lipid emulsion infused separately from dextrose/amino acid/ micronutrient admixture at Y-site)

20% lipid emulsion = 384 mL/d (16 mL/h)

PN volume (dextrose/amino acid/micronutrient admixture) = 2,160 mL (90 mL/h)

Dextrose = 450 g/d

Amino acids = 130 g/d

Potassium chloride = 80 mEq/d (80 mmol/d)

Sodium chloride = 20 mEq/d (20 mmol/d)

Sodium acetate = 60 mEq/d (60 mmol/d)

Sodium phosphate = 20 mmol/d

Calcium gluconate = 10 mEq/d (5 mmol/d)

Magnesium sulfate = 10 mEq/d (5 mmol/d)

Parenteral adult multivitamin = 10 mL/d

Multitrace element (concentrate) = 1 mL/d

7. What recommendations would you have about resuming PN in this patient? Develop a goal PN regimen, as well as a plan to initiate PN, advance PN to goal, and monitor PN therapy while in the hospital.

*Hint: Calculate total calories and protein in the above PN prescription; note amounts of electrolytes (especially phosphate, potassium, magnesium, and sodium), total fluid, and any supplemental vitamins and trace elements; evaluate the patient's fluid needs and assess any abnormal fluid and electrolyte losses (e.g., GI losses); see pp. 1757–1762, Tables 100-3 to 100-5, Table 100-8, and references 1, 2, and 45 in Chapter100 in PPP*

## ⟲ GLOBAL PERSPECTIVE

The refeeding syndrome is a constellation of metabolic derangements that can occur in patients who are malnourished or who have had a prolonged period of inadequate nutrition with significant weight loss. Refeeding syndrome can lead to serious complications, including death, and it is one of the few true emergencies associated with nutrition support. In developing countries or areas where malnutrition is prevalent and nutrient and vitamin deficiencies are common, refeeding syndrome could be a significant concern if the person were to receive a more abundant source of nutrition (orally or parenterally). These individuals with severe protein and calorie malnutrition

may be more likely to have underlying vitamin and trace element deficiencies that could complicate or worsen symptoms of refeeding syndrome (e.g., thiamine, folic acid, vitamin $B_{12}$, vitamin D, iron, selenium, zinc, copper).

This could be especially concerning in growing children with poor body protein and energy reserves and pregnant women who have added energy and nutrient demands. A good rule of thumb in individuals with moderate-to-severe malnutrition is to "start low and go slow" when initiating any type of nutrition whether PN, enteral nutrition, or oral diet. This slow-and-gradual approach is essential to avoid the complications of refeeding syndrome that may severely affect the cardiac, respiratory, neurologic, and neuromuscular systems. It is also important to provide aggressive supplementation of electrolytes and vitamins, *before* initiating nutrition, and regularly as needed during nutrition advancement guided by serum electrolyte concentrations and clinical status.

## CASE SUMMARY

- The patient is exhibiting signs and symptoms consistent with refeeding syndrome. Even though he may not have the traditional marasmic appearance (i.e., "skin and bone"), he has experienced dramatic weight loss and has had little or no nutrition intake for approximately 10 days. Individuals at risk for refeeding syndrome should be first identified, and electrolyte supplementation provided immediately with supportive treatment provided when necessary to avoid comorbidities and possibly death. Individuals who exhibit signs and symptoms of refeeding syndrome should have nutrition support stopped until symptoms and electrolyte abnormalities are corrected. A specific prevention and treatment plan should be outlined.

- After electrolyte abnormalities are corrected and symptoms have improved/resolved, PN should be restarted very cautiously, and a treatment plan should be developed to avoid signs and symptoms of refeeding syndrome from recurring.

- The patient also has type 2 DM, and is NPO with a complete small bowel obstruction. Therefore, a plan must be developed to adequately treat hyperglycemia while he is NPO and receiving PN in the hospital.

**For more information on the care plan and facilitator's guide please visit http://www.mhpharmacotherapy.com.**

# 103 Obesity

Maqual R. Graham

## CASE LEARNING OBJECTIVES

- Identify parameters utilized to diagnose obesity and other objective information that indicates the severity of disease
- Identify desired therapeutic goals for patients who are obese
- Recommend appropriate nonpharmacologic and pharmacologic therapeutic interventions for obese patients
- Implement a monitoring plan that will assess both the efficacy and safety of therapy initiated
- Educate the patient about the disease state and associated risks, appropriate lifestyle modifications, and drug therapy options necessary for effective treatment

## PATIENT PRESENTATION

### Chief Complaint

"I will be 60 years old very soon. I am tired of being tired. I want more energy; I want to feel young again."

### History of Present Illness

Joseph Michelson is a 59-year-old male patient presenting to the Cardiovascular Disease Risk Reduction Clinic for an initial evaluation. He was referred by his primary care provider for aggressive weight management. The patient states that he rarely eats healthy, even though his wife continually suggests healthier food choices. He prefers to eat meals high in fat and carbohydrates. He defines himself as a meat and potato type of guy. He snacks on corn and potato chips several times per day. He usually follows his salty snack with sweet-tasting foods, such as cookies or candy. He rarely consumes fruit. He drinks a glass of orange juice every morning. Throughout the day, he generally craves soda that is usually dark in color and caffeinated. Because of his work schedule, he finds it difficult to exercise. If he does have time to exercise in the evening, he lacks motivation. He has lost weight many times in the past. Each drop in weight resulted in him feeling more energetic and thus he appears ready to lose weight.

### Past Medical History

HTN diagnosed 5 years ago
GERD diagnosed 10 years ago

### Family History

Father had CHD and died following a second MI at age 63. Mother is alive at age 89 with type 2 DM and hypothyroidism.

He has 3 sisters and 1 brother who are all alive. His brother was recently hospitalized with cardiac chest pain (age 61).

### Social History

The patient is married and lives with his wife of 41 years. He has 2 children (ages 35 and 39). He owns a small business that specializes in floor covering.

### Tobacco/Alcohol/Substance Use

The patient denies tobacco use. He occasionally drinks alcohol, 1–2 beers on the weekend. No current or past illicit drug use.

### Allergies/Intolerances/Adverse Drug Events

None

### Medications (Current)

Metoprolol 25 mg PO twice daily
Diltiazem 360 mg PO once daily
Aspirin 325 mg PO once daily
Ranitidine 150 mg PO twice daily

### Review of Systems

▸ *General*

The patient has gained 10 lb (4.5 kg) in the last year.

▸ *Skin*

No rashes or other skin changes

> ### HEENT

Hearing good; (−) tinnitus; (−) infections. The patient reports two mild colds in the last year.

> ### Neck

(−) Lumps, goiter

> ### Respiratory

(−) Cough, wheezing, SOB

> ### Cardiovascular

(−) Dyspnea, chest pain, palpitations

> ### Gastrointestinal

Appetite good; (−) nausea, vomiting; (+) daily bowel movements. Occasional reflux symptoms following very high fat meals

> ### Urinary

(−) Change in urinary frequency, hematuria

> ### Neurologic

(−) Syncope; (−) loss of consciousness

## Physical Examination

> ### General

Well-developed, middle-aged male in no acute distress

> ### Vital Signs

BP 132/74 mm Hg, P 58 bpm, RR 12 rpm, T 96.8°F (36.0°C)

Weight 225 lb (102.3 kg)

Height 65 in. (165.1 cm)

Waist circumference 46.5 in. (118 cm)

Pain 0/10

> ### Skin

(−) Lesions; nails without clubbing or cyanosis

> ### HEENT

PERRLA, EOMI; (−) sinus tenderness; TM appears normal bilaterally; oral mucosa pink

> ### Neck and Lymph Nodes

Neck supple; (−) lymphadenopathy; trachea midline; (−) enlarged thyroid, (−) thyroid nodules; (−) carotid bruits

> ### Chest

Clear to auscultation bilaterally

> ### Cardiovascular

Regular rhythm, bradycardic, (−) $S_3$ or $S_4$

> ### Abdomen

Nontender, nondistended, bowel sounds active in all four quadrants, no masses detected

> ### Neurology

CNs II–XII intact; strength 5/5; normal gait; (−) Romberg, normal reflexes

> ### Extremities

Warm and without edema bilaterally

> ### Genitourinary

Examination deferred

> ### Rectal

Examination deferred

## Laboratory Tests

### Fasting

| | Conventional Units | SI Units |
|---|---|---|
| Na | 140 mEq/L | 140 mmol/L |
| K | 4.6 mEq/L | 4.6 mmol/L |
| Cl | 106 mEq/L | 106 mmol/L |
| $CO_2$ | 24 mEq/L | 24 mmol/L |
| BUN | 12 mg/dL | 4.3 mmol/L |
| SCr | 0.9 mg/dL | 80 µmol/L |
| Glu | 96 mg/dL | 5.3 mmol/L |
| Ca | 9.7 mg/dL | 2.43 mmol/L |
| Lipase | 26 U/L | 0.43 µkat/L |
| Amylase | 36 U/L | 0.60 µkat/L |
| Hgb | 14.9 g/dL | 149 g/L; 9.25 mmol/L |
| Hct | 44% | 0.44 |
| WBC | $5.4 \times 10^3/mm^3$ | $5.4 \times 10^9/L$ |
| Platelets | $156 \times 10^3/\mu L$ | $156 \times 10^9/L$ |
| AST | 29 U/L | 0.48 µkat/L |
| ALT | 38 U/L | 0.63 µkat/L |
| TSH | 1.498 µIU/mL | 1.498 mIU/L |
| Total cholesterol | 286 mg/dL | 7.40 mmol/L |
| LDL cholesterol | 201 mg/dL | 5.20 mmol/L |
| HDL cholesterol | 31 mg/dL | 0.80 mmol/L |
| Triglycerides | 272 mg/dL | 3.07 mmol/L |

## Assessment

A 59-year-old obese male in need of reduced cardiovascular disease (CVD) risk

## TARGETED QUESTIONS

1. How would you classify this patient's BMI?

   *Hint: See Table 102-1 in PPP*

2. Does this patient have a high-risk waist circumference?

   *Hint: See Table 102-2 and p. 1797 in PPP*

3. Does this patient have CV risk factors, and if so, which one(s)?

   *Hint: See Table 102-3 in PPP*

4. Is this patient a candidate for weight loss, and if so, what is the initial weight loss goal?

   *Hint: See p. 1797 in PPP*

5. Is nonpharmacologic therapy, pharmacologic therapy, or both recommended for this patient?

   *Hint: See pp. 1798–1804 in PPP*

6. What patient parameters need to be assessed when this patient returns for follow-up?

   *Hint: See pp. 1804–1806 in PPP*

## FOLLOW-UP

The patient has returned for all scheduled follow-up assessment visits in the CVD risk reduction clinic. By the 6-month follow-up visit, the patient's weight was reduced by 10 lb (4.5 kg). His waist circumference is now 45.5 in. (116 cm). He appears compliant with the therapy previously recommended. He feels a little more energetic; however, he wishes that he was closer to his weight loss goal.

7. Should the initial therapeutic recommendations be altered, and if so, how?

   *Hint: See pp. 1804–1806 in PPP*

## ⊙ GLOBAL PERSPECTIVE

Energy imbalance, or energy intake greater than energy expenditure, is a key factor in the development of obesity. The longer the imbalance occurs, the greater the extent of obesity. Height and weight can easily be assessed anytime a patient–provider interaction occurs. From these two parameters, BMI can be determined. Waist circumference should also be evaluated as well as presence of other comorbidities and CV risk factors. Weight reduction, maintaining weight loss, and preventing weight gain are the general therapeutic goals for obese patients. Controlling related risks is an additional goal in the management of obesity. Lifestyle changes (dietary modification, increased physical activity, and behavioral therapy), drug treatment, surgery, or a combination of strategies are necessary for meeting desired outcomes. Frequent monitoring is necessary to determine the success or failure of the treatment plan.

## CASE SUMMARY

- JM is a Class 2 obese patient with a high-risk waist circumference and CV risk factors that include male gender and age 45 years or older, HTN, high LDL cholesterol, and low HDL cholesterol.

- Lifestyle changes are recommended to reduce his weight by 22 lb (10 kg) in 6 months at a rate of 1–2 lb (0.45–0.9 kg)/wk.

- Aggressive management of related risks (BP, LDL cholesterol, and HDL cholesterol) is necessary for overall effective treatment of the obese patient.

For more information on the care plan and facilitator's guide please visit http://www.mhpharmacotherapy.com.

# Appendix A: Conversion Factors and Anthropometrics*

## CONVERSION FACTORS

### SI Units

SI (*le Systéme International d'Unités*) units are used in many countries to express clinical laboratory and serum drug concentration data. Instead of using units of mass (e.g., micrograms), the SI system uses moles (mol) to represent the amount of a substance. A molar solution contains 1 mole (the molecular weight of the substance in grams) of the solute in 1 L of solution. The following formula is used to convert units of mass to moles (mcg/mL to $\mu$mol/L or, by substitution of terms, mg/mL to mmol/L or ng/mL to nmol/L).

▶ *Micromoles per Liter*

Micromoles per liter ($\mu$mol/L)

$$= \frac{\text{drug concentration (mcg/mL)} \times 1{,}000}{\text{molecular weight of drug (g/mol)}}$$

▶ *Milliequivalents*

An equivalent weight of a substance is the weight that will combine with or replace 1 g of hydrogen; a milliequivalent is 1/1,000 of an equivalent weight.

### Milliequivalents per Liter

Milliequivalents per liter (mEq/L)

$$= \frac{\text{weight of salt (g)} \times \text{valence of ion} \times 1{,}000}{\text{molecular weight of salt}}$$

$$\text{Weight of salt (g)} = \frac{\text{mEq/L} \times \text{molecular weight of salt}}{\text{valence of ion} \times 1{,}000}$$

| Approximate Milliequivalents: Weight Conversions for Selected Ions | | |
|---|---|---|
| **Salt** | **mEq/g Salt** | **mg Salt/ mEq** |
| Calcium carbonate ($CaCO_3$) | 20.0 | 50.0 |
| Calcium chloride ($CaCl_2 \cdot 2H_2O$) | 13.6 | 73.5 |
| Calcium gluceptate ($Ca[C_7H_{13}O_8]_2$) | 4.1 | 245.2 |
| Calcium gluconate ($Ca[C_6H_{11}O_7]_2 \cdot H_2O$) | 4.5 | 224.1 |
| Calcium lactate ($Ca[C_3H_5O_3]_2 \cdot 5H_2O$) | 6.5 | 154.1 |
| Magnesium gluconate ($Mg[C_6H_{11}O_7]_2 \cdot H_2O$) | 4.6 | 216.3 |
| Magnesium oxide ($MgO$) | 49.6 | 20.2 |
| Magnesium sulfate ($MgSO_4$) | 16.6 | 60.2 |
| Magnesium sulfate ($MgSO_4 \cdot 7H_2O$) | 8.1 | 123.2 |
| Potassium acetate ($K[C_2H_3O_2]$) | 10.2 | 98.1 |
| Potassium chloride ($KCl$) | 13.4 | 74.6 |
| Potassium citrate ($K_3[C_6H_5O_7] \cdot H_2O$) | 9.2 | 108.1 |
| Potassium iodide ($KI$) | 6.0 | 166.0 |
| Sodium acetate ($Na[C_2H_3O_2]$) | 12.2 | 82.0 |
| Sodium acetate ($Na[C_2H_3O_2] \cdot 3H_2O$) | 7.3 | 136.1 |
| Sodium bicarbonate ($NaHCO_3$) | 11.9 | 84.0 |
| Sodium chloride ($NaCl$) | 17.1 | 58.4 |
| Sodium citrate ($Na_3[C_6H_5O_7] \cdot 2H_2O$) | 10.2 | 98.0 |
| Sodium iodide ($NaI$) | 6.7 | 149.9 |
| Sodium lactate ($Na[C_3H_5O_3]$) | 8.9 | 112.1 |
| Zinc sulfate ($ZnSO_4 \cdot 7H_2O$) | 7.0 | 143.8 |

*This appendix contains information from Appendices 1 and 2 of Smith KM, Riche DM, Henyan NN (eds). Clinical Drug Data, 11th ed. New York: McGraw-Hill, 2010:1239–1246; With permission.

| Valences and Atomic/Molecular Weights of Selected Ions | | | |
|---|---|---|---|
| **Substance** | **Electrolyte** | **Valence** | **Atomic/ Molecular Weight** |
| Calcium | $Ca^{2+}$ | 2 | 40.1 |
| Chloride | $Cl^-$ | 1 | 35.5 |
| Magnesium | $Mg^{2+}$ | 2 | 24.3 |
| Phosphate | $HPO_4^-$ (80%) | 1.8 | $96.0^a$ |
| (pH = 7.4) | $H_2PO_4^-$ (20%) | | 97.0 |
| Potassium | $K^+$ | 1 | 39.1 |
| Sodium | $Na^+$ | 1 | 23.0 |
| Sulfate | $SO_4^-$ | 2 | $96.0^a$ |

$^a$The atomic/molecular weight of phosphorus is only 31; that of sulfur is only 32.1.

## Anion Gap

The anion gap is the concentration of plasma anions not routinely measured by laboratory screening. It is useful in the evaluation of acid–base disorders. The anion gap is greater with increased plasma concentrations of endogenous species (e.g., phosphate, sulfate, lactate, and ketoacids) or exogenous species (e.g., salicylate, penicillin, ethylene glycol, ethanol, and methanol). The formulas for calculating the anion gap are as follows:

$$\text{Anion gap} = (Na^+ + K^+) - (Cl^- + HCO_3^-)$$

or

$$\text{Anion gap} = Na^+ - (Cl^- + HCO_3^-)$$

where the expected normal value for the first equation is 11 to 20 mmol/L and for the second equation is 7 to 16 mmol/L. Note that there is a variation in the upper and lower limits of the normal range.

## Temperature

Fahrenheit to Centigrade: $(°F - 32) \times 5/9 = °C$
Centigrade to Fahrenheit: $(°C \times 9/5) + 32 = °F$
Centigrade to Kelvin: $°C + 273 = °K$

## Calories

1 calorie = 1 kilocalorie = 1,000 calories = 4.184 kilojoules (kJ)
1 kilojoule = 0.239 calories = 0.239 kilocalories = 239 calories

## Weights and Measures

### ▶ Metric Weight Equivalents

1 kilogram (kg) = 1,000 grams
1 gram (g) = 1,000 milligrams
1 milligram (mg) = 0.001 gram
1 microgram (mcg, μg) = 0.001 milligram
1 nanogram (ng) = 0.001 microgram
1 picogram (pg) = 0.001 nanogram
1 femtogram (fg) = 0.001 picogram

### ▶ Metric Volume Equivalents

1 liter (L) = 1,000 milliliters
1 deciliter (dL) = 100 milliliters
1 milliliter (mL) = 0.001 liter
1 microliter (μL) = 0.001 milliliter
1 nanoliter (nL) = 0.001 microliter
1 picoliter (pL) = 0.001 nanoliter
1 femtoliter (fL) = 0.001 picoliter

### ▶ Apothecary Weight Equivalents

1 scruple (℈) = 20 grains (gr)
60 grains (gr) = 1 dram (ʒ)
8 drams (ʒ) = 1 ounce (℥)
1 ounce (℥) = 480 grains (gr)
12 ounces (℥) = 1 pound (lb)

### ▶ Apothecary Volume Equivalents

60 minims (m) = 1 fluidram (fl ʒ)
8 fluidrams (fl ʒ) = 1 fluid ounce (fl ℥)
1 fluid ounce (fl ℥) = 480 minims (m)
16 fluid ounces (fl ℥) = 1 pint (pt)

### ▶ Avoirdupois Equivalents

1 ounce (oz) = 437.5 grains
16 ounces (oz) = 1 pound (lb)

### ▶ Weight/Volume Equivalents

1 mg/dL = 10 mcg/mL
1 mg/dL = 1 mg%
1 ppm = 1 mg/L

### ▶ Conversion Equivalents

1 gram (g) = 15.43 grains (gr)
1 grain (gr) = 64.8 milligrams (mg)
1 ounce (℥) = 31.1 grams (g)
1 ounce (oz) = 28.35 grams (g)
1 pound (lb) = 453.6 grams (g)
1 kilogram (kg) = 2.2 pounds (lb)
1 milliliter (mL) = 16.23 minims (m)
1 minim (m) = 0.06 milliliter (mL)
1 fluid ounce (fl oz) = 29.57 milliliters (mL)
1 pint (pt) = 473.2 milliliters (mL)
1 US gallon = 3.78 liters (L)
1 Canadian gallon = 4.55 liters (L)
0.1 milligram = 1/600 grain
0.12 milligram = 1/500 grain
0.15 milligram = 1/400 grain
0.2 milligram = 1/300 grain
0.3 milligram = 1/200 grain
0.4 milligram = 1/150 grain
0.5 milligram = 1/120 grain
0.6 milligram = 1/100 grain
0.8 milligram = 1/80 grain
1 milligram = 1/65 grain

► *Metric Length Conversion Equivalents*

2.54 cm = 1 inch
30.48 cm = 1 foot
1 m = 3.28 feet
1.6 km = 1 mile

# ANTHROPOMETRICS

## Creatinine Clearance Formulas

► *Formulas for Estimating Creatinine Clearance in Patients with Stable Renal Function*

### Cockcroft-Gault Formula

Adults (age 18 years and older)[1]:

$$CrCl\ (men) = \frac{(140 - age) \times weight}{SCr \times 72}$$

$$CrCl\ (women) = 0.85 \times above\ value^*$$

where CrCl is creatinine clearance (in mL/min), SCr is serum creatinine (in mg/dL [or μmol/L divided by 88.4]), age is in years, and weight is in kilograms.

* Some studies suggest that the predictive accuracy of this formula for women is better *without* the correction factor of 0.85.

### Traub-Johnson Formula

Children (age 1–18 years)[2]:

$$CrCl = \frac{0.48 \times height \times BSA}{SCr \times 1.73}$$

where BSA is body surface area (in m[2]), CrCl is creatinine clearance (in mL/minute), SCr is serum creatinine (in mg/dL [or μmol/L divided by 88.4]), and height is in centimeters.

► *Formula for Estimating Creatinine Clearance From a Measured Urine Collection*

$$CrCl\ (mL/minute) = \frac{U \times V}{P \times T}$$

where $U$ is the concentration of creatinine in a urine specimen in mg/dL, $V$ is the volume of urine in mL, $P$ is the concentration of creatinine in serum at the midpoint of the urine collection period in mg/dL, and $T$ is the time of the urine collection period in minutes (e.g., 6 hours = 360 minutes; 24 hours = 1,440 minutes). Procedures for obtaining urine specimens should stress the importance of complete urine collection during the collection time period.

► *MDRD Formula for Estimating Glomerular Filtration Rate (From the Modification of Diet in Renal Disease Study)[3]*

Conventional calibration MDRD equation (used only with those creatinine methods that have *not* been recalibrated to be traceable to isotope dilution mass spectrometry [IDMS])
For creatinine in mg/dL:

$$X = 186\ creatinine^{-1.154} \times age^{-0.203} \times constant$$

For creatinine in μmol/L:

$$X = 32,788 \times creatinine^{-1.154} \times age^{-0.203} \times constant$$

where $X$ is the glomerular filtration rate (GFR), constant for white men is 1 and for women is 0.742, and constant for African Americans is 1.21. Creatinine levels in μmol/L can be converted to mg/dL by dividing by 88.4.

► *IDMS-Traceable MDRD Equation (Used Only With Creatinine Methods That Have Been Recalibrated to Be Traceable to IDMS)*

For creatinine in mg/dL:

$$X = 175 \times creatinine^{-1.154} \times age^{-0.203} \times constant$$

For creatinine in μmol/L:

$$X = 175 \times (creatinine/88.4)^{-1.154} \times age^{-0.203} \times constant$$

where $X$ is the GFR, constant for white men is 1 and for women is 0.742, and constant for African Americans is 1.21.

## Ideal Body Weight

IBW is the weight expected for a nonobese person of a given height. The IBW formulas below and various life insurance tables can be used to estimate IBW. Dosing methods described in the literature may use IBW as a method in dosing obese patients.

**Adults (age 18 years and older)[4]:**

IBW (men) = 50 + (2.3 × height in inches over 5 ft)
IBW (women) = 45.5 + (2.3 × height in inches over 5 ft)

where IBW is in kilograms.

**Children (age 1–18 years)[2] under 5 feet tall:**

$$IBW = \frac{height^2 \times 1.65}{1,000}$$

where IBW is in kilograms and height is in centimeters.

**Children (age 1–18 years) 5 feet or taller:**

IBW (males) = 39 + (2.27 × height in inches over 5 ft)
IBW (females) = 42.2 + (2.27 × height in inches over 5 ft)

where IBW is in kilograms.

## REFERENCES

1. Cockcroft DW, Gault MH. Prediction of creatinine clearance from serum creatinine. Nephron 1976;16:31–41.
2. Traub SI, Johnson CE. Comparison of methods of estimating creatinine clearance in children. Am J Hosp Pharm 1980;37:195–201.
3. Levey AS, Bosch JP, Lewis JB, et al. A more accurate method to estimate glomerular filtration rate from serum creatinine: A new prediction equation. Modification of Diet in Renal Disease Study Group. Ann Intern Med 1999;130:461–470.
4. Devine BJ. Gentamicin therapy. Drug Intell Clin Pharm 1974;8:650–655.

# Appendix B: Common Laboratory Tests

The following table is an alphabetical listing of some common laboratory tests and their reference ranges for adults as measured in plasma or serum (unless otherwise indicated). Reference values differ among laboratories, so readers should refer to the published reference ranges used in each institution. For some tests, both the Système International Units and Conventional Units are reported.

| Laboratory Test | Conventional Units | Conversion Factor | Système International Units |
|---|---|---|---|
| Acid phosphatase | | | |
|   Male | 2–12 U/L | 16.7 | 33–200 nkat/L |
|   Female | 0.3–9.2 U/L | 16.7 | 5–154 nkat/L |
| Activated partial thromboplastin time (aPTT) | 25–40 sec | | |
| Adrenocorticotropic hormone (ACTH) | 15–80 pg/mL or ng/L | 0.2202 | 3.3–17.6 pmol/L |
| Alanine aminotransferase (ALT, SGPT) | 7–53 U/L | 0.01667 | 0.12–0.88 μkat/L |
| Albumin | 3.5–5.0 g/dL | 10 | 35–50 g/L |
| Albumin:creatinine ratio (urine) | | 0.113 | |
|   Normal | Less than 30 mg/g creatinine | | Less than 3.4 mg/mmol creatinine |
|   Microalbuminuria | 30–300 mg/g creatinine | | 3.4–34 mg/mmol creatinine |
|   Proteinuria | Greater than 300 mg/g creatinine | | Greater than 34 mg/mmol creatinine |
| or | or | | |
| Normal | | | |
|   Male | Less than 18 mg/g creatinine | 0.113 | Less than 2.0 mg/mmol creatinine |
|   Female | Less than 25 mg/g creatinine | 0.113 | Less than 2.8 mg/mmol creatinine |
| Microalbuminuria | | | |
|   Male | 18–180 mg/g creatinine | 0.113 | 2.0–20 mg/mmol creatinine |
|   Female | 25–250 mg/g creatinine | 0.113 | 2.8–28 mg/mmol creatinine |
| Proteinuria | | | |
|   Male | Greater than 180 mg/g creatinine | 0.113 | Greater than 20 mg/mmol creatinine |
|   Female | Greater than 250 mg/mmol creatinine | 0.113 | Greater than 28 mg/mmol creatinine |
| Alcohol | | | |
|   See under Ethanol | | | |
| Aldosterone | | | |
|   Supine | Less than 16 ng/dL | 27.7 | Less than 444 pmol/L |
|   Upright | Less than 31 ng/dL | 27.7 | Less than 860 pmol/L |
| Alkaline phosphatase | | | |
|   10–15 years | 130–550 IU/L | 0.01667 | 2.17–9.17 μkat/L |
|   16–20 years | 70–260 IU/L | 0.01667 | 1.17–4.33 μkat/L |
|   Greater than 20 years | 38–126 IU/L | 0.01667 | 0.63–2.10 μkat/L |
| α-Fetoprotein (AFP) | Less than 15 ng/mL | 1 | Less than 15 mcg/L |
| α-1-Antitrypsin | 80–200 mg/dL | 0.01 | 0.8–2.0 g/L |

*(Continued)*

| Laboratory Test | Conventional Units | Conversion Factor | Système International Units |
|---|---|---|---|
| Amikacin, therapeutic | | | |
|   Peak | 15–30 mg/L | 1.71 | 25.6–51.3 µmol/L |
|   Trough | Less than or equal to 8 mg/L | 1.71 | Less than or equal to 13.7 µmol/L |
| Amitriptyline | 80–200 ng/mL or mcg/L | 3.605 | 288–721 nmol/L |
| Ammonia (plasma) | 15–56 mcg $NH_3$/dL | 0.5872 | 9–33 µmol $NH_3$/L |
| Amylase | 25–115 U/L | 0.01667 | 0.42–1.92 µkat/L |
| Androstenedione | 50–250 ng/dL | 0.0349 | 1.7–8.7 nmol/L |
| Angiotensin-converting enzyme | 15–70 units/L | 16.67 | 250–1167 nkat/L |
| Anion gap | 7–16 mEq/L | 1 | 7–16 mmol/L |
| Anti–double-stranded DNA (anti-ds DNA) | Negative | | |
| Anti-HAV | Negative | | |
| Anti-HBc | Negative | | |
| Anti-HBs | Negative | | |
| Anti-HCV | Negative | | |
| Anti-Sm antibody | Negative | | |
| Antinuclear antibody (ANA) | Negative | | |
| Apolipoprotein A-1 | | | |
|   Male | 95–175 mg/dL | 0.01 | 0.95–1.75 g/L |
|   Female | 100–200 mg/dL | 0.01 | 1.0–2.0 g/L |
| Apolipoprotein B | | | |
|   Male | 50–110 mg/dL | 0.01 | 0.5–1.10 g/L |
|   Female | 50–105 mg/dL | 0.01 | 0.5–1.05 g/L |
| Aspartate aminotransferase (AST, SGOT) | 11–47 IU/L | 0.01667 | 0.18–0.78 µkat/L |
| $\beta_2$-Microglobulin | Less than 0.2 mg/dL | 10 | Less than 2 mg/L |
| Bicarbonate | 22–26 mEq/L | 1 | 22–26 mmol/L |
| Bilirubin | | | |
|   Total | 0.3–1.1 mg/dL | 17.1 | 5.1–18.8 µmol/L |
|   Direct | 0–0.3 mg/dL | 17.1 | 0–5.1 µmol/L |
|   Indirect | 0.1–1.0 mg/dL | 17.1 | 1.7–17.1 µmol/L |
| Bleeding time | 3–7 minutes | 60 | 180–420 seconds |
| Blood gases (arterial) | | | |
|   pH | 7.35–7.45 | 1 | 7.35–7.45 |
|   $Po_2$ | 80–105 mm Hg | 0.133 | 10.6–14.0 kPa |
|   $Pco_2$ | 35–45 mm Hg | 0.133 | 4.7–6.0 kPa |
|   $HCO_3$ | 22–26 mEq/L | 1 | 22–26 mmol/L |
|   $O_2$ saturation | Greater than or equal to 95% | 0.01 | Greater than or equal to 0.95 |
| Blood urea nitrogen (BUN) | 8–25 mg/dL | 0.357 | 2.9–8.9 mmol/L |
| B-type natriuretic peptide (BNP) | 0–99 pg/mL | 1 | 0–99 ng/L |
| | | 0.289 | 0–29 pmol/L |
| BUN-to-creatinine ratio | 10:1–20:1 | | |
| C-peptide | 0.51–2.70 ng/mL | 331 | 170–894 pmol/L |
| | | 0.331 | 0.17–0.89 nmol/L |
| C-reactive protein | Less than 0.8 mg/dL | 10 | Less than 8 mg/L |
| CA-125 | Less than 35 units/mL | 1 | Less than 35 kU/L |

*(Continued)*

| Laboratory Test | Conventional Units | Conversion Factor | Système International Units |
|---|---|---|---|
| CA 15–3 | Less than 30 units/mL | 1 | Less than 30 kU/L |
| CA 19–9 | Less than 37 units/mL | 1 | Less than 37 kU/L |
| CA 27.29 | Less than 38 units/mL | 1 | Less than 38 kU/L |
| Calcium | | | |
| Total | 8.6–10.3 mg/dL | 0.25 | 2.15–2.58 mmol/L |
| | 4.3–5.16 mEq/L | 0.50 | 2.15–2.58 mmol/L |
| Ionized | 4.5–5.1 mg/dL | 0.25 | 1.13–1.28 mmol/L |
| | 2.26–2.56 mEq/L | 0.50 | 1.13–1.28 mmol/L |
| Carbamazepine, therapeutic | 4–12 mg/L | 4.23 | 17–51 µmol/L |
| Carboxyhemoglobin (nonsmoker) | Less than 2% | 0.01 | Less than 0.02 |
| Carcinoembryonic antigen (CEA) | | | |
| Nonsmokers | Less than 2.5 ng/mL | 1 | Less than 2.5 mcg/L |
| Smokers | Less than 5 ng/mL | 1 | Less than 5 mcg/L |
| CD4 lymphocyte count | 31–61% of total lymphocytes | 0.01 | 0.31–0.61 of total lymphocytes |
| CD8 lymphocyte count | 18–39% of total lymphocytes | 0.01 | 0.18–0.39 of total lymphocytes |
| Cerebrospinal fluid (CSF) | | | |
| Pressure | 75–175 mm $H_2O$ | | |
| Glucose | 40–70 mg/dL | 0.0555 | 2.2–3.9 mmol/L |
| Protein | 15–45 mg/dL | 0.01 | 0.15–0.45 g/L |
| White blood cell (WBC) count | Less than 10/mm³ | 1 | Less than $10 \times 10^6$/L |
| Ceruloplasmin | 18–45 mg/dL | 10 | 180–450 mg/L |
| Chloride | 97–110 mEq/L | 1 | 97–110 mmol/L |
| Cholesterol | | | |
| Desirable | Less than 200 mg/dL | 0.0259 | Less than 5.18 mmol/L |
| Borderline high | 200–239 mg/dL | 0.0259 | 5.18–6.19 mmol/L |
| High | Greater than or equal to 240 mg/dL | 0.0259 | Greater than or equal to 6.2 mmol/L |
| Chorionic gonadotropin ($\beta$-hCG) | Less than 5 mIU/mL | 1 | Less than 5 IU/L |
| Clozapine, minimum trough | 300–350 ng/mL or mcg/L | 3.06 | 918–1,071 nmol/L |
| | | 0.00306 | 0.92–1.07 µmol/L |
| $CO_2$ content | 22–30 mEq/L | 1 | 22–30 mmol/L |
| Complement component 3 (C3) | 70–160 mg/dL | 0.01 | 0.70–1.60 g/L |
| Complement component 4 (C4) | 20–40 mg/dL | 0.01 | 0.20–0.40 g/L |
| Copper | 70–150 mcg/dL | 0.157 | 11–24 µmol/L |
| Cortisol (fasting, morning) | 5–25 mcg/dL | 27.6 | 138–690 nmol/L |
| Cortisol (free, urinary) | 10–100 mcg/d | 2.76 | 28–276 nmol/day |
| Creatine kinase | | | |
| Male | 30–200 IU/L | 0.01667 | 0.50–3.33 µkat/L |
| Female | 20–170 IU/L | 0.01667 | 0.33–2.83 µkat/L |
| MB fraction | 0–7 IU/L | 0.01667 | 0.0–0.12 µkat/L |
| Creatinine clearance (CrCl) (urine) | 85–135 mL/min/1.73 m² | 0.00963 | 0.82–1.30 mL/s/m² |

*(Continued)*

| Laboratory Test | Conventional Units | Conversion Factor | Système International Units |
|---|---|---|---|
| Creatinine | | | |
|   Male 4–20 years | 0.2–1.0 mg/dL | 88.4 | 18–88 µmol/L |
|   Female 4–20 years | 0.2–1.0 mg/dL | 88.4 | 18–88 µmol/L |
|   Male (adults) | 0.7–1.3 mg/dL | 88.4 | 62–115 µmol/L |
|   Female (adults) | 0.6–1.1 mg/dL | 88.4 | 53–97 µmol/L |
| Cyclosporine | | | |
|   Renal, cardiac, liver, or pancreatic transplant | 100–400 ng/mL or mcg/L | 0.832 | 83–333 nmol/L |
| Cryptococcal antigen | Negative | | |
| D-dimers | Less than 250 ng/mL | 1 | Less than 250 mcg/L |
| Desipramine | 75–300 ng/mL or mcg/L | 3.75 | 281–1125 nmol/L |
| Dexamethasone suppression test (DST) (overnight), 8:00 am cortisol | Less than 5 mcg/dL | 27.6 | Less than 138 nmol/L |
| DHEAS (dehydroepiandrosterone sulfate) | | | |
|   Male | 170–670 mcg/dL | 0.0272 | 4.6–18.2 µmol/L |
|   Female | | | |
|     Premenopausal | 50–540 mcg/dL | 0.0272 | 1.4–14.7 µmol/L |
|     Postmenopausal | 30–260 mcg/dL | 0.0272 | 0.8–7.1 µmol/L |
| Digoxin, therapeutic (heart failure) | 0.5–0.8 ng/mL or mcg/L | 1.28 | 0.6–1.0 nmol/L |
|   Therapeutic (atrial fibrillation) | 0.8–2.0 ng/mL or mcg/L | 1.28 | 1.0–2.6 nmol/L |
| Erythrocyte count (blood) | | | |
|   See under red blood cell (RBC) count | | | |
| Erythrocyte sedimentation rate (ESR) | | | |
|   Westergren | | | |
|     Male | 0–20 mm/h | | |
|     Female | 0–30 mm/h | | |
|   Wintrobe | | | |
|     Male | 0–9 mm/h | | |
|     Female | 0–15 mm/h | | |
| Erythropoietin | 2–25 mIU/mL | 1 | 2–25 IU/L |
| Estradiol | | | |
|   Male | 10–36 pg/mL | 3.67 | 37–132 pmol/L |
|   Female | 34–170 pg/mL | 3.67 | 125–624 pmol/L |
| Ethanol, legal intoxication (depends on location) | Greater than or equal to 50–100 mg/dL | 0.217 | Greater than or equal to 10.9–21.7 mmol/L |
| | Greater than or equal to 0.05–0.1% | 217 | Greater than or equal to 10.9–21.7 mmol/L |
| Ethosuccimide, therapeutic | 40–100 mg/L or mcg/mL | 7.08 | 283–708 µmol/L |
| Factor VIII or factor IX | | | |
|   Severe hemophilia | Less than 1 IU/dL | 0.01 | Less than 0.01 IU/mL |
|   Moderate hemophilia | 1–5 IU/dL | 0.01 | 0.01–0.05 IU/mL |
|   Mild hemophilia | Greater than 5 IU/dL | 0.01 | Greater than 0.05 IU/mL |
|   Usual adult levels | 60 to 140 IU/dL | 0.01 | 0.60–1.40 IU/mL |

*(Continued)*

| Laboratory Test | Conventional Units | Conversion Factor | Système International Units |
|---|---|---|---|
| Ferritin | | | |
|     Male | 20–250 ng/mL | 1 | 20–250 mcg/L |
|     Female | 10–150 ng/mL | 1 | 10–150 mcg/L |
| Fibrin degradation products (FDP) | 2–10 mg/L | | |
| Fibrinogen | 200–400 mg/dL | 0.01 | 2.0–4.0 g/L |
| Folate (plasma) | 3.1–12.4 ng/mL | 2.266 | 7.0–28.1 nmol/L |
| Folate (RBC) | 125–600 ng/mL | 2.266 | 283–1,360 nmol/L |
| Follicle-stimulating hormone (FSH) | | | |
|     Male | 1–7 mIU/mL | 1 | 1–7 IU/L |
|     Female | | | |
|         Follicular phase | 1–9 mIU/mL | 1 | 1–9 IU/L |
|         Midcycle | 6–26 mIU/mL | 1 | 6–26 IU/L |
|         Luteal phase | 1–9 mIU/mL | 1 | 1–9 IU/L |
|         Postmenopausal | 30–118 mIU/mL | 1 | 30–118 IU/L |
| Free thyroxine index ($FT_4I$) | 6.5–12.5 | | |
| Gamma glutamyltransferase (GGT) | 0–30 IU/L | 0.01667 | 0–0.50 µkat/L |
| Gastrin (fasting) | 0–130 pg/mL | 1 | 0–130 ng/L |
| Gentamicin, therapeutic (traditional dosing) | | | |
|     Peak | 4–10 mg/L | 2.09 | 8.4–21 µmol/L |
|     Trough | Less than or equal to 2 mg/L | 2.09 | Less than or equal to 4.2 µmol/L |
| Globulin | 2.3–3.5 g/dL | 10 | 23–35 g/L |
| Glucose (fasting, plasma) | 65–109 mg/dL | 0.0555 | 3.6–6.0 mmol/L |
| Glucose, 2-hour postprandial blood (PPBG) | Less than 140 mg/dL | 0.0555 | Less than 7.8 mmol/L |
| Granulocyte count | $1.8–6.6 \times 10^3/mm^3$ | $10^6$ | $1.8–6.6 \times 10^9/L$ |
| Growth hormone (fasting) | | | |
|     Male | Less than 5 ng/mL | 1 | Less than 5 mcg/L |
|     Female | Less than 10 ng/mL | 1 | Less than 10 mcg/L |
| Haptoglobin | 60–270 mg/dL | 0.01 | 0.6–2.7 g/L |
| Hepatitis B surface antigen, extracellular form (HBeAg) | Negative | | |
| Hepatitis B surface antigen (HbsAg) | Negative | | |
| Hepatitis B virus (HBV) DNA | Negative | | |
| Hematocrit | | | |
|     Male | 40.7–50.3% | 0.01 | 0.407–0.503 |
|     Female | 36.1–44.3% | 0.01 | 0.361–0.443 |
| Hemoglobin (blood) | | | |
|     Male | 13.8–17.2 g/dL | 10 | 138–172 g/L |
| | | 0.621 | 8.56–10.68 mmol/L |
|     Female | 12.1–15.1 g/dL | 10 | 121–151 g/L |
| | | 0.621 | 7.51–9.36 mmol/L |
| Hemoglobin $A_{1c}$ | 4.0–6.0% | 0.01 | 0.04–0.06 |
| | | $a$ | 20–42 mmol/mol hemoglobin |

*(Continued)*

| Laboratory Test | Conventional Units | Conversion Factor | Système International Units |
|---|---|---|---|
| Heparin | | | |
|    Via protamine titration method | 0.2–0.4 units/mL | | |
|    Via antifactor Xa assay | 0.3–0.7 units/mL | | |
| High-density lipoprotein (HDL) cholesterol | Greater than 35 mg/dL | 0.0259 | Greater than 0.91 mmol/L |
| Homocysteine | 3.3–10.4 µmol/L | | |
| Ibuprofen | | | |
|    Therapeutic | 10–50 mcg/mL | 4.85 | 49–243 µmol/L |
|    Toxic | Greater than or equal to 100 mcg/mL | 4.85 | Greater than or equal to 485 µmol/L |
| Imipramine, therapeutic | 100–300 ng/mL or mcg/L | 3.57 | 357–1,071 nmol/L |
| Immunoglobulin A (IgA) | 85–385 mg/dL | 0.01 | 0.85–3.85 g/L |
| Immunoglobulin G (IgG) | 565–1,765 mg/dL | 0.01 | 5.65–17.65 g/L |
| Immunoglobulin M (IgM) | 53–375 mg/dL | 0.01 | 0.53–3.75 g/L |
| Insulin (fasting) | 2–20 µU/mL or mU/L | 7.175 | 14.35–143.5 pmol/L |
| International normalized ratio (INR), therapeutic | 2.0–3.0 (2.5–3.5 for some indications) | | |
| Iron | | | |
|    Male | 45–160 mcg/dL | 0.179 | 8.1–28.6 µmol/L |
|    Female | 30–160 mcg/dL | 0.179 | 5.4–28.6 µmol/L |
| Iron-binding capacity (total) | 220–420 mcg/dL | 0.179 | 39.4–75.2 µmol/L |
| Iron saturation | 15–50% | 0.01 | 0.15–0.50 |
| Itraconazole | | | |
|    Trough, therapeutic | 0.5–1 mcg/mL | 1 | 0.5–1 mg/L |
| Lactate (plasma) | 0.7–2.1 mEq/L | 1 | 0.7–2.1 mmol/L |
| | 6.3–18.9 mg/dL | 0.111 | 0.7–2.1 mmol/L |
| Lactate dehydrogenase (LDH) | 100–250 IU/L | 0.01667 | 1.67–4.17 µkat/L |
| Lead | Less than 25 mcg/dL | 0.0483 | Less than 1.21 µmol/L |
| Leukocyte count | $3.8–9.8 \times 10^3/mm^3$ | $10^6$ | $3.8–9.8 \times 10^9/L$ |
| Lidocaine, therapeutic | 1.5–6.0 mcg/mL or mg/L | 4.27 | 6.4–25.6 µmol/L |
| Lipase | Less than 100 IU/L | 0.01667 | 1.67 µkat/L |
| Lithium, therapeutic | 0.5–1.25 mEq/L | 1 | 0.5–1.25 mmol/L |
| Low-density lipoprotein (LDL) cholesterol | | | |
|    Target for very high-risk patients | Less than 70 mg/dL | 0.0259 | Less than 1.81 mmol/L |
|    Target for high-risk patients (optimal) | Less than 100 mg/dL | 0.0259 | Less than 2.59 mmol/L |
|    Desirable | Less than 130 mg/dL | 0.0259 | Less than 3.36 mmol/L |
|    Borderline high risk | 130–159 mg/dL | 0.0259 | 3.36–4.11 mmol/L |
|    High risk | Greater than or equal to 160 mg/dL | 0.0259 | Greater than or equal to 4.14 mmol/L |
| Luteinizing hormone (LH) | | | |
|    Male | 1–8 mIU/mL | 1 | 1–8 IU/L |
|    Female | | | |
|       Follicular phase | 1–12 mIU/mL | 1 | 1–12 IU/L |
|       Midcycle | 16–104 mIU/mL | 1 | 16–104 IU/L |

*(Continued)*

| Laboratory Test | Conventional Units | Conversion Factor | Système International Units |
|---|---|---|---|
| Luteal phase | 1–12 mIU/mL | 1 | 1–12 IU/L |
| Postmenopausal | 16–66 mIU/mL | 1 | 16–66 IU/L |
| Lymphocyte count | $1.2–3.3 \times 10^3/mm^3$ | $10^6$ | $1.2–3.3 \times 10^9/L$ |
| Magnesium | 1.3–2.2 mEq/L | 0.5 | 0.65–1.10 mmol/L |
| | 1.58–2.68 mg/dL | 0.411 | 0.65–1.10 mmol/L |
| Mean corpuscular volume (MCV) | $80.0–97.6~\mu m^3$ | 1 | 80.0–97.6 fL |
| Mononuclear cell count | $0.2–0.7 \times 10^3/mm^3$ | $10^6$ | $0.2–0.7 \times 10^9/L$ |
| Nortriptyline, therapeutic | 50–150 ng/mL or mcg/L | 3.797 | 190–570 nmol/L |
| Osmolality (serum) | 275–300 mOsm/kg | 1 | 275–300 mmol/kg |
| Osmolality (urine) | 250–900 mOsm/kg | 1 | 250–900 mmol/kg |
| Parathyroid hormone (PTH), intact | 10–60 pg/mL or ng/L | 0.107 | 1.1–6.4 pmol/L |
| PTH, N-terminal | 8–24 pg/mL or ng/L | | |
| PTH, C-terminal | 50–330 pg/mL or ng/L | | |
| Phenobarbital, therapeutic | 15–40 mcg/mL or mg/L | 4.31 | $65–172~\mu mol/L$ |
| Phenytoin, therapeutic | 10–20 mcg/mL or mg/L | 3.96 | $40–79~\mu mol/L$ |
| Phosphate | 2.5–4.5 mg/dL | 0.323 | 0.81–1.45 mmol/L |
| Platelet count | $140–440 \times 10^3/mm^3$ | $10^6$ | $140–440 \times 10^9/L$ |
| Potassium (plasma) | 3.3–4.9 mEq/L | 1 | 3.3–4.9 mmol/L |
| Prealbumin (adult) | 19.5–35.8 mg/dL | 10 | 195–358 mg/L |
| Primidone, therapeutic | 5–12 mcg/mL or mg/L | 4.58 | $23–55~\mu mol/L$ |
| Procainamide, therapeutic | 4–10 mcg/mL or mg/L | 4.25 | $17–42~\mu mol/L$ |
| Progesterone | | | |
| Male | 13–97 ng/dL | 0.0318 | 0.4–3.1 nmol/L |
| Female | | | |
| Follicular phase | 15–70 ng/dL | 0.0318 | 0.5–2.2 nmol/L |
| Luteal phase | 200–2,500 ng/dL | 0.0318 | 6.4–79.5 nmol/L |
| Prolactin | Less than 20 ng/mL | 1 | Less than 20 mcg/L |
| Prostate-specific antigen (PSA) | Less than 4 ng/mL | 1 | Less than 4 mcg/L |
| Protein, total | 6.0–8.0 g/dL | 10 | 60–80 g/L |
| Prothrombin time (PT) | 10–12 second | | |
| Quinidine, therapeutic | 2–5 mcg/mL or mg/L | 3.08 | $6.2–15.4~\mu mol/L$ |
| Radioactive iodine uptake (RAIU) | Less than 6% in 2 hours | | |
| Red blood cell (RBC) count (blood) | | | |
| Male | $4–6.2 \times 10^6/mm^3$ | $10^6$ | $4–6.2 \times 10^{12}/L$ |
| Female | $4–6.2 \times 10^6/mm^3$ | $10^6$ | $4–6.2 \times 10^{12}/L$ |
| Pregnant | | | |
| Trimester 1 | $4–5 \times 10^6/mm^3$ | $10^6$ | $4–5 \times 10^{12}/L$ |
| Trimester 2 | $3.2–4.5 \times 10^6/mm^3$ | $10^6$ | $3.2–4.5 \times 10^{12}/L$ |
| Trimester 3 | $3–4.9 \times 10^6/mm^3$ | $10^6$ | $3–4.9 \times 10^{12}/L$ |
| Postpartum | $3.2–5 \times 10^6/mm^3$ | $10^6$ | $3.2–5 \times 10^{12}/L$ |
| Red blood cell distribution width (RDW) | 11.5–14.5% | 0.01 | 0.115–0.145 |

*(Continued)*

| Laboratory Test | Conventional Units | Conversion Factor | Système International Units |
|---|---|---|---|
| Reticulocyte count | | | |
|    Male | 0.5–1.5% of total RBC count | 0.01 | 0.005–0.015 |
|    Female | 0.5–2.5% of total RBC count | 0.01 | 0.005–0.025 |
| Retinol-binding protein (RBP) | 2.7–7.6 mg/dL | 10 | 27–76 mg/L |
| Rheumatoid factor (RF) titer | Negative | | |
| Salicylate, therapeutic | 150–300 mcg/mL or mg/L | 0.00724 | 1.09–2.17 mmol/L |
| | 15–30 mg/dL | 0.0724 | 1.09–2.17 mmol/L |
| Sirolimus (renal transplant) | 4–20 ng/mL | 1 | 4–20 mcg/L |
| | | 1.094 | 4–22 nmol/L |
| Sodium | 135–145 mEq/L | 1 | 135–145 mmol/L |
| Tacrolimus | | | |
|    Renal, cardiac, liver, or pancreatic transplant | 5–20 ng/mL | 1 | 5–20 mcg/L |
| | | 1.24 | 6.2-24.8 nmol/L |
| Testosterone (total) | | | |
|    Men | 300–950 ng/dL | 0.0347 | 10.4–33.0 nmol/L |
|    Women | 20–80 ng/dL | 0.0347 | 0.7–2.8 nmol/L |
| Testosterone (free) | | | |
|    Men | 9–30 ng/dL | 0.0347 | 0.31–1.04 nmol/L |
|    Women | 0.3–1.9 ng/dL | 0.0347 | 0.01–0.07 nmol/L |
| Theophylline | | | |
|    Therapeutic | 5–15 mcg/mL or mg/L | 5.55 | 28–83 µmol/L |
|    Toxic | 20 mcg/mL or mg/L or more | 5.55 | 111 µmol/L or more |
| Thiocyanate | Toxic level unclear; units are mcg/mL or mg/L | 17.2 | µmol/L |
| Thrombin time | 20–24 second | | |
| Thyroglobulin | Less than 42 ng/mL | 1 | Less than 42 mcg/L |
| Thyroglobulin antibodies | Negative | | |
| Thyroxine-binding globulin (TBG) | 1.2–2.5 mg/dL | 10 | 12–25 mcg/L |
| Thyroid-stimulating hormone (TSH) | 0.35–6.20 µIU/mL | 1 | 0.35–6.20 mIU/L |
| TSH receptor antibodies (TSHRab) | 0–1 units/mL | | |
| Thyroxine ($T_4$) | | | |
|    Total | 4.5–12.0 mcg/dL | 12.87 | 58–154 nmol/L |
|    Free | 0.7–1.9 ng/dL | 12.87 | 9.0–24.5 pmol/L |
| Thyroxine index, free ($FT_4I$) | 6.5–12.5 | | |
| TIBC—see Iron binding capacity (total) | | | |
| Tobramycin, therapeutic (traditional dosing) | | | |
|    Peak | 4–10 mcg/mL or mg/L | 2.14 | 8.6–21.4 µmol/L |
|    Trough | Less than or equal to 2 mcg/mL or mg/L | 2.14 | Less than or equal to 4.3 µmol/L |
| Transferrin | 200–430 mg/dL | 0.01 | 2.0–4.3 g/L |
| Transferrin saturation | 30–50% | 0.01 | 0.30–0.50 |
| Triglycerides (fasting) | Less than 160 mg/dL | 0.0113 | Less than 1.81 mmol/L |
| Triiodothyronine ($T_3$) | 45–132 ng/dL | 0.0154 | 0.0.69–2.03 nmol/L |
| Triiodothyronine ($T_3$) resin uptake | 25–35% | | |

*(Continued)*

| Laboratory Test | Conventional Units | Conversion Factor | Système International Units |
|---|---|---|---|
| Uric acid | 3–8 mg/dL | 59.48 | 178–476 µmol/L |
| Urinalysis (urine) | | | |
| pH | 4.8–8.0 | | 4.8–8.0 |
| Specific gravity | 1.005–1.030 | | |
| Protein | Negative | | |
| Glucose | Negative | | |
| Ketones | Negative | | |
| RBC | 1–2 per low-power field | | |
| WBC | Less than 5 per low-power field | | |
| Valproic acid, therapeutic | 50–100 mcg/mL or mg/L | 6.93 | 346–693 µmol/L |
| Vancomycin, therapeutic | | | |
| Peak | 20–40 mcg/mL or mg/L | 0.690 | 14–28 µmol/L |
| Trough | 10–20 mcg/mL or mg/L | 0.690 | 7–14 µmol/L |
| Trough for central nervous system infections | 15–20 mcg/mL or mg/L | 0.690 | 10–14 µmol/L |
| Vitamin A (retinol) | 30–95 mcg/dL | 0.0349 | 1.05–3.32 µmol/L |
| Vitamin $B_{12}$ | 180–1,000 pg/mL | 0.738 | 133–738 pmol/L |
| Vitamin $D_3$, 125-dihydroxy | 20–76 pg/mL | 2.4 | 48–182 pmol/L |
| Vitamin $D_3$, 25-hydroxy | 10–50 ng/mL | 2.496 | 25–125 nmol/L |
| Vitamin E (a-tocopherol) | 0.5–2.0 mg/dL | 23.22 | 12–46 µmol/L |
| WBC count | $4–10 \times 10^3/mm^3$ | $10^6$ | $4–10 \times 10^9/L$ |
| WBC differential (peripheral blood) | | | |
| Polymorphonuclear neutrophils (PMNs) | 50–65% | 0.01 | 0.50–0.65 |
| Bands | 0–5% | 0.01 | 0–0.05 |
| Eosinophils | 0–3% | 0.01 | 0–0.03 |
| Basophils | 1–3% | 0.01 | 0.01–0.03 |
| Lymphocytes | 25–35% | 0.01 | 0.25–0.35 |
| Monocytes | 2–6% | 0.01 | 0.02–0.06 |
| WBC differential (bone marrow) | | | |
| PMNs | 3–11% | 0.01 | 0.03–0.11 |
| Bands | 9–15% | 0.01 | 0.09–0.15 |
| Metamyelocytes | 9–25% | 0.01 | 0.09–0.25 |
| Myelocytes | 8–16% | 0.01 | 0.08–0.16 |
| Promyelocytes | 1–8% | 0.01 | 0.01–0.08 |
| Myeloblasts | 0–5% | 0.01 | 0–0.05 |
| Eosinophils | 1–5% | 0.01 | 0.01–0.05 |
| Basophils | 0–1% | 0.01 | 0–0.01 |
| Lymphocytes | 11–23% | 0.01 | 0.11–0.23 |
| Monocytes | 0–1% | 0.01 | 0–0.01 |
| Zinc | 60–150 mcg/dL | 0.153 | 9.2–23.0 µmol/L |

[a]Hemoglobin $A_{1c}$ (mmol/mol hemoglobin) = (Hemoglobin $A_{1c}$ (%) − 2.15) × 10.929.

This table is a modification of the Medical Algorithms Project (Chapter 40), unit conversions of the following Excel worksheets: Conversion of Conventional to SI units: Blood Chemistries; Conversion of Conventional to SI units: Urine Chemistries; Conversion of Conventional to SI units: Hematology and Coagulation; and Conversion of Conventional to SI units: Therapeutic Drug Monitoring.

Other references (conventional and SI units from the preceding table were double-checked against the following references and modified as needed):

A–Z Health Guide from WebMD. Medical Tests: Brain Natriuretic Peptide (BNP) Test. Available at http://www.webmd. com/heart-disease/brain-natriuretic-peptide-bnp-test?page=2; accessed October 28, 2011.

proBNP ©2005 Roche Diagnostics Roche Diagnostics GmbH, D-68298 Mannheim.

Jacobs, D.S., Oxley, D.K., DeMott, W.R. (Eds.). (2001) Laboratory Test Handbook (5th ed.). Hudson OH: Lexi-Comp, Inc.

Young, D.S., Huth, E.J. (Eds.). (1998) SI units for clinical measurement. Philadelphia, PA: American College of Physicians.

Reviewed and updated by: Edward W. Randell.

# Appendix C: Common Medical Abbreviations

These are the abbreviations used commonly in medical practice both in verbal communication and in the medical record.

| | |
|---|---|
| A&O | alert and oriented |
| A&O×3 | awake (or alert) and oriented to person, place, and time |
| A&O×4 | awake (or alert) and oriented to person, place, time, and situation |
| A&P | active and present; anterior and posterior; assessment and plans; auscultation and percussion |
| A&W | alive and well |
| $A_{1c}$ | hemoglobin $A_{1c}$ |
| AA | aplastic anemia; alcoholics anonymous |
| AAA | abdominal aortic aneurysm |
| AAO | awake, alert, and oriented |
| AAO×3 | awake and orientated to time, place, and person |
| ABC | absolute band counts; absolute basophil count; apnea, bradycardia, and cytology; aspiration, biopsy, and cytology; artificial beta cells |
| Abd | abdomen |
| ABG | arterial blood gases |
| ABO | blood group system (A, AB, B, and O) |
| ABP | arterial blood pressure |
| ABW | actual body weight |
| ABx | antibiotics |
| AC | before meals (*ante cibos*) |
| ACE | angiotensin-converting enzyme |
| ACE-I | angiotensin-converting enzyme inhibitor |
| ACLS | advanced cardiac life support |
| ACS | acute coronary syndromes |
| ACTH | adrenocorticotropic hormone |
| AD | Alzheimer's disease; right ear (*auris dextra*) |
| ADA | American Diabetes Association; adenosine deaminase |
| ADE | adverse drug effect (or event) |
| ADH | antidiuretic hormone |
| ADHD | attention-deficit hyperactivity disorder |
| ADL | activities of daily living |
| ADR | adverse drug reaction |
| AF | atrial fibrillation |
| AFB | Acid-fast bacillus; aortofemoral bypass; aspirated foreign body |

| | |
|---|---|
| AFEB | afebrile |
| AI | aortic insufficiency |
| AIDS | acquired immune deficiency syndrome |
| AKA | above-knee amputation; alcoholic ketoacidosis; all known allergies; also known as |
| AKI | acute kidney injury |
| ALFT | abnormal liver function test |
| ALL | acute lymphoblastic leukemia; acute lymphocytic leukemia |
| ALP | alkaline phosphatase |
| ALS | amyotrophic lateral sclerosis |
| ALT | alanine transaminase (SGPT); alanine aminotransferase |
| AMA | against medical advice; American Medical Association; antimitochondrial antibody |
| AMI | acute myocardial infarction |
| AML | acute myelogenous leukemia |
| Amp | ampule |
| ANA | antinuclear antibody |
| ANC | absolute neutrophil count |
| ANLL | acute nonlymphocytic leukemia |
| AODM | adult-onset diabetes mellitus |
| AOM | acute otitis media |
| AP | anteroposterior |
| APAP | acetaminophen (acetyl-*p*-aminophenol) |
| aPTT | activated partial thromboplastin time |
| ARB | angiotensin receptor blocker |
| ARC | AIDS-related complex |
| ARD | acute respiratory disease; adult respiratory disease; antibiotic removal device; aphakic retinal detachment |
| ARDS | adult respiratory distress syndrome |
| ARF | acute renal failure; acute respiratory failure; acute rheumatic fever |
| AROM | active range of motion |
| AS | left ear (*auris sinistra*) |
| ASA | aspirin (acetylsalicylic acid) |
| ASCVD | arteriosclerotic cardiovascular disease |
| ASD | atrial septal defect |
| ASH | asymmetric septal hypertrophy |
| ASHD | arteriosclerotic heart disease |

| | | | |
|---|---|---|---|
| AST | aspartate transaminase (SGOT); aspartate aminotransferase | CI | Cardiac index |
| ATG | antithymocyte globulin | CIWA | Clinical Institute Withdrawal Assessment |
| ATN | acute tubular necrosis | CK | creatine kinase |
| AU | each ear (*auris uterque*) | CKD | chronic kidney disease |
| AV | arteriovenous; atrioventricular; auditory visual | CLL | chronic lymphocytic leukemia |
| AVR | aortic valve replacement | CM | costal margin |
| BBB | bundle branch block; blood–brain barrier | CMG | cystometrogram |
| BC | blood culture | CML | chronic myelogenous leukemia |
| BCOP | Board Certified Oncology Pharmacist | CMV | cytomegalovirus |
| BCP | birth control pill | CN | cranial nerve |
| BCPP | Board Certified Psychiatric Pharmacist | CNS | central nervous system |
| BCPS | Board Certified Pharmacotherapy Specialist | C/O | complains of |
| BE | barium enema | CO | cardiac output; carbon monoxide |
| BG | blood glucose | COLD | chronic obstructive lung disease |
| bid | twice daily (*bis in die*) | COPD | chronic obstructive pulmonary disease |
| BKA | below-knee amputation | CP | chest pain; cerebral palsy |
| BM | bone marrow; bowel movement; an isoenzyme of creatine phosphokinase | CPAP | continuous positive airway pressure |
| | | CPK | creatine phosphokinase (BB, MB, and MM are isoenzymes) |
| BMC | bone marrow cells | | |
| BMD | bone mineral density | CPP | cerebral perfusion pressure |
| BMI | body mass index | CPR | cardiopulmonary resuscitation |
| BMP | basic metabolic panel | CrCl | creatinine clearance |
| BMR | basal metabolic rate | CRF | chronic renal failure; corticotropin-releasing factor |
| BMT | bone marrow transplantation | | |
| BP | blood pressure | CRH | corticotropin-releasing hormone |
| BPD | bronchopulmonary dysplasia | CRI | chronic renal insufficiency; catheter-related infection |
| BPH | benign prostatic hyperplasia | | |
| bpm | beats per minute | CRNA | Certified Registered Nurse Anesthetist |
| BR | bed rest | CRNP | Certified Registered Nurse Practitioner |
| BS | bowel sounds; breath sounds; blood sugar | CRP | C-reactive protein |
| BSA | body surface area | CRTT | Certified Respiratory Therapy Technician |
| BUN | blood urea nitrogen | CSF | cerebrospinal fluid; colony-stimulating factor |
| Bx | biopsy | CT | computed tomography; chest tube |
| C&S | culture and sensitivity | cTnI | cardiac troponin I |
| CA | cancer; calcium | CTZ | chemoreceptor trigger zone |
| CABG | coronary artery bypass grafting | CV | cardiovascular |
| CAD | coronary artery disease | CVA | cerebrovascular accident |
| CAH | chronic active hepatitis | CVC | central venous catheter |
| CAM | complementary and alternative medicine | CVP | central venous pressure |
| CAPD | continuous ambulatory peritoneal dialysis | Cx | culture; cervix |
| CBC | complete blood count | CXR | chest x-ray |
| CBD | common bile duct | CYP | cytochrome P450 |
| CBG | capillary blood gas; corticosteroid-binding globulin | D&C | dilatation and curettage |
| | | $D_5W$ | 5% dextrose in water |
| CC | chief complaint | DBP | diastolic blood pressure |
| CCA | calcium channel antagonist | D/C | discontinue; discharge |
| CCB | calcium channel blocker | DCC | direct-current cardioversion |
| CCE | clubbing, cyanosis, edema | DI | diabetes insipidus |
| CCK | cholecystokinin | DIC | disseminated intravascular coagulation |
| CCU | coronary care unit | Diff | differential |
| CF | cystic fibrosis | DJD | degenerative joint disease |
| CFS | chronic fatigue syndrome | DKA | diabetic ketoacidosis |
| CFU | colony-forming unit | dL | deciliter |
| CHD | coronary heart disease | DM | diabetes mellitus |
| CHF | congestive heart failure; chronic heart failure | DNA | deoxyribonucleic acid |
| | | DNR | do not resuscitate |
| CHO | carbohydrate | DO | Doctor of osteopathy |

| | |
|---|---|
| DOA | dead on arrival; date of admission; duration of action |
| DOB | date of birth |
| DOE | dyspnea on exertion |
| DOT | directly observed therapy |
| DPGN | diffuse proliferative glomerulonephritis |
| DPI | dry powder inhaler |
| DRE | digital rectal examination |
| DRG | diagnosis-related group |
| DS | double strength |
| d/t | due to |
| DTP | diphtheria–tetanus–pertussis |
| DTR | deep tendon reflex |
| DVT | deep vein thrombosis |
| Dx | diagnosis |
| EBV | Epstein-Barr virus |
| EC | enteric coated |
| ECF | extracellular fluid |
| ECG | electrocardiogram |
| ECHO | echocardiogram |
| ECT | electroconvulsive therapy |
| ED | emergency department |
| EEG | electroencephalogram |
| EENT | eyes, ears, nose, throat |
| EF | ejection fraction |
| EGD | esophagogastroduodenoscopy |
| EIA | enzyme immunoassay |
| ECG | electrocardiogram |
| EMG | electromyogram |
| EMT | Emergency Medical Technician |
| Endo | endotracheal, endoscopy |
| EOMI | extraocular movements (or muscles) intact |
| EPO | erythropoietin |
| EPS | extrapyramidal symptoms |
| ER | emergency room |
| ERCP | endoscopic retrograde cholangiopancreatography |
| ERT | estrogen replacement therapy |
| ESKD | end-stage kidney disease |
| ESLD | end-stage liver disease |
| ESR | erythrocyte sedimentation rate |
| ESRD | end-stage renal disease |
| ET | endotracheal |
| EtOH | ethanol |
| FB | finger breadth; foreign body |
| FBS | fasting blood sugar |
| FDA | Food and Drug Administration |
| FEF | forced expiratory flow rate |
| $FEV_1$ | forced expiratory volume in 1 second |
| FFP | fresh-frozen plasma |
| FH | family history |
| $FiO_2$ | fraction of inspired oxygen |
| FOBT | fecal occult blood test |
| FPG | fasting plasma glucose |
| FPIA | fluorescence polarization immunoassay |
| FSH | follicle-stimulating hormone |
| FTA | fluorescent treponemal antibody |

| | |
|---|---|
| $FT_4$ | free thyroxine |
| F/U | follow-up |
| FUO | fever of unknown origin |
| Fx | fracture |
| g | gram |
| G-CSF | granulocyte colony-stimulating factor |
| G6PD | glucose-6-phosphate dehydrogenase |
| GB | gallbladder |
| GBS | group B *Streptococcus*; Guillain-Barré syndrome |
| GC | gonococcus |
| GDM | gestational diabetes mellitus |
| GE | gastroesophageal; gastroenterology |
| GERD | gastroesophageal reflux disease |
| GFR | glomerular filtration rate |
| GGT | γ-glutamyl transferase |
| GGTP | γ-glutamyl transpeptidase |
| GI | gastrointestinal |
| GM-CSF | granulocyte-macrophage colony-stimulating factor |
| GN | glomerulonephritis; graduate nurse |
| gr | grain |
| GT | gastrostomy tube |
| gtt | drops (*guttae*) |
| GTT | glucose tolerance test |
| GU | genitourinary |
| GVHD | graft-versus-host disease |
| GVL | graft-versus-leukemia |
| Gyn | gynecology |
| H&H, H/H | hemoglobin and hematocrit |
| H&P | history and physical examination |
| HA | headache |
| HAART | highly active antiretroviral therapy |
| HAMD | Hamilton Rating Scale for Depression |
| HAV | Hepatitis A virus |
| Hb, hgb | hemoglobin |
| HbAlc | glycosylated hemoglobin (hemoglobin Alc) |
| HBIG | hepatitis B immune globulin |
| HBP | high blood pressure |
| HBsAg | hepatitis B surface antigen |
| HBV | hepatitis B virus |
| HC | hydrocortisone, home care |
| HCG | human chorionic gonadotropin |
| $HCO_3$ | bicarbonate |
| Hct | hematocrit |
| HCTZ | hydrochlorothiazide |
| HCV | hepatitis C virus |
| HD | Hodgkin's disease; hemodialysis |
| HDL | high-density lipoprotein |
| HEENT | head, eyes, ears, nose, and throat |
| HF | heart failure |
| HFA | hydrofluoroalkane |
| H flu | *Hemophilus influenzae* |
| HGH | human growth hormone |
| HH | hiatal hernia |
| Hib | *Hemophilus influenzae* type b |
| HIT | heparin-induced thrombocytopenia |

| | | | |
|---|---|---|---|
| HIV | human immunodeficiency virus | IVP | intravenous pyelogram; intravenous push |
| HJR | hepatojugular reflux | JODM | juvenile-onset diabetes mellitus |
| HLA | human leukocyte antigen; human lymphocyte antigen | JRA | juvenile rheumatoid arthritis |
| | | JVD | jugular venous distension |
| HMG-CoA | hydroxy-methylglutaryl coenzyme A | JVP | jugular venous pressure |
| H/O | history of | K | potassium |
| HOB | head of bed | kcal | kilocalorie |
| HPA | hypothalamic–pituitary axis | KCl | potassium chloride |
| hpf | high-power field | KOH | potassium hydroxide |
| HPI | history of present illness | KUB | kidney, ureter, and bladder |
| HR | heart rate | KVO | keep vein open |
| $H_2RA$ | $H_2$ receptor antagonist | L | liter |
| HRSD | Hamilton Rating Scale for Depression | LABA | long-acting beta agonist |
| HRT | hormone-replacement therapy | LAD | left anterior descending; left axis deviation |
| HS | at bedtime (*hora somni*) | LAO | left anterior oblique |
| HSV | herpes simplex virus | LBBB | left bundle branch block |
| HTN | hypertension | LBP | low-back pain |
| Hx | history | LDH | lactate dehydrogenase |
| I&D | incision and drainage | LDL | low-density lipoprotein |
| I&O, I/O | intake and output | LE | lower extremity |
| IBD | inflammatory bowel disease | LES | lower esophageal sphincter |
| IBW | ideal body weight | LFT | liver function test |
| ICD | implantable cardioverter defibrillator | LHRH | luteinizing hormone-releasing hormone |
| ICP | intracranial pressure | LLE | left lower extremity |
| ICS | intercostal space; inhaled corticosteroid | LLL | left lower lobe |
| ICU | intensive care unit | LLQ | left lower quadrant (abdomen) |
| ID | identification; infectious disease | LMD | local medical doctor |
| IDDM | insulin-dependent diabetes mellitus | LMP | last menstrual period |
| IFN | interferon | LMWH | low-molecular-weight heparin |
| Ig | immunoglobulin | LOS | length of stay |
| IgA | immunoglobulin A | LP | lumbar puncture |
| IgD | immunoglobulin D | LPN | Licensed Practical Nurse |
| IHD | ischemic heart disease | LPT | Licensed Physical Therapist |
| IJ | internal jugular | LR | Lactated Ringer's |
| IM | intramuscular; infectious mononucleosis | LS | lumbosacral |
| INH | isoniazid | $LT_4$ | levothyroxine |
| INR | international normalized ratio | LUE | left upper extremity |
| IOP | intraocular pressure | LUL | left upper lobe |
| IP | intraperitoneal | LUQ | left upper quadrant |
| IPG | impedance plethysmography | LUTS | lower urinary tract symptoms |
| IPN | interstitial pneumonia | LVH | left ventricular hypertrophy |
| IRB | institutional review board | MAP | mean arterial pressure |
| ISA | intrinsic sympathomimetic activity | MAR | medication administration record |
| ISH | isolated systolic hypertension | MB-CK | a creatine kinase isoenzyme |
| IT | intrathecal | mcg | microgram |
| ITP | idiopathic thrombocytopenic purpura | MCH | mean corpuscular hemoglobin |
| IU | international units (this can be dangerous abbreviation because it may be read as "IV" for "intravenous") | MCHC | mean corpuscular hemoglobin concentration |
| | | MCV | mean corpuscular volume |
| | | MD | Doctor of Medicine |
| IUD | intrauterine device | MDI | metered-dose inhaler |
| IV | intravenous; Roman numeral four; symbol for class 4 controlled substances | MDRD | modification of diet in renal disease |
| | | MEFR | maximum expiratory flow rate |
| IVC | inferior vena cava; intravenous cholangiogram | mEq | milliequivalent |
| IVDA | intravenous drug abuse | mg | milligram |
| IVDU | injection drug use; intravenous drug use | MHC | major histocompatibility complex |
| | | MI | myocardial infarction; mitral insufficiency |
| IVF | intravenous fluids | | |
| IVIG | intravenous immunoglobulin | MIC | minimum inhibitory concentration |

| | |
|---|---|
| mL | milliliter |
| MM | multiple myeloma; an isoenzyme of creatine phosphokinase |
| MMR | measles–mumps–rubella; midline malignant reticulosis |
| MOM | milk of magnesia |
| MPV | mean platelet volume |
| m/r/g | murmur/rub/gallop |
| MRI | magnetic resonance imaging |
| MRSA | methicillin-resistant *Staphylococcus aureus* |
| MRSE | methicillin-resistant *Staphylococcus epidermitis* |
| MS | mental status; mitral stenosis; musculoskeletal; multiple sclerosis; morphine sulfate |
| MSE | mental status exam |
| MSW | Master of Social Work |
| MTD | maximum tolerated dose |
| MTX | methotrexate |
| MVA | motor vehicle accident |
| MVI | multivitamin |
| MVR | mitral valve replacement; mitral valve regurgitation |
| MVS | mitral valve stenosis; motor, vascular, and sensory |
| N&V | nausea and vomiting |
| NAD | no acute (or apparent) distress |
| N/C | noncontributory; nasal cannula |
| NG | nasogastric |
| NGT | nasogastric tube; normal glucose tolerance |
| NIDDM | non–insulin-dependent diabetes mellitus |
| NIH | National Institutes of Health |
| NKA | no known allergies |
| NKDA | no known drug allergies |
| NHDA | nonketotic hyperosmolar acidosis |
| NL | normal |
| NOS | not otherwise specified |
| NPN | nonprotein nitrogen |
| NPO | nothing by mouth (*nil per os*) |
| NS | normal saline solution (0.9% sodium chloride solution); neurosurgery |
| NSAID | nonsteroidal antiinflammatory drug |
| NSR | normal sinus rhythm |
| NSS | normal saline solution |
| NTG | nitroglycerin |
| NT/ND | nontender, nondistended |
| NVD | nausea/vomiting/diarrhea; neck vein distension; neovascularization of the disk; neurovesicle dysfunction; nonvalvular disease |
| N&V | nausea and vomiting |
| NYHA | New York Heart Association |
| O&P | ova and parasites |
| OA | osteoarthritis |
| OB | obstetrics |
| OCD | obsessive-compulsive disorder |
| OD | right eye (*oculus dexter*) |
| OGTT | oral glucose tolerance test |
| OPV | Oral poliovirus vaccine |

| | |
|---|---|
| OR | operating room |
| OR×1 | oriented to time |
| OR×2 | oriented to time and place |
| OR×3 | oriented to time, place, and person |
| OS | left eye (*oculus sinister*) |
| OSA | obstructive sleep apnea |
| OT | occupational therapy |
| OTC | over the counter |
| OU | each eye (*oculus uterque*) |
| P | pulse; plan; percussion; pressure |
| P&A | percussion and auscultation |
| P&T | peak and trough |
| PA | physician assistant; posteroanterior; pulmonary artery |
| PAC | premature atrial contraction |
| $Paco_2$ | arterial carbon dioxide tension |
| $Pao_2$ | arterial oxygen tension |
| PAOP | pulmonary artery occlusion pressure |
| PC | after meals (*post cibum*) |
| PCA | patient-controlled analgesia |
| PCI | percutaneous coronary intervention |
| PCKD | polycystic kidney disease |
| PCN | penicillin |
| PCP | *Pneumocystis carinii* pneumonia (also known as *Pneumocystis jirovecii* pneumonia); pneumocystis pneumonia; primary care physician; phencyclidine |
| PCWP | pulmonary capillary wedge pressure |
| PDE | paroxysmal dyspnea on exertion |
| PE | physical examination; pulmonary embolism |
| PEEP | positive end-expiratory pressure |
| PEFR | peak expiratory flow rate |
| PEG | percutaneous endoscopic gastrostomy; polyethylene glycol |
| Peg-IFN | pegylated interferon |
| PERL | pupils equal, react to light |
| PERRLA | pupils equal, round, and reactive to light and accommodation |
| PERRRLA | pupils equal, round, regular, and react to light and accommodation |
| PET | positron emission tomography |
| PFT | pulmonary function test |
| pH | hydrogen ion concentration |
| PH | past history; personal history; pinhole; poor health; pubic hair; public health |
| PHx | past history |
| PharmD | Doctor of Pharmacy |
| PID | pelvic inflammatory disease |
| PJD | *Pneumocystis jirovecii* pneumonia (also known as *Pneumocystis carinii* pneumonia) |
| PKU | phenylketonuria |
| PMH | past medical history |
| PMI | past medical illness; point of maximal impulse |
| PMN | polymorphonuclear leukocyte |
| PMS | premenstrual syndrome |
| PND | paroxysmal nocturnal dyspnea |

| | |
|---|---|
| Po | by mouth (*per os*) |
| Po$_2$ | partial pressure of oxygen |
| POAG | primary open-angle glaucoma |
| POD | postoperative day |
| PPBG | postprandial blood glucose |
| ppd | packs per day |
| PPI | proton pump inhibitor |
| PPN | peripheral parenteral nutrition |
| PR | per rectum |
| PRBC | packed red blood cell |
| PRERLA | pupils round, equal, react to light and accommodation |
| PRN | when necessary, as needed (*pro re nata*) |
| PSA | prostate-specific antigen |
| PSH | past surgical history |
| PST | paroxysmal supraventricular tachycardia |
| PSVT | paroxysmal supraventricular tachycardia |
| PT | prothrombin time; physical therapy; patient |
| PTA | prior to admission; percutaneous transluminal angioplasty |
| PTCA | percutaneous transluminal coronary angioplasty |
| PTE | pulmonary thromboembolism |
| PTH | parathyroid hormone |
| PTSD | posttraumatic stress disorder |
| PTT | partial thromboplastin time |
| PUD | peptic ulcer disease |
| PVC | premature ventricular contraction |
| PVD | peripheral vascular disease |
| PVR | peripheral vascular resistance |
| PVT | paroxysmal ventricular tachycardia |
| q | every (*quaque*) |
| QA | quality assurance |
| qday | every day (*quaque die*) |
| QI | quality improvement |
| qid | four times daily (*quater in die*) |
| QNS | quantity not sufficient |
| qod | every other day |
| QOL | quality of life |
| QS | quantity sufficient |
| QTc | corrected QT interval |
| R&M | routine and microscopic |
| R&R | rate and rhythm |
| RA | rheumatoid arthritis; right atrium |
| RAAS | renin–angiotensin–aldosterone system |
| RBC | red blood cell |
| RCA | right coronary artery |
| RCM | right costal margin |
| RDA | Recommended Daily Allowance |
| RDS | respiratory distress syndrome |
| RDW | red blood cell distribution width |
| REM | rapid eye movement; recent event memory |
| RES | reticuloendothelial system |
| RF | rheumatoid factor; renal failure; rheumatic fever |
| Rh | rhesus factor in blood |
| RHD | rheumatic heart disease |
| RLE | right lower extremity |
| RLL | right lower lobe |
| RLQ | right lower quadrant |
| RML | right middle lobe |
| RN | Registered Nurse |
| RNA | ribonucleic acid |
| R/O | rule out |
| ROM | range of motion |
| ROS | review of systems |
| RPh | Registered Pharmacist |
| RR | respiratory rate; recovery room |
| RRR | regular rate and rhythm |
| RRT | Registered Respiratory Therapist |
| RSV | respiratory syncytial virus |
| RT | radiation therapy |
| RUE | right upper extremity |
| RUL | right upper lobe |
| RUQ | right upper quadrant |
| RVH | right ventricular hypertrophy |
| S$_1$ | first heart sound |
| S$_2$ | second heart sound |
| S$_3$ | third heart sound (ventricular gallop) |
| S$_4$ | fourth heart sound (atrial gallop) |
| SA | sinoatrial |
| SABA | short-acting beta agonist |
| SAD | seasonal affective disorder |
| SAH | subarachnoid hemorrhage |
| Sao$_2$ | arterial oxygen percent saturation |
| SBE | subacute bacterial endocarditis |
| SBFT | small bowel follow-through |
| SBGM | self-blood glucose monitoring |
| SBO | small bowel obstruction |
| SBP | systolic blood pressure |
| SC | subcutaneous; subclavian |
| SCr | serum creatinine |
| SEM | systolic ejection murmur |
| SG | specific gravity |
| SGOT (AST) | serum glutamic oxaloacetic transaminase (aspartate transaminase) |
| SGPT (ALT) | serum glutamic pyruvic transaminase (alanine transaminase) |
| SH | social history |
| SIADH | syndrome of inappropriate antidiuretic hormone secretion |
| SIDS | sudden infant death syndrome |
| SJS | Stevens-Johnson syndrome |
| SL | sublingual |
| SLE | systemic lupus erythematosus |
| SMA-6 | sequential multiple analyzer for sodium, potassium, $CO_2$, chloride, glucose, and BUN |
| SMA-7 | sequential multiple analyzer for sodium, potassium, $CO_2$, chloride, glucose, BUN, and creatinine |
| SMA-12 | sequential multiple analyzer for glucose, BUN, uric acid, calcium, phosphorous, total protein, albumin, cholesterol, total bilirubin, alkaline phosphatase, SGOT, and LDH |

| | | | |
|---|---|---|---|
| SMA-23 | includes the entire SMA-12 plus sodium, potassium, $CO_2$, chloride, direct bilirubin, triglyceride, SGPT, indirect bilirubin, R fraction, and BUN/creatinine ratio | tid | three times daily (*ter in die*) |
| | | TLC | therapeutic lifestyle changes |
| | | TMJ | Temporomandibular joint |
| | | TMP-SMX | trimethoprim–sulfamethoxazole |
| SMBG | self-monitoring of blood glucose | TNTC | too numerous to count |
| SNF | skilled nursing facility | TOD | target organ damage |
| SNS | sympathetic nervous system | TPN | total parenteral nutrition |
| SOB | shortness of breath; see order book; side of bed | TPR | temperature, pulse, respiration |
| S/P | status post | T PROT | total protein |
| SPF | sun protection factor | TSH | thyroid-stimulating hormone |
| SQ | subcutaneous | TURP | transurethral resection of the prostate |
| SSKI | saturated solution of potassium iodide | Tx | treat, treatment |
| SSRI | selective serotonin reuptake inhibitor | UA | urinalysis, uric acid |
| STAT | immediately; at once | UC | ulcerative colitis |
| STEMI | ST-segment elevated myocardial infarction | UE | upper extremity |
| STD | sexually transmitted disease | UFH | unfractionated heparin |
| SV | stroke volume | UGI | upper gastrointestinal |
| SVC | superior vena cava | UOQ | upper outer quadrant |
| SVRI | systemic vascular resistance index | UPT | urine pregnancy test |
| SVR | supraventricular rhythm; systemic vascular resistance | URI | upper respiratory infection |
| | | USP | United States Pharmacopeia |
| SVT | supraventricular tachycardia | UTI | urinary tract infection |
| SW | social worker | UV | ultraviolet |
| Sx | signs | VF | ventricular fibrillation |
| T | temperature | VLDL | very low-density lipoprotein |
| $T_3$ | triiodothyroxine | VO | verbal order |
| $T_4$ | thyroxine | VOD | veno-occlusive disease |
| T&A | tonsillectomy and adenoidectomy | $V_A/Q$ | ventilation–perfusion |
| T&C | type and crossmatch | VRE | vancomycin-resistant enterococcus |
| TB | tuberculosis | VS | vital signs |
| TBG | thyroid-binding globulin | VSS | vital signs stable |
| TBI | total-body irradiation; traumatic brain injury | VT | ventricular tachycardia |
| TBW | total body weight | VTE | venous thromboembolism |
| T bili | total bilirubin | WA | while awake |
| TCA | tricyclic antidepressant | WBC | white blood cell (count) |
| TCN | tetracycline | W/C | wheelchair |
| Tdap | tetanus, diphtheria, acellular pertussis vaccine | WDWN | well-developed, well-nourished |
| TEE | transesophageal echocardiogram | WHO | World Health Organization |
| TFT | thyroid function test | WNL | within normal limits |
| TG | triglyceride | W/U | workup |
| TIA | transient ischemic attack | yo | year old |
| TIBC | total iron-binding capacity | y | year |

# Appendix D: Glossary

Acanthosis nigricans: Increased thickness and hyperpigmentation of the outer cell layers of the skin; typically observed at areas of flexure.

Acaricide: A chemical that kills mites and ticks.

Acetaldehyde: Metabolic by-product of alcohol; hepatotoxic.

Acetylcholine: Neurotransmitter responsible for transmitting messages between certain nerve cells in the brain.

Achalasia: Disorder in which the esophageal sphincter is impaired, preventing normal swallowing and often causing reflux of contents and a feeling that something is caught in the throat.

Achlorhydria: Absence of free hydrochloric acid in the stomach.

Acidemia: An increase in the hydrogen ion concentration of the blood or a fall below normal in pH.

Acidosis: Any pathologic state that leads to acidemia.

Acinar cells: Exocrine glands of the pancreas that secrete digestive enzymes.

Acromegaly: A pathologic condition characterized by excessive production of growth hormone during adulthood after epiphyseal (long bone) fusions have completed.

Action potential: A rapid change in the polarity of the voltage of a cell membrane from negative to positive and back to negative; a wave of electrical discharge that travels across a cell membrane.

Acute coronary syndromes: Ischemic chest discomfort at rest most often accompanied by ST-segment elevation, ST-segment depression, or T-wave inversion on the 12-lead electrocardiogram; further, it is caused by plaque rupture and partial or complete occlusion of the coronary artery by thrombus. Acute coronary syndromes include myocardial infarction and unstable angina. Former terms used to describe types of acute coronary syndromes include Q-wave myocardial infarction, non–Q-wave myocardial infarction, and unstable angina.

Acute disorder: An acid-base disturbance that has been present for minutes to hours.

Acute kidney injury: Spectrum of acute changes in kidney function ranging from minor changes to those requiring renal replacement therapy.

Acute otitis media: Inflammation of the middle ear accompanied by fluid in the middle ear space and signs or symptoms of an acute ear infection.

Acute tubular necrosis: Form of acute kidney injury that results from toxic or ischemic injury to the cells in the proximal tubule of the kidney.

Adenoma: A nonmalignant tumor of the epithelial tissue that is characterized by glandular structures.

Adenomatous polyposis coli gene: A tumor suppressor gene (see definition) that is one of the first genes mutated in the development of colon cancer. Patients with familial adenomatous polyposis are born with this gene mutated.

Adjuvant chemotherapy: Treatment given after the primary treatment that is designed to eliminate any remaining cancer cells that are undetectable with the goal of improving survival. Adjuvant therapy for cancer usually refers to surgery followed by chemotherapy or radiation.

Adjuvant therapy: Treatment which follows the primary modality with the intent of reducing the risk of disease relapse and prolonging survival. The ultimate goal is to cure patients who would not otherwise be cured by the primary modality alone.

Adnexal: Adjacent or appending as the fallopian tubes and ovaries are to the uterus.

Adrenalectomy: Surgical removal of an adrenal gland.

Adrenocorticotropic hormone: A hormone secreted by the anterior pituitary that controls secretion of cortisol from the adrenal glands. Also referred to as corticotropin.

Adverse drug reaction: Any unexpected, unintended, undesired, or excessive response to a medication that may require discontinuing the medication, changing the medication, or modifying the dose (except for minor dosage adjustments); necessitates admission to the hospital; prolongs stay in a healthcare facility; necessitates supportive treatment; significantly complicates diagnosis; negatively affects prognosis; or results in temporary or permanent harm, disability, or death.

Aeroallergen: An airborne substance that causes an allergic response.

Afterload: The force against which a ventricle contracts that is contributed to by the vascular resistance, especially of the arteries, and by the physical characteristics (mass and viscosity) of the blood.

Ageism: Discrimination against aged persons.

Air embolus: An obstruction in a small blood vessel caused by air that is introduced into a blood vessel and is carried through the circulation until it lodges in a smaller vessel.

Aldosterone: A hormone produced in and secreted by the zona glomerulosa of the adrenal cortex. Aldosterone acts on the kidneys to reabsorb sodium and excrete potassium. It is also a part of the renin-angiotensin-aldosterone system that regulates blood pressure and blood volume.

Alkalemia: A decrease in the hydrogen ion concentration of the blood or a rise above normal in pH.

Alkalosis: Any pathologic state that leads to alkalemia.

Allogeneic: A transplant taking cells from one person and donating them to another.

Allogeneic HSCT: In the setting of stem cell transplantation, the scenario in which the donor is genetically similar but not identical to the recipient. The donor is usually a sibling or a matched related donor.

Allograft: Tissue or organ transplanted from a donor of the same species but different genetic makeup; recipient's immune system must be suppressed to prevent rejection of the graft.

Allograft survival: After the transplant procedure, when the transplanted organ continues to have some degree of function, from excellent to poor.

Allorecognition: Recognition of the foreign antigens present on the transplant organ or the donor's antigen presenting cells.

Alopecia: Hair loss.

Amenorrhea: Abnormal cessation or absence of menses.

Ampulla of Vater: Dilation of the duodenal wall at the opening of the fused pancreatic and common bile ducts.

Amyloid: Any of a group of chemically diverse proteins which are composed of linear nonbranching aggregated fibrils.

Anaphylactic/anaphylaxis: Immediate, severe, potentially fatal hypersensitivity reaction induced by an antigen.

Anaphylactoid: An anaphylactic-like reaction, similar in signs and symptoms but not mediated by IgE. The drug causing this reaction produces direct release of inflammatory mediators by a pharmacologic effect.

Anastomosis: The connection of two hollow organs to restore continuity after resection.

Androgen: A steroid hormone, such as testosterone or androsterone, that controls the development and maintenance of masculine characteristics.

Anemia: A reduction below normal in the concentration of hemoglobin in the body that results in a reduction of the oxygen-carrying capacity of the blood.

Anemia of chronic kidney disease: A decline in red blood cell production caused by a decrease in erythropoietin production by the progenitor cells of the kidney. As kidney function declines in chronic kidney disease, erythropoietin production also declines, resulting in decreased red blood cell production. Other contributing factors include iron deficiency and decreased red blood cell life span caused by uremia.

Anergy: A reduction or lack of an immune response to a specific antigen.

Angina: Discomfort in the chest or adjacent areas caused by decreased blood and oxygen supply to the myocardium (myocardial ischemia).

Angina pectoris: Severe constricting pain in the chest, often radiating from the precordium to a shoulder (usually left) and down the arm, due to ischemia of the heart muscle usually caused by a coronary disease.

Angioedema: Swelling similar to urticaria (hives), but the swelling occurs beneath the skin instead of on the surface. Angioedema is characterized by deep swelling around the eyes and lips and sometimes of the hands and feet. If it proceeds rapidly, it can lead to airway obstruction and suffocation, and it should therefore be treated as a medical emergency.

Angiogenesis: The formation of new blood vessels; tumors require angiogenesis to grow and spread. Antiangiogenesis drugs attempt to block this process, thereby preventing tumor growth.

Angiography: Examination of the blood vessels using x-rays after injection of a radiopaque substance.

Anorexia: The loss of appetite, especially as a result of disease.

Antiangiogenic: Preventing or inhibiting the formation and differentiation of blood vessels.

Anticoagulant: Any substance that inhibits, suppresses, or delays the formation of blood clots. These substances occur naturally and regulate the clotting cascade. Several anticoagulants have been identified in a variety of animal tissues and have been commercially developed for medicinal use.

Antimicrobial prophylaxis: Use of an antimicrobial to prevent an infection.

Antiproteinase: A substance that inhibits the enzymatic activity of a proteinase.

Anuria: Urine output of less than 50 mL over 24 hours.

Apoptosis: Programmed cell death as signaled by the nuclei in normally functioning cells when age or state of cell health and condition dictates.

Arcuate scotoma: An arc-shaped area of blindness in the field of vision.

Arthrocentesis: Puncture and aspiration of a joint. Certain drugs can be injected into the joint space for a local effect.

Arthus reaction: Local inflammatory response due to deposition of immune complexes in tissues.

Articular: Related to a joint or joints.

Ascites: Accumulation of fluid within the peritoneal cavity.

Asterixis: A flapping tremor of the arms and hands that is seen in patients with end-stage liver disease.

Astringent: A substance that causes tissues to constrict, resulting in a drying effect of the skin.

Atelectasis: Decreased or absent air in a partial or entire lung, with resulting loss of lung volume.

Atherosclerosis: Accumulation of lipids, inflammatory cells, and cellular debris in the subendothelial space of the arterial wall.

Atopy: A genetic predisposition to develop type I hypersensitivity reactions against common environmental antigens. Commonly seen in patients with allergic rhinitis, asthma, and atopic dermatitis.

Atresia: Congenital absence of a normal opening or normally patent lumen.

Attenuate: Render less virulent.

Auto-induction: The process of a drug increasing or inducing its own metabolism.

Autologous: A transplant using one's own stem cells.

Autologous HSCT: In the setting of stem cell transplantation, the scenario in which the donor and recipient are the same person.

Automaticity: Ability of a cardiac fiber or tissue to spontaneously initiate depolarizations.

Azoospermic: Having no living spermatozoa in the semen, or failure of spermatogenesis.

B2 microglobulin: A low-molecular-weight protein that may be elevated in multiple myeloma.

Bacille Calmette-Guérin: A tuberculosis vaccine prepared from an attenuated strain of the closely related species *Mycobacterium bovis*, used for immunization against tuberculosis in many countries, but not in the United States.

Bacteriuria: Presence of bacteria in urine.

Barium enema: A diagnostic test using an x-ray examination to view the lower gastrointestinal tract (colon and rectum) after rectal administration of barium sulfate, a chalky liquid contrast medium.

Barrett's esophagus: Disorder in which the cells of the lower esophagus are damaged, most often a result of long-standing reflux.

Bence-Jones proteins: Free light chains of immunoglobulins found in the urine.

Bilateral salpingo-oophorectomy: Surgical excision (removal) of both ovaries.

Bile acids: The organic acids in bile. Bile is the yellowish-brown or green fluid secreted by the liver and discharged into the duodenum where it aids in the emulsification of fats, increases peristalsis, and retards putrefaction; contains sodium glycocholate and sodium taurocholate, cholesterol, biliverdin and bilirubin, mucus, fat, lecithin, and cells and cellular debris.

Biliary sludge: A deposit of tiny stones or crystals made up of cholesterol, calcium bilirubinate, and other calcium salts. The cholesterol and calcium bilirubinate crystals in biliary sludge can lead to gallstone formation.

Biopsy: A procedure that involves obtaining a tissue specimen for microscopic analysis to establish a precise diagnosis.

Bladder hypotonicity: Inability of the detrusor muscle of the bladder to contract when the bladder is full.

Blast: An immature cell.

Blastopore: A fungal spore produced by budding.

Blood dyscrasias: Any abnormality in the blood or bone marrow's cellular components such as low white or red blood cell count or low platelets.

Blood urea nitrogen (BUN): A waste product in the blood produced from the breakdown of dietary proteins. The kidneys filter blood to remove urea and maintain homeostasis; a decline in kidney function results in an increase in BUN.

Body mass index: A calculation utilized to correct weight changes for height and is a direct calculation regardless of gender. It is the result of the weight in kilograms divided by the height in meters squared. If nonmetric measurements are used, it is the result of the weight in pounds multiplied by 703 and then that quantity divided by the product of height in inches squared.

Bone remodeling: The constant process of bone turnover involving bone resorption followed by bone formation.

Bouchard's nodes: Hard, bony enlargement of the proximal interphalangeal (middle) joint of a finger or toe.

Brachial plexus: Collection of nerves that arises from the spine at the base of the neck from nerves that supply parts of the shoulder, arm, forearm, and hand.

Brachytherapy: A procedure in which radioactive material sealed in needles, seeds, wires, or catheters is placed directly into or near a tumor. Also called internal radiation, implant radiation, or interstitial radiation therapy.

Bronchiectasis: Chronic condition of one or more bronchi or bronchioles marked by irreversible dilatation and destruction of the bronchial walls.

Bronchoalveolar lavage: Diagnostic procedure in which a scope is passed through the nose or mouth into the lungs and fluid is squirted into an area of lung, then recollected for examination.

Bullectomy: Surgical removal of one or more bullae (air spaces in the lung measuring more than 1 cm in diameter in the distended state).

Bursitis: An inflammation of the bursa, the fluid-filled sac near the joint where tendons and muscles pass over bone.

Cachexia: Weight loss, wasting of muscle, loss of appetite, and general debility that can occur with cancer. Anorexia may or may not be present.

Capillary leak: Loss of intravascular volume into the interstitial space within the body.

Carcinoembryonic antigen: A protein normally seen during fetal development. When elevated in adults, it suggests the presence of colorectal and other cancers. Normal level range is less than 2.5 ng/mL (less than 2.5 mcg/L) in nonsmokers but can be elevated in smokers and other nonmalignant conditions such as pancreatitis.

Carcinogenesis: Production or origin of cancer.

Carcinoma: A malignant growth that arises from epithelium, found in skin or the lining of body organs. Carcinomas tend to infiltrate into adjacent tissue and spread to distant organs.

Carcinomatosis: Condition of having widespread dissemination of carcinoma (cancer) in the body.

Cardiac cachexia: Physical wasting with loss of weight and muscle mass caused by cardiac disease; a wasting syndrome that causes weakness and a loss of weight, fat, and muscle.

Cardiac index: Cardiac output normalized for body surface area (cardiac index = cardiac output/body surface area).

Cardiac output: The volume of blood ejected from the left side of the heart per unit of time [cardiac output (L/min) = stroke volume × heart rate].

Cardiac remodeling: Genome expression resulting in molecular, cellular, and interstitial changes and manifested clinically as changes in size, shape, and function of the heart resulting from cardiac load or injury.

Carotid: The two main arteries in the neck.

Carotid bruit: Abnormal sound heard when auscultating a carotid artery caused by turbulent blood flow usually due to the presence of atherosclerotic plaques.

Carotid intima-media thickness: A measurement of the surface between the intima and media. This is a well-validated measure of the progression of atherosclerosis. Increasing measurements over time correlate with increasing atherosclerosis, whereas a decrease in the measurement is indicative of atherosclerotic regression.

Caseating granulomas: A central soft, dry, crumbly cheese-like necrotic mass bordered by giant multinucleated cells, and surrounded by epithelioid cell aggregates, lymphocytes, and fibroblasts.

Cavitary lesions: A spherical, air-containing lesion found on radiograph or computer tomography. The lesion usually has a thick wall and can be found within an area of a surrounding infiltrate or mass.

CCR5 inhibitor: A drug that prevents the binding of HIV to the coreceptor CCR5 on the host cell surface, thereby inhibiting viral entry into the cell.

Cephalic: Of or relating to the head.

Cervicitis: Inflammation of the cervix.

Chemoprevention: The use of drugs, vitamins, or other agents to reduce the risk of, or delay the development or recurrence of, cancer.

Chemoreceptor trigger zone: Located in the area postrema of the fourth ventricle of the brain, it is exposed to cerebrospinal fluid and blood and is easily stimulated by circulating toxins to induce nausea and vomiting.

Chemosis: Edema of the bulbar conjunctiva.

Cheyne-Stokes respiration: Pattern of breathing with gradual increase in depth (and sometimes in rate) to a maximum, followed by a decrease resulting in apnea; the cycles ordinarily are 30 seconds to 2 minutes in duration, with 5 to 30 seconds of apnea.

Chimeric: Composed of parts from different origins.

Chloasma: Melasma characterized by irregularly shaped brown patches on the face and other areas of the skin, often seen during pregnancy or associated with the use of oral contraceptives.

Cholecystitis: Inflammation of the gallbladder.

Cholelithiasis: Formation of stones in the gallbladder.

Cholestasis: Reduced or lack of flow of bile, or obstruction of bile flow.

Cholesteatoma: A mass of keratinized epithelial cells and cholesterol resembling a tumor that forms in the middle ear or mastoid region.

Cholinesterase inhibitors: A class of medications used in the treatment of Alzheimer's disease which prevent the breakdown of acetylcholine.

Chronic disorder: An acid-base disturbance that has been present for hours to days.

Chronic kidney disease: A progressive, irreversible decline in kidney function that occurs over a period of several months to years.

Chronic stable angina: Manifestation of ischemic heart disease that typically results when an atherosclerotic plaque progresses to occlude at least 70% of a major coronary artery. Patients typically present with a sensation of chest pressure or heaviness that is provoked by exertion and relieved with rest or sublingual nitroglycerin.

Chronotropic: Pertaining to the heart rate.

Chvostek's sign: A tap on the patient's facial nerve adjacent to the ear produces a brief contraction of the upper lip, nose, or side of the face.

Chylothorax: The presence of lymphatic fluid (chyle) in the pleural cavity.

Circulatory shock: A condition wherein the circulatory system is inadequately supplying oxygen and vital metabolic substrates to cells throughout the body.

Cirrhosis: Progressive scarring of the liver resulting in nonfunctional hepatocytes.

Clinical cure: Resolution of signs and symptoms of a disease.

Clonal expansion: An immunologic response in which lymphocytes stimulated by antigen proliferate and amplify the population of relevant cells.

Closed comedo: A plugged follicle of sebum, keratinocytes, and bacteria that remains beneath the surface of the skin. Also referred to as a "whitehead."

Clotting cascade: A series of enzymatic reactions by clotting factors leading to the formation of a blood clot. The clotting cascade is initiated by several thrombogenic substances. Each reaction in the cascade is triggered by the preceding one and the effect is amplified by positive feedback loops.

Clotting factor: Plasma proteins found in the blood that are essential to the formation of blood clots. Clotting factors circulate in inactive forms but are activated by their predecessor in the clotting cascade or a thrombogenic substance. Each clotting factor is designated by a Roman numeral (e.g., Factor VII) and by the letter "a" when activated (e.g., Factor VIIa).

Clubbing: Proliferation of soft tissues, especially in the nail bed, which results in thickening and widening of finger and toe extremities.

Coalescence: Fusion of smaller lipid emulsion particles forming larger particles, resulting in destabilization of the emulsion.

Coitus: Sexual intercourse.

Collateral damage: Use of an antimicrobial agent that leads to an increase in colonization and infections with multidrug-resistant organisms in a population setting.

Colloids: Intravenous fluids composed of water and large-molecular-weight molecules used to increase volume in patients with hypovolemic shock via increased intravascular oncotic pressure.

Colon cancer: A disease in which cells in the lining of the colon become malignant and proliferate without control. Often referred to as colorectal cancer to include cancer cells found in the rectum.

Colonoscopy: A visual examination of the colon using a lighted, lens-equipped, flexible tube (colonoscope) inserted into the rectum.

Colony-forming units: The number of microorganisms that form colonies when cultured and is indicative of the number of viable microorganisms in a sample.

Combined modality: Use of two or more different treatment strategies such as systemic chemotherapy (i.e., cyclophosphamide plus doxorubicin; recently, non–anthracycline-containing regimens have also been shown to be effective) plus radiation to "consolidate" local-regional control of the tumor, and surgery such as modified radical mastectomy (breast conserving surgery has been performed with good results but established guidelines are limited by small numbers, lack of randomized trials, and absence of long-term follow-up).

Comedolytic: An agent that is able to break up or destroy a comedo.

Comorbidities: Multiple disease states occurring concurrently in one patient.

Compartment syndrome: The compression of nerves and blood vessels within an enclosed space.

Complete remission: Disappearance of all previously identifiable disease.

Complete response: In cancer, disappearance of all targeted lesions.

Complex regimen: Taking medications 3 or more times per day, or 12 or more doses per day.

Complicated disorder: The presence of two or more distinct acid-base disorders.

Congenital adrenal hyperplasia: A rare inherited condition resulting from a deficiency in cortisol and aldosterone synthesis with resulting excess androgen production. The clinical presentation depends on the variant of the condition but typically manifests as abnormalities in sexual development and/or adrenal insufficiency.

Conjunctivitis: Inflammation of the conjunctiva.

Conjunctivitis medicamentosa: A drug-induced form of allergic conjunctivitis resulting from overuse of topical ocular vasoconstrictors.

Consolidation: A type of high-dose chemotherapy given as the second phase (after induction) of a treatment regimen for leukemia.

Contiguous: Describes two structures that are in close contact, or located next to each other.

Convection: The movement of dissolved solutes across a semipermeable membrane by applying a pressure gradient to the fluid transport.

Convulsion: Uncontrolled muscle movement that may or may not result from abnormal electrical activity in the brain.

Cor pulmonale: Right-sided heart failure caused by lung disease.

Corneal arcus: Accumulation of lipid on the cornea.

Coronary artery bypass graft: Surgical intervention to improve coronary blood flow by removing a vein from the leg and attaching one end to the aorta and the other end to the coronary artery distal to the atherosclerotic plaque. Alternatively, an artery from the inside of the chest wall may be used to bypass the coronary occlusion.

Coronary artery disease: Narrowing of one or more of the major coronary arteries, most commonly by atherosclerotic plaques. May be referred to as coronary heart disease.

Coronary heart disease: Narrowing of one or more of the major coronary arteries, most commonly by atherosclerotic plaques. May be referred to as coronary artery disease.

Corpus luteum: The small yellow endocrine structure that develops within a ruptured ovarian follicle and secretes progesterone and estrogen.

Corticotropin-releasing hormone: A hormone released by the hypothalamus that stimulates release of adreno-corticotropic hormone by the anterior pituitary gland.

Cortisol: An adrenal gland hormone responsible for maintaining homeostasis of carbohydrate, protein, and fat metabolism.

Cosyntropin: A synthetic version of adrenocorticotropic hormone.

Counterirritant: A substance that elicits a superficial inflammatory response with the objective of reducing inflammation in deeper, adjacent structures.

Creaming: Aggregation of lipid emulsion particles that then migrate to the surface of the emulsion; can be reversed with mild agitation.

Creatine kinase, creatine kinase myocardial band: Creatine kinase (CK) enzymes are found in many isoforms, with varying concentrations depending on the type of tissue. Creatine kinase is a general term used to describe the nonspecific total release of all types of CK, including that found in skeletal muscle (MM), brain (BB), and heart (MB). Creatine kinase MB is released into the blood from necrotic myocytes in response to infarction and is a useful laboratory test for diagnosing myocardial infarction. If the total CK is elevated, then the relative index (RI), or fraction of the total that is composed of CK-MB, is calculated as follows:

$$RI = (CK\text{-}MB/CK\ total) \times 100$$

A RI greater than 2 is typically diagnostic of infarction.

Creatinine: A waste product in the blood produced from the breakdown of protein by-products generated by muscle in the body or ingested in the diet. The kidneys filter blood to remove creatinine and maintain homeostasis; a decline in kidney function results in an increase in creatinine.

Creatinine clearance: Rate at which creatinine is filtered across the glomerulus; estimate of glomerular filtration rate.

Crepitus: A grating sound or sensation typically produced by friction between bone-on-cartilage or bone-on-bone contact.

Cross-allergenicity: Sensitivity to one drug and then reacting to a different drug with a similar chemical structure.

Crypt abscess: Neutrophilic infiltration of the intestinal glands (Crypts of Lieberkuhn); a characteristic finding in patients with ulcerative colitis.

Crystalloids: Intravenous fluids composed of water and electrolytes (e.g., sodium chloride, etc.) used as intravascular volume expanders for patients with hypovolemic shock.

Culture-negative IE: Implies acute endocardial damage with negative blood cultures. It is common in patients treated with antibiotics before blood cultures are obtained.

Cure: Disease-free period, which may vary by tumor type or disease state, exceeding an arbitrary duration of time. For breast cancer, this period exceeds 15 years from the end of treatment; for acute leukemia, the period is 5 years. [Note: By this definition, dormant viable tumor cells may still be present even in patients who are deemed cured.]

Cutis laxa: Hyperflaccidity of the skin with loss of elasticity.

Cyanosis: Bluish discoloration of the skin and mucous membranes due to lack of oxygenation.

Cyclic citrullinated peptide: A circular peptide (a ring of amino acids) containing the amino acid citrulline. Autoantibodies directed against cyclic citrullinated peptide provide the basis for a test of importance in rheumatoid arthritis.

Cyclooxygenase: An enzyme that catalyzes the conversion of arachidonic acid to prostaglandins and consists of two isoforms, generally abbreviated COX-1 and COX-2.

Cystitis: Inflammation of urinary bladder.

Cystocele: Hernial protrusion of the bladder, usually through the vaginal wall.

Cytokines: Regulatory proteins, such as interleukins and lymphokines, that are released by cells of the immune system and act as intercellular mediators in the generation of an immune response. Soluble glycoproteins released by the immune system which act through specific receptors to regulate immune responses.

Cytomegalovirus (CMV) disease: This is the term used when patients who are already infected with CMV present with the classic associated symptoms that resemble a viral infection and may include fever, malaise, arthralgias and others.

Cytomegalovirus (CMV) infection: This is the term used when a patient has anti-CMV antibodies in the blood, when CMV antigens are detected in infected cells, or when the virus is isolated from a culture.

Deep vein thrombosis: A disorder of thrombus formation causing obstruction of a deep vein in the leg, pelvis, or abdomen.

Delirium: Transient brain syndrome presenting as disordered attention, cognition, psychomotor behavior, and perception.

Dementia: Loss of brain function that occurs with certain diseases. It affects memory, thinking, judgment, and behavior.

Dennie-Morgan line: A line or fold below the lower eyelids; associated with atopy.

Dermatophytes: Any microscopic fungus that grows on the skin, scalp, nails, or mucosa but does not invade deeper tissues.

Desensitization: A method to reduce or eliminate an individual's negative reaction to a substance or stimulus.

Desquamation: Peeling or shedding of the epidermis (superficial layer of the skin) in scales or flakes.

Detumescence: The return of the penis to a flaccid state.

Dialysate: The physiologic solution used during dialysis to remove excess fluids and waste products from the blood.

Dialysis: The process of removing fluid and waste products from the blood across a semipermeable membrane to maintain fluid, electrolyte, and acid-base balance in patients with kidney failure.

Diaphoresis: Perspiration.

Diarthrodial joint: A freely moveable joint (e.g., knee, shoulder). Contrast with amphiarthrodial joint (a slightly movable joint; e.g., vertebral joint) and synarthrodial joint (an unmovable joint; e.g., fibrous joint).

Diastolic dysfunction: Abnormal filling of the ventricles during diastole.

Diffusion: The movement of a solute across the dialyzer membrane from an area of higher concentration (usually the blood) to a lower concentration (usually the dialysate).

2,3-Diphosphoglycerate: A compound in red blood cells that affects oxygen binding to and release from hemoglobin.

Direct current cardioversion: The process of administering a synchronized electrical shock to the chest, the purpose of which is to simultaneously depolarize all of the myocardial cells, resulting in restoration of normal sinus rhythm.

Directly observed therapy: Directly observing patients while taking their anti-tuberculosis medication to ensure compliance.

Disease-free survival: Length of time after treatment during which no disease is found.

Disease progression: In cancer, at least a 20% increase in the sum of the longest diameter of target lesions from baseline, including new lesions discovered during treatment.

Disseminated idiopathic skeletal hyperostosis: Excessive bone formation at skeletal sites subject to stress, generally where tendons and ligaments attach to bone.

DNA mismatch repair genes: Genes that identify and correct errors in DNA base pairs during DNA replication. Mutations in the genes can lead to cancer by allowing abnormal cells to continue to grow.

Down-regulation: The process of reducing or suppressing a response to a stimulus.

Drusen: Tiny yellow or white deposits of extracellular material in the eye.

Ductus arteriosus: Shunt connecting the pulmonary artery to the aortic arch that allows most of the blood from the right ventricle to bypass fetal lungs.

Duodenal: The first of three parts of the small intestine.

Dysarthria: Speech disorder due to weakness or incoordination of speech muscles; speech is slow, weak, and imprecise.

Dyslipidemia: Elevation of the total cholesterol, low-density lipoprotein cholesterol, or triglyceride concentrations or a decrease in high-density lipoprotein cholesterol concentration in the blood.

Dysmenorrhea: Crampy pelvic pain occurring with or just prior to menses. "Primary" dysmenorrhea implies pain in the setting of normal pelvic anatomy, while "secondary" dysmenorrhea is secondary to underlying pelvic pathology.

Dyspareunia: Pain during or after sexual intercourse.

Dysphagia: Difficulty in swallowing.

Dysphonia: Impairment of the voice or difficulty speaking.

Dysphoria: An unhappy or depressed feeling.

Dyspnea: Shortness of breath or difficulty breathing.

Dyssynergic defecation: A lack of coordination between the pelvic floor muscles and the anal sphincter.

Dysuria: Difficulty or pain in urination.

Ebstein's anomaly: Congenital heart defect in which the opening of the tricuspid valve is displaced toward the apex of the right ventricle of the heart.

Eburnation: A condition in which bone or cartilage becomes hardened and denser.

Ecchymosis: Passage of blood from ruptured blood vessels into subcutaneous tissue causing purple discoloration of the skin.

Ectopic pregnancy: Presence of a fertilized ovum outside of the uterine cavity.

Effector cells: Cells that become active in response to initiation of the immune response.

Ejection fraction: The fraction of the volume present at the end of diastole that is pushed into the aorta during systole.

Electrocardiogram: A noninvasive recording of the electrical activity of the heart.

Electroencephalogram: A test that measures and records electrical activity in the brain.

Embolectomy: Surgical removal of a clot or embolism.

Embolism: The sudden blockage of a vessel caused by a blood clot or foreign material which has been brought to the site by the flow of blood.

Embolization: The process by which a blood clot or foreign material dislodges from its site of origin, flows in the blood, and blocks a distant vessel.

Emesis: See vomiting.

Endarterectomy: Removal of a thrombus from the carotid artery.

Endometritis: Inflammation of the endometrium.

Endoscopic evaluation: General term used to describe the visual inspection of the inside of hollow organs with an endoscope; used mainly for diagnostic purposes; refers to procedures such as gastroscopy, duodenoscopy, colonoscopy, sigmoidoscopy, and others.

Endoscopy: A diagnostic tool used to examine the inside of the body using a lighted, flexible instrument called an endoscope.

Endothelial cell: A single layer of cells surrounding the lumen of arteries.

End-stage liver disease: Liver failure that is usually accompanied by complications such as ascites or hepatic encephalopathy.

Engraftment: The process by which transplanted stem cells begin to grow and reproduce in the recipient to produce functioning leukocytes, erythrocytes, and platelets.

Enteral nutrition: Delivery of nutrients via the gastrointestinal tract, either by mouth or by feeding tube.

Enterobacteriaceae: A family of enteric gram-negative bacilli, e.g., *Escherichia coli* or *Klebsiella pneumoniae*.

Enterocytes: Cells lining the small intestine.

Enthesitis: Inflammation of the sites where tendons, ligaments, or fascia attach to bone.

Enuresis: Incontinence at night.

Enzyme-linked immunosorbent assay: A solid phase in the form of a microtiter plate or bead to which HIV antigen is attached. The antigen may be either a preparation of lysed whole virus or a combination of recombinant viral antigens.

Epilepsy: The propensity for a patient to have repeated, unprovoked seizures.

Epistaxis: A nosebleed.

Erectile dysfunction: Condition defined as the inability to achieve or maintain an erection sufficient for sexual intercourse.

Erythema multiforme: A rash characterized by papular (small raised bump) or vesicular lesions (blisters), and reddening or discoloration of the skin often in concentric zones about the lesion.

Erythematous: Flushing of the skin caused by dilation of capillaries. Erythema is often a sign of inflammation and infection.

Erythropoiesis stimulating agents: Agents developed by recombinant DNA technology that have the same biologic activity as endogenous erythropoietin to stimulate erythropoiesis (red blood cell production) in the bone marrow. The currently available agents in the United States are epoetin alfa and darbepoetin alfa.

Erythropoietin: A hormone primarily produced by the progenitor cells of the kidney that stimulates red blood cell production in the bone marrow. Lack of this hormone leads to anemia.

Esophageal varices: Dilated blood vessels in the esophagus.

Essential fatty acid deficiency: Deficiency of linoleic acid, linolenic acid, and/or arachidonic acid, characterized by hair loss, thinning of skin, and skin desquamation. Long-chain fatty acids include trienes (containing 3 double-bonds [e.g., 5,8,11-eicosatrienoic acid {or Mead acid}, trienoic acids]) and tetraenes (containing 4 double-bonds [e.g., arachidonic acid]). Biochemical evidence of essential fatty acid deficiency includes a triene-to-tetraene ratio greater than 0.2 and low linoleic or arachidonic acid plasma concentrations.

Euphoria: A feeling of happiness and excitement.

Event-free survival: This term refers to the length of time after treatment that a person remains free of certain negative events.

Evoked potential testing: A procedure in which sensory nerve pathways are stimulated, and the time lapse to electrical response in the corresponding area of the brain is measured.

Exanthem: Eruption of the skin.

Exfoliative dermatitis: Severe inflammation of the entire skin surface due to a reaction to certain drugs.

Exploratory laparotomy: Surgical incision into the abdominal cavity, performed to examine the abdominal organs and cavity in search of an abnormality and diagnosis.

External beam radiotherapy: Treatment by radiation emitted from a source located at a distance from the body. Also called beam therapy and external beam therapy.

Extra-abdominal: Outside of the abdominal cavity.

Extraction ratio: Fraction of the drug entering the liver in the blood which is irreversibly removed.

Extrapyramidal symptoms: Adverse drug effects of medications such as phenothiazines; includes dystonia (involuntary muscle contractions), tardive dyskinesia (repetitive, involuntary movements), and akathisia (motor restlessness or anxiety).

Facultative: Biologic term meaning "optional." A facultative intracellular pathogen can optionally survive intracellularly even if it is typically an extracellular pathogen.

Facultative anaerobe: An organism that makes adenosine triphosphate by aerobic respiration if oxygen is present, but switches to fermentation under anaerobic conditions.

Felty's syndrome: An extraarticular manifestation of rheumatoid arthritis associated with splenomegaly and neutropenia.

Fibrin: An insoluble protein that is one of the principal ingredients of a blood clot. Fibrin strands bind to one another to form a fibrin mesh. The fibrin mesh often traps platelets and other blood cells.

Fibrinolysis: A normal ongoing process that dissolves fibrin and results in removal of small blood clots; hydrolysis of fibrin.

Fibroadenoma: A benign neoplasm which commonly occurs in breast tissue and is derived from glandular epithelium.

Fibrosis: Formation of tissue containing connective tissues formed by fibroblasts as part of tissue repair or as a reactive process.

Fistula: Abnormal connection between two internal organs (e.g., arteriovenous fistula is a connection between an artery and a vein), or between an internal organ and the exterior or skin (e.g., enterocutaneous fistula is a connection between the intestine and the skin).

Floppy iris syndrome: Alpha-adrenergic antagonists cause relaxation of the iris and papillary constriction. This complicates cataract surgery. Also known as the small pupil syndrome.

Flow cytometry: A technology used to study characteristics of individual cells in a suspension.

Fluorescence in situ hybridization: A laboratory technique used to look at genes or chromosomes in cells and tissues. Pieces of DNA that contain a fluorescent dye are made in the laboratory and added to cells or tissues on a glass slide. When these pieces of DNA bind to specific genes or areas of chromosomes on the slide, they light up when viewed under a microscope with a special light.

Foam cell: Lipid-laden white blood cell.

Forced expiratory volume in 1 second: The volume of air that a patient can blow out in the first second of forced exhalation after taking a maximal breath.

Forced vital capacity: The maximum volume of air that can be forcibly exhaled after taking a maximal breath.

Fragility fracture: A fracture resulting from a fall from standing height or less amount of trauma.

Frailty: Excess demand imposed on reduced capacity; a common biologic syndrome in the elderly.

Frank-Starling mechanism: One of the mechanisms by which the heart can increase cardiac output.

Fremitus: A palpable vibration, as felt by the hand placed on the chest during coughing or speaking.

Friable: Easily crumbled, pulverized, or reduced to powder.

Friction: Risk factor for pressure ulcers that is created when a patient is dragged across a surface, which can lead to superficial skin damage.

Fructooligosaccharides: Polymers of fructose that reach the colon undigested and are broken down there to short-chain fatty acids by bacterial enzymes.

Functional gastrointestinal disorder: A term used to describe symptoms occurring in the gastrointestinal tract in the absence of a demonstrated pathologic condition; the clinical product of psychosocial factors and altered intestinal physiology involving the brain–gut interrelationship.

Gadolinium: An intravenous contrast agent used with magnetic resonance imaging.

Gallstone (cholelithiasis): A solid formation in the gallbladder or bile duct composed of cholesterol and bile salts.

Gastrectomy: Surgical excision of part or all of the stomach.

Gastric bypass: A surgical procedure for weight loss that elicits its effectiveness through malabsorption and volume limitation. The procedure involves full partitioning of the proximal gastric segment into a jejunal loop.

Gastritis: Chronic or acute inflammation of the lining of the stomach.

Gastroenteritis: Inflammation of the gastrointestinal tract causing nausea, vomiting, diarrhea, and fever; sometimes referred to as the stomach flu although not related to influenza.

Gastroplasty: A surgical procedure for weight loss that elicits its effectiveness through gastric volume limitation. The procedure involves partial partitioning at the proximal gastric segment with the placement of a gastric outlet stoma of fixed diameter.

Gastroschisis: Inherited congenital abdominal wall defect in which the intestines and sometimes other organs develop outside the fetal abdomen through an opening in the abdominal wall.

Gastrostomy: Operative placement of a new opening into the stomach, usually associated with feeding tube placement.

Geniculate nucleus: The portion of the brain that processes visual information from the optic nerve and relays it to the cerebral cortex.

Genotype: The genetic constitution of an individual.

Geriatric syndrome: Age-specific presentations or differential diagnoses, including visual and hearing impairment, malnutrition and weight loss, urinary incontinence, gait impairment and falls, osteoporosis, dementia, delirium, sleep problems, and pressure ulcers; commonly seen conditions in elder patients.

Gigantism: A condition of abnormal size or overgrowth of the entire body or of any of its parts.

Glasgow Coma Scale: A scale for evaluating level of consciousness after central nervous system injury (evaluates eye opening and verbal and motor responsiveness).

Glomerular filtration rate: The volume of plasma that is filtered by the glomerulus per unit time, usually expressed as mL/min or mL/min/1.73 m$^2$, which adjusts the value for body surface area. This is the primary index used to describe overall renal function.

Glomerulonephritis: Glomerular lesions that are characterized by inflammation of the capillary loops of the glomerulus. These lesions are generally caused by immunologic, vascular or other idiopathic diseases. Leads to high blood pressure and possible loss of kidney function.

Glutamate: Primary excitatory neurotransmitter in the central nervous system involved in memory, learning, and neuronal plasticity.

Gonioscopy: Examination of the anterior chamber angle. A gonioprism or Goldman lens are used to perform gonioscopic evaluation.

Graft versus host disease: A complication of stem cell transplantation where the donor's cells attack the host's tissue.

Graft versus tumor effect: The phenomenon by which transplanted donor cells recognize host malignant cells as foreign and thus eradicate the malignant cells through immunologic mechanisms.

Granulomas: Unique inflammatory response composed of macrophages, giant cells and other cells of the immune response to wall off infectious pathogens perceived as foreign but cannot be eliminated.

Gummatous: A tumor of rubbery consistency that is characteristic of the tertiary stage of syphilis.

Gut-associated lymphoid tissue: Lymphoid tissue, including Peyer's patches, found in the gut that are important for providing localized immunity to pathogens.

Haptenation: The process where a drug, usually of low molecular weight, is bound to a carrier protein or cell and becomes immunogenic.

Health literacy: Degree to which individuals have the capacity to obtain, process, and understand basic health information and services needed to make appropriate health decisions.

Heberden's nodes: Hard, bony enlargement of the distal interphalangeal (terminal) joint of a finger or toe.

Hemarthrosis: Blood in the joint space.

Hematemesis: The vomiting of blood.

Hematochezia: Bright red blood per rectum.

Hematogenous: Spread through the blood.

Hematuria: Presence of blood or red blood cells in urine.

Hemiparesis: Weakness on one side of the body.

Hemisensory deficit: Loss of sensation on one side of the body.

Hemithorax: A single side of the trunk between the neck and the abdomen in which the heart and lungs are situated.

Hemoptysis: The expectoration of blood or blood-tinged sputum from the larynx, trachea, bronchi, or lungs.

Hemorrhagic conversion: Conversion of an ischemic stroke into a hemorrhagic stroke.

Hemostasis: Cessation of bleeding through natural (clot formation or construction of blood vessels), artificial (compression or ligation), or surgical means.

Heparin-induced thrombocytopenia: A clinical syndrome of IgG antibody production against the heparin-platelet factor 4 complex occurring in approximately 1% to 5% of patients exposed to either heparin or low-molecular-weight heparin. Heparin-induced thrombocytopenia results in excess production of thrombin, platelet aggregation, and thrombocytopenia (due to platelet clumping), often leading to venous and arterial thrombosis, amputation of extremities, and death.

Hepatic encephalopathy: Confusion and disorientation experienced by patients with advanced liver disease due to accumulation of ammonia in the bloodstream.

Hepatic steatosis: Accumulation of fat in the liver.

Hepatocellular carcinoma: Cancer of the liver.

Hepatojugular reflex: Distention of the jugular vein induced by pressure over the liver; it suggests insufficiency of the right heart.

Hepatorenal syndrome: Acute kidney injury resulting from decreased perfusion in cirrhosis.

Hepatosplenomegaly: An enlarged liver and spleen secondary to leukemic infiltration.

Hepatotoxicity: Toxicity to the liver causing damage to liver cells.

Herniation: Protrusion of the brain through the cranial wall.

Heterotopic: Placing a transplanted organ into an abnormal anatomic location.

Heterozygous: Having different alleles at a gene locus.

Hirschsprung's disease: A congenital abnormality where the ganglia in sections of the large intestine do not develop, resulting in chronic constipation and possibly obstruction; the severity of the condition can range from mild to severe.

Hirsutism: Excessive body and facial hair, especially in the female.

Histocompatibility: The examination of human leukocyte antigen differences between a donor and a recipient in order to determine if the recipient is more likely to accept, rather than reject, a graft from that particular donor.

HIV genotype: A type of resistance testing for HIV where a patient's blood sample is obtained, their HIV RNA is sequenced, and mutations that have developed which may confer resistance to antiretrovirals are reported.

HIV phenotype: A type of resistance testing for HIV where a patient's blood sample is obtained, and the patient's HIV genes that encode for reverse transcriptase and protease are removed and placed in an HIV viral vector. This viral vector is replicated in a cell culture system with varying concentrations of antiretrovirals. A drug concentration-viral inhibition curve is developed and the concentration needed to inhibit 50% of the patient's virus is reported. This is used to predict resistance versus susceptibility.

HIV virtual phenotype: A database of matching HIV genotypes and phenotypes is developed. When an HIV genotype for a patient is obtained, the database is used to predict the patient's phenotype based on their actual genotype using matches that occur in the database.

Homeostenosis: Impaired capability to withstand stressors and decreased ability to maintain physiologic and psychosocial homeostasis; a state commonly found in the elderly.

Homozygous: Having identical alleles at a gene locus.

Hormone-receptor positive breast cancer: Tumors that appear to grow in the presence of estrogens; likewise, anti-estrogen therapy or estrogen deprivation strategies lead to tumor regression.

Hospice: The provision of palliative care during the last 6 months of life as defined by federal guidelines.

Hot flashes: A feeling of warmth that is commonly accompanied by skin flushing and mild to severe perspiration.

Human leukocyte antigens (HLA): Groups of genes found on the major histocompatibility complex which contain cell-surface antigen presenting proteins. The body uses HLA to distinguish between self cells and nonself cells.

Humoral: Products secreted into the blood or body fluids.

Hydramnios: Increased amniotic fluid.

Hyperalgesia: An exaggerated intensity of pain sensation.

Hypercalcemia: Excessive amount of calcium in the blood.

Hypercalciuria: Excessive amount of calcium in the urine.

Hypercapnia: Abnormally high concentration of carbon dioxide in the blood.

Hypercoagulable state: A disorder or state of excessive or frequent thrombus formation; also known as thrombophilia.

Hyperemesis gravidarum: A rare disorder of severe and persistent nausea and vomiting during pregnancy that can result in dehydration, malnutrition, weight loss, and hospitalization.

Hyperglycemic hyperosmolar nonketotic syndrome: Severe increase in serum glucose concentration without the production of ketones, leading to an increase in serum osmolality and symptoms such as increased thirst, increased urination, weakness, fatigue, confusion, and in severe cases, convulsions and/or coma.

Hyperopia: Farsightedness.

Hyperpigmentation: A common darkening of the skin which occurs when an excess of melanin forms deposits in the skin.

Hyperplasia: An abnormal or unusual increase in the cells of a body part.

Hyperprolactinemia: A medical condition of elevated serum prolactin characterized by prolactin serum concentrations greater than 20 ng/mL (20 mcg/L) in men or 25 ng/mL (25 mcg/L) in women.

Hypertrichosis: Excessive growth of hair.

Hypertrophy: An increase in the size of the cells in a tissue or organ.

Hypogammaglobinemia: Reduced levels of antibodies.

Hypogonadism: A medical condition resulting from or characterized by abnormally decreased functional activity of the gonads, with retardation of growth and sexual development. Associated with testosterone deficiency resulting from either testicular or pituitary/hypothalamic diseases. Presenting symptoms differ according to the timing of disease onset in relation to puberty.

Hypopituitarism: A clinical disorder characterized by complete or partial deficiency in pituitary hormone production.

Hypovolemic shock: Circulatory shock caused by severe loss of blood volume and/or body water.

Hypoxemia: Deficiency of oxygen in the blood.

Hysterectomy: Excision of the uterus.

Immune reconstitution inflammatory syndrome: A condition in AIDS patients or other types of immunosuppression where paradoxical worsening of the infection is observed as the immune system begins to recover due to increasing inflammation at the site of infection.

Immunogenicity: The property that gives a particular substance the ability to provoke an immune response.

Immunoglobulin G index: The ratio of immunoglobulin G to protein in the serum or cerebrospinal fluid.

Immunophenotype: The process of identification and quantitation of cellular antigens through flourochrome-labeled monoclonal antibodies.

Immunotherapy: Treatment of a disease by stimulating the body's own immune system.

Impedance pH monitoring: Detects gastroesophageal reflux based on changes in resistance to electrical current flow between two electrodes when a liquid and/or gas bolus moves between them. It can detect both acid and nonacid reflux.

Implantable cardioverter-defibrillator: A device implanted into the heart transvenously with a generator implanted subcutaneously in the pectoral area that provides internal electrical cardioversion of ventricular tachycardia or defibrillation of ventricular fibrillation.

Index patient: The patient originally diagnosed with a disease.

Indirect immunofluorescence assay: HIV-infected T-lymphocytes are fixed onto a microscope slide, covered with the blood sample to be tested, incubated under heat, and washed. If antibodies to HIV are bound to the fixed viral antigens, they will remain on the slide. FITC-conjugated anti-human globulin is then added, incubated, and washed. If the sample contains antibodies to HIV, the cells will show a bright, fluorescent membrane under the microscope.

Induction: Treatment designed to be used as the first step in eliminating the leukemic burden.

Infarction: The formation of an infarct, an area of tissue death due to a local lack of oxygen.

Initiation: It occurs in cancer when a carcinogenic substance encounters a normal cell to produce genetic damage, and results in a mutated cell.

Inotropic: Relating to or influencing the force of muscular contractions.

Insulin-like growth factor-I: An anabolic peptide that acts as a direct stimulator of cell proliferation and growth in all body cells.

Integrase strand transfer inhibitor: A drug that prevents the enzyme integrase from allowing the HIV RNA to incorporate into the host cell genome.

International normalized ratio (INR): The ratio of the patient's clotting time to the clinical laboratory's mean reference value; normalized by raising it to the international sensitivity index (ISI) power to account for differences in thromboplastin reagents. Therefore: INR = (Patient's prothrombin time/laboratory's mean normal prothrombin time)[ISI].

Intima: The inner layer of the wall of an artery or vein.

Intraarticular: Administered to or occurring in the space within joints.

Intraabdominal: Within the abdominal cavity.

Intraperitoneal: Within the peritoneal cavity.

Intrathecal: Within the meninges of the spinal cord.

Intravenous pyelogram: After intravenous administration of radiocontrast media, an x-ray of kidneys, ureters, bladder, and urethra is performed, which provides information on anatomic aspects (size, shape, location, axis) and function of these organs.

Intravesicular: Administration directly into the bladder through the urethra.

Intussusception: The prolapse of one part of the intestine into the lumen of an immediately adjoining part.

Iontophoresis: Introduction of a medication into tissue through use of an electric current.

Ipsilateral: Occurring on the same side.

Ischemic heart disease: Imbalance between myocardial oxygen supply and oxygen demand.

Jejunal: A section of the small intestine connecting the duodenum to the ileum.

Jejunostomy: Operative placement of a new opening into the jejunum, usually associated with feeding tube placement.

Kegel exercises: Specific exercises that strengthen the pelvic floor muscles and help to prevent and treat stress incontinence.

Keratinization: The sloughing of epithelial cells in the hair follicle.

Keratinocyte: The epidermal cell that synthesizes keratin; makes up 95% of all epidermal cells; commonly called "skin cells."

Keratitis: Infection of the cornea.

Keratoconjunctivitis sicca: Ocular surface disease caused by dysfunctional tear film; also known as Sjogren's syndrome or dry eye syndrome.

Kindling: A process of inducing epilepsy in a laboratory animal by repeated, low-level electrical stimulation of specific areas of the brain.

Koebner phenomenon: The occurrence of psoriatic lesions due to skin trauma.

Korotkoff sounds: The noise heard over an artery by auscultation when pressure over the artery is reduced below the systolic arterial pressure.

KRAS: Protein involved in normal cell signaling processes (product of KRAS gene).

Kyphosis: Abnormal curvature of the spine resulting in protrusion of the upper back; hunchback.

$\beta$-Lactam allergy: Allergy to the $\beta$-lactam family, namely penicillins and cephalosporins, but may also include carbapenems.

Lactose intolerance: An inability to digest milk and some dairy products, resulting in abnormal bloating, cramping, and diarrhea; caused by enzymatic lactase deficiency.

Lag-ophthalmos: Poor closure of the upper eyelid.

Lamina cribrosa: A series of perforated sheets of connective tissue that the optic nerve passes through as it exits the eye.

Laminectomy: Excision of the posterior arch of a vertebra to relieve pressure on the spinal cord.

Laparoscopic: Abdominal exploration or surgery employing a type of endoscope called laparoscope.

Laparotomy: Surgical opening of the abdominal cavity.

Latent tuberculosis (TB) infection: Infection with *Mycobacterium tuberculosis* has occurred but the disease is not active. Patients with latent tuberculosis are not infectious, and it is not possible to get TB from someone with latent tuberculosis.

Lentigines: Plural of lentigo—a small, flat, tan to dark brown or black, macular melanosis on the skin which looks like a freckle but is histologically distinct. Lentigines do not darken on exposure to sunlight, freckles do.

Leukocytoclastic: The breaking up of white blood cells.

Leukopenia: A condition where the number of circulating white blood cells are abnormally low due to decreased production of new cells, possibly in conjunction with medication toxicities.

Leukostasis: An abnormal intravascular leukocyte aggregation and clumping seen in leukemia patients. The brain and the lungs are the two most frequent organs involved.

Lhermitte's sign: Tingling or shock-like sensation passing down the arms or trunk when the neck is flexed.

Libido: Conscious or unconscious sexual desire.

Ligament of Treitz: Landmark in the proximal portion of the jejunum beyond which it is preferred that postpyloric feedings be delivered for minimization of aspiration.

Light chain assay: A highly sensitive assay that determines the ratio of serum free light chain kappa to lambda.

Linea nigra: Dark vertical line that appears on the abdomen during pregnancy.

Lipoprotein lipase: Enzyme located in the capillary endothelium involved in the breakdown of intravenous lipid emulsion particles.

Liver biopsy: A procedure whereby tissue is removed from the liver and used to determine the severity of liver damage.

Luteolysis: Death of the corpus luteum.

Lymphadenectomy: Surgical excision of lymph nodes.

Lymphangitis: Inflammation of lymphatic channels.

Lymphatic: The network of vessels carrying tissue fluids.

Lymphoproliferative: Of or related to the growth of lymphoid tissue.

Maceration: The softening or breaking down of a solid by leaving it immersed in a liquid.

Macrophages: Large scavenger cell.

Macula: The central portion of the retina.

Maculopapular: A rash that contains both macules and papules. A macule is a flat discolored area of the skin, and a papule is a small raised bump. A maculopapular rash is usually a large area that is red, and has small, confluent bumps.

Major malformation: A defect that has either cosmetic or functional significance to the child.

Mastalgia: Tenderness of the breast.

Matrix metalloproteinases: Any of a group of enzymes, normally located in the extracellular space of tissue, that function to break down proteins (e.g., collagen), and require zinc or calcium atoms as cofactors for enzymatic activity.

Meatal stenosis: Abnormal narrowing or closing of the urethral opening, which slows urination or causes a change in the direction of the urinary stream.

Meconium: The first intestinal discharge or "stool" of a newborn infant, usually green in color and consisting of epithelial cells, mucus, and bile.

Media: The middle layer of the wall of an artery or vein.

Melanosis: Excessive pigmentation of the skin due to a disturbance in melanin pigmentation; also called melanism.

Melasma: Dark skin discoloration.

Melena: Abnormally dark black, tarry feces containing blood (usually from gastrointestinal bleeding).

Menarche: The onset of cyclic menstrual periods in a woman.

Meninges: Covering of the brain consisting of three layers.

Menopause: Permanent cessation of menses following the loss of ovarian follicular activity.

Menorrhagia: Menstrual blood loss of greater than 80 mL per cycle or menstrual cycles lasting greater than 7 days.

Mesothelioma: A benign or malignant tumor affecting the lining of the chest or abdomen. Commonly caused by exposure to asbestos fibers.

Metabolic acidosis: A condition in the blood and tissues that is a consequence of an accumulation of lactic acid resulting from tissue hypoxia and anaerobic metabolism.

Metabolic alkalosis: Alkalosis that is caused by an increase in the concentration of alkaline compounds (typically bicarbonate).

Metabolic syndrome: Constellation of cardiovascular risk factors related to hypertension, abdominal obesity, dyslipidemia, and insulin resistance diagnosed by the presence of at least three of the following criteria: increased waist circumference, elevated triglyceride concentrations, decreased high-density lipoprotein (HDL) cholesterol or active treatment to raise HDL cholesterol, elevated blood pressure or active treatment with antihypertensive therapy, or elevated fasting glucose or active treatment for diabetes.

Metastasis: Plural is metastases. Cancer that has spread from the original site of the tumor.

Micelles: A microscopic particle of digested fat and cholesterol.

Microalbuminuria: Urinary excretion of small but abnormal amounts of albumin. Confirmed spot urine albumin to creatinine ratio of 30 to 300 mg/g (3.4 to 34 mg/mmol creatinine) is consistent with microalbuminuria. Considered an early sign of chronic kidney disease.

Micrognathia: Abnormal smallness of the jaws.

Micrometastasis: Deposits of tumor cells in distant organs that cannot be detected by any imaging techniques available.

Microsatellite instability: Unstable sequences of repeating DNA caused by deficiencies in the normal DNA repair process.

Microvascular pulmonary emboli: An obstruction in the small blood vessels in the lung caused by material (e.g., blood clot, fat, air, foreign body) that is carried through the circulation until it lodges in another small vessel.

Minimal residual disease: A quantitative assessment of subclinical remnant of leukemic burden remaining at the end of the initial phase of treatment (induction) when a patient may appear to be in a complete morphologic remission.

Minimum inhibitory concentration: The lowest concentration of an antimicrobial agent that inhibits visible bacterial growth after approximately 24 hours.

Minor malformation: A defect that has neither cosmetic nor functional significance to the child.

Mixed disorder: See Complicated disorder.

Miosis: Pupil constriction.

Mobilization: The release of stem cells into the peripheral blood from the bone marrow compartment for the purposes of collecting these stem cells (in anticipation of stem cell transplantation).

Mobitz type I: A type of second-degree AV nodal blockade.

Mobitz type II: A type of second-degree AV nodal blockade.

Moebius syndrome: Extremely rare congenital neurologic disorder which is characterized by facial paralysis and affects eye movement.

Monocytes: A variety of white blood cells.

Monoparesis: Slight or incomplete paralysis affecting a single extremity or part of one.

Monosodium urate: A crystallized form of uric acid that can deposit in joints leading to an inflammatory reaction and the symptoms of gout.

Morphology: The science of structure and form of cells without regard to function.

Mucosa-associated lymphoid tissue: Lymphoid tissue in the gut that samples luminal antigens and delivers them to the systemic lymph system.

Mucositis: Inflammation of mucous membranes, typically within the oral and esophageal mucosa. Usually associated with certain chemotherapy agents and radiation therapy involving mucosal area.

Mucous colitis: A condition of the mucous membrane of the colon characterized by pain, constipation, or diarrhea (sometimes alternating), and passage of mucus or mucous shreds.

Muscularis mucosa: The thin layer of smooth muscle found in most parts of the gastrointestinal tract.

Mydriasis: Pupil dilation.

Myelin: A protein and phospholipid sheath that surrounds the axons of certain neurons. Myelinated nerves conduct impulses more rapidly than nonmyelinated nerves.

Myeloablative preparative regimen: Radiation and/or chemotherapy that destroys bone marrow activity in preparation for a stem cell transplant. Patients will not likely recover bone marrow function without an infusion of "rescue" autologous or allogeneic stem cells.

Myelodysplastic syndrome: A disease in which the bone marrow does not function properly.

Myelosuppression: Reduction in white blood cells, red blood cells, and platelets caused by bone marrow suppression.

Myocarditis: Inflammation of the muscular wall of the heart.

Myoglobinuria: The presence of myoglobin in urine.

Myonecrosis: Necrotic damage to muscle tissue.

Myopathy: Any disease of the muscle causing weakness, pain, and tenderness.

Myringotomy: A surgical incision in the tympanic membrane to relieve pressure and drain fluid from the middle ear.

Nasal scotoma: An area of blindness in the nasal portion of peripheral vision.

Nascent: Immature.

Nasolacrimal occlusion: The closing of the tear duct to decrease systemic absorption of a drug.

Nausea: The subjective feeling of a need to vomit.

Necrosectomy: Surgical excision of necrotic tissue; debridement.

Necrotizing enterocolitis: Medical condition primarily seen in premature infants, where portions of the bowel undergo necrosis Nelson syndrome: A condition characterized by the aggressive growth of a pituitary tumor and hyperpigmentation of the skin.

Neoadjuvant chemotherapy: Chemotherapy or radiation therapy given prior to primary surgical treatment. In cancer, it is often used to downstage the tumor to a resectable stage.

Neoadjuvant therapy: Therapeutic strategy that precedes primary treatment modality (usually surgery). The goals are to "down-stage" tumors so that the surgical field is smaller or to transform a patient from a nonsurgical candidate to one that is. Neoadjuvant therapy may improve overall survival. Strategies usually involve the use of systemic therapy with or without radiation.

Neovascular maculopathy: Proliferation of blood vessels in the macula.

Nephrolithiasis: A condition marked by the presence of renal calculi (stones) in the kidney or urinary system.

Nephron: The working unit of the kidney that filters blood to remove fluid, toxins, and drugs. Each kidney contains approximately 1 million nephrons.

Nephrostomy: Insertion of a catheter through the skin into the renal pelvis to bypass ureteral obstruction and facilitate urine drainage.

Neuralgia: Pain which extends along the course of one or more nerves.

Neuritis: Inflammation of a nerve.

Neutralizing antibodies: Antibodies that develop in response to a therapeutic agent that decrease the efficacy of the agent.

Nidus: A central point or focus consisting of a fibrin matrix (in the case of infective endocarditis), where bacteria are able to accumulate and multiply, allowing for formation of an infected vegetation.

Nitric oxide: An endogenous vasodilator.

NMDA-receptor antagonist: A medication used in the treatment of Alzheimer's disease. It blocks the *N*-methyl-D-aspartate receptors and protects cells against excess glutamate.

Nociceptors: Receptors for pain caused by injury from physical stimuli (mechanical, electrical, or thermal) or chemical stimuli (toxins); located in the skin, muscles, or in the walls of the viscera.

Nocturia: Excessive urination at night.

Nodules: When seen with rheumatoid arthritis, nodules are subcutaneous knobs over bony prominences or extensor surfaces.

Nonbacterial thrombotic endocarditis: Endocarditis caused by noninfectious vegetations.

Nonmyeloablative preparative regimen: Radiation and/or chemotherapy that does not completely eradicate host bone marrow activity; host bone marrow activity is suppressed but may recover after approximately 4 weeks, even in the absence of "rescue" allogeneic stem cells.

Nonnucleoside reverse transcriptase inhibitor (NNRTI): A noncompetitive inhibitor of the viral reverse transcriptase enzyme by binding to the active site of the enzyme itself, rather than by terminating the enzymatic product. NNRTIs are only active against HIV-1.

Nonpolyposis: Absence of polyps.

Nonprotein kilocalorie-to-nitrogen ratio: Numerical value derived from dividing kilocalories from carbohydrate plus fat by the number of grams of nitrogen in the diet.

Non–ST-segment elevation: A type of myocardial infarction (MI) that is limited to the subendocardial myocardium and is smaller and less extensive than an ST-segment MI, and usually there is no pathologic Q wave on the electrocardiogram.

Normochromic: Being normal in color; referring especially to red blood cells.

Normocytic: Normal size especially referring to red blood cells.

Nuchal rigidity: Neck stiffness.

Nuclear factor kappa B (Nf-kappa-B): Regulates cytokine production.

Nucleoside reverse transcriptase inhibitor (NRTI)/nucleotide reverse transcriptase inhibitor (NtRI): A modified version of a naturally occurring nucleoside or nucleotide that prevents HIV replication by interfering with the function of the viral reverse transcriptase enzyme. The nucleoside/nucleotide analog causes early termination of the proviral DNA chain. For activity, an NRTI requires three phosphorylation steps once inside the cell, whereas a NtRI has a phosphate group attached and needs only two phosphorylation steps inside the cell for activity.

Nulliparity: Condition of not having given birth to a child.

Nystagmus: Rapid involuntary eye movement.

Obliterative bronchiolitis: Inflammation of the bronchioles (the small elements of the tracheobronchial tree) characterized by obliteration and/or permanent narrowing of the airways.

Off-label use: Use of a medication outside the scope of its approved, labeled use.

Oiling out: Continued coalescence of lipid emulsion particles, resulting in irreversible separation of the emulsion (also called "breaking" or "cracking" of the emulsion).

Oligoanovulation: The condition of having few to no ovulatory menstrual cycles.

Oligoclonal bands: Small discrete bands in the γ-globulin region of fluid electrophoresis.

Oligohydramnios: Decreased amniotic fluid.

Oligomenorrhea: Abnormally light or infrequent menstruation.

Oliguria: Reduced urine output; usually defined as less than 400 mL in 24 hours or less than 0.5 mL/kg/h.

Omentumectomy: Excision of the double fold of peritoneum attached to the stomach and connecting it with abdominal viscera (omentum).

Oncogene: Genes that cause transformation of normal cells into cancer cells by promoting uncontrolled cell growth and multiplication leading to tumor formation.

Open comedo: A plugged follicle of sebum, keratinocytes, and bacteria that protrudes from the surface of the skin and appears black or brown in color. Also referred to as a "blackhead."

Opsonization: The process by which an antigen is altered so as to become more readily and more efficiently engulfed by phagocytes.

Optic neuritis: Usually monocular central visual acuity loss and ocular/periorbital pain caused by demyelination of the optic nerve.

Oral rehydration solution: A liquid preparation, commercially prepared or made at home using common ingredients according to a formula developed by the World Health Organization, designed to replace fluid loss in persons with diarrhea.

Orchiectomy: The surgical removal of the testicles.

Orthopnea: Difficulty in breathing that occurs when lying down and is relieved upon changing to an upright position.

Orthostasis: Characterized by a drop in blood pressure when standing up from sitting or lying down, often causing lightheadedness and dizziness.

Orthotopic: Placing a transplanted organ into the normal anatomic location.

Osmolality: A measure of the number of osmotically active particles per unit solution, independent of the weight or nature of the particle.

Osmolar gap: The difference between the measured serum osmolality and the calculated serum osmolality.

Osteoblasts: Cells involved in bone formation; "builders of bone."

Osteoclasts: Cells involved in bone resorption; "creators of cavities."

Osteomalacia: Softening of the bones.

Osteonecrosis: Death of bone tissue.

Osteopenia: Reduced bone density or mass, which can lead to osteoporosis.

Osteophytes: Bony outgrowths (also called bone spurs) into the joint space.

Osteoporosis: Disease of the bones characterized by a loss of bone tissue, resulting in brittle, weak bones that are susceptible to fracture (porous bones).

Ostomy: Surgical operation where part of the abdominal wall is opened and part of the intestine is connected to the opening for intestinal draining (e.g., colostomy, ileostomy).

Otitis media with effusion: Fluid in the middle ear space with no signs or symptoms of an acute infection.

Ovulation: Periodic ripening and rupture of mature follicle and the discharge of ovum from the cortex of the ovary.

Pacemaker: A mass of fibers that possess actual or potential automaticity which initiates and determines the rate of spontaneous depolarizations.

Palliative care: The active, total care of patients whose disease is not responsive to curative treatment.

Palliative chemotherapy: Treatment given to control the symptoms of an incurable cancer.

Pancolitis: Inflammation that involves the majority of the colon in patients with inflammatory bowel disease.

Pancreatic pseudocysts: A cyst-like space not lined by epithelium and contained within the pancreas.

Pancreatitis: Inflammation of the pancreas.

Panhypopituitarism: A state in which the secretion of all anterior pituitary hormones is inadequate or absent.

Pannus: Inflamed synovial tissue that invades and destroys articular structures.

Paracentesis: Removal of (ascitic) fluid from the peritoneal space.

Paracentral scotoma: Blind spots near the center of the visual field.

Parenchyma: Specific cells or tissue of an organ.

Parenteral nutrition: Delivery of nutrients via the intravenous route.

Paroxysmal: Intermittent occurrence, initiating suddenly and spontaneously, lasting minutes to hours, and terminating suddenly and spontaneously.

Partial response: In cancer, at least a 30% decrease in the sum of the longest diameter of target lesions from baseline.

Patient survival: After the transplant procedure, the survival of the transplant recipient, without regard to the function or survival of the allograft.

Peak expiratory flow: The maximum flow rate of air leaving the lungs upon forced exhalation.

Pelvic inflammatory disease: Inflammation of the endometrium, uterine tubes, and pelvic peritoneum; often due to a sexually transmitted infection.

Percutaneous coronary intervention: A minimally invasive procedure whereby access to the coronary arteries is obtained through the femoral artery up the aorta to the coronary os. Contrast media is used to visualize the coronary artery stenosis using a coronary angiogram. A guidewire is used to cross the stenosis and a small balloon is inflated and/or stent is deployed to break up atherosclerotic plaque and restore coronary artery blood flow. The stent is left in place to prevent acute closure and restenosis of the coronary artery. Newer stents are coated with antiproliferative drugs, such as paclitaxel and sirolimus, which further reduce the risk of restenosis of the coronary artery.

Percutaneous endoscopic gastrostomy: Gastric feeding tube placed via endoscopic technique.

Percutaneous endoscopic jejunostomy: Jejunal feeding tube placed via endoscopic technique.

Performance status: An attempt to quantify the ability of a cancer patient to perform daily activities. This is used to determine if and how much chemotherapy they can receive. Patients with good performance status can tolerate more aggressive chemotherapy.

Perihilar: The area surrounding the depression in the medial surface of a lung that forms the opening through which the bronchus, blood vessels, and nerves pass.

Perimenopause: Also known as the climacteric, it is the period of time prior to menopause when hormonal and biologic changes and physical symptoms begin to occur and usually last for 1 year after the last menstrual period. The perimenopausal period may last for an average of 3 to 5 years.

Perimetry: Measurement of the field of vision.

Peripheral artery disease: Atherosclerosis of the peripheral arteries.

Peripheral resistance: The sum of resistance to blood flow offered by systemic blood vessels.

Peritonitis: An acute inflammatory reaction of the peritoneal lining to microorganisms or chemical irritation.

Petechiae: Tiny localized hemorrhages from the small blood vessels just beneath the surface of the skin.

PET scan: A scan that produces images of the body after the injection of a radioactive form of glucose. The scan is often used to detect cancer since tumors use more sugar than normal cells. PET scans may also be used to see how well the tumor is responding to treatment.

Phagocytic cell: A cell that absorbs waste material, harmful microorganisms, or other foreign bodies in the bloodstream and tissues.

Phagocytosis: The process of engulfing and ingesting an antigen by phagocytes.

Pharmacogenomic: The influence of genetic variation on drug response in patients and is used to correlate gene expression with a drug's efficacy or toxicity.

Pharyngitis: Inflammation and/or infection of the pharynx that causes throat pain.

Pheochromocytoma: A tumor arising from chromaffin cells, most commonly found in the adrenal medulla. The tumor causes the adrenal medulla to hypersecrete epinephrine and norepinephrine resulting in hypertension and other signs and symptoms of excessive sympathetic nervous system activity. The tumor is usually benign but may occasionally be cancerous.

Phenotype: The visible properties of an organism that are produced by the interaction of the genotype and the environment.

Phlebitis: Inflammation of a blood vessel (e.g., vein).

Photochemotherapy: The use of phototherapy together with topical or systemic drugs in the treatment of psoriasis.

Photodynamic therapy: Cancer treatment that uses interaction between laser light and a substance that makes the cells more sensitive to light. When light is applied to cells that have been treated with this substance, a chemical reaction occurs and destroys cancer cells.

Photophobia: Intolerance to bright light.

Phototherapy: The use of ultraviolet light applied to the skin, for example in treating psoriasis or neonatal hyperbilirubinemia.

Pilosebaceous unit: A hair follicle and the surrounding sebaceous glands.

Plaques: Extracellular protein deposits of fibrils and amorphous aggregates of b-amyloid protein.

Plasma cell: Antibody producing cells.

Plasmapheresis: A process of separating cells out from the plasma. This process is used to remove the monoclonal antibodies from the blood.

Pleocytosis: A transient increase in the number of leukocytes in a body fluid.

Pleuritis: Inflammation of the lining around the lungs.

Pneumatic otoscopy: A diagnostic technique involving visualization of the tympanic membrane for transparency, position, and color, and its response to positive and negative air pressure to assess mobility.

Pneumothorax: The presence of air in the pleural cavity, often causing part of the lung to collapse.

Podocyte: The epithelial cells that surround the capillaries in the Bowman's capsule and are responsible for filtering blood in the glomerulus of the nephron.

Polycythemia: An abnormal increase in the number of erythrocytes in the blood.

Polypharmacy: Taking multiple medications concurrently.

Polyps: A growth from a mucous membrane commonly found in organs such as the colon, rectum, and the nose. Usually not malignant, these can develop into cancer and require removal once found.

Polyuria: Excessive excretion of urine resulting in profuse micturition.

Portal hypertension: Increased pressure in vessel leading to liver; usually a result of cirrhosis.

Postpyloric feeding: Delivery of nutrients via a tube placed with its tip past the pyloric sphincter separating the stomach from the duodenum.

Prader-Willi syndrome: A genetic disorder characterized by short stature, mental retardation, low muscle tone, abnormally small hands and feet, hypogonadism, and excessive eating leading to extreme obesity.

Predictive factors: Any measurements associated with response to therapy (e.g., over-expression of HER2 increases the likelihood of response to agents targeting the receptor; the same is true for ER).

Preload: The stretched condition of the heart muscle at the end of diastole just before contraction; volume in the left ventricle at the end of diastole estimated by the pulmonary artery occlusion pressure (also known as the pulmonary artery wedge pressure or pulmonary capillary wedge pressure).

Preparative regimen (conditioning regimen): Radiation and/or chemotherapy given to stem cell transplant patients in order to kill malignant cells, create space in the bone marrow compartment, and suppress the immune system of the host in order to prevent graft rejection.

Priapism: A prolonged, painful erection lasting more than 4 hours. Considered a medical emergency.

Primary amenorrhea: Absence of menses by age 15 in the presence of normal secondary sexual development or absence of menses within 5 years of breast development (if occurring prior to age 10).

Primary prevention: The removal or reduction of risk factors before the development of disease.

Prinzmetal's angina: Vasospasm or contraction of the coronary arteries in the absence of significant atherosclerosis. Also referred to as variant angina.

Probiotics: Dietary supplements containing potentially beneficial bacteria that promote health by stimulating optimal mucosal immune responses.

Proctitis: Inflammation confined to the rectum in patients with inflammatory bowel disease.

Progenitor: A primitive cell.

Prognostic factors: Biologic or clinical indicators associated with survival independent of therapy (e.g., over-expression of HER2 is associated with increased risk of relapse and shorter survival).

Progression: In cancer, cell proliferation takes over and the tumor spreads or develops metastases.

Progression-free survival: Length of time that a disease remains stable following treatment.

Progressive primary disease: Tuberculosis infection in which the immune response fails to control multiplication of the tubercle bacilli. The primary focus in the lung enlarges rapidly and spreads.  This occurs in less than 10% of normal adults, but it is more common in children younger than 5 years, and in patients with suppressed immunity.

Prolapse: Protrusion of an organ or part of an organ through an opening, e.g., uterine prolapse occurs when the uterus is displaced downward such that the cervix is within the vaginal opening (first degree), the cervix is outside the opening (second degree), or the entire uterus is outside the opening (third degree).

Promotion: Reversible process in cancer, the environment is altered by carcinogens or other factors to favor the growth of the mutated cell over the normal cell.

Prostaglandin: Any of a large group of biologically active, carbon-20, unsaturated fatty acids that are produced by the metabolism of arachidonic acid through the cyclooxygenase pathway.

Prostatectomy: Surgical removal of the prostate.

Prostatic hyperplasia: Enlargement of the prostate.

Prosthetic-valve endocarditis: Endocarditis that occurs in patients with bioprosthetic or synthetic implanted heart valves.

Protease inhibitor: A drug that acts by inhibiting the viral protease enzyme, which prevents long strands of protein from being cleaved into the smaller proteins that the virus requires for assembly.

Protectant: An agent that forms an occlusive barrier between the skin and surrounding moisture.

Protected specimen brush: Used in bronchoscopy, a brush in the lumen of a tube inside the bronchoscope. The brush is extended into the lung to obtain a sample, then retracted back into the tube for removal from the lung.

Proteinase: Any of numerous enzymes that catalyze the breakdown of proteins (also called protease).

Proteinuria: The presence of measurable amounts of protein (greater than 150 mg/day) in the urine, which is often indicative of glomerular or tubular damage in the kidney.

Proteoglycans: Glycosaminoglycans (mucopolysaccharides) bound to protein chains in covalent complexes. Proteoglycans are present in the extracellular matrix of connective tissue.

Proteasome: An enzyme complex that degrades intracellular proteins.

Proteolysis: The degradation of proteins in damaged tissue.

Prothrombin: A clotting factor that is converted to thrombin; also known as Factor II.

Prothrombin time: A measure of coagulation representing the amount of time required to form a blood clot after the addition of thromboplastin to the blood sample; also known as Quick's test.

Prothrombotic state: A state of high coagulation of the blood.

Protooncogenes: Normal genes that are present in all normal cells and regulate cell function and replication, and through some genetic alteration caused by carcinogens, change into oncogenes.

Pseudohyphae: Elongated forms created by replicating yeast that form buds but do not detach from one another.

Pseudophakic: Presence of an artificial lens placed after cataract extraction.

Pseudopolyps: An area of hypertrophied gastrointestinal mucosa that resembles a polyp and contains nonmalignant cells.

Pulmonary artery catheter: An invasive device used to measure hemodynamic parameters directly, including cardiac output and pulmonary artery occlusion pressure; calculated parameters include stroke volume and systemic vascular resistance.

Pulmonary artery occlusion pressure: A hemodynamic measurement obtained via a catheter placed into the pulmonary artery used to evaluate patient volume status within the left ventricle.

Pulmonary embolism: A disorder of thrombus formation causing obstruction of a pulmonary artery or one of its branches and resulting in pulmonary infarction.

Pulsus paradoxus: A large fall in systolic blood pressure and pulse volume during inspiration or an abnormal variation in pulse volume during respiration in which the pulse becomes weaker with inspiration and stronger with expiration.

Purkinje fiber: Specialized myocardial fibers that conduct impulses from the atrioventricular node to the ventricles.

Purified protein derivative: A mixture of antigens obtained from the culture of M. tuberculosis that can be injected intracutaneously to stimulate the immune system to produce a measurable response.

Purpura: A small hemorrhage of the skin, mucous membrane, or serosal surface.

Purulent: Containing, consisting of, or being pus.

Pyelonephritis: Inflammation of a kidney.

Pyuria: Presence of pus in urine when voided.

Quality indicators: A list of indicator used by long-term care facility administrators and government overseers to identify potential problems in patient care.

Quality of life: Perceived physical and mental health over time.

Radiofrequency catheter ablation: Procedure during which radiofrequency energy is delivered through a catheter positioned at the atrioventricular node for the purpose of destroying one pathway of a reentrant circuit.

Receptor editing: The process by which cells proofread, alter, and re-express modified receptors to become nonautoreactive.

Recombinant activated factor VII: A clotting factor manufactured via recombinant technology used off-label (non–Food and Drug Administration approved) to foster clotting in hemorrhagic shock patients with massive hemorrhage refractory to conventional therapies such as fresh frozen plasma.

Rectal prolapse: Sinking of the rectum through the anal sphincter so that it is visible externally.

Reentry: Circular movement of electrical impulses, a mechanism of many arrhythmias.

Refractory period: The period of time after an impulse is initiated and conducted during which cells cannot be depolarized again.

Regurgitation: A passive process without involvement of the abdominal wall and the diaphragm wherein gastric or esophageal contents move into the mouth.

Remission: An inability to detect the presence of disease.

Renal osteodystrophy (ROD): Altered bone turnover that results from sustained metabolic conditions that occur in chronic kidney disease, including secondary hyperparathyroidism, hyperphosphatemia, hypocalcemia, and vitamin D deficiency. The disease can be characterized by high bone turnover, low bone turnover, or adynamic disease, or may be a mixed disorder.

Renin-angiotensin-aldosterone system: The hormonal system controlled mainly by the kidneys and adrenal glands that regulates blood pressure, blood volume, and electrolyte balance.

Replication capacity: This term is often used interchangeably with the term "viral fitness" and refers to how quickly HIV reproduces or replicates. The slower HIV replicates, the less likely a patient is to have disease progression. A replication capacity may be reported on a resistance test. It is reported as a percentage of the median replication rate for drug-sensitive (wild-type) HIV strains.

Resorption: The process of bone breakdown by osteoclasts.

Respiratory acidosis: Acidosis that is caused by an accumulation of carbon dioxide.

Respiratory alkalosis: Alkalosis that is caused by a loss of carbon dioxide.

Restenosis: Renarrowing of the coronary artery after a percutaneous intervention to improve coronary blood flow.

Retching: A process that follows nausea and consists of diaphragm, abdominal wall, and chest wall contractions and spasmodic breathing against a closed glottis.

Reticulocytes: Immature blood cells that mature into erythrocytes.

Reticuloendothelial system: Phagocytic cells excluding granulocytes; widely distributed throughout the body.

Retrograde ejaculation: Flow of ejaculate into the bladder instead of antegrade out of the urethra.

Rhabdomyolysis: Destruction of skeletal muscle.

Rheumatic fever: An acute inflammatory disease involving the joints, heart, skin, brain, and other tissues caused by an immune response to streptococcal infection in genetically susceptible people, particularly in children.

Rheumatoid factors: Antibodies reactive with the Fc region of IgG.

Rhinosinusitis: Inflammation of the mucous membranes in the nose and sinuses.

Rhonchi: Abnormal, rumbling sounds heard on auscultation of an obstructed airway. They are more prominent during expiration and may clear somewhat on coughing.

Rouleaux formation: The stacking of red blood cells on a peripheral smear when diluted.

Rubefacients: A substance that produces redness of the skin.

Salicylism: A toxic syndrome caused by excessive doses of acetylsalicylic acid (aspirin), salicylic acid, or any other salicylate product. Signs and symptoms may include severe headache, nausea, vomiting, tinnitus (ringing in the ears), confusion, increased pulse, and increased respiratory rate.

Scarlatiniform rash: Bright, scarlet-colored skin eruption that occurs in patches over the entire body with eventual peeling as a result of streptococcal infection.

Scleritis: Inflammation of the outer layer of the eyeball.

Scoliosis: A congenital lateral curvature of the spine.

Secondary amenorrhea: Absence of menses for 3 cycles or 6 months in a previously menstruating woman.

Secondary hyperparathyroidism: Increased secretion of parathyroid hormone from the parathyroid glands caused by hyperphosphatemia, hypocalcemia, and vitamin D deficiency that results from decreased kidney function. Secondary hyperparathyroidism can lead to bone disease (renal osteodystrophy).

Secondary transmission: Transferring a disease from the primary source to another person.

Seizure: A sudden electrical disturbance in the brain that results from a population of neurons rapidly and repetitively firing in a rhythmic and synchronous pattern for seconds to minutes.

Semiology: The clinical symptoms and presentation of a seizure.

Sentinel lymph node: Refers to the first (axillary) node that picks up dye injected into the tumor.

Sera: Pertaining to human serum.

Seropositive: Showing a positive reaction to a test on blood serum for a disease.

Serum sickness: A group of symptoms caused by a delayed immune response to certain medications. Arthralgias, fever, malaise, and urticaria may develop usually 7 to 14 days after exposure to the causative antigen.

Shear stress: Risk factor for pressure ulcers that is generated when the head of a patient's bed is elevated and can cause deeper blood vessels to crimp, leading to ischemia.

Sick sinus syndrome: Idiopathic sinus node dysfunction leading to symptomatic sinus bradycardia.

Sigmoidoscopy: A visual inspection of the sigmoid colon and rectum with a flexible tube called a sigmoidoscope.

Simple disorder: The presence of a single acid-base disorder, with or without compensation.

Sjögren's syndrome: A chronic autoimmune disease characterized by dry eyes and dry mouth.

Sleep apnea: The temporary stopping of breathing during sleep; can be caused by narrowing of the airways resulting from swelling of soft tissue.

Slit-lamp biomicroscope: An instrument that allows for the microscopic examination of the cornea, anterior chamber lens, and posterior chamber.

Somatic hypermutation: The occurrence of multiple point mutations.

Somatotrope: Growth hormone producing cells in the anterior pituitary

Spastic colon: A synonym for irritable bowel syndrome.

Spasticity: A motor disorder characterized by an increase in muscle tone with exaggerated tendon jerks, resulting from hyperexcitability of the stretch reflex.

Spectrum of activity: A qualitative term that describes the number of different bacterial species that are susceptible to an antimicrobial regimen. Generally, broad-spectrum activity refers to regimens that possess activity against many bacterial species, whereas narrow-spectrum therapy refers to activity against a few bacterial species.

Sphincter of Oddi: Structure through which the common bile duct empties bile and pancreatic secretions into the duodenum.

Spirometry: Measurement by means of a spirometer of the air entering and leaving the lungs.

Splenomegaly: An enlarged spleen secondary to leukemic infiltration.

Sprain: An overstretching of supporting ligaments that results in a partial or complete tear of the ligament.

Sputum culture: A sputum sample obtained from the lower respiratory tract is placed into a container that contains substances to promote, in this case, mycobacterial growth. Positive results indicate live mycobacteria, which can be tested for susceptibility to drugs.

Sputum smear: A sputum sample obtained from the lower respiratory tract, spread on a glass slide, and stained for examination under a microscope. Used to identify the presence of microorganisms.

Stable disease: In cancer, neither sufficient shrinkage to qualify for partial response nor sufficient increase to qualify for progressive disease.

Staging: Analysis that provides a semiquantitative estimate of tumor burden, which is not only of prognostic importance, but also has important implications regarding appropriate treatment options.

Steatohepatitis: A severe form of liver disease caused by fat deposition in the liver, characterized by hepatic inflammation that may rapidly progress to liver fibrosis and cirrhosis.

Steatorrhea: Excessive loss of fat in stool.

Steatosis: Excessive fat accumulation. Fat deposition in liver.

Stenosis: Blockage of an artery.

Stenting: Placement of a stent to allow blood flow through an artery.

Stereotactic radiosurgery: Radiation technique that uses a large number of narrow, precisely aimed, highly focused beams of ionizing radiation. The beams are aimed from many directions circling the head and meet at a specific point.

Stevens-Johnson syndrome: A severe expression of erythema multiforme (also known as erythema multiforme major). It typically involves the skin and the mucous membranes with the potential for severe morbidity and even death.

Stomatitis: Inflammation of mucous membranes in the mouth.

Strain: Damage to the muscle fibers or tendon without tearing of the ligament.

Striae: Linear, atrophic, pinkish or purplish, scarlike lesions that later become white (striae albicantes, lineae albicantes), which may occur on the abdomen, breasts, buttocks, and thighs. They are due to weakening of the elastic tissues; commonly called stretch marks.

Stricture: An area of narrowing or constriction in the gastrointestinal tract due to buildup of fibrotic tissue; often a result of long-standing inflammation.

Stroke volume: The amount of blood ejected from the heart during systole.

ST-segment elevation: A type of myocardial infarction that typically results in an injury that transects the thickness of the myocardial wall. Following an ST-elevation myocardial infarction, pathologic Q waves are frequently seen on the electrocardiogram, indicating transmural myocardial infarction.

Subchondral: Situated beneath and supporting cartilage.

Subtrochanteric: Below the trochanter (the bony protrusion at the end of the femur where the hip and thigh muscles attach).

Surgical site infection: Infections occurring at or near the surgical incision within 30 days of the operation; up to 1 year if a prosthesis is implanted.

Suspending agent: An additive used in the compounding of oral liquid medications to suspend drug particles throughout a liquid and enables resuspension of particles by agitation (e.g., shaking well).

Synechia: Adhesions or the abnormal attachment of the iris to another structure. Peripheral anterior synechia refers to occurrence of synechia with the trabecular meshwork.

Synovitis: Inflammation of the synovial membrane, often in combination with pain and swelling of the affected joint.

Synovium: The membrane lining the internal surfaces of the joint.

Systolic dysfunction: An abnormal contraction of the ventricles during systole.

Tachycardia: Abnormally fast heart rate.

Tachyphylaxis: Rapid decreasing response to a drug or other physiologically active agent after a few doses.

Tachypnea: Abnormally fast respiratory rate.

Tangles: Twisted fibers of a protein, tau, that build up inside cells.

Telangiectasia: Permanent dilation of preexisting small blood vessels (capillaries, arterioles, venules), usually in the skin or mucous membranes which presents as a coarse or fine red line.

Tendonitis: Inflammation of the tendon.

Tenesmus: Difficulty with bowel evacuation despite the urgency to defecate.

Tenosynovitis: Inflammation of the tendon sheath.

Teratogenic potential: The ability of an agent to cause harm or malformations to a fetus or embryo. Medications are assigned pregnancy categories based on their teratogenic potential.

Terminal secretions: The noise produced by the oscillatory movements of secretions in the upper airways in association with the inspiratory and expiratory phases of respiration. It is also known as "death rattle."

Thelarche: The onset of breast development in women.

Third spacing: Fluid accumulation in the interstitial space disproportionate to the intracellular and extracellular fluid spaces.

Thoracentesis: Removal of fluid that is present in the pleural space. Common procedure to determine what caused the fluid accumulation.

Thrombin: An enzyme formed from prothrombin which converts fibrinogen to fibrin. It is the principal driving force in the clotting cascade.

Thrombocytopenia: A condition where the number of circulating platelets are abnormally low due to decreased production of new cells, possibly secondary to medication toxicities.

Thrombocytosis: Increased number of platelets in the blood.

Thrombogenesis: The process of forming a blood clot.

Thrombolysis: The process of enzymatically dissolving or breaking apart a blood clot.

Thrombolytic: An enzyme that dissolves or breaks apart blood clots.

Thrombophlebitis: Inflammation of a blood vessel (e.g., vein) associated with the stimulations of clotting and formation of a thrombus (or blood clot).

Thromboplastin: A substance that triggers the coagulation cascade. Tissue factor is a naturally occurring thromboplastin and is used in the prothrombin time test.

Thrombosis: A condition in which blood changes from a liquid to a solid state and produces a blood clot.

Thrombotic thrombocytopenic purpura: Condition characterized by formation of small clots within the circulation resulting in the consumption of platelets and a low platelet count.

Thrombus: Blood clot attached to the vessel wall and consisting of platelets, fibrin, and clotting factors. A thrombus may partially or completely occlude the lumen of a blood vessel compromising blood flow and oxygen delivery to distal tissue.

Thyroiditis: Inflammation of the thyroid gland.

Tocolytic: Medication used to suppress premature labor.

Tonometry: A method by which the cornea is indented or flattened by an instrument. The pressure required to achieve corneal indentation or flattening is a measure of intraocular pressure.

Topoisomerase: Enzymes that temporarily alter supercoiled DNA by cutting the DNA, causing the DNA to relax the supercoil during DNA replication. Topoisomerase inhibitors prevent the DNA from sealing the cut which causes DNA strand breakage.

Torsade de pointes: Very rapid ventricular tachycardia characterized by a gradually changing QRS complex in the ECG; may change into ventricular fibrillation.

Toxic epidermal necrolysis: A life-threatening skin disorder characterized by blistering and peeling of the top layer of skin.

Toxoid: A modified bacterial exotoxin that has lost toxicity.

Tracheal aspirate: Suctioning of secretions from the trachea.

Transesophageal echocardiogram: Procedure used to generate an image of the heart via sound waves, via a probe introduced into the esophagus (rather than the traditional transthoracic view) in order to obtain a better image of the left atrium.

Transformation (conversion): Mutated cell becomes malignant.

Transient ischemic attack: Focal neurologic deficit lasting less than 24 hours where symptoms resolve completely.

Translocation: Movement of bacteria and endotoxin from the intestinal lumen through the gut mucosa and into the lymphatic and systemic circulation.

Transmural: Across the wall of an organ or structure; in the case of Crohn's disease, inflammation may extend through all four layers of the intestinal wall.

Tubal ligation: Surgical process of tying up the fallopian tubes to prevent passage of ova from the ovaries to the uterus.

Tumor suppressor genes: Genes that normally restrain cell growth but, when missing or inactivated by mutation, allow cells to grow uncontrolled and tumors to form.

Tuberoeruptive xanthomas: Small yellow-red raised papules usually presenting on the elbows, knees, back, and buttocks.

Tubulointerstitial: Involving the tubules or interstitial tissue of the kidneys.

Tumor lysis syndrome: A syndrome resulting from cytotoxic therapy, occurring generally in aggressive, rapidly proliferating lymphoproliferative disorders. It is characterized by combinations of hyperuricemia, lactic acidosis, hyperkalemia, hyperphosphatemia, and hypocalcemia.

T2-weighted magnetic resonance imaging: A setting of the magnetic resonance imaging machine that shows water as a bright signal.

Tympanocentesis: Puncture of the tympanic membrane with a needle to aspirate middle ear fluid.

Tympanostomy tube: Small plastic or metal tube inserted in the eardrum to keep the middle ear aerated and improve hearing in patients with chronic middle ear effusion.

Uhthoff's phenomenon: Acute worsening of multiple sclerosis symptoms on exposure to heat because high body temperatures may exceed the capacitance of the demyelinated nerve and conduction may fail.

Ultrafiltration: The movement of plasma water across a semipermeable membrane.

Uncomplicated disorder: See Simple disorder.

Uremia: A condition that results from accumulation of metabolic waste products and endogenous toxins in the body resulting from impaired kidney function. Symptoms of uremia include nausea, vomiting, weakness, loss of appetite, and mental confusion.

Urethral stricture: Narrowing of the urethral lumen by scar tissue. This could result from trauma, inflammation, infection, or instrumentation.

Uricosuric: Pertaining to, characterized by, or promoting renal excretion of uric acid.

Urosepsis: Sepsis resulting from a urinary source.

Urticaria: Itchy, raised, swollen areas on the skin. Also known as hives.

Uveitis: An inflammation of the uvea. Uveal structures include the iris, the ciliary body, and the choroids.

Vagal maneuvers: Stimulate the activity of the parasympathetic nervous system, which inhibits atrioventricular nodal conduction. Examples of vagal maneuvers include cough, carotid sinus massage, and Valsalva.

Vagotomy: A surgical procedure that blocks vagal (cholinergic) stimulation to the stomach.

Valsalva maneuver: Vagal maneuver; patient bears down against a closed glottis, as if they were having a bowel movement.

Variceal bleeding: Varices are weak collateral blood vessels that are friable and rupture easily; often observed in the esophagus or stomach.

Vasculitis: Inflammation of the walls of blood vessels.

Vasomotor symptoms: Menopausal symptoms that include both hot flashes and night sweats.

Vasopressors: Medications that cause constriction of blood vessels, increase in vascular resistance, and increase in blood pressure.

Vasospasm: Narrowing (constriction) of a blood vessel causing a reduction in blood flow.

Ventilation/perfusion ratio ($V_A$/Q): A comparison of the proportion of lung tissue being ventilated by inhaled air to the rate of oxygenation of pulmonary blood.

Ventricular depolarization: Change in the membrane potential of a ventricular myocyte, resulting in loss of polarization. Under normal conditions, depolarization of ventricular myocytes is followed by ventricular contraction.

Vertigo: Sensation of spinning or feeling out of balance.

Vesicants: A chemical or agent that causes significant tissue damage if extravasation occurs during IV administration.

Virilization: Production or acquisition of virilism, which is masculine characteristics.

Volvulus: Twisting of the intestine causing obstruction and possible necrosis.

Vomiting: A reflexive rapid and forceful oral expulsion of upper gastrointestinal contents due to powerful and sustained contractions in the abdominal and thoracic musculature.

Waist circumference: A practical tool to measure the abdominal fat in patients with a BMI of less than 35.

Western blot analysis: The "gold standard" for HIV diagnostic testing. Disrupted virus is purified, gel-electrophoresed to separate by molecular weight to form bands corresponding to the nine HIV antigens, and blotted onto a membrane support. HIV serum antibodies from the patient are allowed to bind to proteins in the membrane support. If HIV antibodies from the patient are bound, the bands will change color. The test is considered reactive if 2 of the 3 major bands (p24, gp41, and/or gp120/160) change color. The test is nonreactive if no viral bands are visible.

White coat hypertension: A persistently elevated average office blood pressure of greater than 140/90 mm Hg and an average awake ambulatory reading of less than 135/85 mm Hg.

Wilson's disease: A disorder of copper metabolism, characterized by cirrhosis of the liver and neurologic manifestations.

Xanthoma: Firm raised nodules composed of lipid-containing histocytes.

Xerostomia: Dry mouth resulting from decreased salivary secretion.

ZAP-70 expression: An intracellular tyrosine kinase found in CLL B-cells.

Zymogen: An inactive protein precursor of an enzyme that is converted into an active form.

Six pharmacotherapy careplans based on cases in the book have been provided so the student will have a better understanding of the structure and content of typical careplans. Note that some information has been left out of these examples so you will not have all the 'answers' for your own workup of these cases. As discussed in Chapter 1, the careplan forms are meant to be a guide in structuring your thoughts and information, and there is no single correct way to do it. As you gain more experience, developing the elements of the care plan will become more intuitive. Remember, your most important job is to provide the best possible drug therapy for the patient.

# 28 Euvolemic Hyponatremia: Example Careplan with Missing Data

Mark A. Malesker          Lee E. Morrow          Vijay Gogineni

## PATIENT DATABASE FORM

| | | |
|---|---|---|
| **Patient Name:** Albert Buterol | **Patient ID:** 09921234 | **Location:** ICU |
| **Physician:** Dr. Pepper | **Pharmacy:** | |
| **Age (or Date of Birth):** 89 yo | **Race:** Caucasian | **Sex:** Male |
| **Height:** 71 in. (180 cm) | **Weight:** 155.5 lb (70.7 kg) | |
| **Date of Admission/Initial Visit:** 6/15/2012 | **Occupation:** Retired Factory Worker | |

### Allergies/Intolerances/ADRs

❑ No known drug allergies/ADRs

❑ Not known/inadequate information

| Drug: | Reaction: |
|---|---|
| Antihistamines | Unknown |
| Sulfa | Unknown |
| Tramadol | Unknown |
| Amitriptyline | Unknown |
| | |
| | |
| | |
| | |
| | |
| | |

### HPI, PMH, FH, SH, etc...

MI, post-PCI

Pacemaker for bradycardia

HTN

Enlarged prostate with frequent UTIs

Quit smoking 10 yr ago

Denies alcohol and illicit drug use

**Medications prior to admission:**

HCTZ 50 mg PO daily

Celecoxib 200 mg PO daily

Finasteride 5 mg PO daily

Pantoprazole 40 mg PO daily

Cotrimoxazole PO twice daily

Lorazepam 1 mg PO q 8 h PRN anxiety

Latanoprost eyedrops both eyes at bedtime

| Prioritized Medical Problem List | Medication Profile |
|---|---|
| Intracranial pressure | Nicardipine IV infusion to keep systolic BP <160 mm Hg |
| | Codeine 15–30 mg IV q 8 h as needed for cough |
| Euvolemic hyponatremia | 3% NaCl initiate at 15 mL/h |
| _____ | Piperacillin–tazobactam 3.375 g IV q 6 h |
| | Levofloxacin 500 mg IV q 24 h |
| | Vancomycin 1 g IV q 24 h |
| HTN | Nicardipine IV drip to keep BP <160 mm Hg |
| History of GERD/stress ulcer prophylaxis | Pantoprazole 40 mg IV daily |
| Nausea/vomiting | Metoclopramide 10 mg IV q 6 h as needed |
| Verification of medication allergies, intolerances | |

The form is from *ASHP National Clinical Skills Competition Case Documents*, Copyright 2009, American Society of Health-System Pharmacists, Bethesda, MD (www.ashp.org). Adapted with permission.

| Vital Signs, Laboratory Data, and Diagnostic Test Results | | | |
| --- | --- | --- | --- |
| Date | 6/16/2012 at 0600 | 6/16/2012 at 2000 | 6/17/2012 at 0745 |
| **Weight (lb/kg)** | 155.5 (70.7) | | |
| **Temperature (°C)** | 37.4 | 36.5 | |
| **Blood pressure (mm Hg)** | 148/83 | 147/60 | |
| **Pulse** | 120 | 71 | |
| **Respiratory rate** | 19 | 20 | |
| **Na** 135–145 mEq/L (135–145 mmol/L) | 119 | 125 | 129 |
| **K** 3.3–4.9 mEq/L (3.3–4.9 mmol/L) | 3.7 | 3.6 | 4.1 |
| **Cl** 97–110 mEq/L (97–110 mmol/L) | 84 | 84 | 87 |
| **$CO_2/HCO_3$** 22–26 mEq/L (22–26 mmol/L) | 27 | 27 | 23 |
| **BUN** 8–25 mg/dL (2.9–8.9 mmol/L) | 16 (5.7) | 26 (9.3) | 20 (7.1) |
| **Creatinine (adult)** Male 0.7–1.3 mg/dL; female 0.6–1.1 mg/dL (male 62–115 μmol/L; female 53–97 μmol/L) | 1.0 (88) | 1.0 (88) | 1.3 (115) |
| **Creatinine clearance (adult)** 85–135 mL/min (1.42–2.25 mL/s) | | | |
| **Glucose (fasting)** 65–109 mg/dL (3.6–6.0 mmol/L) | 186 (10.3) | 171(9.5) | 160 (8.9) |
| **Total Ca** 8.6–10.3 mg/dL (2.15–2.58 mmol/L) | 8.3 (2.08) | 8.5 (2.13) | 8.6 (2.15) |
| **Mg** 1.3–2.2 mEq/L (0.65–1.10 mmol/L) | | | |
| **$PO_4$** 2.5–4.5 mg/dL (0.81–1.45 mmol/L) | | | |
| **Hemoglobin** Male 13.8–17.2 g/dL; female 12.1–15.1 g/dL (male 138–172 g/L; female 121–151 g/L; male 8.57–10.68 mmol/L; female 7.51–9.38 mmol/L) | 12.9 (129; 8.01) | | |
| **Hematocrit** Male 40.7–50.3%; female 36.1–44.3% (male 0.407–0.503; female 0.361–0.443) | 31.2 (0.312) | | |
| **MCV** 80.0–97.6 μm³ (80.0–97.6 fL) | | | |
| **WBC** 4–10 × 10³/mm³ (4–10 × 10⁹/L) | 12.9 | | |
| **Differential** | | | |
| **Platelet** 140–440 × 10³/mm³ (140–440 × 10⁹/L) | 182 | | |
| **Albumin** 3.5–5.0 g/dL (35–50 g/L) | 4 (40) | | |
| **Total bilirubin** 0.3–1.1 mg/dL (5.1–18.8 μmol/L) | | | |
| **Direct bilirubin** 0–0.3 mg/dL (0–5.1 μmol/L) | | | |
| **AST** 11–47 IU/L (0.18–0.78 μkat/L) | | | |
| **ALT** 7–53 IU/L (0.12–0.88 μkat/L) | | | |
| **Alk phos (adult)** 38–126 IU/L (0.63–2.10 μkat/L) | | | |

| Vital Signs, Laboratory Data, and Diagnostic Test Results | | | |
|---|---|---|---|
| **Plasma osmolality**<br>273–300 mOsm/kg (273–300 mmol/kg) | | 265 | |
| **Urine osmolality**<br>250–900 mOsm/kg (250–900 mmol/kg) | 475 | | |
| **Urine sodium**<br>20–250 mEq/L (20–250 mmol/L) | <20 | | |

| Notes |
|---|
| |
| |
| |
| |
| |
| |
| |
| |
| |

## DRUG THERAPY PROBLEM WORKSHEET

| Type of Problem | Possible Causes | Problem List | Notes |
|---|---|---|---|
| Correlation between drug therapy and medical problems | Drugs without obvious medical indications | Home medications latanoprost, celecoxib, pantoprazole, lorazepam | |
| | Medications unidentified | | |
| | Untreated medical conditions | | |
| Need for additional drug therapy | New medical condition requiring new drug therapy | Hyponatremia, _____ | |
| | Chronic disorder requiring continued drug therapy | | |
| | Condition best treated with combination drug therapy | | |
| | May develop new medical condition without prophylactic or preventative therapy or premedication | | |
| Unnecessary drug therapy | Medication with no valid indication | | |
| | Condition caused by accidental or intentional ingestion of toxic amount of drug or chemical | | |
| | Medical problem(s) associated with use of or withdrawal from alcohol, drug, or tobacco | | |
| | Condition is better treated with nondrug therapy | | |
| | Taking multiple drugs when single agent as effective | | |
| | Taking drug(s) to treat an avoidable adverse reaction from another medication | | |
| Appropriate drug selection | Current regimen not usually as effective as other choices | | |
| | Current regimen not usually as safe as other choices | | |
| | Therapy not individualized to patient | | |
| Wrong drug | Medical problem for which drug is not effective | | |
| | Patient has risk factors that contraindicate use of drug | | |
| | Patient has infection with organisms resistant to drug | | |
| | Patient refractory to current drug therapy | | |
| | Taking combination product when single agent appropriate | | |
| | Dosage form inappropriate | | |
| | Medication error | | |
| Drug regimen | PRN use not appropriate for condition | | |
| | Route of administration/dosage form/mode of administration not appropriate for current condition | | |
| | Length or course of therapy not appropriate | | |
| | Drug therapy altered without adequate therapeutic trial | | |
| | Dose or interval flexibility not appropriate | | |
| Dose too low | Dose or frequency too low to produce desired response in this patient | | |
| | Serum drug level below desired therapeutic range | | |
| | Timing of antimicrobial prophylaxis not appropriate | | |
| | Medication not stored properly | | |
| | Medication error | | |

**DRUG THERAPY PROBLEM WORKSHEET**

| Type of Problem | Possible Causes | Problem List | Notes |
|---|---|---|---|
| Dose too high | Dose or frequency too high for this patient | | |
| | Serum drug level above the desired therapeutic range | | |
| | Dose escalated too quickly | | |
| | Dose or interval flexibility not appropriate for this patient | | |
| | Medication error | | |
| Therapeutic duplication | Receiving multiple agents without added benefit | | |
| Drug allergy/ adverse drug events | History of allergy or ADE to current (or chemically related) agents | Sulfa allergy—verify celecoxib and HCTZ | |
| | Allergy or ADE history not in medical records | | |
| | Patient not using alert for severe allergy or ADE | | |
| | Symptoms or medical problems that may be drug induced | | |
| | Drug administered too rapidly | | |
| | Medication error, actual or potential | | |
| Interactions (drug–drug, drug–disease, drug–nutrient, drug–laboratory test) | Effect of drug altered due to enzyme induction/ inhibition from another drug patient is taking | | |
| | Effect of drug altered due to protein-binding alterations from another drug patient is taking | | |
| | Effect of drug altered due to pharmacodynamic change from another drug patient is taking | | |
| | Bioavailability of drug altered due to interaction with another drug or food | | |
| | Effect of drug altered due to substance in food | | |
| | Patient's laboratory test altered due to interference from a drug the patient is taking | | |
| Failure to receive therapy | Patient did not adhere with the drug regimen | | |
| | Drug not given due to medication error | | |
| | Patient did not take due to high drug cost/lack of insurance | | |
| | Patient unable to take oral medication | | |
| | Patient has no IV access for IV medication | | |
| | Drug product not available | | |
| Financial impact | The current regimen is not the most cost-effective | | |
| | Patient unable to purchase medications/no insurance | Unknown | |
| Patient knowledge of drug therapy | Patient does not understand the purpose, directions, or potential side effects of the drug regimen | Patient unresponsive | |
| | Current regimen not consistent with the patient's health beliefs | Unknown | |

# PHARMACOTHERAPY CARE PLAN

| Medical Problem List | Current Drug Regimen | Drug Therapy Problems | Therapy Goals, Desired Endpoints | Therapeutic Recommendations | Rationale | Therapeutic Alternatives | Monitoring |
|---|---|---|---|---|---|---|---|
| Euvolemic hyponatremia | ——— | May be due to ——— | Return sodium to within normal limits; no further increase in ICP; correct serum Na no faster than 0.5 mEq/L/h (0.5 mmol/L/h) or max of 12 mEq (12 mmol) in 24 h | ——— | Need for acute management due to compromised neuro status; 1 L of 3% sodium chloride will correct the sodium by about 9 mEq (9 mmol) in this patient; avoid too-rapid correction and risk of osmotic myelinolysis syndrome | ——— ——— | Monitor electrolytes q 2–4 h to ensure you do not correct the sodium by more than 12 mEq (12 mmol) q 24 h |
| | | | | After the patient recovers from head trauma, investigate the cause of euvolemic hyponatremia and treat accordingly | | Conivaptan IV, but unclear safety and efficacy in neurotrauma patient. Tolvaptan PO is an option for chronic SIADH | |
| Hypokalemia | ——— | May be due to HCTZ | Serum K >4.0 mEq/L (>4.0 mmol/L) in critically ill patients | ——— | Unable to give PO; risk of hypokalemia-related complications in critically ill patients | K phosphate, K acetate if hypophosphatemic or acidotic | ——— |
| Pneumonia | ——— | ——— | Cure infection | ——— | Broad coverage since critically ill, pneumonia; history not clear | Carbapenem, third-generation cephalosporin | CBC, CXR q 24 h; ABGs q 6 h |
| HTN | HCTZ | ——— | ——— | Nicardipine IV infusion | Improves cerebral perfusion | ——— | BP, neurochecks q 1 h |
| | | | | When recovered from head trauma, reassess HTN regimen | | | |
| Nausea/vomiting | ——— | ——— | Prevent vomiting-related increased ICP | Metoclopramide 10 mg IV q 6 h PRN | ——— | ——— | ——— |
| Hx GERD/stress ulcer prophylaxis | ——— | ——— | No stress ulcer bleeding | Pantoprazole 40 mg q 24 h | Stress ulcer prophylaxis indicated in head trauma, mechanical ventilation | | CBC; hemoccult; NG suction fluid |

**PATIENT EDUCATION SUMMARY**

**Notes**

- Patient is unresponsive at this time.

# 35 Parkinson's Disease: Example Careplan with Missing Data

Jack J. Chen

## PATIENT DATABASE FORM

| | | |
|---|---|---|
| **Patient Name:** Oliver Covey | **Patient ID:** 01892500 | **Location:** Neurologist's Office |
| **Physician:** | **Pharmacy:** | |
| **Age (or Date of Birth):** 62 yo | **Race:** Caucasian | **Sex:** Male |
| **Height:** 71 in. (180 cm) | **Weight:** 180 lb (81.8 kg) | |
| **Date of Admission/Initial Visit:** 10/20/2012 | **Occupation:** Agricultural Irrigation Consultant | |

### Allergies/Intolerances/ADRs

❏ No known drug allergies/ADRs

❏ Not known/inadequate information

| Drug: | Reaction: |
|---|---|
| Sulfonamides | Rash |
| | |
| | |
| | |
| | |

### HPI, PMH, FH, SH, etc...

| |
|---|
| BPH × 1 yr |
| GERD × 1 yr |
| Hyperlipidemia × 5 yr |
| Nephrolithiasis in the past |
| Tonsillectomy |
| Tennis player |
| |
| |

| Prioritized Medical Problem List | Medication Profile |
|---|---|
| Parkinson's disease | |
| | |
| | |
| BPH | Silodosin 8 mg PO q 24 h |
| | |
| GERD | Omeprazole 20 mg PO q 24 h |
| | |
| _____ | Simvastatin 20 mg PO q 24 h |
| | |
| | Multivitamin one tablet PO q 24 h |
| | |
| | |

The form is from *ASHP National Clinical Skills Competition Case Documents*, Copyright 2009, American Society of Health-System Pharmacists, Bethesda, MD (www.ashp.org). Adapted with permission.

| Vital Signs, Laboratory Data, and Diagnostic Test Results | | | |
|---|---|---|---|
| **Date** | 09/20/2012 | | |
| **Weight (lb/kg)** | 178 (80.9) | | |
| **Temperature (°C)** | 36.2 | | |
| **Blood pressure (mm Hg)** | 126/74 | | |
| **Pulse** | 77 | | |
| **Respiratory rate** | 15 | | |
| **Na**<br>135–145 mEq/L (135–145 mmol/L) | 140 | | |
| **K**<br>3.3–4.9 mEq/L (3.3–4.9 mmol/L) | 4.0 | | |
| **Cl**<br>97–110 mEq/L (97–110 mmol/L) | 99 | | |
| **$CO_2$/$HCO_3$**<br>22–26 mEq/L (22–26 mmol/L) | 29 | | |
| **BUN**<br>8–25 mg/dL (2.9–8.9 mmol/L) | 14 (5.0) | | |
| **Creatinine (adult)**<br>Male 0.7–1.3 mg/dL; female 0.6–1.1 mg/dL (male 62–115 μmol/L;<br>  female 53–97 μmol/L) | 1 (88) | | |
| **Creatinine clearance (adult)**<br>85–135 mL/min (1.42–2.25 mL/s) | 81.6 (1.36) | | |
| **Glucose (fasting)**<br>65–109 mg/dL (3.6–6.0 mmol/L) | 90 (5.0) | | |
| **Total Ca**<br>8.6–10.3 mg/dL (2.15-2.58 mmol/L) | 9.5 (2.38) | | |
| **Mg**<br>1.3–2.2 mEq/L (0.65–1.10 mmol/L) | 2.2 (1.10) | | |
| **$PO_4$**<br>2.5–4.5 mg/dL (0.81–1.45 mmol/L) | 3.5 (1.13) | | |
| **Hemoglobin**<br>Male 13.8–17.2 g/dL; female 12.1–15.1 g/dL (male 138–172 g/L;<br>  female 121–151 g/L; male 8.57–10.68 mmol/L; female 7.51–9.38 mmol/L) | 16.4 (164; 10.18) | | |
| **Hematocrit**<br>Male 40.7–50.3%; female 36.1–44.3% (male 0.407–0.503;<br>  female 0.361–0.443) | 48.7 (0.487) | | |
| **MCV**<br>80.0–97.6 μm$^3$ (80.0–97.6 fL) | 86.4 | | |
| **WBC**<br>4–10 × 10$^3$/mm$^3$ (4–10 × 10$^9$/L) | 8.5 | | |
| **Differential** | | | |
| **Platelet**<br>140–440 × 10$^3$/mm$^3$ (140–440 × 10$^9$/L) | 300 | | |
| **Albumin**<br>3.5–5.0 g/dL (35–50 g/L) | 3.7 (37) | | |
| **Total bilirubin**<br>0.3–1.1 mg/dL (5.1–18.8 μmol/L) | | | |
| **Direct bilirubin**<br>0–0.3 mg/dL (0–5.1 μmol/L) | | | |
| **AST**<br>11–47 IU/L (0.18–0.78 μkat/L) | | | |
| **ALT**<br>7–53 IU/L (0.12–0.88 μkat/L) | | | |
| **Alk phos (adult)**<br>38–126 IU/L (0.63–2.10 μkat/L) | | | |

| Vital Signs, Laboratory Data, and Diagnostic Test Results | | | |
|---|---|---|---|
| **Total cholesterol**<br><200 mg/dL (<5.17 mmol/L) | 180 (4.65) | | |
| **LDL cholesterol**<br><130 mg/dL (<3.36 mmol/L) | 100 (2.59) | | |
| **HDL cholesterol**<br>>35 mg/dL (>0.91 mmol/L) | 38 (0.98) | | |

| Notes |
|---|
| |
| |
| |
| |
| |
| |
| |
| |

## DRUG THERAPY PROBLEM WORKSHEET

| Type of Problem | Possible Causes | Problem List | Notes |
|---|---|---|---|
| Correlation between drug therapy and medical problems | Drugs without obvious medical indications | | |
| | Medications unidentified | | |
| | Untreated medical conditions | | |
| Need for additional drug therapy | New medical condition requiring new drug therapy | Parkinson's disease | |
| | Chronic disorder requiring continued drug therapy | | |
| | Condition best treated with combination drug therapy | | |
| | May develop new medical condition without prophylactic or preventative therapy or premedication | | |
| Unnecessary drug therapy | Medication with no valid indication | | |
| | Condition caused by accidental or intentional ingestion of toxic amount of drug or chemical | | |
| | Medical problem(s) associated with use of or withdrawal from alcohol, drug, or tobacco | | |
| | Condition is better treated with nondrug therapy | | |
| | Taking multiple drugs when single agent as effective | | |
| | Taking drug(s) to treat an avoidable adverse reaction from another medication | | |
| Appropriate drug selection | Current regimen not usually as effective as other choices | | |
| | Current regimen not usually as safe as other choices | | |
| | Therapy not individualized to patient | | |
| Wrong drug | Medical problem for which drug is not effective | | |
| | Patient has risk factors that contraindicate use of drug | | |
| | Patient has infection with organisms resistant to drug | | |
| | Patient refractory to current drug therapy | | |
| | Taking combination product when single agent appropriate | | |
| | Dosage form inappropriate | | |
| | Medication error | | |
| Drug regimen | PRN use not appropriate for condition | | |
| | Route of administration/dosage form/mode of administration not appropriate for current condition | | |
| | Length or course of therapy not appropriate | | |
| | Drug therapy altered without adequate therapeutic trial | | |
| | Dose or interval flexibility not appropriate | | |
| Dose too low | Dose or frequency too low to produce desired response in this patient | | |
| | Serum drug level below desired therapeutic range | | |
| | Timing of antimicrobial prophylaxis not appropriate | | |
| | Medication not stored properly | | |
| | Medication error | | |
| Dose too high | Dose or frequency too high for this patient | | |
| | Serum drug level above the desired therapeutic range | | |
| | Dose escalated too quickly | | |
| | Dose or interval flexibility not appropriate for this patient | | |
| | Medication error | | |

## DRUG THERAPY PROBLEM WORKSHEET

| Type of Problem | Possible Causes | Problem List | Notes |
|---|---|---|---|
| Therapeutic duplication | Receiving multiple agents without added benefit | | |
| Drug allergy/ adverse drug events | History of allergy or ADE to current (or chemically related) agents | | |
| | Allergy or ADE history not in medical records | Any allergies or ADEs other than sulfonamides? | |
| | Patient not using alert for severe allergy or ADE | | |
| | Symptoms or medical problems that may be drug induced | Any previous use of neuroleptics, metoclopramide, or other dopamine receptor-blocking agents? | |
| | Drug administered too rapidly | | |
| | Medication error, actual or potential | | |
| Interactions (drug–drug, drug–disease, drug–nutrient, drug–laboratory test) | Effect of drug altered due to enzyme induction/ inhibition from another drug patient is taking | | |
| | Effect of drug altered due to protein-binding alterations from another drug patient is taking | | |
| | Effect of drug altered due to pharmacodynamic change from another drug patient is taking | | |
| | Bioavailability of drug altered due to interaction with another drug or food | Multivitamin may contain $Fe^{++}$. If carbidopa/levodopa is initiated, $Fe^{++}$ will reduce levodopa bioavailability by 50% | If carbidopa/levodopa therapy is selected, make sure the patient is educated about proper times to administer |
| | Effect of drug altered due to substance in food | | |
| | Patient's laboratory test altered due to interference from a drug the patient is taking | | |
| Failure to receive therapy | Patient did not adhere with the drug regimen | | |
| | Drug not given due to medication error | | |
| | Patient did not take due to high drug cost/lack of insurance | | |
| | Patient unable to take oral medication | | |
| | Patient has no IV access for IV medication | | |
| | Drug product not available | | |
| Financial impact | The current regimen is not the most cost-effective | | |
| | Patient unable to purchase medications/no insurance | Insurance coverage not known | If a branded drug is initiated, can provide drug samples to see if the drug is effective and tolerated |
| Patient knowledge of drug therapy | Patient does not understand the purpose, directions, or potential side effects of the drug regimen | Patient's background understanding of anti-PD medications unknown | Educate the patient and caregiver about purpose, directions, and potential side effects of drug regimen |
| | Current regimen not consistent with the patient's health beliefs | Cultural beliefs not known | |

# PHARMACOTHERAPY CARE PLAN

| Medical Problem List | Current Drug Regimen | Drug Therapy Problems | Therapy Goals, Desired Endpoints | Therapeutic Recommendations | Rationale | Therapeutic Alternatives | Monitoring |
|---|---|---|---|---|---|---|---|
| Parkinson's Disease | ___ | ___ | Improve motor symptoms (tremor, rigidity, slowness). Allow the patient to continue to enjoy his tennis game | ___ ___ Avoid medications that may worsen symptoms (dopamine blockers) | Appropriate for mild-severity PD. Well-tolerated and once-daily administration No anticholinergic due to BPH | Dopamine agonist such as pramipexole or ropinirole. Titrated to maintenance dose as per package insert. Pramipexole and ropinirole immediate-release available as generic, so may be more cost effective | Rasagiline is well tolerated. Monitor for nausea. Self-monitor symptoms (tennis game); return to neurologist 2 mo  If dopamine agonist, monitor for: ___ ___ |
| BPH | Silodosin 8 mg PO q 24 h | ___ | Improve urinary voiding dysfunction | ___ ___ ___ | ___ ___ ___ | Other $\alpha_1$-receptor blockers, 5a- reductase inhibitors, combination therapy | Monitor for side effects such as dizziness, orthostatic hypotension, sexual dysfunction |
| GERD | Omeprazole 20 mg PO q 24 h | ___ | No GERD symptoms | ___ ___ ___ | ___ ___ ___ | ___ ___ ___ | ___ ___ |
| ___ | Simvastatin 20 mg PO q 24 h | ___ | ___ ___ ___ | Continue with current regimen. Provide healthy lifestyle (diet, exercise) recommendations | LDL and HDL are at goal | ___ ___ ___ | Recheck lipid panel in 3 mo |

## PATIENT EDUCATION SUMMARY

### Notes

**Parkinson's Disease**

- The reason for taking this medication called rasagiline is to replace or enhance the dopamine that your brain is not producing in adequate amounts. In doing so, your movement should get better.
- Take this medication once a day as your physician directed.
- If you experience stomach upset or nausea while taking this medication, take it with _____.
- If you miss a dose, _____.
- You should begin to feel better within _____ wk of starting this medication, maybe sooner.
- This is a very well-tolerated medication, and these problems will not occur if you take the medication as directed.
- Call your physician immediately if you experience any effects that you believe might be a side effect.
- Since there is no cure for Parkinson's disease, you will likely need to take this medication indefinitely.

**Benign Prostatic Hypertrophy**

- Continue with your drug regimen as long as it is controlling your symptoms. If you have any questions, consult with your primary care physician.

**Gastroesophageal Reflux Disease**

- Continue with your drug regimen as long as it is controlling your symptoms. If you have any questions, consult with your primary care physician.

**Hyperlipidemia**

- Your total cholesterol and LDL (the "bad") cholesterol is in control. Your HDL (the "good") cholesterol is adequate. You will need periodic blood tests to make sure your lipid levels are still controlled and to assess for side effects.
- If you notice any muscle pains not explained by exercise, notify your physician.
- Continue with your drug regimen and remember to keep a healthy diet, keep exercising, and avoid using tobacco, and consume alcohol in moderation.
- If you have questions, consult with your primary care physician.

# 44 Anxiety: Example Careplan with Missing Data

Sheila Botts

## PATIENT DATABASE FORM

| | | |
|---|---|---|
| **Patient Name:** Angela Brown | **Patient ID:** 00869702 | **Location:** Physician's Office |
| **Physician:** | **Pharmacy:** Wal-Mart | |
| **Age (or Date of Birth):** 32 yo | **Race:** Caucasian | **Sex:** Female |
| **Height:** 65 in. (165 cm) | **Weight:** 145 lb (65.9 kg) | |
| **Date of Admission/Initial Visit:** 12/2/2012 | **Occupation:** Art Teacher | |

### Allergies/Intolerances/ADRs

❏ No known drug allergies/ADRs

❏ Not known/inadequate information

| Drug: | Reaction: |
|---|---|
| Fluoxetine | Agitation and anxiety |
| | |
| | |
| | |
| | |

### HPI, PMH, FH, SH, etc...

| |
|---|
| Depression 3 yr ago after death of father |
| Migraine headache diagnosed 5 yr ago |
| Sibling treated for anxiety with citalopram |

| Prioritized Medical Problem List | Medication Profile |
|---|---|
| Panic disorder with agoraphobia | Diazepam 5 mg PO PRN |
| Depressive symptoms | |
| Migraine headaches | Zolmitriptan 2.5 mg PO PRN |
| EtOH use | |
| Muscle aches, ? due to anxiety | Ibuprofen 400 mg PO PRN |
| Tachycardia, ? due to anxiety | |

The form is from *ASHP National Clinical Skills Competition Case Documents*, Copyright 2009, American Society of Health-System Pharmacists, Bethesda, MD (www.ashp.org). Adapted with permission.

| Vital Signs, Laboratory Data, and Diagnostic Test Results | | | |
|---|---|---|---|
| **Date** | 12/1/2012 | | |
| **Weight (lb/kg)** | 145 (65.9) | | |
| **Temperature (°C)** | 37.1 | | |
| **Blood pressure (mm Hg)** | 118/76 | | |
| **Pulse** | 88 | | |
| **Respiratory rate** | 18 | | |
| **Na** <br> 135–145 mEq/L (135–145 mmol/L) | 142 | | |
| **K** <br> 3.3–4.9 mEq/L (3.3–4.9 mmol/L) | 4.1 | | |
| **Cl** <br> 97–110 mEq/L (97–110 mmol/L) | 100 | | |
| **$CO_2$/$HCO_3$** <br> 22–26 mEq/L (22–26 mmol/L) | 24 | | |
| **BUN** <br> 8–25 mg/dL (2.9–8.9 mmol/L) | 10 (3.6) | | |
| **Creatinine (adult)** <br> Male 0.7–1.3 mg/dL; female 0.6–1.1 mg/dL (male 62–115 μmol/L; <br> female 53–97 μmol/L) | 0.7 (62) | | |
| **Creatinine clearance (adult)** <br> 85–135 mL/min (1.42–2.25 mL/s) | | | |
| **Glucose (fasting)** <br> 65–109 mg/dL (3.6–6.0 mmol/L) | 98 (5.4) | | |
| **Total Ca** <br> 8.6–10.3 mg/dL (2.15–2.58 mmol/L) | | | |
| **Mg** <br> 1.3–2.2 mEq/L (0.65–1.10 mmol/L) | | | |
| **$PO_4$** <br> 2.5–4.5 mg/dL (0.81–1.45 mmol/L) | | | |
| **Hemoglobin** <br> Male 13.8–17.2 g/dL; female 12.1–15.1 g/dL (male 138–172 g/L; <br> female 121–151 g/L; male 8.57–10.68 mmol/L; <br> female 7.51–9.38 mmol/L) | 14.5 (145; 9.00) | | |
| **Hematocrit** <br> Male 40.7–50.3%; female 36.1–44.3% (male 0.407–0.503; <br> female 0.361–0.443) | 42 (0.42) | | |
| **MCV** <br> 80.0–97.6 μm³ (80.0–97.6 fL) | | | |
| **WBC** <br> $4$–$10 \times 10^3$/mm³ ($4$–$10 \times 10^9$/L) | 6.8 | | |
| **Differential** | | | |
| **Platelet** <br> $140$–$440 \times 10^3$/mm³ ($140$–$440 \times 10^9$/L) | | | |
| **Albumin** <br> 3.5–5.0 g/dL (35–50 g/L) | | | |
| **Total bilirubin** <br> 0.3–1.1 mg/dL (5.1–18.8 μmol/L) | | | |
| **Direct bilirubin** <br> 0–0.3 mg/dL (0–5.1 μmol/L) | | | |
| **AST** <br> 11–47 IU/L (0.18–0.78 μkat/L) | 22 (0.37) | | |
| **ALT** <br> 7–53 IU/L (0.12–0.88 μkat/L) | 28 (0.47) | | |
| **Alk phos (adult)** <br> 38–126 IU/L (0.63–2.10 μkat/L) | 40 (0.67) | | |

| Vital Signs, Laboratory Data, and Diagnostic Test Results | | | |
|---|---|---|---|
| **TSH**<br>0.35–6.20 µU/mL (0.35–6.20 mU/L) | 1.2 | | |
| **Total cholesterol**<br><200 mg/dL (<5.17 mmol/L) | 178 (4.60) | | |
| **LDL cholesterol**<br><130 mg/dL (<3.36 mmol/L) | 89 (2.30) | | |
| **HDL cholesterol**<br>>35 mg/dL (>0.91 mmol/L) | 36 (0.93) | | |

| Notes |
|---|
| Urine drug screen: (+) benzodiazepines |
| Urine pregnancy test (−) |
| ECG report from ER noted sinus tachycardia, otherwise no significant findings |
| |
| |
| |
| |
| |

## DRUG THERAPY PROBLEM WORKSHEET

| Type of Problem | Possible Causes | Problem List | Notes |
|---|---|---|---|
| Correlation between drug therapy and medical problems | Drugs without obvious medical indications | | |
| | Medications unidentified | Supplement use?; other analgesics | |
| | Untreated medical conditions | | |
| Need for additional drug therapy | New medical condition requiring new drug therapy | Panic disorder | Currently receiving diazepam PRN |
| | Chronic disorder requiring continued drug therapy | ? Migraine | |
| | Condition best treated with combination drug therapy | | |
| | May develop new medical condition without prophylactic or preventative therapy or premedication | | |
| Unnecessary drug therapy | Medication with no valid indication | | |
| | Condition caused by accidental or intentional ingestion of toxic amount of drug or chemical | | |
| | Medical problem(s) associated with use of or withdrawal from alcohol, drug, or tobacco | EtOH use increased to control anxiety; may increase depressive symptoms also | |
| | Condition is better treated with nondrug therapy | | |
| | Taking multiple drugs when single agent as effective | | |
| | Taking drug(s) to treat an avoidable adverse reaction from another medication | | |
| Appropriate drug selection | Current regimen not usually as effective as other choices | | |
| | Current regimen not usually as safe as other choices | | |
| | Therapy not individualized to patient | | |
| Wrong drug | Medical problem for which drug is not effective | | |
| | Patient has risk factors that contraindicate use of drug | | |
| | Patient has infection with organisms resistant to drug | | |
| | Patient refractory to current drug therapy | | |
| | Taking combination product when single agent appropriate | | |
| | Dosage form inappropriate | | |
| | Medication error | | |
| Drug regimen | PRN use not appropriate for condition | Panic disorder | |
| | Route of administration/dosage form/mode of administration not appropriate for current condition | | |
| | Length or course of therapy not appropriate | | |
| | Drug therapy altered without adequate therapeutic trial | | |
| | Dose or interval flexibility not appropriate | | |
| Dose too low | Dose or frequency too low to produce desired response in this patient | | |
| | Serum drug level below desired therapeutic range | | |
| | Timing of antimicrobial prophylaxis not appropriate | | |
| | Medication not stored properly | | |
| | Medication error | | |

## DRUG THERAPY PROBLEM WORKSHEET

| Type of Problem | Possible Causes | Problem List | Notes |
|---|---|---|---|
| Dose too high | Dose or frequency too high for this patient | | |
| | Serum drug level above the desired therapeutic range | | |
| | Dose escalated too quickly | | |
| | Dose or interval flexibility not appropriate for this patient | | |
| | Medication error | | |
| Therapeutic duplication | Receiving multiple agents without added benefit | | |
| Drug allergy/ adverse drug events | History of allergy or ADE to current (or chemically related) agents | Fluoxetine | Did not tolerate— starting dose too high, experienced agitation, and anxiety |
| | Allergy or ADE history not in medical records | Other allergies or medication intolerance? | |
| | Patient not using alert for severe allergy or ADE | | |
| | Symptoms or medical problems that may be drug induced | | |
| | Drug administered too rapidly | | |
| | Medication error, actual or potential | | |
| Interactions (drug–drug, drug–disease, drug–nutrient, drug–laboratory test) | Effect of drug altered due to enzyme induction/ inhibition from another drug patient is taking | | |
| | Effect of drug altered due to protein-binding alterations from another drug patient is taking | | |
| | Effect of drug altered due to pharmacodynamic change from another drug patient is taking | Diazepam use with EtOH will increase CNS depression; potential SSRI/ triptan interaction | Diazepam not recommended |
| | Bioavailability of drug altered due to interaction with another drug or food | | |
| | Effect of drug altered due to substance in food | | |
| | Patient's laboratory test altered due to interference from a drug the patient is taking | | |
| Failure to receive therapy | Patient did not adhere with the drug regimen | | |
| | Drug not given due to medication error | | |
| | Patient did not take due to high drug cost/lack of insurance | | |
| | Patient unable to take oral medication | | |
| | Patient has no IV access for IV medication | | |
| | Drug product not available | | |
| Financial impact | The current regimen is not the most cost-effective | | |
| | Patient unable to purchase medications/no insurance | No information on insurance status | |
| Patient knowledge of drug therapy | Patient does not understand the purpose, directions, or potential side effects of the drug regimen | | |
| | Current regimen not consistent with the patient's health beliefs | Health beliefs not known | Discuss treatment preference (pharmacologic vs. nonpharmacologic) with the patient |

| Medical Problem List | Current Drug Regimen | Drug Therapy Problems | Therapy Goals, Desired Endpoints | Therapeutic Recommendations | Rationale | Therapeutic Alternatives | Monitoring |
|---|---|---|---|---|---|---|---|
| Panic disorder | _____ _____ | EtOH and benzodiazepine use; PRN treatment not best | Reduce panic attack frequency and severity; reduce anticipatory anxiety; reduce agoraphobic avoidance | _____ _____ _____ _____ | Antidepressant therapy preferred for chronic treatment; starting dose low to avoid drug-induced anxiety and panic | Switch to another SSRI, SNRI (e.g., venlafaxine), or cognitive behavioral therapy (CBT). May also augment medication with CBT if some benefit with initial medication | Monitor weekly during first month for ADEs (GI, altered sleep, HA, etc.) and improvement in panic symptoms; if patient without considerable reduction in anxiety symptoms at 6–8 wk, consider changing antidepressant or augmentation |
| Depressive symptoms | _____ _____ | _____ _____ _____ | No signs or symptoms of depression | _____ _____ _____ | Antidepressant therapy indicated with comorbid panic disorder and depression; unclear if this patient has major depression, but symptoms expected to improve with treatment | As per panic disorder plan | Assess depressive symptoms at the same time as anxiety symptoms; assess with Physician Health Questionnaire (PH Q-9) or Beck Depression Inventory |
| Migraine Headaches | Zolmitriptan 2.5 mg PO PRN | Frequency of use unknown; responsiveness to ibuprofen? Risk of serotonin syndrome, triptan, SSRI | _____ _____ _____ _____ | Migraine frequency and severity may improve with SSRI treatment of anxiety disorder | | If frequency of headaches increases to warrant prophylactic treatment, consider first-line agent such as propranolol, topiramate, or divalproex | Headache frequency and intensity; signs and symptoms of serotonin syndrome with SSRI and triptan use |

## PHARMACOTHERAPY CARE PLAN

| Medical Problem List | Current Drug Regimen | Drug Therapy Problems | Therapy Goals, Desired Endpoints | Therapeutic Recommendations | Rationale | Therapeutic Alternatives | Monitoring |
|---|---|---|---|---|---|---|---|
| EtOH use | ‒‒<br>‒‒ | ‒‒<br>‒‒ | ‒‒<br>‒‒<br>‒‒ | EtOH use likely to decrease anxiety symptoms improve and sleep restored | ‒‒<br>‒‒<br>‒‒<br>‒‒ | If EtOH use continues or increases, refer to substance-abuse counseling/program | ‒‒<br>‒‒<br>‒‒<br>‒‒ |
| Muscle aches | ‒‒<br>‒‒ | ‒‒<br>‒‒ | ‒‒<br>‒‒ | Continue PRN use as needed; shoulder aches likely to improve with anxiety treatment; nondrug therapy (exercise, yoga, hot baths, massage) | Muscle aches commonly accompany tension associated with severe anxiety | ‒‒<br>‒‒<br>‒‒ | ‒‒<br>‒‒<br>‒‒ |
| Tachycardia | None | ‒‒<br>‒‒ | ‒‒<br>‒‒ | Likely to improve with reduction of anxiety symptoms; if continues to worsen, refer for workup | ‒‒<br>‒‒ | If not severe and ECG normal, no treatment recommended | Reassess at the next clinic visit along with anxiety symptoms; self-monitoring |

## PATIENT EDUCATION SUMMARY

### Notes

**Panic Disorder**

- This medication is being used to reduce your anxiety, fears, and panic attacks. Over time it will also help with worry about having future panic attacks and avoiding places or situations due to anxiety.
- Take this medication once daily as your health care provider directed.
- If you miss a dose, _____.
- You should begin to feel better within _____ weeks of starting this medication, but it may take up to _____ wk for the full benefit. You will initially notice an improvement in your anxiety and sleep. Mood and panic attack reduction may take longer.
- This medication may cause _____. The side effects often go away as the treatment continues. If you experience suicidal thoughts or extreme irritability, you should stop the medication and call your health care provider.
- Do not abruptly discontinue this medication, unless instructed by your health care provider. Abrupt discontinuation can lead to an increase in anxiety symptoms, stomach upset, nausea, diarrhea, and body aches.
- It is very important to keep regular appointments with your health care provider to monitor your therapy so that you can gain the full benefit of this therapy while avoiding potential side effects.

**Migraine Headaches**

- Your migraine headaches may improve with the treatment of your anxiety disorder; however, if your headaches increase, you should inform your health care provider immediately.
- Your antimigraine medication in combination with your anxiety mediaction can result in a rare adverse reaction called serotonin syndrome. Serotonin syndrome occurs rapidly and causes symptoms of _____ _____. If you notice any of these symptoms, you should seek immediate care.

**Depression**

- Your depressive symptoms may be worsened by your alcohol use. Reduction in your daily alcohol consumption to one drink or less may improve your mood. Also, the medication prescribed for your anxiety will also help with depression.
- If your mood worsens or you begin to have suicidal thoughts after starting the medication, you should inform your health care provider immediately.

**EtOH Use**

- Your current alcohol consumption, in response to your anxiety, may worsen your sleep and increase your depression. This amount of alcohol use over time may also put you at risk for other chronic health conditions.
- You are being prescribed medication to reduce your anxiety, which may take a few weeks to work.
- If you are unable to reduce your alcohol use on your own, your provider will help you with other treatment options.

**Muscle Aches**

- Your muscle aches in your shoulders may improve as your anxiety improves.
- Regular exercise, stretching, yoga, massage, and hot baths may also be helpful.

**Tachycardia**

- Your rapid heart rate should improve as your anxiety is reduced.
- Rapid increases in your heart rate may also be a sign of other medical problems or drug interactions and should be reported to your health care provider.
- Relaxation exercises, deep breathing, and meditation may also be helpful.

# 52 Hypothyroidism: Example Careplan with Missing Data

Michael D. Katz

---

### PATIENT DATABASE FORM

| | | |
|---|---|---|
| **Patient Name:** Yi-Ling Wang | **Patient ID:** 01892487 | **Location:** Physician's Office |
| **Physician:** | **Pharmacy:** | **Sex:** Female |
| **Age (or Date of Birth):** 49 yo | **Race:** Chinese | |
| **Height:** 62 in (157.5 cm) | **Weight:** 127.6 lb (58 kg) | |
| **Date of Admission/Initial Visit:** 04/29/2012 | **Occupation:** | |

**Allergies/Intolerances/ADRs**

❏ No known drug allergies/ADRs

❏ Not known/inadequate information

| Drug: | Reaction: |
|---|---|
| Penicillin | Rash |
| | |
| | |
| | |
| | |

**HPI, PMH, FH, SH, etc...**

Iron-deficiency anemia diagnosed 6 mo ago

Depression for 6 mo

Menorrhagia diagnosed 6 mo ago

Osteopenia for 1 yr

| Prioritized Medical Problem List | Medication Profile |
|---|---|
| Hypothyroidism | |
| | |
| _____ versus hypothyroid symptoms | Sertraline 50 mg PO q 24 h |
| | |
| Dyslipidemia, ? due to hypothyroidism | |
| Osteopenia | Calcium carbonate 1,000 mg PO q 12 h |
| | Alendronate 35 mg PO weekly |
| Constipation, ? due to hypothyroidism, medications (Fe++, Ca++) | MOM 30 mL PO q 24 h PRN |
| | Rhubarb (Chinese herb) PRN |
| _____, now resolved | $FeSO_4$ 300 mg PO q 24 h |
| _____, now resolved | Ortho Tri-Cyclen-28 PO q 24 h |
| | Acetaminophen 650 mg PO PRN HA, body aches |

| Vital Signs, Laboratory Data, and Diagnostic Test Results | | | |
|---|---|---|---|
| Date | 04/29/2012 | | |
| Weight (lb/kg) | 127.6 (58) | | |
| Temperature (°C) | 36.2 | | |
| Blood pressure (mm Hg) | 112/76 | | |
| Pulse | 64 | | |
| Respiratory rate | 12 | | |
| Na<br>135–145 mEq/L (135–145 mmol/L) | 142 | | |
| K<br>3.3–4.9 mEq/L (3.3–4.9 mmol/L) | 4.1 | | |
| Cl<br>97–110 mEq/L (97–110 mmol/L) | 100 | | |
| $CO_2/HCO_3$<br>22–26 mEq/L (22–26 mmol/L) | 24 | | |
| BUN<br>8–25 mg/dL (2.9–8.9 mmol/L) | 7 (2.5) | | |
| Creatinine (adult)<br>Male 0.7–1.3 mg/dL; female 0.6–1.1 mg/dL (male 62–115 µmol/L;<br>  female 53–97 µmol/L) | 0.7 (62) | | |
| Creatinine clearance (adult)<br>85–135 mL/min (1.42–2.25 mL/s) | 96 (1.60) | | |
| Glucose (fasting)<br>65–109 mg/dL (3.6–6.0 mmol/L) | 104 (5.8) | | |
| Total Ca<br>8.6–10.3 mg/dL (2.15–2.58 mmol/L) | 9.4 (2.35) | | |
| Mg<br>1.3–2.2 mEq/L (0.65–1.10 mmol/L) | 1.8 (0.90) | | |
| $PO_4$<br>2.5–4.5 mg/dL (0.81–1.45 mmol/L) | 3.8 (1.23) | | |
| Hemoglobin<br>Male 13.8–17.2 g/dL; female 12.1–15.1 g/dL (male 138–172 g/L;<br>  female 121–151 g/L; male 8.57–10.68 mmol/L; female 7.51–9.38 mmol/L) | 13.5 (135; 8.38) | | |
| Hematocrit<br>Male 40.7–50.3%; female 36.1–44.3% (male 0.407–0.503;<br>  female 0.361–0.443) | 39.7 (0.397) | | |
| MCV<br>80.0–97.6 µm³ (80.0–97.6 fL) | 83.0 | | |
| WBC<br>$4–10 \times 10^3/mm^3$ ($4–10 \times 10^9/L$) | 7.6 (7.6) | | |
| Differential | | | |
| Platelet<br>$140–440 \times 10^3/mm^3$ ($140–440 \times 10^9/L$) | | | |
| Albumin<br>3.5–5.0 g/dL (35–50 g/L) | 3.8 (38) | | |
| Total bilirubin<br>0.3–1.1 mg/dL (5.1–18.8 µmol/L) | | | |
| Direct bilirubin<br>0–0.3 mg/dL (0–5.1 µmol/L) | | | |
| AST<br>  11–47 IU/L (0.18–0.78 µkat/L) | | | |
| ALT<br>7–53 IU/L (0.12–0.88 µkat/L) | | | |
| Alk phos (adult)<br>38–126 IU/L (0.63–2.10 µkat/L) | | | |

| Vital Signs, Laboratory Data, and Diagnostic Test Results | | | |
|---|---|---|---|
| **TSH**<br>0.35–6.20 µU/mL (0.35–6.20 mU/L) | 12.8 | | |
| **Free T$_4$**<br>0.7–1.9 ng/dL (9.0–24.5 pmol/L) | 0.71 (9.1) | | |
| **Anti-TPO antibody** | + | | |
| **Total cholesterol**<br><200 mg/dL (<5.18 mmol/L) | 268 (6.93) | | |
| **LDL cholesterol**<br><130 mg/dL (<3.36 mmol/L) | 142 (3.67) | | |
| **HDL cholesterol**<br>>35 mg/dL (>0.91 mmol/L) | 36 (0.93) | | |

| Notes |
|---|
| |
| |
| |
| |
| |
| |
| |
| |
| |

## DRUG THERAPY PROBLEM WORKSHEET

| Type of Problem | Possible Causes | Problem List | Notes |
|---|---|---|---|
| Correlation between drug therapy and medical problems | Drugs without obvious medical indications | | |
| | Medications unidentified | Chinese herbal product | Confirm ingredients |
| | Untreated medical conditions | | |
| Need for additional drug therapy | New medical condition requiring new drug therapy | Overt hypothyroidism | |
| | Chronic disorder requiring continued drug therapy | | |
| | Condition best treated with combination drug therapy | | |
| | May develop new medical condition without prophylactic or preventative therapy or premedication | | |
| Unnecessary drug therapy | Medication with no valid indication | | |
| | Condition caused by accidental or intentional ingestion of toxic amount of drug or chemical | | |
| | Medical problem(s) associated with use of or withdrawal from alcohol, drug, or tobacco | | |
| | Condition is better treated with nondrug therapy | | |
| | Taking multiple drugs when single agent as effective | | |
| | Taking drug(s) to treat an avoidable adverse reaction from another medication | | |
| Appropriate drug selection | Current regimen not usually as effective as other choices | | |
| | Current regimen not usually as safe as other choices | | |
| | Therapy not individualized to patient | | |
| Wrong drug | Medical problem for which drug is not effective | | |
| | Patient has risk factors that contraindicate use of drug | | |
| | Patient has infection with organisms resistant to drug | | |
| | Patient refractory to current drug therapy | | |
| | Taking combination product when single agent appropriate | | |
| | Dosage form inappropriate | | |
| | Medication error | | |
| Drug regimen | PRN use not appropriate for condition | | |
| | Route of administration/dosage form/mode of administration not appropriate for current condition | | |
| | Length or course of therapy not appropriate | | |
| | Drug therapy altered without adequate therapeutic trial | | |
| | Dose or interval flexibility not appropriate | | |
| Dose too low | Dose or frequency too low to produce desired response in this patient | | |
| | Serum drug level below desired therapeutic range | | |
| | Timing of antimicrobial prophylaxis not appropriate | | |
| | Medication not stored properly | | |
| | Medication error | | |
| Dose too high | Dose or frequency too high for this patient | | |
| | Serum drug level above the desired therapeutic range | | |
| | Dose escalated too quickly | | |
| | Dose or interval flexibility not appropriate for this patient | | |
| | Medication error | | |

**DRUG THERAPY PROBLEM WORKSHEET**

| Type of Problem | Possible Causes | Problem List | Notes |
|---|---|---|---|
| Therapeutic duplication | Receiving multiple agents without added benefit | | |
| Drug allergy/ adverse drug events | History of allergy or ADE to current (or chemically related) agents | | |
| | Allergy or ADE history not in medical records | Any allergies or ADEs other than penicillin? | |
| | Patient not using alert for severe allergy or ADE | | |
| | Symptoms or medical problems that may be drug induced | Constipation due to or worsened by $Fe^{++}$ or $Ca^{++}$ | |
| | Drug administered too rapidly | | |
| | Medication error, actual or potential | | |
| Interactions (drug–drug, drug–disease, drug–nutrient, drug–laboratory test) | Effect of drug altered due to enzyme induction/ inhibition from another drug patient is taking | | |
| | Effect of drug altered due to protein-binding alterations from another drug patient is taking | | |
| | Effect of drug altered due to pharmacodynamic change from another drug patient is taking | | |
| | Bioavailability of drug altered due to interaction with another drug or food | _____ | Make sure the patient is educated about proper times to administer |
| | Effect of drug altered due to substance in food | | |
| | Patient's laboratory test altered due to interference from a drug the patient is taking | Assess diet for excess goitrogens | |
| Failure to receive therapy | Patient did not adhere with the drug regimen | Patient's prior adherence not known | |
| | Drug not given due to medication error | | |
| | Patient did not take due to high drug cost/lack of insurance | | |
| | Patient unable to take oral medication | | |
| | Patient has no IV access for IV medication | | |
| | Drug product not available | | |
| Financial impact | The current regimen is not the most cost-effective | | |
| | Patient unable to purchase medications/no insurance | _____ | |
| Patient knowledge of drug therapy | Patient does not understand the purpose, directions, or potential side effects of the drug regimen | | |
| | Current regimen not consistent with the patient's health beliefs | Cultural beliefs not known | |

## PHARMACOTHERAPY CARE PLAN

| Medical Problem List | Current Drug Regimen | Drug Therapy Problems | Therapy Goals, Desired Endpoints | Therapeutic Recommendations | Rationale | Therapeutic Alternatives | Monitoring |
|---|---|---|---|---|---|---|---|
| Hypothyroidism | None | Ca, Fe will be an issue with $LT_4$ | Relieve symptoms (fatigue, cognition, dry skin, constipation); euthyroid state with TSH in target range [0.5–2.5 µU/mL (0.5–2.5 mU/L)] | ___ ___ ___ ___ | Drug of choice; most physiologic treatment; brand name to assure the same product with each refill; less-than-full replacement dose since hypothyroidism state not severe | ___ ___ ___ | Patient to self-monitor s/s daily; repeat TSH in 6 wk; if TSH not in target range, recheck TSH 6–8 wk after each dose change; once $LT_4$ dose stable. check TSH q 6–12 mo, or if clinical status changes; monitor for ADEs |
| ___ | Sertraline 50 mg q 24 h | ___ | No signs or symptoms of depression | ___ ___ ___ | Not clear if the patient has major depression based on information provided | If major depression and not responding to sertraline and $LT_4$, consider changing to alternative antidepressant (venlafaxine, bupropion, etc.) | ___ ___ ___ ___ |
| Dyslipidemia | None | ___ | ___ ___ ___ | LDL likely to reach target when euthyroid, so no lipid-lowering drugs at this point; provide healthy lifestyle (diet, exercise) recommendations | LDL will be reduced with $LT_4$ therapy | If LDL does not reach target after TSH at target, initiate simvastatin 10 mg q HS | |
| Osteopenia | ___ ___ | Ca may interfere with $LT_4$ absorption | ___ ___ | Continue current therapy; take $LT_4$ at least 2 h apart from Ca | Effective treatment; weekly bisphosphonate more convenient than daily | ___ ___ ___ | BMD q 2 yr; self-monitor for ADEs ; follow usual bisphosphonate instructions |

## PHARMACOTHERAPY CARE PLAN

| Medical Problem List | Current Drug Regimen | Drug Therapy Problems | Therapy Goals, Desired Endpoints | Therapeutic Recommendations | Rationale | Therapeutic Alternatives | Monitoring |
|---|---|---|---|---|---|---|---|
| Constipation | Milk of Magnesia 30 mL q 24 h PRN | Not sure what is in Rhubarb; may be due to or worsened by Ca, Fe | Normal bowel movements | _____ _____ _____ _____ | _____ _____ _____ _____ | If not better, add senna two tablets PO bid | _____ _____ _____ |
| | Rhubarb | | | | | | |
| _____ _____ | FeSO$_4$ 300 mg q 24 h | May be worsening constipation; problem may be resolved since menorrhagia improved; Fe may reduce LT$_4$ absorption | _____ _____ _____ | Consider discontinuing Fe | May no longer need Fe since the underlying problem resolved | _____ _____ _____ _____ | Self-monitor menses; CBC q 6 mo |
| _____ _____ | Ortho Tri-Cyclen-28 q 24 h | _____ _____ | Normal menses; prevent Fe deficiency | _____ _____ _____ _____ | _____ _____ _____ _____ | If not effective or ADE develops, alter estrogen and/or progestin component | _____ _____ _____ |

## PATIENT EDUCATION SUMMARY

### Notes

### Hypothyroidism

- The reason for taking this medication (levothyroxine, $LT_4$) is to replace the hormone that your thyroid gland is not producing in adequate amounts. In doing so, your symptoms should disappear and your abnormal laboratory values should return to normal.
- Make sure you receive the same brand of this medication each time the prescription is filled. _____ _____.
- Take this medication once a day exactly as your physician directed.
- Space this medicine from your iron and calcium tablets by _____ h. The iron and calcium tablets may _____ _____.
- While taking this medication with food can decrease the absorption, it is more important to take this medication in a consistent manner in regard to food intake and time of day.
- If you miss a dose, _____ _____.
- You should begin to feel better within 2–3 wk of starting this medication. You will initially notice an improvement in your energy and mood. Other symptoms, such as dry skin, may take longer to disappear.
- Blood tests will need to be checked periodically (every _____ wk) until your physician determines the best dose for you. After that, you will need to have a blood test only once or twice a year unless there is a change in your condition or if the brand of medication is changed.
- If the dose of your medication is too high, you may experience _____. Call your physician if you notice these side effects. Over a long period of time, taking too much of this medication can cause problems with your bones and heart.
- Taking too little of the medication can make you have the same symptoms you started with, plus you can develop hypertension, high cholesterol levels and an increased risk of heart disease. This is a very safe medication, and these problems will not occur if you take the medication as directed and if your thyroid blood tests are checked periodically and stay in the desired range.
- Call your physician immediately if you experience any _____.
- Because your thyroid gland is not producing enough thyroid hormone, you will likely need to take this medication for the rest of your life.
- It is very important to keep regular appointments with your physician to monitor your therapy so that you can gain the full benefit of this therapy while avoiding potential side effects.

### Depression

- Your depression symptoms may be due to your hypothyroidism. If so, those symptoms should improve as your thyroid condition improves with $LT_4$ therapy. The sertraline should be continued until you are instructed to stop taking it.

### Dyslipidemia

- _____.
- You should adopt a healthy lifestyle by improving your diet, exercising, not using tobacco, and using alcohol in moderation.

### Osteopenia

- Take your calcium at least _____ h before or after your $LT_4$ dose.
- Make sure you follow the instructions provided for your alendronate therapy (_____).
- Make sure you participate in weight-bearing exercise at least _____ d/wk.

### Constipation

- Your constipation may improve as your hypothyroidism improves and if your iron tablets are stopped.
- Drinking adequate amounts of liquids and exercise can also help constipation.
- Do not use other laxatives or enemas unless you talk to your physician or pharmacist first.

### History of Fe-Deficiency Anemia

- Since your anemia has resolved and your periods are now normal, you no longer need to take iron.

### Menorrhagia

- _____.
- Do not use tobacco since that could increase your risk of heart attacks.
- If you develop sudden shortness of breath, leg pain, chest pain, loss of vision, severe headache, or abdominal pain, please call your physician immediately.

# 54 Pregnancy: Example Careplan with Missing Data

Ema Ferreira      Caroline Morin      Évelyne Rey

## PATIENT DATABASE FORM

| | | |
|---|---|---|
| **Patient Name:** Loretta Baldwin | **Patient ID:** 467788 | **Location:** Physician's Office |
| **Physician:** Dr. J. Brown (Medical Clinic) | **Pharmacy:** Unknown | |
| **Age (or Date of Birth):** 26 yo | **Race:** Caucasian | **Sex:** Female |
| **Height:** 67 in (170 cm) | **Weight:** 207.2 lb (94.2 kg) | |
| **Date of Admission/Initial Visit:** 09/01/2012 | **Occupation:** Clerk | |

### Allergies/Intolerances/ADRs

❑ No known drug allergies/ADRs

☒ Not known/inadequate information

| Drug: | Reaction: |
|---|---|
| Phenytoin | Unknown reaction at the age of 13 |
| | |
| | |
| | |

### HPI, PMH, FH, SH, etc...

HPI: Pregnancy

PMH: Epilepsy, obesity, chronic headaches, occasional constipation, light nausea

FMH: DM, HTN, obesity, hypothyroidism

| Prioritized Medical Problem List | Medication Profile |
|---|---|
| Epilepsy | Lamotrigine 200 mg PO twice daily; stopped yesterday |
| | Carbamazepine CR 400 mg PO twice daily; stopped yesterday |
| Pregnancy | No folic acid or multivitamins |
| | |
| Urinary tract infection (asymptomatic bacteriuria) | No treatment |
| Chronic headaches | Feverfew herbal tea two to five times a week |
| | Ibuprofen 400 mg PO PRN headache; twice weekly in the last month |
| Light nausea | No medication |
| | |
| Constipation | Milk of Magnesia 30 mL PO once daily as needed |
| | |
| Suboptimal diet | No folic acid or multivitamins |
| Obesity | No medication; poor diet |
| | |

The form is from *ASHP National Clinical Skills Competition Case Documents*, Copyright 2009, American Society of Health-System Pharmacists, Bethesda, MD (www.ashp.org). Adapted with permission.

| Vital Signs, Laboratory Data, and Diagnostic Test Results | | | |
|---|---|---|---|
| Date | 09/01/2012 | | |
| Weight (lb/kg) | 207.2 (94.2) | | |
| Temperature (°C) | 36.2 | | |
| Blood pressure (mm Hg) | 112/76 | | |
| Pulse | 89 | | |
| Respiratory rate | 12 | | |
| Na<br>135–145 mEq/L (135–145 mmol/L) | | | |
| K<br>3.3–4.9 mEq/L (3.3–4.9 mmol/L) | | | |
| Cl<br>97–110 mEq/L (97–110 mmol/L) | | | |
| $CO_2/HCO_3$<br>22–26 mEq/L (22–26 mmol/L) | | | |
| BUN<br>8–25 mg/dL (2.9–8.9 mmol/L) | | | |
| Creatinine (adult)<br>Male 0.7–1.3 mg/dL; female 0.6–1.1 mg/dL (male 62–115 µmol/L;<br>    female 53–97 µmol/L) | 0.63 (56) | | |
| Creatinine clearance (adult)<br>85–135 mL/min (1.42–2.25 mL/s) | | | |
| Glucose (fasting)<br>65–109 mg/dL (3.6–6.0 mmol/L) | 100.9 (5.6) | | |
| Total Ca<br>8.6–10.3 mg/dL (2.15–2.58 mmol/L) | | | |
| Mg<br>1.3–2.2 mEq/L (0.65–1.10 mmol/L) | | | |
| $PO_4$<br>2.5–4.5 mg/dL (0.81–1.45 mmol/L) | | | |
| Hemoglobin<br>Male 13.8–17.2 g/dL; female 12.1–15.1 g/dL (male 138–172 g/L;<br>    female 121–151 g/L; male 8.57–10.68 mmol/L; female<br>    7.51–9.38 mmol/L) | 12.3 (123; 7.63) | | |
| Hematocrit<br>Male 40.7–50.3%; female 36.1–44.3% (male 0.407–0.503;<br>    female 0.361–0.443) | 37.8 (0.378) | | |
| MCV<br>80.0–97.6 µm³ (80.0–97.6 fL) | 82 | | |
| WBC<br>$4–10 \times 10^3/mm^3$ ($4–10 \times 10^9/L$) | 5.4 | | |
| Differential | | | |
| Platelet<br>$140–440 \times 10^3/mm^3$ ($140–440 \times 10^9/L$) | 203 | | |
| Albumin<br>3.5–5.0 g/dL (35–50 g/L) | | | |
| Total bilirubin<br>0.3–1.1 mg/dL (5.1–18.8 µmol/L) | | | |
| Direct bilirubin<br>0–0.3 mg/dL (0–5.1 µmol/L) | | | |
| AST<br>11–47 IU/L (0.18–0.78 µkat/L) | | | |
| ALT<br>7–53 IU/L (0.12–0.88 µkat/L) | | | |

| Vital Signs, Laboratory Data, and Diagnostic Test Results | | | |
|---|---|---|---|
| **Alk phos (adult)**<br>38–126 IU/L (0.63–2.10 μkat/L) | | | |
| **Urine pregnancy test** | + | | |
| **Blood group/Rhesus type** | O⁺ | | |
| **Urinalysis** | Bacteria ++<br>Nitrite + | | |
| **Urine culture** | Results pending | | |
| **Rubella antibody** | + | | |
| **Hepatitis B surface antigen** | − | | |
| **HIV antibody** | − | | |
| **Vaginal culture** | − | | |
| **Lamotrigine level** | Not done | | |
| **Carbamazepine level**<br>4–10 mcg/L (17–42 μmol/L) | 4.2 (18) | | |

| Notes | | | |
|---|---|---|---|
| | | | |

### DRUG THERAPY PROBLEM WORKSHEET

| Type of Problem | Possible Causes | Problem List | Notes |
|---|---|---|---|
| Correlation between drug therapy and medical problems | Drugs without obvious medical indications | Feverfew | |
| | Medications unidentified | | |
| | Untreated medical conditions | Obesity | Dietitian consult required; no drug therapy recommended |
| | | Mild nausea | To evaluate if treatment required |
| Need for additional drug therapy | New medical condition requiring new drug therapy | Pregnancy | Folic acid required |
| | | Mild nausea | To evaluate if treatment required |
| | Chronic disorder requiring continued drug therapy | Epilepsy | To continue treatment |
| | Condition best treated with combination drug therapy | Suboptimal diet | To be evaluated by dietitian for need of vitamins and minerals supplement |
| | May develop new medical condition without prophylactic or preventative therapy or premedication | Pregnancy—prevention of congenital anomalies | Folic acid required |
| | | Asymptomatic bacteriuria: complications include hypertension, preterm labor and acute pyelonephritis | Antibiotic treatment to be prescribed |
| Unnecessary drug therapy | Medication with no valid indication | Feverfew herbal tea | No proven efficacy; no safety data available |
| | Condition caused by accidental or intentional ingestion of toxic amount of drug or chemical | | |
| | Medical problem(s) associated with use of or withdrawal from alcohol, drug, or tobacco | | |
| | Condition is better treated with nondrug therapy | Mild nausea Constipation Obesity | |
| | Taking multiple drugs when single agent as effective | Lamotrigine and carbamazepine | To evaluate if single therapy can be used |
| | Taking drug(s) to treat an avoidable adverse reaction from another medication | | |
| Appropriate drug selection | Current regimen not usually as effective as other choices | | |
| | Current regimen not usually as safe as other choices | _____ | Should be stopped at 26 wk Acetaminophen first choice during pregnancy |
| | Therapy not individualized to patient | | |
| Wrong drug | Medical problem for which drug is not effective | Feverfew herbal tea | No proven efficacy |
| | Patient has risk factors that contraindicate use of drug | | |
| | Patient has infection with organisms resistant to drug | | |
| | Patient refractory to current drug therapy | | |
| | Taking combination product when single agent appropriate | | |
| | Dosage form inappropriate | Feverfew | Formulation and dosage not effective |
| | Medication error | | |

## DRUG THERAPY PROBLEM WORKSHEET

| Type of Problem | Possible Causes | Problem List | Notes |
|---|---|---|---|
| Drug regimen | PRN use not appropriate for condition | Milk of Magnesia PRN | PRN laxative might not be effective for chronic constipation |
| | Route of administration/dosage form/mode of administration not appropriate for current condition | | |
| | Length or course of therapy not appropriate | | |
| | Drug therapy altered without adequate therapeutic trial | | |
| | Dose or interval flexibility not appropriate | | |
| Dose too low | Dose or frequency too low to produce desired response in this patient | | |
| | Serum drug level below desired therapeutic range | _____ | Obtain concentrations if possible |
| | Timing of antimicrobial prophylaxis not appropriate | | |
| | Medication not stored properly | | |
| | Medication error | | |
| Dose too high | Dose or frequency too high for this patient | | |
| | Serum drug level above the desired therapeutic range | | |
| | Dose escalated too quickly | | |
| | Dose or interval flexibility not appropriate for this patient | | |
| | Medication error | | |
| Therapeutic duplication | Receiving multiple agents without added benefit | | |
| Drug allergy/adverse drug events | History of allergy or ADE to current (or chemically related) agents | Phenytoin – reaction unknown | Question patient on allergy |
| | Allergy or ADE history not in medical records | | |
| | Patient not using alert for severe allergy or ADE | | |
| | Symptoms or medical problems that may be drug induced | | |
| | Drug administered too rapidly | | |
| | Medication error, actual or potential | | |
| Interactions (drug–drug, drug–disease, drug–nutrient, drug–laboratory test) | Effect of drug altered due to enzyme induction/inhibition from another drug patient is taking | Interaction between lamotrigine and carbamazepine | _____ _____ |
| | Effect of drug altered due to protein-binding alterations from another drug patient is taking | | |
| | Effect of drug altered due to pharmacodynamic change from another drug patient is taking | | |
| | Bioavailability of drug altered due to interaction with another drug or food | | |
| | Effect of drug altered due to substance in food | | |
| | Patient's laboratory test altered due to interference from a drug the patient is taking | | |
| Failure to receive therapy | Patient did not adhere with the drug regimen | Patient stopped her anticonvulsants | |
| | Drug not given due to medication error | | |
| | Patient did not take due to high drug cost/lack of insurance | | |
| | Patient unable to take oral medication | | |
| | Patient has no IV access for IV medication | | |
| | Drug product not available | | |

## DRUG THERAPY PROBLEM WORKSHEET

| Type of Problem | Possible Causes | Problem List | Notes |
|---|---|---|---|
| Financial impact | The current regimen is not the most cost-effective | | |
| | Patient unable to purchase medications/no insurance | | |
| Patient knowledge of drug therapy | Patient does not understand the purpose, directions, or potential side effects of the drug regimen | Patient does not understand the risk of stopping anticonvulsants | |
| | Current regimen not consistent with the patient's health beliefs | Patient does not know risks of anticonvulsant therapy during pregnancy | |

## PHARMACOTHERAPY CARE PLAN

| Medical Problem List | Current Drug Regimen | Drug Therapy Problems | Therapy Goals, Desired Endpoints | Therapeutic Recommendations | Rationale | Therapeutic Alternatives | Monitoring |
|---|---|---|---|---|---|---|---|
| | Carbamazepine 400 mg CR PO twice daily (stopped yesterday) Lamotrigine 200 mg PO twice daily (stopped yesterday) | Medication stopped | Prevent seizures Prevent pregnancy complications due to seizures | ——— ——— ——— | Seizure control is important during pregnancy Use treatment that controls seizure in this patient | ——— ——— ——— | Seizures Aura Drugs concentrations every trimester if dose is changed or if clinical condition warrants it |
| Pregnancy | None | No prevention of congenital anomalies | Prevent neural tube defects and other congenital anomalies | Start folic acid 4 mg once daily ASAP and continue throughout first trimester | Folic acid reduces the risk of neural tube defects and other congenital anomalies | None | ——— ——— ——— |
| Pregnancy | None | Patient does not understand the risks of disease and drugs | Promote drug compliance and optimal treatment | ——— ——— ——— | Proper counseling will encourage compliance to anticonvulsants | ——— ——— ——— | Interview the patient at follow-up |
| Asymptomatic bacteriuria | None | Treatment required to prevent medical condition | ——— ——— ——— | ——— ——— ——— | Treatment reduces the risk of complications | Cephalexin 250 – 500 mg orally 4 × daily for 7 d | Urinary culture 10 d after the end of treatment or at next prenatal visit and monthly thereafter |
| Nausea | None | ——— | Relief of nausea Ensure absorption of other treatments | Nonpharmacologic methods (i.e., small meals, etc.) Doxylamine and pyridoxine if necessary ——— | ——— ——— ——— | ——— ——— ——— | ——— ——— ——— |

## PHARMACOTHERAPY CARE PLAN

| Medical Problem List | Current Drug Regimen | Drug Therapy Problems | Therapy Goals, Desired Endpoints | Therapeutic Recommendations | Rationale | Therapeutic Alternatives | Monitoring |
|---|---|---|---|---|---|---|---|
| Constipation | Milk of Magnesia 30 mL once daily as needed | Constipation treatment is not optimal | Normal bowel movements<br>Prevention of hemorrhoids | | | Add docusate sodium if constipation persists or | Self-monitor daily |
| Chronic headaches | Ibuprofen 400 mg orally as needed<br>Feverfew herbal tea as needed | Ibuprofen is not an optimal treatment during pregnancy<br>Herbal product has no proven efficacy | | Acetaminophen 500–1,000 mg PO q 6 h as needed (maximum 4 g/24 h)<br>Ibuprofen sporadically as needed (maximum for 48 h and stop at 26 wk pregnancy)<br>Stop feverfew herbal tea | Ibuprofen is associated with:<br>Feverfew should be discontinued since: | Encourage lifestyle changes (rest, avoidance of triggers, etc.) If acetaminophen is not sufficient and if severe headaches, consider adding an opiate (e.g., codeine) | |
| Obesity | | | Healthy diet<br>Healthy weight gain during pregnancy | Dietitian consultation<br>Add vitamin supplements if necessary. Mild-to-moderate exercise | Healthy diet is important during pregnancy for fetal growth<br>Use of drugs to promote weight loss is not recommended during pregnancy | | Weight at each prenatal visit<br>Monitor for anemia<br>Evaluation by dietitian |

## PATIENT EDUCATION SUMMARY

### Notes

### Epilepsy

- Seizure control during pregnancy is important.
- Drug compliance is essential.
- Risk of congenital malformations is of 2–3% in the general population and is increased to approximately 5% with these anticonvulsants (95% chance of having a healthy baby).
- You will have drug concentrations measured regularly to ensure that drugs are at optimal concentrations.

### Pregnancy and Folic Acid

- Folic acid will _____.
- You will need to take a folic acid supplement until at least the end of the _____ trimester.

### Asymptomatic bacteriuria

- Antibiotic will reduce the risk of pregnancy complications
- Treatment has to be completed (7 days)
- Follow-up urinary cultures are important

### Constipation

- Your constipation is worsened by pregnancy.
- It is important to eat a diet _____ in fiber.
- Drinking adequate amounts of liquids and exercise can also help constipation. Some medication are useful and safe during pregnancy.
- Treating and preventing constipation will prevent hemorrhoids that are also common during pregnancy.
- _____ use other laxatives or enemas unless you talk to your health care provider.

### Chronic Headaches

- Regular ibuprofen is not the first choice throughout pregnancy since it can affect _____.
- Regular rest and avoidance of too much caffeine or other triggers is helpful to prevent headaches.
- Use acetaminophen, which is safe throughout pregnancy.
- Talk to your physician or pharmacist if headaches persist despite the use of acetaminophen. (Other treatments are available.)

### Obesity/Suboptimal Diet

- A healthy diet during pregnancy is important.
- A dietitian can evaluate your diet and recommend a program to promote healthy habits.
- You might have to take calcium and iron supplements.
- Healthy weight gain is approximately _____.
- Dieting (with or without drugs) is not recommended during pregnancy.

### Nausea

- _____.
- _____.

# 91  Acute Osteomyelitis: Example Careplan with Missing Data

Melinda M. Neuhauser        Susan L. Pendland

## PATIENT DATABASE FORM

| | | |
|---|---|---|
| **Patient Name:** Sam Cole | **Patient ID:** | **Location:** ED |
| **Physician:** | **Pharmacy:** | |
| **Age (or Date of Birth):** 18 yo | **Race:** Caucasian | **Sex:** Male |
| **Height:** 69 in. (175.3 cm) | **Weight:** 162.8 lb (74 kg) | |
| **Date of Admission/Initial Visit:** 08/03/2012 | **Occupation:** Full-time student; part-time job at movie theater | |

### Allergies/Intolerances/ADRs

❏ No known drug allergies/ADRs
❏ Not known/inadequate information

| Drug: | Reaction: |
|---|---|
| Benadryl | Jittery |
| | |
| | |
| | |
| | |

### HPI, PMH, FH, SH, etc...

Fractured proximal humerus (7 d ago)

Asthma

Allergic rhinitis

| Prioritized Medical Problem List | Medication Profile |
|---|---|
| Acute osteomyelitis | Vancomycin 1500 mg infusion q 12 h |
| _____ | Cephalexin 500 mg one capsule PO q 6 h for 7 d |
| | Ibuprofen 400 mg one tablet PO q 6 h PRN mild-to-moderate arm pain |
| | Hydrocodone/acetaminophen 5/325 mg one tablet PO q 4 h PRN severe arm pain |
| _____ | Fluticasone/salmeterol 250/50 mcg 1 puff twice daily |
| | Albuterol 1 to 2 puffs q 4 h PRN wheezing |
| Allergic rhinitis | Loratadine 10 mg one tablet PO once daily |
| | Fluticasone intranasal spray two puffs each nostril once daily PRN allergies |
| | Acetaminophen 325 mg one to two tablets PRN headaches |

| Vital Signs, Laboratory Data, and Diagnostic Test Results | | | |
|---|---|---|---|
| **Date** | 08/03/2012 | | |
| **Weight (lb/kg)** | 162.8 (74) | | |
| **Temperature (°C)** | 37.9 | | |
| **Blood pressure (mm Hg)** | 117/76 | | |
| **Pulse** | 85 | | |
| **Respiratory rate** | 16 | | |
| **Na**<br>135–145 mEq/L (135–145 mmol/L) | 141 | | |
| **K**<br>3.3–4.9 mEq/L (3.3–4.9 mmol/L) | 3.9 | | |
| **Cl**<br>97–110 mEq/L (97–110 mmol/L) | 101 | | |
| **$CO_2/HCO_3$**<br>22–26 mEq/L (22–26 mmol/L) | 25 | | |
| **BUN**<br>8–25 mg/dL (2.9–8.9 mmol/L) | 5 (1.8) | | |
| **Creatinine (adult)**<br>Male 0.7–1.3 mg/dL; female 0.6–1.1 mg/dL (male 62–115 µmol/L;<br>female 53–97 µmol/L) | 0.5 (44) | | |
| **Creatinine clearance (adult)**<br>85–135 mL/min (1.42–2.25 mL/s) | >120 (>2.00) | | |
| **Glucose (fasting)**<br>65–109 mg/dL (3.6–6.0 mmol/L) | 105 mg (5.8) | | |
| **Total Ca**<br>8.6–10.3 mg/dL (2.15–2.58 mmol/L) | | | |
| **Mg**<br>1.3–2.2 mEq/L (0.65–1.10 mmol/L) | | | |
| **$PO_4$**<br>2.5–4.5 mg/dL (0.81–1.45 mmol/L) | | | |
| **Hemoglobin**<br>Male 13.8–17.2 g/dL; female 12.1–15.1 g/dL (male 138–172 g/L; female<br>121–151 g/L; male 8.57–10.68 mmol/L; female 7.51–9.38 mmol/L) | 15.0 (150; 9.31) | | |
| **Hematocrit**<br>Male 40.7–50.3%; female 36.1–44.3% (male 0.407–0.503;<br>female 0.361–0.443) | 43.7 (0.437) | | |
| **MCV**<br>80.0–97.6 µm$^3$ (80.0–97.6 fL) | | | |
| **WBC**<br>$4–10 \times 10^3/mm^3$ ($4–10 \times 10^9/L$) | 12.1 | | |
| **Differential** | | | |
| **Platelet**<br>$140–440 \times 10^3/mm^3$ ($140–440 \times 10^9/L$) | | | |
| **Albumin**<br>3.5–5.0 g/dL (35–50 g/L) | | | |
| **Total bilirubin**<br>0.3–1.1 mg/dL (5.1–18.8 µmol/L) | | | |
| **Direct bilirubin**<br>0–0.3 mg/dL (0–5.1 µmol/L) | | | |
| **AST**<br>11–47 IU/L (0.18–0.78 µkat/L) | | | |
| **ALT**<br>7–53 IU/L (0.12–0.88 µkat/L) | | | |
| **Alk phos (adult)**<br>38–126 IU/L (0.63–2.10 µkat/L) | | | |

| Vital Signs, Laboratory Data, and Diagnostic Test Results | | | |
|---|---|---|---|
| **ESR**<br>0–20 mm/h (0–5.6 μm/s) | 119 (33.1) | | |
| **CRP**<br><0.8 mg/dL (<8 mg/L) | 68 (680) | | |

| Notes |
|---|
| Microbiology: |
| Blood culture (×2): Pending |
| Bone biopsy: Gram stain shows Gram-positive cocci in clusters; culture is pending |
| |
| Imaging: |
| *Magnetic resonance imaging (MRI):* Positive for increased uptake in left proximal humerus |
| |

## DRUG THERAPY PROBLEM WORKSHEET

| Type of Problem | Possible Causes | Problem List | Notes |
|---|---|---|---|
| Correlation between drug therapy and medical problems | Drugs without obvious medical indications | | |
| | Medications unidentified | Sinus medication | _____ |
| | Untreated medical conditions | | |
| Need for additional drug therapy | New medical condition requiring new drug therapy | Acute osteomyelitis | Discontinue oral cephalexin |
| | Chronic disorder requiring continued drug therapy | | |
| | Condition best treated with combination drug therapy | | |
| | May develop new medical condition without prophylactic or preventative therapy or premedication | | |
| Unnecessary drug therapy | Medication with no valid indication | | |
| | Condition caused by accidental or intentional ingestion of toxic amount of drug or chemical | | |
| | Medical problem(s) associated with use of or withdrawal from alcohol, drug, or tobacco | | |
| | Condition is better treated with nondrug therapy | | |
| | Taking multiple drugs when single agent as effective | | |
| | Taking drug(s) to treat an avoidable adverse reaction from another medication | | |
| Appropriate drug selection | Current regimen not usually as effective as other choices | | |
| | Current regimen not usually as safe as other choices | | |
| | Therapy not individualized to patient | | |
| Wrong drug | Medical problem for which drug is not effective | | |
| | Patient has risk factors that contraindicate use of drug | | |
| | Patient has infection with organisms resistant to drug | | |
| | Patient refractory to current drug therapy | | |
| | Taking combination product when single agent appropriate | | |
| | Dosage form inappropriate | | |
| | Medication error | | |
| Drug regimen | PRN use not appropriate for condition | Intranasal corticosteroid | Change from PRN to daily |
| | Route of administration/dosage form/mode of administration not appropriate for current condition | | |
| | Length or course of therapy not appropriate | | |
| | Drug therapy altered without adequate therapeutic trial | | |
| | Dose or interval flexibility not appropriate | | |
| Dose too low | Dose or frequency too low to produce desired response in this patient | | |
| | Serum drug level below desired therapeutic range | | |
| | Timing of antimicrobial prophylaxis not appropriate | | |
| | Medication not stored properly | | |
| | Medication error | | |
| Dose too high | Dose or frequency too high for this patient | | |
| | Serum drug level above the desired therapeutic range | | |
| | Dose escalated too quickly | | |
| | Dose or interval flexibility not appropriate for this patient | | |
| | Medication error | | |

## DRUG THERAPY PROBLEM WORKSHEET

| Type of Problem | Possible Causes | Problem List | Notes |
|---|---|---|---|
| Therapeutic duplication | Receiving multiple agents without added benefit | | |
| Drug allergy/ adverse drug events | History of allergy or ADE to current (or chemically related) agents | | |
| | Allergy or ADE history not in medical records | | |
| | Patient not using alert for severe allergy or ADE | | |
| | Symptoms or medical problems that may be drug induced | | |
| | Drug administered too rapidly | | |
| | Medication error, actual or potential | | |
| Interactions (drug–drug, drug–disease, drug–nutrient, drug–laboratory test) | Effect of drug altered due to enzyme induction/ inhibition from another drug patient is taking | | |
| | Effect of drug altered due to protein-binding alterations from another drug patient is taking | | |
| | Effect of drug altered due to pharmacodynamic change from another drug patient is taking | | |
| | Bioavailability of drug altered due to interaction with another drug or food | | |
| | Effect of drug altered due to substance in food | | |
| | Patient's laboratory test altered due to interference from a drug the patient is taking | | |
| Failure to receive therapy | Patient did not adhere with the drug regimen | In the past, several acute asthma exacerbations secondary to nonadherence to asthma medications | _____ _____ |
| | Drug not given due to medication error | | |
| | Patient did not take due to high drug cost/lack of insurance | | |
| | Patient unable to take oral medication | | |
| | Patient has no IV access for IV medication | | |
| | Drug product not available | | |
| Financial impact | The current regimen is not the most cost-effective | | |
| | Patient unable to purchase medications/no insurance | Health insurance coverage through father | |
| Patient knowledge of drug therapy | Patient does not understand the purpose, directions, or potential side effects of the drug regimen | | |
| | Current regimen not consistent with the patient's health beliefs | Cultural beliefs not known | |

## PHARMACOTHERAPY CARE PLAN

| Medical Problem List | Current Drug Regimen | Drug Therapy Problems | Therapy Goals, Desired Endpoints | Therapeutic Recommendations | Rationale | Therapeutic Alternatives | Monitoring |
|---|---|---|---|---|---|---|---|
| Acute osteomyelitis | None (new diagnosis) | _____ _____ _____ | Eradicate infection and prevent recurrence | _____ _____ _____ Achieve steady-state vancomycin trough concentration of 15–20 mcg/mL (10.4–13.8 µmol/L) with goal $AUC_{24}$/MIC of >350–400 | Appropriate therapy | Alternatives include – Daptomycin – Linezolid – TMP/SMX in combination with oral rifampin | Monitor BUN/SCr, vancomycin troughs, CPR, and ESR weekly Monitor for: _____ _____ _____ |
| _____ _____ | Ibuprofen 400 mg one tablet PO q 6 h PRN mild-to-moderate arm pain; Hydrocodone/acetaminophen 5/325 mg one tablet q 4 h PRN severe arm pain; Cephalexin 500 mg one capsule PO q 6 h for 7 d | _____ _____ _____ | Reduce symptoms of pain | Change ibuprofen to 400 mg one tablet q 6 h with food for 48 h and then switch to PRN; Continue hydrocodone/acetaminophen 5/325 mg PO PRN for pain not controlled with ibuprofen; Discontinue cephalexin | _____ _____ _____ | Dosage modification of ibuprofen and/or hydrocodone/acetaminophen; If severe pain, consider oxycodone/acetaminophen | |
| Asthma | Fluticasone/salmeterol 250/50 mcg one puff twice daily; Albuterol 1 to 2 puffs q 4 h PRN wheezing | _____ _____ _____ | Reduce symptoms, maintain normal pulmonary function, and prevent acute exacerbations | _____ _____ _____ | Patient asymptomatic when adheres to the current regimen | Dosage modification of fluticasone/salmeterol | Self-monitor symptoms (dyspnea, cough, SOB); Pulmonary function tests |
| Allergic rhinitis | Loratadine 10 mg one tablet PO once daily; Fluticasone intranasal spray 2 puffs each nostril once daily PRN allergies; Acetaminophen 325 mg 1 to 2 tablets PO PRN headaches | Unidentified sinus medication; need to identify ingredients | Reduce symptoms | _____ Change fluticasone to scheduled once daily rather than PRN _____ | Fluticasone therapy will be optimized if utilized as scheduled rather than PRN | Different agent within the class of second-generation antihistamines or intranasal corticosteroids; Decongestants _____ | _____ _____ |

## PATIENT EDUCATION SUMMARY

### Notes

**Acute Osteomyelitis**

- The reason for taking the intravenous antibiotic is to: _____
  _____.

- It is extremely important that you receive the antibiotic exactly as prescribed by your health care provider and for as long as prescribed by health care provider. It is very important that you do not miss a single dose of your antibiotic. The bacteria causing the infection may become resistant to the medication you are taking and could result in treatment failure.

- Blood tests will need to be done weekly to help the health care provider determine if your infection is responding to the antibiotic or if changes need to be made in either the drug or the dose.

- You should begin to feel better in _____
  _____.

- It is important to keep regularly scheduled appointments with your health care provider so that your infection and response to therapy can be carefully monitored.

**Asthma**

- It is important that you use the fluticasone/salbuterol inhaler every morning and every evening. If you take the medication twice daily as directed, your breathing should improve and you should have fewer visits to the emergency department for your asthma.

- _____.

- _____.

- Ask your friends not to smoke when you are with them and tell them how it worsens your breathing.

**Allergic Rhinitis**

- Your nasal spray should work better if you use it every day. If you use it daily for 3 wk and your allergy symptoms are still present, contact your health care provider.

- _____.

**Fractured Proximal Humerus**

- Take the pain medication exactly as your health care provider directed. If your pain increases or has not decreased in 2 or 3 d, contact your health care provider.

- Avoid taking too much acetaminophen (Tylenol). _____.